Pediatric Orthopaedics

Volume Two

Volume Two

Pediatric Orthopaedics

Edited by

WOOD W. LOVELL, M.D.
Medical Director
Scottish Rite Hospital
Atlanta, Georgia

and

ROBERT B. WINTER, M.D.
Professor of Orthopaedic Surgery
University of Minnesota Medical School
Twin Cities Scoliosis Center, and
Medical Director
Gillette Children's Hospital
Minneapolis, Minnesota

With 32 Contributors

J. B. Lippincott Company
Philadelphia • Toronto

Copyright © 1978, by J. B. Lippincott Company

This book is fully protected by copyright, and, with the exception of brief excerpts for review, no part of it may be reproduced
in any form, by print, photoprint, microfilm, or any other
means, without written permission from the publisher.

ISBN 0-397-50391-1
Library of Congress Catalog Card Number 78-12546

Printed in the United States of America

3 5 4 2

Library of Congress Cataloging in Publication Data

Main entry under title:

Pediatric orthopaedics.

    Includes index.
    1. Pediatric orthopedia.   I. Lovell, Wood W.
II. Winter, Robert B.
RD732.3.C48P43   617.3   78-12546
ISBN 0-397-50391-1

Contributors

Henry H. Banks, M.D.

Professor and Chairman, Department of Orthopedic Surgery, Tufts University School of Medicine, and Orthopedic Surgeon-in-Chief, New England Medical Center Hospitals, Boston, Massachusetts

Anthony J. Bianco, Jr., M.D., M.S.

Professor of Orthopaedic Surgery, Mayo Medical School, and Consultant in Pediatric Orthopaedics, Mayo Clinic, Rochester, Minnesota

Walter P. Bobechko, M.D.

Assistant Professor of Surgery, University of Toronto, and Chief of Orthopaedic Surgery, Hospital for Sick Children, Toronto, Ontario

Charles A. Bonnett, M.D.

Assistant Clinical Professor of Surgery (Orthopedics), University of Southern California School of Medicine, Los Angeles, California, and Chief, Spinal Deformity Service, Rancho Los Amigos Hospital, Downey, California

Joyce D. Brink, M.D.

Associate Clinical Professor of Pediatrics, University of Southern California School of Medicine, Los Angeles, California, and Chief, Department of Pediatrics, Rancho Los Amigos Hospital, Downey, California

David M. Brown, M.D.

Professor, Departments of Pediatrics, Laboratory Medicine, and Pathology, University of Minnesota Medical School, Minneapolis, Minnesota

Wilton H. Bunch, M.D., Ph.D.

Professor and Chairman, Department of Orthopedics, Loyola University of Chicago Stritch School of Medicine, Maywood, Illinois

Jonathan Cohen, M.D.

Professor of Orthopedic Surgery, Tufts University School of Medicine, Boston, Massachusetts

Sherman S. Coleman, M.S., M.D.

Professor of Orthopedic Surgery, University of Utah College of Medicine, and Chief Surgeon, Shriners Hospital for Crippled Children, Salt Lake City, Utah

Henry R. Cowell, M.D.

Associate Surgeon-in-Chief and Director of Clinical Research, Alfred I. duPont Institute, Wilmington, Delaware

James C. Drennan, M.D.

Assistant Professor, Department of Surgery (Orthopaedic), University of Connecticut School of Medicine, Farmington, Connecticut; Assistant Clinical Professor, Department of Orthopedic Surgery, Yale University School of Medicine, New Haven, Connecticut; and Director of Orthopaedics, Newington Children's Hospital, Newington, Connecticut

J. William Fielding, M.D.

Clinical Professor of Orthopedic Surgery, Columbia University College of Physicians and Surgeons, and Director of Orthopedic Surgery, St. Luke's Hospital, New York, New York

Robert E. Florin, M.D.

Assistant Professor of Surgery (Neurological), University of Southern California School of Medicine, Los Angeles, California, and Consulting Neurological Surgeon, Rancho Los Amigos Hospital, Downey, California

Paul P. Griffin, M.D.

Professor and Chairman, Department of Orthopedics and Rehabilitation, Vanderbilt University School of Medicine, Nashville, Tennessee

Virginia Guess, M.A., R.P.T.

Formerly Physical Therapy Supervisor, Rancho Los Amigos Hospital, Downey, California

Richard J. Hawkins, M.D.

Clinical Assistant Professor of Orthopaedic Surgery, University of Western Ontario Faculty of Medicine, St. Joseph's Hospital, London, Ontario

Robert N. Hensinger, M.D.

Associate Professor, Department of Surgery, Section of Orthopaedics, University of Michigan Medical School, Ann Arbor, Michigan

M. Mark Hoffer, M.D.

Assistant Clinical Professor of Orthopedics and Pediatrics, University of Southern California School of Medicine, Los Angeles, California, and Chief, Children's Orthopedic Surgery, Rancho Los Amigos Hospital, Downey, California

S. Henry LaRocca, M.D.

Associate Professor of Orthopaedic Surgery, Tulane University School of Medicine, New Orleans, Louisiana

Wood W. Lovell, M.D.

Medical Director, Scottish Rite Hospital, Atlanta, Georgia

Newton C. McCollough III, M.D.

Professor and Acting Chairman, Department of Orthopedics and Rehabilitation, University of Miami School of Medicine, and Chief of Pediatric Orthopedics, University of Miami Hospital, Miami, Florida

G. Dean MacEwen, M.D.

Professor of Orthopaedic Surgery, Jefferson Medical College of Thomas Jefferson University, Philadelphia, Pennsylvania, and Medical Director, Alfred I. duPont Institute, Wilmington, Delaware

John S. Marsh, M.D.

Assistant Clinical Professor of Surgery (Neurological), University of Southern California School of Medicine, Los Angeles, California

Peter L. Meehan, M.D.

Director of Pediatric Orthopaedic Education, Scottish Rite Hospital, Atlanta, Georgia

Margaret Mitani, O.T.R.

Occupational Therapy Supervisor, Rancho Los Amigos Hospital, Downey, California

Colin F. Moseley, M.D.

Lecturer, University of Toronto, and Orthopaedic Surgeon, Hospital for Sick Children and Ontario Crippled Children's Centre, Toronto, Ontario

Kurt M. W. Niemann, M.D.

John D. Sherrill Professor of Orthopaedic Surgery and Director, Division of Orthopaedic Surgery, University of Alabama School of Medicine, Birmingham, Alabama

Charles T. Price, M.D.

Division of Pediatric Surgery, Jewett Orthopaedic Clinic, Winter Park, Florida

Paul L. Ramsey, M.D.

Clinical Associate Professor of Orthopedic Surgery, Indiana University School of Medicine, Indianapolis, Indiana

Daniel C. Riordan, M.D.

Professor of Clinical Orthopaedics, Tulane University School of Medicine; Professor of Clinical Orthopaedics, Louisiana State University School of Medicine in New Orleans, Louisiana; and Consultant in Hand Surgery, Shriners Hospital for Crippled Children, Shreveport, Louisiana

Marvin B. Rothenberg, M.D.

Director, Growth and Metabolic Clinic, Scottish Rite Hospital, Atlanta, Georgia

Frank H. Stelling III, M.D.

Associate Clinical Professor of Orthopaedic Surgery, Medical University of South Carolina College of Medicine, Charleston, South Carolina; Assistant Clinical Professor of Orthopaedic Surgery, Duke University School of Medicine, Durham, North Carolina; and Chief Surgeon, Shriners Hospital for Crippled Children, Greenville, South Carolina

Robert E. Tooms, M.D.

Associate Clinical Professor, Department of Orthopedic Surgery, University of Tennessee Center for the Health Sciences, and Campbell Clinic, Memphis, Tennessee

Robert B. Winter, M.D.

Professor of Orthopaedic Surgery, University of Minnesota Medical School, Twin Cities Scoliosis Center, and Medical Director, Gillette Children's Hospital, Minneapolis, Minnesota

Contents

VOLUME ONE

Index

VOLUME TWO

Index

15 *The Cervical Spine*

J. William Fielding, M.D., Robert Hensinger, M.D., and Richard J. Hawkins, M.D.

BASILAR IMPRESSION

Basilar impression (or basilar invagination) is a deformity of the bones of the base of the skull at the margin of the foramen magnum. The floor of the skull appears to be indented by the upper cervical spine, and therefore the tip of the odontoid is more cephalad, sometimes protruding into the opening of the foramen magnum, and it may encroach upon the brain stem. This increases the risk of neurologic damage from injury, circulatory embarrassment, or impairment of cerebrospinal fluid flow. Chamberlain[3] in 1939 first called attention to the clinical significance of this anomaly with this vivid description.

"The changes shown by the roentgenogram give the impression of softening of the base of the skull and moulding through the force of gravity. It is as though the weight of the head has caused the ears to approach the shoulders, while the cervical spine, refusing to be shortened, has pushed the floor of the posterior fossa upward into the brain space."

The terms "platybasia" and "basilar impression" are often used as synonyms, but they are not related anatomically or pathologically. Platybasia has *no clinical significance;* it is merely an anthropologic term used to denote *flattening* of the angle formed by the intersection of the plane of the anterior fossa with the plane of the clivus. Basilar impression, which is *invagination* in the region of the foramen magnum, does have clinical significance. Patients with symptomatic basilar impression are seldom found to have an associated platybasia.

There are two types of basilar impression: (1) primary basilar impression is a congenital abnormality often associated with other vertebral defects, such as atlanto-occipital fusion, hypoplasia of the atlas, bifid posterior arch of the atlas, odontoid abnormalities, and Klippel-Feil syndrome; and (2) secondary basilar impression is a developmental condition usually attributed to softening of the osseous structures at the base of the skull with the deformity developing later in life. This is occasionally seen in conditions such as osteomalacia, rickets, Paget's disease,[5] osteogenesis imperfecta, renal osteodystrophy, rheumatoid arthritis and ankylosing spondylitis.

Roentgenographic Findings

Basilar impression is difficult to assess roentgenographically, and many measurement schemes have been proposed. Those most commonly used are Chamberlain's,[3] McGregor's,[11] and McRae's lines in the lateral roentgenogram (Fig. 15-1) and in the anteroposterior projection, Fischgold-Metzger's line[6] (Fig. 15-2). Chamberlain's line[3] (a line drawn from the dorsal marginal hard palate to the posterior lip of the foramen magnum) is seldom used, as the posterior lip of the foramen magnum (opisthion) is difficult to define on a standard roentgenogram (Fig. 15-3A), and is often itself invaginated in basilar impressions. McGregor's[11] (a line drawn from the upper surface

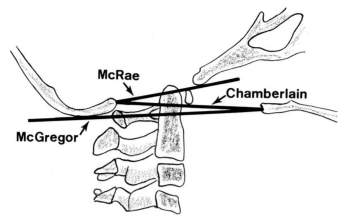

FIG. 15-1. Lateral craniometry. The drawing indicates the three lines used to determine basilar impressions. Chamberlain's line (1939) is drawn from the posterior lip of the foramen magnum (opisthion) to the dorsal margin of the hard palate. McGregor's line (1948) is drawn from the upper surface of the posterior edge of the hard palate to the most caudad point of the occipital curve of the skull. McRae's line (1953) defines the opening of the foramen magnum. McGregor's line is the best method for screening, as the bony landmarks can be clearly defined at all ages on a routine lateral roentgenogram.

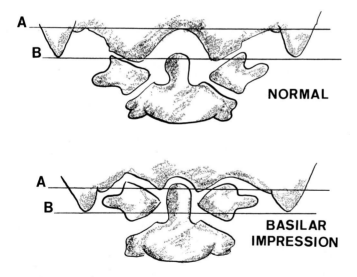

NORMAL

BASILAR IMPRESSION

FIG. 15-2. Anterior craniometry. Fischgold and Metzger (1952) noted that in the normal skull a line joining the lower poles of the mastoid processes (B) passes through the tip of the odontoid. Due to the variability in the size of mastoid processes this was further refined to a line drawn between the digastric grooves (A). These lines are best visualized on an anteroposterior transoral tomogram. Although this is the most accurate method for assessing basilar impression, its routine use is impractical and expensive.

of the posterior edge of the hard palate to the most caudal point of the occipital curve of the skull) is easier to identify (Fig. 15-1, 15-3B), and it is therefore preferable. The position of the tip of the odontoid is measured in relation to this base line, and a distance of 4.5 mm. above McGregor's line is considered to be on the extreme edge of normality.[11] However, Hinck's study of normal variations demonstrated a wide range of normality, as well as difference between males and females.[9] McRae's line defines the opening of the foramen magnum and is derived from his observation that if

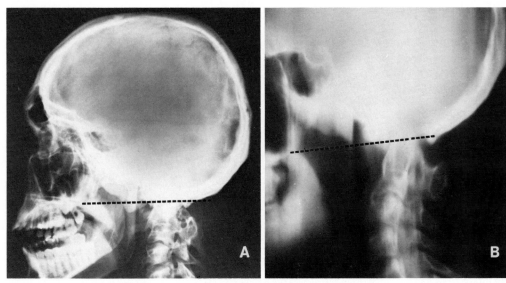

FIG. 15-3. A 15-year-old male with history of an unusual gait and a recent episode of unconsciousness after mild head trauma. *(A)* Routine lateral roentgenogram suggests that the odontoid is displaced proximally into the opening of the foramen magnum. *(B)* Lateral laminogram demonstrates that there is fusion of C1 to the occiput (occipitalization of C1) and that the tip of the odontoid is well above McGregor's line, it is projecting into the opening of the foramen magnum (McRae's line).

the tip of the odontoid lies below the opening of the foramen magnum, the patient will probably be asymptomatic. McRae's line is an accurate guide in the clinical assessment of patients with basilar impression.[9]

A criticism of the lateral lines (McGregor's and Chamberlain's) is that the hard palate is not actually a part of the skull and it may be distorted by an abnormal facial configuration or a highly arched palate, quite independent of a cranial-vertebral anomaly. In addition, the patient may have an abnormally long or short odontoid or an abnormality of the axis or occipital facets, which can diminish the value of the measurements. As a consequence, Fischgold and Metzger[6] described a more accurate method to assess basilar impression based on a line drawn between the two digastric grooves (junction of the medial aspect of the mastoid process at the base of the skull) on an anteroposterior laminographic view of the skull (Fig. 15-2). In the normal skull, this line will pass well above the odontoid tip (10.7 mm.) and the atlanto-occipital joints (11.6 mm.).[9]

In summary, McGregor's line is the best method for routine screening, as the landmarks can be clearly defined at all ages on a routine lateral roentgenogram. More elaborate measurements (Fischgold-Metzger's digastric line) are generally reserved for the patient whose routine examination or clinical findings may suggest the presence of an occipitocervical anomaly. McRae's line is a helpful guide in assessing the clinical significance of basilar impression.

Clinical Findings

Patients with basilar impresssion frequently have a deformity of the skull or neck (a short neck in 78 per cent, asymmetry of the face or skull, or torticollis in 68 per cent).[4] These physical findings are often found in patients without basilar impression (Klippel-Feil syndrome, occipitalization) and are not considered pathognomonic.

The symptoms (or lack of them) even in severe basilar impression are difficult to explain.[4] Basilar impression is frequently associated with anomalous neurologic conditions, such as the Arnold-Chiari malformation[4] and syringomyelia, which can further cloud the clinical picture. Symptoms are generally due to crowding of the neural structures at the level of the foramen magnum, particularly the medulla oblongata. There is an unusually high incidence of basilar impression in northeast Brazil, and the work of DeBarros[4] has been helpful in delineating the symptoms and signs. Patients who were symptomatic with pure basilar impression had the dominant complaints of motor and sensory disturbances, and 85 per cent had weakness and paresthesia of the limbs. In contrast, those patients who are symptomatic with pure Arnold-Chiari malformation were more likely to have cerebellar and vestibular disturbances (unsteadiness of gait, dizziness, and nystagmus). In both conditions, there may be impingement of the lower cranial nerves as they emerge from the medulla oblongata, particularly the trigeminal (V), glossopharyngeal (IX), vagus (X), and hypoglossal (XIII).[4] Headache and pain in the nape of the neck, in the distribution of the greater occipital nerve, is a common finding.[4]

Posterior encroachment may cause blockage of the aqueduct of Silvius, and the presenting symptoms may be from increased intercranial pressure or hydrocephalus.[4, 11] Compression of the cerebellum with vestibular involvement or herniation of the cerebellar tonsils (the Arnold-Chiari malformation) is a frequent finding,[4] leading to vertical or lateral nystagmus in 65 per cent of cases. These symptoms may not be due to direct pressure from the posterior rim of the foramen magnum, but rather they may be caused from a thickened band of dura not visible on plain roentgenograms, prompting several authors to recommend routine myelographic evaluation.

There is a high incidence of vertebral artery anomalies in basilar impression and atlanto-occipital fusion.[2] In addition, the vertebral arteries may be compressed as they pass through the crowded foramen magnum causing symptoms suggestive of vertebral arterial insufficiency, such as dizziness, seizures, mental deterioration, and syncope.[2, 11] These symptoms may occur alone or in combination with those of spinal cord compression.[2, 4, 8, 11] Michie[10] and Bach[1] have theorized that one explanation

for the frequent association of syringomyelia or syringobulbia and basilar impression, is that the vertebral arteries and the anterior spinal artery are compromised in the region of the foramen magnum, with subsequent degeneration of the spinal cord and medulla. Unfortunately, arteriographic studies are not available to confirm this interesting thesis.

Although this condition is congenital, many patients do not develop symptoms until the second or third decade of life.[4] This may be due to a gradually increasing instability from ligamentous laxity due to aging, similar to the delayed myelopathies reported following atlantoaxial dislocations or the increasing instability of C1 and C2 in patients with odontoid agenesis.[7] These individuals often develop premature cervical osteoarthritis as found in the family studies by Gunderson.[8] Chamberlain[3] and others have theorized that the young developing brain might be more tolerant to compressive effects, later proving deleterious to older tissues. Similarly, arteriosclerotic changes in the vertebral arteries may make these vessels more susceptible to minor constrictions. The symptoms frequently occur in older patients in whom a congenital anomaly would not ordinarily be considered. Patients with this malformation have been mistakenly diagnosed as having multiple sclerosis, posterior fossa tumors, amyotrophic lateral sclerosis, or traumatic injury. It is therefore important to survey this area whenever such a diagnosis is considered and this malformation is in any way suspected.

Treatment

Treatment depends on the cause of the symptoms, often requiring the combined talents of the orthopaedist, neurosurgeon, neurologist, and radiologist. It is quite possible to have a severe basilar impression without neurologic symptoms, and a search for associated conditions must be conducted. If the symptoms are predominantly due to anterior impingement from a hypermobile odontoid, stabilization of the occipitocervical junction, in extension, may be required. If the odontoid cannot be reduced, an anterior excision can be considered, preceded by stabilization in extension.[11a] Posterior impingement usually requires suboc-

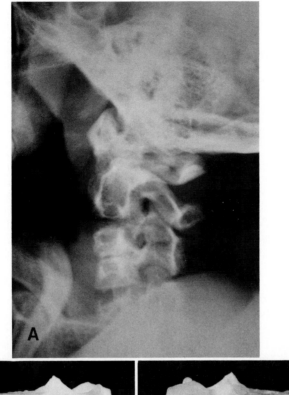

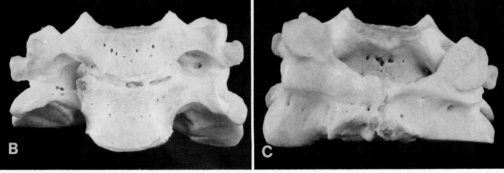

FIG. 15-4. Sixteen-year-old male with the Klippel-Feil syndrome and myelodysplasia. *(A)* Lateral roentgenogram of the cervical spine demonstrates a congenital block vertebrae of C3-C4. The patient subsequently expired from the complications of chronic renal disease. *(B)* Postmortem specimen of C3-C4—anterior view, *(C)* posterior view. The specimen demonstrates complete fusion of C3-C4. Remnants of the cartilaginous vertebral end-plates can be visualized both in the specimen and in the roentgenograms.

cipital craniectomy and decompression of the posterior ring of C1 and possibly C2, coupled with posterior stabilization. Most authors suggest opening the dura to look for a tight posterior dural band.[4] These are generalizations regarding treatment and appropriate references should be consulted in the evaluation of individual patients.

KLIPPEL-FEIL SYNDROME (CONGENITAL SYNOSTOSIS OF THE CERVICAL VERTEBRAE, BREVICOLLIS)

In 1912, Klippel and Feil[30] published the first complete description of clinical aspects and pathology of this condition. Their atten-

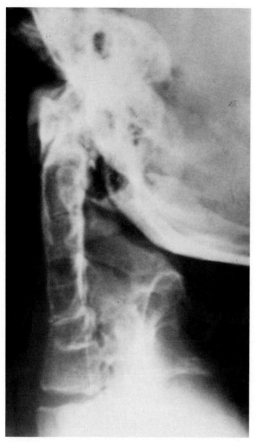

Fig. 15-5. Lateral roentgenogram of a 16-year-old male with the Klippel-Feil syndrome demonstrates a complete fusion of the cervical spine and an abnormal atlantoaxial articulation.

Table 15-1. Abnormalities Associated With the Klippel-Feil Syndrome

Common	Percentage
Scoliosis	60
Renal abnormalities	35
Sprengel's deformity	30
Deafness	30
Synkinesia	20
Congenital heart disease	14
Less Common	
Ptosis	
Duane's contracture	
Lateral rectus palsy	
Facial nerve palsy	
Syndactyly	
Hypoplastic thumb	
Upper extremity hypoplasia	

tion was attracted to a patient who had the unusual clinical findings of marked shortening of the neck, a low posterior hairline, and severe restriction of neck motion. The patient died and at the postmortem examination they discovered a complete fusion of the cervical vertebrae. Subsequently, Feil was able to collect 13 additional examples and published a thesis in 1919 which included his findings from this larger group and a review of the literature. The term "Klippel-Feil syndrome" in its present usage refers to all patients with congenital fusion of the cervical vertebrae, whether it involve two segments, congenital block vertebrae (Fig. 15-4), or the entire cervical spine (Fig. 15-5). Feil originally suggested a system of clas-

sification based on the extent and type of the cervical fusion. However, with the exception of the area of genetics,[19, 23] this classification has not proven to be clinically useful. Rather, as additional patients were discovered and roentgenographic techniques improved, it became apparent that certain anomalies of the occipitocervical junction (see atlanto-occipital fusion, p. 556; basilar impression, p. 533; and abnormalities of the odontoid, p. 548) should be considered separately from the original syndrome. Although these conditions occur commonly in conjunction with fusion of the lower cervical vertebrae, their significance is dependent upon how they influence the atlantoaxial joint. Their prognostic and therapeutic implications are distinctly different and they occur with sufficient frequency to warrant individual analysis.

Congenital cervical fusion is the result of failure of the normal segmentation of the cervical somites during the third to eighth week of life. With the exception of a few patients in whom this condition is inherited,[23, 24] the etiology is as yet undetermined. It is important to note that the effect of this embryologic abnormality is not limited to the cervical spine. The entire organism may be adversely influenced. Patients with the Klippel-Feil syndrome, even those with minor cervical lesions, may have other less

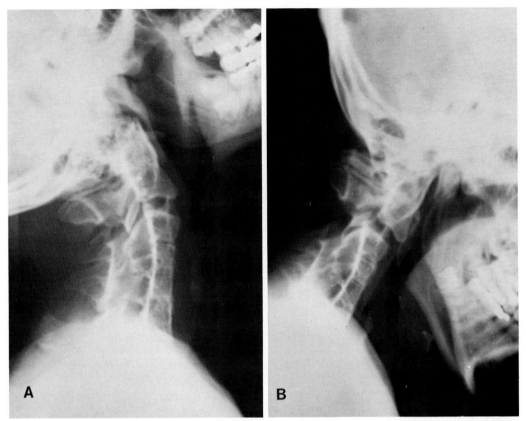

Fig. 15-6. *(A and B)*. Eighteen-year-old female with the Klippel-Feil syndrome demonstrating flexion-extension of the cervical spine. The majority of her neck motion occurs at the C3-C4 disc space. Clinically the patient is able to maintain 90° of flexion-extension. At present the patient is asymptomatic, but with aging this hypermobile articulation may become grossly unstable.

apparent or even occult defects in the genitourinary,[26, 32, 42] nervous,[14, 15] and cardiopulmonary systems,[13, 36, 39] and even hearing loss.[26, 33, 41, 44] Many of these "hidden" abnormalities may be more detrimental to the patient's general well-being than the obvious deformity of the neck. In the review by Hensinger and his associates, a high incidence of related congenital anomalies was found[26] (Table 15-1), emphasizing that all patients with the Klippel-Feil syndrome should be thoroughly investigated.

Clinical Appearance

The classical clinical description of the syndrome is a triad—low posterior hairline, short neck, and limitation of neck motion—but less than one half of the patients have all three signs.[26] Their presence is directly related to the degree of cervical spine involvement. Clinically, the most consistent finding is limitation of neck motion.[23] However, if fewer than three vertebrae are fused, or if only the lower cervical segments are fused, the patient generally has no detectable limitation.[23] In addition, many patients with marked cervical involvement are able to compensate with hypermobility at the unfused joints and to maintain a deceptively good range of motion.[26] Several of our patients have 90° of flexion-extension, occurring at the only open interspace (Fig. 15-6). Generally, flexion-extension is better preserved than rotation or lateral bend.

Shortening of the neck, unless extreme, is a subtle finding. Similarly, the low posterior

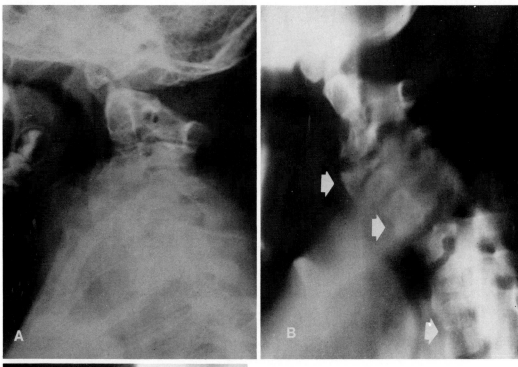

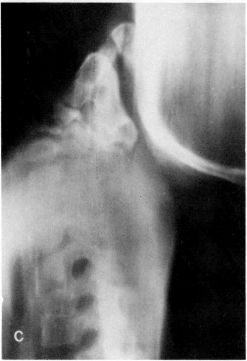

FIG. 15-7. Six-year-old male with the Klippel-Feil syndrome. *(A)* Routine lateral roentgenogram of the cervical spine. Overlapping shadows from the shoulder and occiput obscure much of the cervical spine. *(B)* Lateral laminogram in flexion demonstrates an anterior hemivertebrae *(arrow)*, probably C4, and congenital fusion of C2-C3, C6-C7, and T3-T4. *(C)* Lateral laminogram in extension demonstrates absence of the posterior ring of Cl and an unstable C1-C2 articulation. Flexion-extension laminographic views are helpful in providing the information necessary to evaluate children with severe deformity, particularly if vertebral instability is suspected.

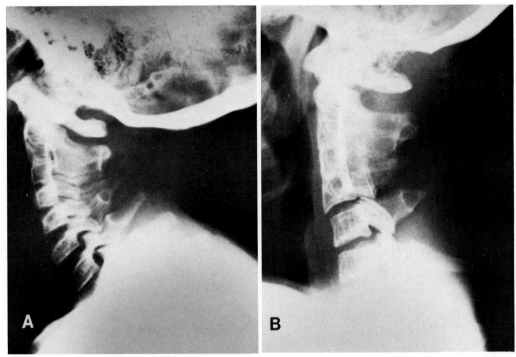

FIG. 15-8. Maturation of the cervical fusion in a patient with the Klippel-Feil syndrome. *(A)* Roentgenogram at age 6 demonstrates posterior fusion of the lamina and spinous process and incomplete fusion of the vertebral bodies. *(B)* At age 19, fusion of the vertebral bodies of C2 to C5 is now complete. In children, narrowing of the cervical disc spaces cannot always be appreciated, as ossification of the vertebral bodies is not completed until adolescence. The unossified cartilage endplates can give the false impression of a normal disc space.

hairline is not constant. Less than 20 per cent of patients with the Klippel-Feil syndrome have obvious facial asymmetry, torticollis, or webbing of the neck.[23, 26] When extreme, webbing of the neck is called "pterygium colli," and it consists of large skin folds extending from the mastoid to the acromion.[22] The underlying muscles may be involved, but surgical release generally does not result in improved neck motion.

Sprengel's deformity occurs in 25 to 35 per cent, unilaterally or bilaterally.[19, 23, 26, 32, 43] At the third week of gestation, the scapula develops from mesodermal tissue high in the neck at the level of C4. It descends into the thoracic position by the eighth week, or approximately at the same time that Klippel-Feil lesion is thought to occur.[19, 23] Therefore, it is logical to expect a significant relation between these two anomalies. Occasionally there is a bony bridge between the cervical spine and scapula, an omovertebral bone. Its removal may permit an increase in neck and shoulder motion.

Probably for the same embryologic reasons, other clinical findings are occasionally found (Table 15-1)—ptosis of the eye, Duane's contracture (contracture of the lateral rectus muscle[23]), lateral rectus palsy, facial nerve palsy, and a cleft or high-arched palate. Abnormalities of the upper extremities include syndactyly, hypoplastic thumb, supernumerary digits, and hypoplasia of the upper extremity. Abnormalities of the lower extremities are infrequent.

Roentgenographic Features

In the severely involved child, an adequate roentgenographic evaluation can be difficult. Fixed bony deformities frequently prevent proper positioning, and

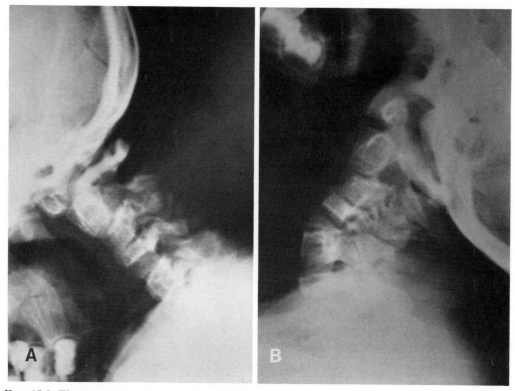

FIG. 15-9. Three-year-old with the Klippel-Feil syndrome and congenital scoliosis. Lateral flexion-extension roentgenograms of the cervical spine *(A and B)* demonstrate that neck motion occurs predominantly between C4-C5. Flexion-extension views are helpful in determining the type and extent of congenital fusion in the young child.

overlapping shadows from the mandible, occiput, or foramen magnum may obscure the upper vertebrae (Fig. 15-7). In this situation, flexion-extension laminographic views are quite helpful in providing the information necessary to evaluate the deformity. If vertebral instability is suspected, the study should be augmented by cineradiography. Knowledge of the normal variations in cervical spine mobility in children noted in the work of Cattell and Filtzer,[17] and Sullivan and his associates[45] helps in evaluating the Klippel-Feil patient.

Aside from vertebral synostosis, flattening and widening of the involved vertebral bodies and absent disc spaces are the most common findings. Hypoplasia of the disc space or remnants of it can often be seen (Fig. 15-5). In the young child, narrowing of the cervical disc space cannot always be ap-

preciated, as the ossification of the vertebral body is incomplete and the unossified endplates may give the false impression of a normal disc space (Fig. 15-8). However, with continued growth the ossification of the vertebral bodies is completed and the fusion becomes obvious. If fusion is suspected in a child, it may be confirmed by flexion-extension views (Fig. 15-9). Juvenile rheumatoid arthritis, rheumatoid spondylitis, and infection can mimic the roentgenographic findings, but usually the clinical history and physical examination indicate the correct diagnosis.

Posterior element fusion usually parallels that of the vertebral bodies. In the young child, particular attention should be paid to the laminae, as fusion posteriorly is often more apparent than anteriorly in early life[26] (Fig. 15-10). Narrowing of the spinal canal, if it occurs, is usually in adult life and due to degenerative changes (osteoarthritic spurs) or hypermobility.[18] Enlargement of the cervical canal is uncommon and if found, it suggests the presence of conditions such as syringomyelia, hydromyelia, or the Arnold-Chiari malformation.[38] The intervertebral foramina are usually smooth in contour, but they are frequently smaller than normal and oval rather than circular in shape.

All of these defects may extend into the upper thoracic spine, particularly in the severely involved patient. A disturbance of the upper thoracic spine on a routine chest roentgenogram may be the first clue to an unrecognized cervical synostosis. It should be a routine when evaluating a high thoracic congenital scoliosis that the roentgenographic evaluation include lateral views of the cervical spine.

Associated Conditions

Scoliosis is the most frequent anomaly found in association with this syndrome.[26, 32] Sixty per cent of these patients have a significant degree of scoliosis (greater than 15° by the Cobb method).[26] The majority of these patients require treatment and should be followed through the growth years. The roentgenographic examinations should include lateral views of the spine, as an increasing kyphosis may make the need for treatment of the scoliosis more urgent. If the deformity is recognized early, many children can be successfully controlled with standard spinal orthotics such as the Milwaukee brace. At present, the majority of these patients have required posterior spinal stabilization, in part due to late recognition.[15, 21, 26, 32]

Of interest is the frequent occurrence of progressive scoliosis in the normal-appearing vertebrae below the primary congenital curve. If only the congenitally involved segments are examined in follow-up, an increasing compensatory scoliosis in the lower vertebrae may not be recognized and its significance may not be appreciated until serious deformity results.

Documented progression of scoliosis, whether in the congenitally distorted elements or the compensatory curve below, demands immediate and appropriate treat-

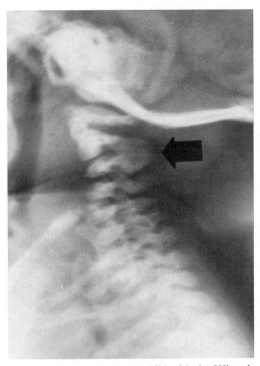

FIG. 15-10. A 3-month-old child with the Klippel-Feil syndrome. The roentgenograms demonstrate posterior fusion of the lamina of C2-C3 *(arrow)*. In the young child, particular attention should be paid to the laminae, as fusion posteriorly is often more apparent than anteriorly in early life.

ment to prevent serious additional deformity. Scoliosis in the thoracic area should not be allowed to progress beyond 55° by the Cobb method in the erect position, as further increase will seriously compromise pulmonary function.[13, 26] More subtle occult abnormalities can lead to respiratory difficulty in some Klippel-Feil patients. Abnormal rib spacing, congenital fusion of the ribs, and deformed costovertebral joints may inhibit full expansion of the rib cage during respiration.[12] Although not causing an angular deformity, fusion of the thoracic vertebrae may decrease the size of the thoracic cage. The spondylothoracic dwarf may represent a severe form of this problem, leading to early respiratory death.[37] In addition, Krieger[31] has recently reported on the relationship of occult respiratory dysfunction and craniovertebral anomalies. He notes that in addition to the obvious problems of bony impingement or traction upon the brain stem, these patients may have subtle hydrocephalus, which may adversely affect respiratory function.

This information has particular application when cervical distraction devices are contemplated in the treatment of scoliosis (halo-femoral or halo-pelvic traction). When considering use of such devices, the physician should be aware that children with the Klippel-Feil syndrome may be more susceptible to neurologic or vascular injury and that the presence of cervical anomalies may preclude the use of cervical distraction.[26]

Renal Abnormalities. In the Klippel-Feil syndrome, over one-third of the children can be expected to have a significant urinary tract anomaly. These anomalies are often asymptomatic in the young, and an intravenous pyelogram should be a routine procedure for these children.[26] The most frequent abnormality is unilateral absence of a kidney. Other abnormalities include a double collecting system, renal ectopia, a horseshoe kidney, and hydronephrosis from ureteral-pelvic obstruction. Two of 50 patients in our series developed severe pyelonephritis in their remaining kidney, requiring renal transplantation.[26] Indeed, in Klippel and Feil's original case report, the patient died from nephritis.[30]

Cardiovascular Abnormalities. The literature notes the association of the Klippel-Feil syndrome with congenital heart disease (4.2 to 14%).[21, 26, 36, 39] The most common lesion reported has been an interventricular septal defect occurring alone or in combination with other defects, such as a patent ductus arteriosus and abnormal positioning of the heart and aorta.

Deafness. The association of hearing impairment and even deafness in the Klippel-Feil syndrome (over 30%) has been reported in the otology literature;[28, 33, 41, 44] however, it is seldom mentioned in orthopaedic reports.[26, 32] Other defects include absence of the auditory canal and microtia.

Jalladeau is credited with the first report of deafness.[28] Stark noted that detailed audiologic data is not yet available, and the precise defect is often not known.[44] There is no characteristic audiologic anomaly, and all types of hearing loss (conductive, sensory-neural, and mixed) have been described. These patients should have an audiometric test when they are discovered. The relationship between hearing loss and speech-language retardation is well documented, and early detection of hearing impairment can reduce the retardation by permitting early initiation of speech and language training.[44]

Mirror Motions (Synkinesia). Synkinesia consists of involuntary paired movements of the hands and occasionally the arms. The patient is unable to move one hand without similar reciprocal motion of the opposite hand. Mirror motion was first described by Bauman, who found it present in four of six patients with the Klippel-Feil syndrome.[15] This condition has been found to occur occasionally in normal preschool children and patients with cerebral palsy or Parkinson's disease. However, the majority of patients afflicted with this problem have the Klippel-Feil syndrome.[19] Approximately 20 per cent demonstrate mirror motions clinically.[26] Baird, in examining 13 patients with the Klippel-Feil syndrome using electromyography, found ten patients with electrically detectable paired motion in the opposite extremity.[14] This suggests that many patients may be subclinically affected and may be more clumsy at two-handed activities.

The etiology of synkinesia is unknown, but it appears to be a separate congenital neurologic defect not due to bony impingement or irritation of the spinal cord. The examination of two autopsy specimens suggests that the clinical findings are due to inadequate or incomplete decussation of the pyramidal tracts in conjunction with a dysrhaphic cervical spinal cord.[12, 25] As a consequence, cerebral control over the upper extremities must follow less direct pathways located in the extrapyramidal system, and the afflicted patient requires more extensive practice to disassociate the movements of the individual extremities.

Synkinesia is most pronounced in the young child, particularly those under 5 years of age. Fortunately, the condition tends to decrease with age. Occupational therapy has been helpful in teaching the patient control over the extremities, or at least in disguising the reciprocal motion to a tolerable cosmetic level. Still, many patients may find discriminating two-handed activity difficult,[40] such as playing the piano, typing, sewing, or ladder climbing.

Symptoms

With the exception of the anomalies that involve the atlantoaxial joint, there are no symptoms that can be directly attributed to the fused cervical vertebrae. All symptoms commonly associated with the Klippel-Feil syndrome originate at the open segments where the remaining free articulations may become compensatorily hypermobile. Due to the increased demands placed on these joints or in response to trauma, this hypermobility can lead to frank instability or to early degenerative arthritis.[43] Symptoms may then arise from two sources: (1) mechanical symptoms due to irritation of the joint, and (2) neurologic symptoms due to root irritation or spinal cord compression. Patients who have a short-segment fusion are less likely to develop symptoms,[23] as the loss of motion is adequately compensated by the remaining free segments. Patients with synostosis of the lower cervical spine are at less risk, as the limitation is minimal and can be adequately compensated by the more normally mobile joints above. The majority of patients who develop symptoms are in the second or third decade,[23] suggesting that the instability is in part a function of time with increasing ligament laxity.

Neurologic symptoms are generally localized to the head, neck, and upper extremities, and result from direct irritation or impingement of the cervical nerve roots with radicular symptoms in the upper extremities.[35] The symptoms usually can be localized to the hypermobile joints adjacent to the fused segments. There may be constriction and narrowing of the nerve root at the foramen from osteophytic spurring.[35] If joint instability is progressive or if there is appropriate trauma, the spinal cord may be involved to varying degrees, from mild spasticity, hyperreflexia, and muscular weakness to sudden complete quadriplegia following minor trauma.[23, 24, 27, 35, 43,]

Patterns of Cervical Motion. One can gain insight into the problem of instability by reviewing the lateral flexion-extension films of the Klippel-Feil patient. The type or pattern

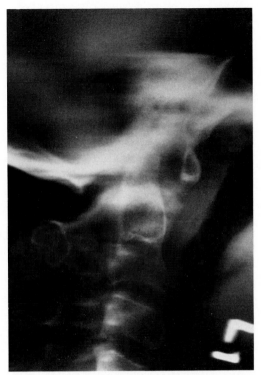

FIG. 15-11. Twenty-three-year-old male with the Klippel-Feil syndrome, ataxic gait, hyperreflexia and a history of several episodes of unconsciousness. Lateral laminographic view of the cervical spine and base of the skull demonstrates a C2-C3 fusion and fusion of the ring of C1 to the opening of the foramen magnum (occipitalization). The odontoid is hypermobile. Patients with this pattern of fusion are at great risk. With aging, the odontoid may become hypermobile and the space available for the spinal cord posteriorly may be compromised.

of cervical motion is dependent upon the location and extent of the fused cervical vertebrae. Those with fusion of the lower cervical vertebrae or with more than two disc spaces between fused segments seem to be at low risk for serious problems, There are, however, three high-risk patterns of cervical spinal motion which potentially have a poor prognosis, either from late instability or degenerative osteoarthritis.

Pattern 1 is fusion of C2 and C3 with occipitalization of the atlas (Fig. 15-11). Complications associated with this pattern were first reported by McRae[34] (1953), and they

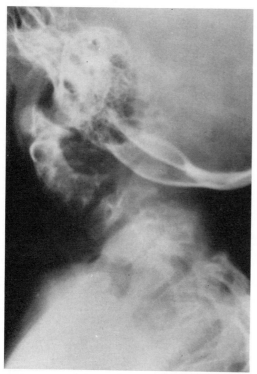

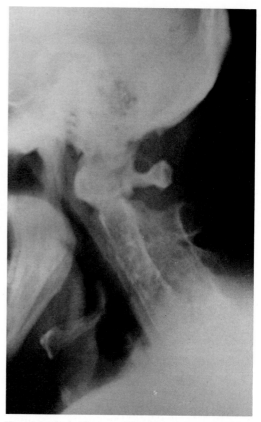

FIG. 15-12. Twelve-year-old female with the Klippel-Feil syndrome. A long segment of cervical fusion (C2-C6) and an abnormal occipitocervical articulation are shown. This pattern could be viewed as a more elaborate variation of the C2-C3 pattern of McRae. The force of flexion-extension and rotation are concentrated in the area of the abnormal occipitocervical junction. These patients may be at risk for developing instability with aging.

FIG. 15-13. A 45-year-old male with the Klippel-Feil syndrome. The patient has complete fusion of C2 to C7. Flexion-extension occurs only at the atlantoaxial articulation. The patient has no symptoms referable to the neck, despite two previous serious falls. This pattern appears to be relatively safe, as the normal occipitocervical junction serves as a protection from late instability.

have received substantial support in the literature.[24] Flexion-extension is concentrated in the area of C1 and C2. With aging, an odontoid can become hypermobile and may dislocate posteriorly, narrowing the spinal canal and compromising the spinal cord and brain stem.

Pattern 2 is a long fusion with an abnormal occipitocervical junction (Fig. 15-12). This is similar to the C2-C3 fusion of McRae and could be reviewed as a more elaborate variation. The force of flexion-extension and rotation is concentrated in the area of the abnormal odontoid or poorly developed ring of C1 which cannot withstand the wear and tear of aging. It is important to differentiate this pattern from the patient with a long fusion and a normal C1-C2 articulation (Fig. 15-13), which is usually compatible with a normal life expectancy.

Pattern 3 is a single open interspace between two fused segments (Fig. 15-14). In this situation, cervical spine motion is concentrated at the single open articulation. In some patients this hypermobility may lead to frank instability or degenerative osteoarthritis.[24, 35, 43] This pattern can be easily recognized, as the cervical spine appears to angle or hinge at the open segment.

Treatment

The minimally involved patient with the Klippel-Feil syndrome can be expected to lead a normal active life with no or only minor restrictions or symptoms. Many of the severely involved patients can enjoy the same good prognosis if early and appropriate treatment is instituted when needed. This is particularly applicable in the area of associated scoliosis and renal abnormalities. Prevention of further deformity or complications can be of great benefit to the patient.

At present, treatment modalities for the cervical spine anomalies are quite limited. Those patients with major areas of cervical synostosis or high-risk patterns of cervical spinal motion should be strongly advised to avoid activities that place stress on the cervical spine. In these patients, the mobile articulations are under greater mechanical demands and are less capable of protecting the patient against traumatic insults.

As has been discussed, sudden neurologic compromise or death following minor trauma has been reported in the Klippel-Feil syndrome and usually is due to disruption at the hypermobile articulation.[24, 35, 43] The role of prophylactic surgical stabilization in the asymptomatic patient has not yet been defined. There is no satisfactory answer to when the risk of instability warrants further reduction of neck motion.

For the symptomatic patient with mechanical problems, the usual treatment measures for degenerative osteoarthritis are applicable and include traction, cervical collar, and analgesics. Symptoms which suggest neurologic compromise need careful consideration and evaluation by a neurologist, neurosurgeon, and orthopaedist. The exact area of irritation must be determined prior to surgical intervention. Attempts should be made preoperatively to obtain reduction of the bony architecture prior to surgical stabilization. The physician must be mindful that there are other associated abnormalities both in the brain stem and in the spinal cord itself which may be contributing to the symptoms.

Treatment of cosmetic aspects of this deformity has met with limited success. Occasionally children with the fixed torticollis posture may be improved with bracing. However, this requires long-term applica-

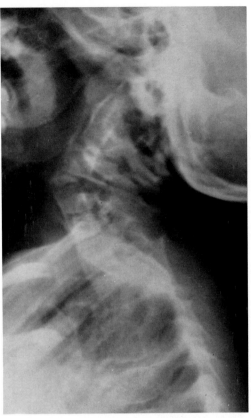

FIG. 15-14. Open interspace between two fused segments. A 7-year-old child with the Klippel-Feil syndrome has flexion-extension motion of the neck occurring primarily at one interspace. The cervical spine appears to angle or hinge at this point. This is a worrisome pattern, as wear and tear of aging may lead to early degenerative change or instability and narrowing of the spinal canal.

tion and excellent patient cooperation. Surgical correction of the bony deformity by direct means such as wedge osteotomy is not recommended. Occasionally carefully selected patients who have cervical congenital scoliosis may obtain some correction and improvement of appearance by use of the halo cast combined with posterior cervical fusion. Bonala described a method of rib resection to attain apparent increase in neck length and motion.[16] However, this procedure is an extensive surgical experience and is a great risk to the patient. No subsequent reports have appeared in the literature.

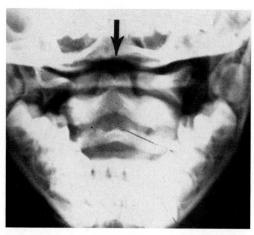

FIG. 15-15. An anteroposterior open-mouth projection demonstrates the V-shaped "dens bicornis." This is normally present as such until age 3 years. (From Fielding, J. W.: Selected observations on the cervical spine in the child. *In* Ahstrom, J. P., Jr. (ed.): Current Practice in Orthopaedic Surgery, Vol. 5. St. Louis, C. V. Mosby, 1973.)

Soft-tissue procedures, Z-plasty, and muscle resection may achieve cosmetic improvement in properly selected patients.[32] These procedures generally do not increase neck motion, and the scars may be extensive, particularly in the patient with a large skin web. A common problem is implanting hair-bearing skin to the top of the shoulders. Scapuloplasty of the Sprengel's deformity can provide some cosmetic improvement, and increased shoulder motion, but no increase in cervical spine motion.

CONGENITAL ANOMALIES OF THE ODONTOID (DENS)

Development of the Odontoid

The body of the odontoid is derived from the mesenchyme of the first cervical sclerotome and is actually the centrum of the first cervical vertebra, which, during development, becomes separated from the atlas to fuse with the remainder of the axis.[68, 79, 81, 84, 86] The apex of the odontoid process is derived from the mesenchyme of the most caudad occipital sclerotome or

proatlas. Ossification of these two segments of the odontoid then proceeds along separate lines.

Between the first and fifth prenatal month, the dens begins to ossify from two centers, one on each side of the midline. By birth, they have fused into a single mass.[47, 49, 55] Occasionally, the right and left halves of the odontoid are not fused at birth and a longitudinal midline cleft may be seen. At birth, the tip of the odontoid has not ossified, is V-shaped, and is known as a *dens bicornis* (Fig. 15-15). A separate ossification center within the V, known as a "summit ossification center" or *ossiculum terminale,* usually appears at age 3 and fuses with the remainder of the dens by age 12.[47, 49, 76, 84] Catell and Filtzer[50] found an ossiculum terminale to be present in 26 per cent of 70 normal children aged 5 to 11.

An ossiculum terminale may never appear or it may occasionally fail to fuse with the dens. It is then called *ossiculum terminale persistens* (Fig. 15-16): It is occasionally discernible as either a cyst or an area of increased density. These developmental anomalies are of little clinical significance.[53, 84] Sherk and Nicholson,[81] however, report a rare case of quadraplegia and death in a mongoloid female directly attributable to atlantoaxial instability secondary to an ossiculum terminale. This is the only such report, since the ossiculum terminale is usually firmly bound to the main body of the dens by cartilage and, consequently, it is not the source of instability.

At birth, the dens is separated from the body of the axis by a cartilaginous band, which represents the epiphyseal growth plate. This epiphyseal plate does not run across the base of the dens at the level of the superior articular facets of the axis, but it lies well below this level within the body of the axis. Therefore, the part of the odontoid below the articular facets contributes to the body of the axis. On the open-mouth view, the odontoid fits like a "cork in a bottle," lying sandwiched between the neural arches (Fig. 15-17). This epiphyseal line is present in nearly all children at age 3, 50 per cent of children by age 4, and absent in most by age 6.[50, 55] It rarely persists into adolescence and only exceptionally does it persist into adulthood. If present, it is not seen at the

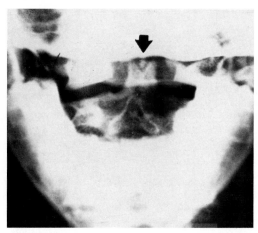

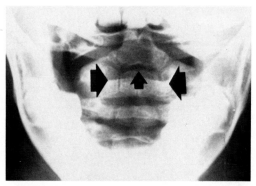

FIG. 15-17. An anteroposterior open-mouth projection demonstrates the horizontal epiphyseal growth plate lying well within the body of the axis, below the level of the superior articular facets. The odontoid fits like a "cork in a bottle" sandwiched between the neural arches *(large arrows)*. These epiphyseal lines disappear by age 6 years. (From Fielding, J. W.: Selected observations on the cervical spine in the child. In Ahstrom, J. P., Jr. (ed.): Current Practice in Orthopaedic Surgery, vol. 5. St. Louis, C. V. Mosby, 1973.)

FIG. 15-16. This anteroposterior open-mouth view demonstrates "ossiculum terminale" or the "summit ossification center," which usually appears at age 3 years and fuses to the remainder of the odontoid by age 12 years. Beyond age 12, it is termed "ossiculum terminale persistens." (From Fielding, J. W.: Selected observations on the cervical spine in the child. *In* Ahstrom, J. P., Jr. (ed.): Current Practice in Orthopaedic Surgery, Vol. 5, St. Louis, C. V. Mosby, 1973.)

base of the dens where a fracture would be anticipated, but it lies well below the level of the superior articular facets within the body of the axis.

Congenital anomalies of the odontoid can lead to an unstable atlantoaxial complex with potential neurological sequelae and even death due to cord pressure. Several gradations or variations of anomalies of the odontoid exist, ranging from *aplasia* (complete absence), to *hypoplasia* (partial absence), and to *os odontoideum* (Fig. 15-18). Associated regional malformations may occur but, unlike many congenital anomalies, they are rare.[48, 78, 84]

Definitions

Aplasia or agenesis of the odontoid is a complete absence of development. Hypoplasia is a partially developed odontoid ranging in size from a short, stubby, peg-like projection to an odontoid of almost normal size. Os odontoideum is an anomaly in which the odontoid process is divided by a wide trans-

verse gap, leaving the apical segment without support from the base.[73, 86]

Frequency

The frequency of these anomalies is unknown, and like many anomalies that may be asymtomatic, they are probably more common than appreciated. They are often incidental findings or are seen in patients sustaining trauma or symptoms sufficient to requiring roentgenographic investigation.

In our experience, aplasia is extremely rare. McRae[71] noted that there was no proven case of odontoid aplasia at the Montreal Neurological Institute up to 1960. Many previous reports have confused aplasia for hypoplasia and, probably, as previously emphasized, aplasia has been a misnomer, since it almost never describes an associated absence of the portion below the articular facets which contributes to the body of the axis. Hypoplasia and os odontoideum are infrequently reported and can be considered rare.[62, 66, 74, 78, 86] With recent awareness, however, these lesions are being recognized more commonly than past literature might indicate.

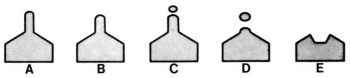

FIG. 15-18. Illustrations of gradations for odontoid anomalies: *(A)* normal odontoid; *(B)* hypoplastic odontoid; *(C)* ossiculum terminale; *(D)* os odontoideum; *(E)* aplastic odontoid.

In such conditions as mongolism, Morquio's syndrome, Klippel-Feil syndrome, and some skeletal dysplasias, odontoid anomalies in association with ligamentous laxity producing atlantoaxial instability are much more common than in the general population.[51, 52, 67, 72, 81, 82, 84]

Etiology

A congenital or developmental etiology of these anomalies has always been assumed. Hypoplasia and os odontoideum can be acquired secondary to trauma or, rarely, infection.[46, 54, 56, 60, 70, 76, 86] Four cases of "os odontoideum" have been reported which developed several years after trauma where a normal odontoid was initially present. This has led to the assumption that some cases of os odontoideum or hypoplasia may be due to an unrecognized fracture to the base or damage to the epiphyseal plate of the odontoid during the first few years of life. This insult could compromise the blood supply to the developing dens, resulting in either partial failure or complete absorption.

It is probable that both congenital or developmental and posttraumatic forms of hypoplasia and os odontoideum do exist. It is thought that failure of fusion of the apex of the odontoid (derived from the proatlas) to the main body of the atlas (derived from the first cervical sclerotome) results in the developmental form of os odontoideum.

The distinction of aplasia or hypoplasia from os odontoideum is somewhat academic since both usually lead to atlantoaxial instability. The clinical signs, symptoms, and treatment are similar. The only distinctive features are roentgenographic.

Roentgenographic Features

Recommended roentgenographic views are open-mouth anteroposterior and lateral, in addition to tomograms. Tomograms are of value since plain films do not always show the anomaly. Flexion-extension movements for lateral flexion-extension films should be conducted voluntarily by the patient, particularly those with neurologic deficits. The degree of anterior or posterior displacement of C1 on C2 should be documented. With odontoid anomalies, measurements must be taken from a line projected superiorly from the anterior border of the body of the axis to the posterior border of the anterior arch of the atlas. A measurement greater than 4mm. should be considered pathologic. The space available for the cord also should be determined in these cases.

Cineradiography has been valuable for understanding odontoid anomalies, particularly those with atlantoaxial instability. Most children with these lesions have a predominance of either anterior or posterior instability, but both can exist together. Myelography is seldom necessary since the pathology is usually obvious. Occasionally, vertebral angiography is helpful.

Normal Variations

At birth, the normal odontoid can be visualized in the lateral view with its epiphyseal plate. A mistaken impression of hypoplasia may be present with a lateral extension roentgenogram, since the anterior arch of the atlas may slide upwards and actually protrude beyond the ossified tip of the dens, especially in the very young (Fig. 15-19).

Aplasia

This extremely rare anomaly may be recognized from birth onwards and is best seen in the open-mouth view, sometimes difficult to obtain in infancy. The diagnostic feature is the absence of the basilar portion of the

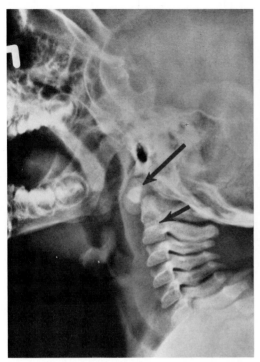

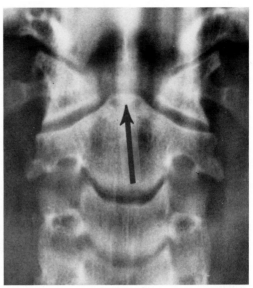

FIG. 15-20. An anteroposterior tomogram of odontoid hypoplasia. This is the commonest form, presenting with a short stubby peg of odontoid, which projects above the level of the superior articular facets of the axis. (From Fielding, J. W., and Hawkins, R. J.: Roentgenographic diagnosis of the injured neck. *In* AAOS Instructional Course Lectures, vol. 25. St. Louis, C. V. Mosby, 1976.)

FIG. 15-19. Lateral extended view of a 4-year-old child demonstrates the presence of a normal high-riding anterior arch of the atlas, giving the mistaken impression of hypoplasia of the odontoid. The short arrow points to the remnant of the epiphyseal plate, which disappears by age 6 years. (From Fielding, J. W., and Hawkins, R. J.: Roentgenographic diagnosis of the injured neck. *In* AAOS Instructional Course Lectures, vol. 25. St. Louis, C. V. Mosby, 1976.)

odontoid, which normally dips down into and contributes to the body of the axis. This basilar portion is well below the level of the superior articular facets of the axis. The lateral view is of little help to distinguish this anomaly from hypoplasia.

Hypoplasia

The commonest form of hypoplasia presents with a short, stubby peg of odontoid projecting just above the lateral facet articulations (Fig. 15-20). Tomograms are necessary to confirm whether an os odontoideum is present in addition to the hypoplasia.

Os Odontoideum

Os odontoideum may be overlooked without tomograms (Fig. 15-21). It appears as a radiolucent oval or round ossicle with a smooth dense border of bone. It may be of variable size, located usually in the position of the normal odontoid tip (orthotopic) or near the basioccipital bone in the area of the foramen magnum, where it may fuse with the clivus (dystopic).[84] The base of the dens is almost invariably hypoplastic.

It may be difficult to differentiate between os odontoideum and nonunion following an odontoid fracture.[70, 86] With a nonunion following a fractured odontoid, there is a narrow line of separation at the base of the odontoid, which may have either irregular or smooth edges of variable cortical thickness. The preservation of the normal shape and size of the dens on the anteroposterior view is an important distinguishing feature. With os odontoideum, the gap between the os and the hypoplastic dens is wide. It usually lies well above the level of the superior articular facets of the axis. The os generally does not preserve the normal shape or size of the odontoid, being usually half the size,

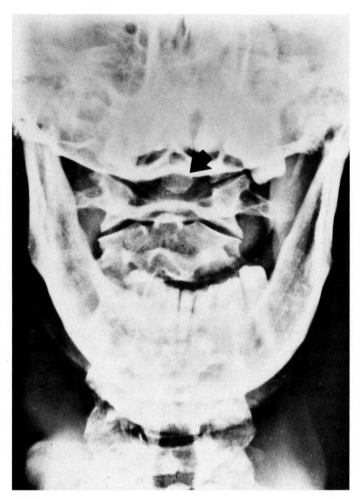

FIG. 15-21. An anteroposterior tomogram of os odontoideum. The arrow points at the small round ossicle with its smooth border lying well above the remaining hypoplastic dens. (From Fielding, J. W., Hawkins, R. J., and Ratzan, S. A.: Spine fusion for atlanto-axial instability. J. Bone Joint Surg., *58A*: 405, 1976.)

rounded or oval, and having a smooth uniform cortex. If the os is in the area of the foramen magnum, there is little diagnostic problem.

The free ossicle of the os odontoideum usually appears fixed to the anterior arch of the atlas and moves with it in flexion and extension (Fig. 15-22). Of the 12 patients that we have fused, seven displayed predominantly anterior and four predominantly posterior instability while one was grossly unstable in all directions.[58] The average displacement was 9.6 mm.

There is controversy regarding the presence of associated bony anomalies in the area of the hypoplastic dens or os odontoideum. In our experience, these changes are occasionally present, but with improved awareness they will undoubtedly be found with increasing frequency. The posterior arch of C1 may be hypoplastic while the anterior arch is hypertrophied.[62, 64] If the posterior ring of C1 is narrow and there is abnormal anterior displacement of C1, there is less available space for the cord. Hence, there is an increased danger of neurologic sequelae.

Clinical Findings

Odontoid hypoplasia and os odontoideum present with similar clinical findings, usually those secondary to instability with displacement of the atlas on the axis. In our experience, the average age at diagnosis has

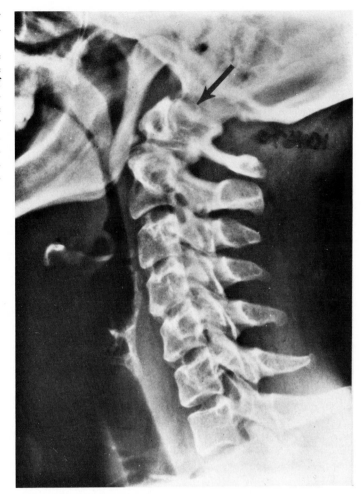

Fig. 15-22. Lateral view showing posterior displacement of the axis on the atlas. The arrow demonstrates the "os" which is bound to the hypertrophied anterior arch of the atlas. Note also the hypoplastic posterior ring of the atlas, which is occasionally present. (From Fielding, J. W., Hawkins, R. J., and Ratzan, S. A.: Spine fusion for atlanto-axial instability, J. Bone Joint Surg., *58A*:405, 1976.)

been 24 years.[58] Others report an average age at diagnosis of 30 years.[62] These problems are uncommonly diagnosed in infancy, although we have seen cases in children less than 3 years of age. On review of the literature, males significantly outnumber females.[58, 66, 70, 71, 74, 78, 86]

Congenital anomalies of the odontoid can be incidental findings in patients who have roentgenograms taken following trauma to the neck. This trauma may initiate atlantoaxial instability or precipitate symptoms in an already compromised, previously asymptomatic atlantoaxial joint. Patients may present clinically with no symptoms (incidental diagnosis); local neck symptoms (neck pain, torticollis, headache); transitory episodes of paresis following trauma; my-elopathies (cord compression),[83, 85] cervical and brain stem ischemia due to vertebral artery compression (seizures, syncope, vertigo, visual disturbances); and death.

Neurologic manifestations are recognized with increasing frequency. Although accurate statistics are not available, we believe that a significant percentage, probably greater than 50 per cent of patients, either have or will develop neurologic problems of some kind.[48, 58, 78] Sudden death has been reported.[78] Neurologic signs and symptoms are varied. Weakness and loss of balance are common complaints. Upper motor neuron signs and proprioceptive and sphincter disturbances are relatively common. Rarely, syncope, vertigo and seizures exist due to vertebral artery insufficiency.[59, 77]

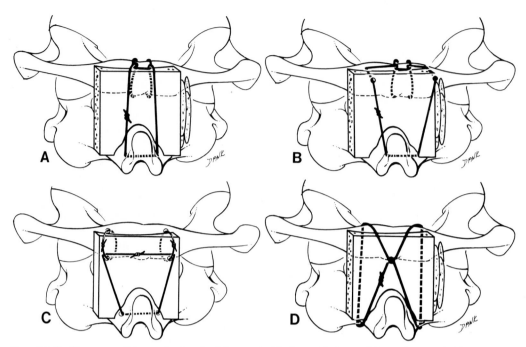

Fig. 15-23. Four possible methods of wiring to hold the graft in position. (From Fielding, J. W., Hawkins, R. J., and Ratzan, S. A.: Spine fusion for atlanto-axial instability. J. Bone Joint Surg., *58A*:403, 1976.)

Treatment

Patients with congenital anomalies of the odontoid lead a precarious existence. The concern is that a trivial insult superimposed on an already weakened and compromised structure may be catastrophic. It is our experience that patients with these problems either have or develop gross atlantoaxial instability and, with it, the possibility of progressive myelopathies, or even death.

Patients with local symptoms or transient myelopathies may expect recovery, at least temporarily.[69, 74, 77] Cervical traction or plaster immobilization may be helpful in such circumstances. Surgical stabilization is indicated if: there is neurologic involvement (even if it is transient); there is instability of greater than 5 mm. anteriorly or posteriorly; there is progressive instability, or if there are persistent neck complaints.

Considerable controversy exists as to the role of prophylactic stabilization in asymptomatic patients with instability.[61, 63, 69, 74] The safety of stability and with it the

ability to lead a normal active life must cause one to weigh the possible complications of surgery against the catastrophic dangers of instability with secondary cord pressure. In the pediatric age group, it may be difficult or impossible to curtail activity, even in the presence of marked instability.[80] In our experience, 14 such patients fused from C1 to C2 are stable and pain free and lead active lives.[58] When fusion is undertaken, regardless of the indication, preoperative skull traction may be required to achieve reduction which may have to be continued during surgery and postoperatively until transfer to a suitable immobilization device.[20, 29, 65, 74]

If upper cervical spine fusion is to be undertaken for atlantoaxial instability secondary to congenital anomalies of the odontoid, Klippel-Feil syndrome, or for bony anomalies at the occipitocervical junction, etc., the approach we recommend is generally posterior. With simple atlantoaxial instability associated with congenital anomalies, atlantoaxial arthrodesis, by the

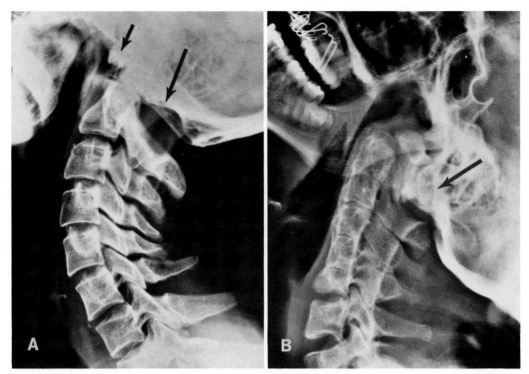

FIG. 15-24. *(A)* Lateral projection of an adult demonstrates complete assimilation of the atlas to the base of the occiput. The small arrow demonstrates the remnant of the anterior arch of the atlas and the larger arrow demonstrates the remnant of the posterior arches of the atlas. Although not wholly visualized, the odontoid is projecting into the foramen magnum. *(B)* Lateral projection of an adolescent demonstrates assimilation of the posterior arches of the atlas *(arrow)* to the base of the occiput. There is associated marked posterior displacement of the atlas on the axis with odontoid hypoplasia. The diagnosis is Klippel-Feil syndrome, as demonstrated by the fused vertebrae.

Gallie technique, is recommended (Fig 15-23). When there are associated bony anomalies at the occipitocervical junction, the fusion may have to be extended up to the occiput. Nonunion is rare in the upper cervical area, and the patient is often rehabilitated to a normal, active life with full participation in sporting events. In performing over 25 fusions of the above nature in childhood and adolescence, we have encountered no major problems.

The technique of surgery with the Gallie fusion involves the use of 22-gauge wire to hold the graft on the posterior arches of the atlas and the axis. In the younger children, the wire may be eliminated, but we have used the wire in children as young as 6 years of age with no problems. The graft is taken from the iliac crest and, for the Gallie fusion,

is shaped as shown in Fig 15-23. If the fusion is extended to the occiput, cortical and cancellous strips are layed along the denuded posterior aspects of the occiput, C1 and C2. Caution must be taken only to expose the bony elements to be fused, because in children there is a great danger of migration of the fusion mass.

Postoperatively, we prefer the use of a Minerva jacket, which can usually be applied at 7 to 14 days and is left on for about 6 weeks followed by use of a brace for an additional 6-week period. If there is gross instability of neurologic deficiencies, traction may need to be continued in the postoperative period for about 6 weeks, followed by use of a brace. With rotary fixation, traction might have to be continued for a 6-week period postoperatively to maintain as much correction as possible while fusion is occurring.

Summary

Although congenital anomalies of the odontoid are uncommon, the importance of recognition lies in their potential to produce serious sequelae due to atlantoaxial instability. Hypoplasia and os odontoideum present either asymptomatically, with transient or permanent neurologic deficits, with persistent neck complaints, or with sudden death. Diagnosis is confirmed with tomography, and flexion-extension stress films are necessary to determine the presence and degree of atlantoaxial instability. Cineradiography is very helpful to appreciate the underlying pathology.

When there is instability, neurologic compromise, and persistent neck complaints, atlantoaxial arthrodesis is favored. Preoperative traction may be necessary for reduction. Prophylactic stabilization in asymptomatic unstable patients is also suggested.

OCCIPITOCERVICAL SYNOSTOSIS

Occipitocervical synostosis, which may be partial or complete, is a congenital union between the atlas and the base of the occiput (Fig. 15-24). Synonyms include assimilation of the atlas, occipitocervical fusion, and occipitalization of the atlas. It ranges from total incorporation of the atlas into the occipital bone to a bony or even fibrous band uniting one small area of the atlas to the occiput. Basilar impression is commonly associated with occipitocervical synostosis; other associated anomalies include Klippel-Feil syndrome, occipital vertebrae, and condylar hypoplasia.[101]

Occipitocervical synostosis, basilar impression, and odontoid anomalies are the commonest developmental malformations of the occipitocervical junction. Incidence ranges from 1.4 to 2.5 per 1,000 children, with sexes being equally affected.[93, 101]

Development of the Occipitocervical Area

Developmental anomalies and malformations are commonest at the lower and upper transitional ends of the spinal column. Bony abnormalities of the atlas, axis, and occiput are called "occipital" or "suboccipital" dysplasias.[102] These include errors of segmentation, aplasias, hypoplasias, dysplasias, and dysrhaphic phenomena, listed in Table 15-2.[101]

The basilar portion of the occiput along with lateral masses and posterior arches of the atlas are derived from the mesenchyme of the most caudad occipital sclerotome or proatlas.[101] Ossiculum terminale and the ossicle of os odontoideum also arise from this sclerotome. These areas of primitive mesenchyme separate or segment from each other during growth of the fetus and then chondrify as distinct units. The anterior arch of the atlas arises from a separate embryologic segment known as the hypochordal bow.

Ossification of the atlas proceeds from paired centers—one for each of the lateral masses. These progress posteriorly into the neural arches, which are fully ossified at birth except for a gap of 5 to 9 mm. posteriorly that closes by the fourth year. In the neonate, the anterior arch of the atlas is not visible. This area most commonly ossifies from a single center which appears during the first year of life and fuses to the remainder of the atlas by the third year.[87, 89, 91, 101]

Since segmentation precedes ossification and most anomalies, particularly occipitocervical synostosis, occur long before ossification, Hadley prefers to describe this lesion as nonsegmentation or failure of segmentation rather than fusion.[92]

Roentgenographic Findings

Standard roentgenograms of this area can be difficult to interpret. Tomograms may be necessary to clarify the pathology.[102] Most commonly, the anterior arch of the atlas is assimilated into the occiput. In this instance, the atlas is displaced posteriorly relative to the occiput, usually in association with a hypoplastic posterior arch. There is varying loss of height of the atlas, allowing the odontoid to project upward into the foramen magnum and creating a primary basilar impression.[103]

The position of the odontoid relative to the foramen magnum was described under the section on basilar impression, page 533. McRae[95, 96] measured the distance from the

Table 15-2. Scheme of Developmental Errors in the Occipitocervical Region

Manifestation of Vertebrae	*Developmental Error*
Basilar impression ⎫ Condylar hypoplasia ⎬ *Assimilation of atlas* ⎭	Primary malformation of occipital bone
Aplasia of arch of atlas Clefts in arch of atlas Atlanto-axial fusion Irregular segmentation of atlas and axis	Malformations of atlas
Persistent ossiculum terminale *Os odontoideum* *Dysplasia, hypoplasia and aplasia of dens* Spina bifida of axis Fusion C2-C3	Malformations of axis

From von Torklus, D. and Gehle, W.: The Upper Cervical Spine. New York, Grune & Stratton, 1975.

posterior aspect of the odontoid to either the posterior arch of the atlas or the posterior lip of the foramen magnum, whichever was closer. He stated that a neurological deficit would be present if this distance was less than 19 mm. This distance should be determined in flexion, since this position most dramatically reduces the space available for the cord.

Flexion-extension stress films will often show posterior displacement of the odontoid from the anterior arch of the atlas as much as 12 mm.[96] Associated atlantoaxial instability has been reported to eventually develop in 50 per cent of patients.[101] This is determined by measuring the distance from the anterior border of the odontoid to the posterior aspect of the anterior arch of the atlas. Greater than 4 mm. in young children who probably have considerable cartilage present and 3 mm. in older children and adults is considered pathologic.[87, 89, 90] The odontoid may be misshapen or occasionally directed posteriorly. There is a high association (reportedly as high as 70 per cent) of congenital fusion between C2 and C3. Other congenital malformations, such as basilar impression, occipital vertebrae, and condylar hypoplasia may be present. These probably arise from a similar developmental defect that produced the occipital cervical synostosis.

Myelography is a useful adjunct to visualize the fairly common posterior encroachment on the upper cervical cord or medulla by a constricting band of dura. This band may groove the spinal cord with resultant neurologic findings. Herniation of the cerebellar tonsils may also be demonstrated by a myelographic block at the level of the foramen magnum.[14]

Clinical Findings

The majority of patients have an appearance much like that in the Klippel-Feil syndrome, with a short broad neck, low hairline, torticollis, high scapula and restricted neck movements.[88, 96, 100, 101] The skull may be deformed and shaped like a "tower skull." Kyphosis and scoliosis are frequent occurrences. Other occasionally seen associated anomalies include dwarfism, funnel chest, pes cavus, syndactylies, jaw anomalies, cleft palate, congenital ear deformities, hypospadius and, occasionally, genitourinary tract defects.

Neurologic symptoms do not usually begin until the age of 40 or 50 years, but they can present during childhood. They progress in a slow, unrelenting manner and may be initiated by traumatic or inflammatory processes. It is rare that symptoms begin dramatically, but they have been reported even as a cause of instant death.[92] It is difficult to explain why neurologic problems develop so late and progress so slowly in these individuals. It may be that the frequently associated atlantoaxial instability progresses with age and the resultant added demands that are placed upon it, producing gradual spinal cord or vertebral artery compromise.

McRae[96] suggests that the key to development of neurologic manifestations lies with the odontoid and its position—an indication of the degree of actual or relative basilar impression. If the odontoid lies below the foramen magnum, the patient is usually asymptomatic.[94] However, with the decrease in vertical height of the atlas, the odontoid may project well into the foramen magnum producing brain stem pressure—a fact well documented by autopsy.[88, 95]

Anterior compression of the brain stem from the backward-projecting odontoid is most common. This produces a variety of findings, depending on the location and degree of pressure. Pyramidal tract signs and symptoms (spasticity, hyperreflexia, muscle weakness and wasting and gait disturbances) are most common, but cranial nerve involvement (diplopia, tinnitus, dysphagia, and auditory disturbances) may be seen less commonly. Compression from the posterior lip of the foramen magnum or the constricting band of dura may disturb the posterior columns, resulting in loss of proprioception, vibration, and tactile discrimination. Nystagmus, a common occurrence, is probably due to posterior cerebellar compression.

Vascular disturbances from vertebral artery involvement may occasionally result in syncope, seizures, vertigo and unsteady gait, among other signs and symptoms of brain stem ischemia.

Disturbed mechanics of the cervical spine may result in a dull aching pain in the posterior occiput and neck with episodic neck stiffness and torticollis. Tenderness noted in the area of the posterior scalp may be due to irritation of the greater occipital nerve.

The following most common signs and symptoms occur, with decreasing frequency: pain in the occiput and neck, vertigo, unsteady gait, paresis of the limbs, paresthesias, speech disturbances, hoarseness, double vision, syncope, auditory noise or disturbance, and interference with swallowing.[101] These all may be manifestations of underlying atlantoaxial instability which, as an isolated lesion, may produce neck pain, headaches, and neurologic deficits from cord or root irritation and, rarely, sudden death.[91, 102]

Treatment

Management of this fortunately uncommon problem may be hazardous. Unlike anomalies of the odontoid, surgical intervention carries a much higher risk of morbidity and mortality.[88, 97, 102]

Nonoperative methods such as cervical collars, braces, plaster, and traction should be attempted initially in some of these patients. These methods are often helpful in those patients with persistent complaints of head and neck pain, and they are particularly helpful if symptoms follow minor trauma or infection. If neurologic deficits are present, immobilization may only achieve temporary relief. Patients presenting with evidence of a compromised situation in the upper cervical area must take precautions not to expose themselves to undue trauma.

With cord signs and symptoms due to an unstable atlantoaxial complex, a C1-C2 fusion is suggested with preliminary traction to attempt reduction, if necessary. If reduction is possible and there are no neurologic signs, surgical intervention carries an improved prognosis.[88, 91, 102]

Posterior signs and symptoms and myelographic evidence of bony or dural compression, depending upon the degree of neurologic involvement, may be indications for a posterior decompression. Results from this vary from complete remission of symptoms to increased neurologic deficits and even death.[88, 97, 103]

CONGENITAL MUSCULAR TORTICOLLIS (CONGENITAL WRYNECK)

This is a common condition usually discovered in the first 6 to 8 weeks of life. The deformity is due to contracture of the sternocleidomastoid muscle, with the head tilted toward the involved side and the chin rotated toward the contralateral shoulder (Fig. 15-25A). If the infant is examined within the first 4 weeks of life, a mass or "tumor" is usually palpable in the neck.[109] It is generally a nontender, soft enlargement which is mobile beneath the skin and attached to or located within the body of the sterno-

FIG. 15-25. A 6-month-old infant with right-sided congenital muscular torticollis. *(A)* Note the rotation of the skull and asymmetry and flattening of the face on the side of the contracted sternocleidomastoid. *(B)* The same patient with the head resting on glass and photographed from below. Note how the face conforms to the surface. When the child sleeps, usually prone, it is more comfortable to have the affected side down, and consequently the face remodels to conform to the bed.

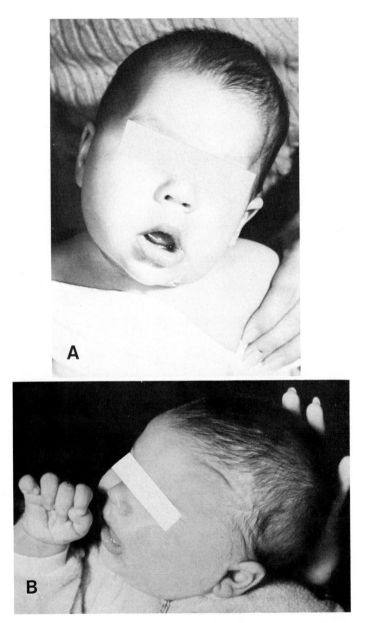

cleidomastoid muscle. The mass attains maximum size within the first month of life and then gradually regresses. If the child is examined after 4 to 6 months of age, the mass is usually absent, and the contracture of the sternocleidomastoid muscle and the torticollis posture are the only clinical findings. The mass is frequently unrecognized and was undetected in 80 per cent of Bianco's patients.[106]

If the condition is progressive, deformities of the face and skull can result, and they are usually apparent within the first year. Flattening of the face on the side of the contracted sternocleidomastoid muscle may be particularly impressive (Fig. 15-25A). The deformity is probably due to the position the child assumes when sleeping (Fig. 15-25B). Children in the United States generally sleep prone,[104] and in this position it is

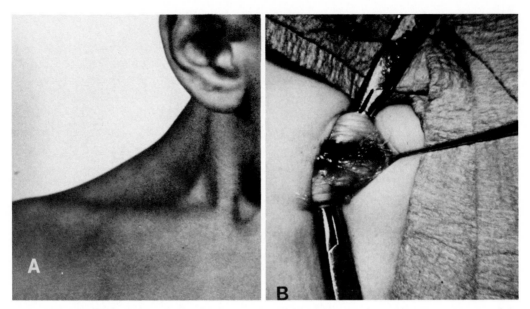

FIG. 15-26. *(A)* Clinical appearance of a 6-year-old child with torticollis. Note the appearance of the two heads of the sternocleidomastoid. *(B)* Operative exposure of the same patient demonstrating complete replacement with fibrous tissue of the two heads of the sternocleidomastoid.

more comfortable for them to have the affected side down. As a consequence, the face remodels to conform to the bed. In children who sleep supine, reverse modeling of the contralateral aspect of the skull is evident. If the condition remains untreated during the growth years, the level of the eyes and ears becomes distorted and may result in considerable cosmetic deformity.

Etiology

At present, congenital muscular torticollis is believed to be the result of local trauma to the soft tissues of the neck at the time of delivery. Birth records of affected children demonstrate a preponderance of breech or difficult forceps deliveries or primiparous births.[109, 110] However, it should be noted that the deformity has occurred following otherwise normal deliveries and has been reported in infants born by caesarian section.[109, 110] Microscopic examinations of resected surgical specimens and experimental work with dogs[105] suggest that the lesion is due to occlusion of the venous outflow of the sternocleidomastoid muscle. This results in edema, degeneration of muscle fibers, and eventually fibrosis of the muscle body.

Coventry[106] suggests that the clinical deformity is related to the ratio of fibrosis to remaining functional muscle. If sufficient normal muscle is present, the sternocleidomastoid will stretch with growth and the child will probably not develop the torticollis posture, whereas if there is a predominance of fibrosis, there is very little elastic potential. There are two additional factors which as yet are not explained. In three out of four children, the lesion is on the right side,[109, 110] and 20 per cent of the children with congenital muscular torticollis have congenital dysplasia of the hip.[107] Roentgenograms of the cervical spine should be obtained to rule out congenital anomaly of the cervical spine.

Treatment

Conservative Measures. Excellent results can be obtained in the majority of patients with conservative measures.[106, 109, 110] Ninety per cent of Coventry's patients responded to stretching exercises alone.[106] Exercises are performed by the parent, with guidance from the physical therapist and physician. Standard maneuvers include positioning of the ear opposite the contracted

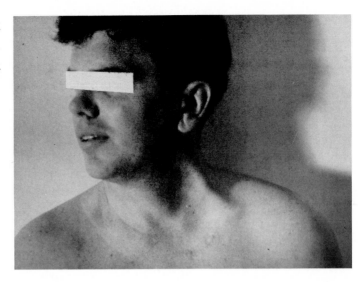

FIG. 15-27. A 23-year-old male who has undergone release of the sternocleidomastoid. The patient has a residual fascial band and slight restriction of neck motion.

muscle to the shoulder, and touching the chin to the shoulder on the affected side. It must be emphasized that when adequate stretching has been obtained in the neutral position, these maneuvers should be repeated with the head hyperextended. This will achieve maximum stretching and prevent residual contractures. Additional treatment measures include positioning of the crib and toys so that the neck will be stretched when the infant is trying to reach and grasp.

Surgery. If conservative measures are unsuccessful, surgical intervention is required. The surgery should be performed prior to school age, usually after the patient has achieved adequate size and health to tolerate an elective general anesthesia. The timing of such procedures is of little importance, as a good (but not perfect) cosmetic result can be obtained as late as 12 years of age.[106] Asymmetry of the skull and face will correct as long as adequate growth potential remains after the deforming pull of the sternocleidomastoid is removed.[106]

Surgery consists of resection of a portion of the distal sternocleidomastoid muscle. The surgeon should remove at least a 1-cm. segment of the tendon to guard against anomalous reattachment and recurrence of the deformity. A transverse incision is made low in the neck to coincide with a normal skin fold.[111] It is important not to place the incision near or over the clavicle, as scars in this area tend to spread and are cosmetically unacceptable. The most common postoperative complaint is disfiguring scars.[110, 111] The two heads of the sternocleidomastoid are identified and both are sectioned (Fig. 15-26). It is important to release the investing fascia about the sternocleidomastoid, as this too is frequently contracted. Rotation of the chin and head at this point generally reveals the adequacy of the surgery, and palpation of the neck demonstrates any extraneous tight bands or aberrant contracted muscles that could lead to a partial recurrence or incomplete correction (Fig. 15-27).[108] Rarely, an accessory incision is required to section the muscle at its insertion on the mastoid process. The whole muscle should not be excised, as this may lead to reverse torticollis[110] or additional deformity from asymmetry in neck contour.

The postoperative regimen includes passive stretching exercises in the same manner as those done preoperatively. They should begin as soon as the patient can tolerate manipulation of the neck. Occasionally head traction at night, particularly with an older child, is helpful. Bracing or casting is generally not needed, and these are difficult to apply. Results of surgery have been uniformly good with a low incidence of complications or recurrence, and nearly all patients are pleased with the result.[106, 109, 110] Slight restriction of neck motion and anomalous reattachment occurs frequently,[110, 111] but generally they are unnoticed by the patient. If the patient is young, the facial asymmetry can be expected to resolve completely unless there is persistence of the torticollis, particularly from residual fascial bands.[110]

TORTICOLLIS DUE TO BONY ANOMALIES

The diagnostic dilemma of childhood torticollis is often compounded by the inability to obtain satisfactory roentgenograms, particularly in the presence of a painful neck. A differential diagnosis of the main causes of torticollis as well as a list of bony anomaly causes of torticollis are listed below.

Congenital Torticollis

Congenital torticollis caused by bony anomalies can be termed "skeletal wryneck." Gyorgyi[126] examined 20 cases of

---

Differential Diagnosis of Torticollis

Congenital

    Occipitocervical anomalies
    Pterygium colli (skin web)
    Congenital muscular torticollis

Acquired

    Neurogenic
        Spinal cord tumors
        Cerebellar tumors (posterior fossa)
        Syringomyelia
        Ocular dysfunction
        Bulbar palsies

    Traumatic

        Subluxations
        Dislocations
        Fractures

    Inflammatory

        Cervical adenitis
        Tuberculosis
        Rheumatoid arthritis

    Idiopathic

        Atlantoaxial rotary displacement
            Subluxation
            Fixation

Torticollis Due to Bony Anomalies

Congenital anomalies of the craniocervical junction

    Klippel-Feil syndrome
    Atlantooccipital synostosis (unilateral)
    Basilar impression (unilateral)
    Odontoid anomalies
        Aplasia
        Hypoplasia
        Os odontoideum
    Occipital vertebra
    Asymmetry of occipital condyles (hypoplasia)

Acquired anomalies of the craniocervical junction

    Traumatic
        Subluxations
        Dislocations
        Fractures
    Inflammatory
        Rheumatoid arthritis
    Idiopathic
        Atlantoaxial rotary displacement
            Subluxation
            Fixation

---

congenital torticollis and found the following coexisting anomalies: spondylosis, asymmetrical facet joints, basilar impression, atlantoaxial dislocation, assimilation of the atlas, and deformities of the odontoid process. He noted that early spondylosis was a feature of congenital torticollis and in 40 per cent there was a history of a breach presentation.

Many occipitocervical malformations present with torticollis. Debauros[4] noted that 68 per cent had basilar impression, most commonly unilaterally. Approximately 20 per cent of patients with Klippel-Feil syndrome have associated torticollis.[122, 127] With asymmetrical development of the occipital condyles, the head tilt may result in a torticollis unless compensated for by a tilt of the lower cervical spine as that which occurs in the milder forms.[122]

Roentgenographic Features. Roentgenographic interpretation of congenital torticollis may be difficult because of the fixed abnormal head position and the restricted motion. Laminograms are often necessary. Flexion-extension stress films and cineradiography are often helpful to confirm open interspaces and associated atlantoaxial instability. The bony anomalies that may be present in congenital torticollis are documented under sections on occipitocervical synostosis, odontoid anomalies, Klippel-Feil syndrome, and basilar impression.

The clinical picture may be varied but the appearance is usually consistent—a short broad neck, low hairline, and torticollis.[135, 136, 145, 150] Motion, particularly rotation and tilt depending on the underlying pathology, may be markedly restricted or surprisingly good. Unlike muscular torticollis, the sternocleidomastoid muscle on the "short" side is not contracted or in spasm.[112]

Symptoms usually do not appear until well into adulthood, they are slowly progressive, and they are not always characteristic of a particular anomaly. The most common symptoms are occipital or neck pain, giddiness and vertigo, often aggravated or produced by certain head movements. Other neurologic manifestations are listed in other sections of this chapter.[135, 136]

Treatment. Nonoperative measures are usually preferred and are safer. The torticollis is a fixed bony deformity, hence little can be done to achieve correction. Immobilization with a neck collar or brace may be helpful for transient symptomatology following trauma or infection.

With atlantoaxial instability, particularly when neurologic signs and symptoms are present, fusion may be warranted. With posterior encroachment, usually from the foramen magnum, and corresponding signs and symptoms, posterior decompression may become necessary, but the risk of such surgical intervention is significant.[150]

Atlantoaxial Rotary Displacement

This is probably one of the commonest causes of childhood torticollis, yet the confusing terminology surrounding these problems indicates a lack of understanding of the underlying pathology. Terms used include rotary dislocation,[113] rotary deformity,[114] rotational subluxation,[132] rotary fixation,[41] and spontaneous hyperemic dislocation.[146]

"Atlantoaxial rotary subluxation" is probably the most accepted term to describe the common childhood torticollis. Almost invariably these children recover spontan-

eously or with minimal treatment. "Subluxation" may be misleading, since these cases usually present within the normal range of motion of the atlantoaxial joint. "Rotary displacement" would be a more appropriate and descriptive term. The onset of these problems may be spontaneous, associated with trivial trauma, or may follow an upper respiratory tract infection.

Rarely, these deformities persist, and the patients present with a resistant, unresolving torticollis best described by the term "atlantoaxial rotary fixation" or "fixed atlantoaxial displacement." This problem may also occur within the normal range of motion, the cause of which remains obscure. It may, however, occur in association with anterior shift of the atlas on the axis or in association with fractures of C1 and C2.

Gradations exist between this very mild, easily correctable rotary subluxation and the severe fixation. Complete atlantoaxial rotary dislocation has rarely been reported in surviving patients.[123] Rotary displacements are characteristically a pediatric problem, but they may occasionally occur in adulthood.

Rotary displacement may be associated with ligamentous deficiency leading to atlantoaxial instability. Fatalities have been reported from uncontrolled rotation of C1 on C2.[113, 141, 143, 148, 149]

We have seen one such patient in which the autopsy revealed that C1 rotated across the canal of C2, crushing the cord. Although rare, neurologic deficits may be associated with rotary displacements, particularly with associated anterior displacement.[128, 130, 132, 151] Catastrophies from vertebral artery compromise have also been reported.[139, 147]

Etiology and Mechanism. Rotary displacement may occur spontaneously following trivial or major trauma or following an upper respiratory tract infection. Indeed, several mechanisms may be responsible for the underlying pathology.

Rarely, it may be associated with anterior displacement of the atlas on the axis, indicating extensive ligamentous involvement. Associated fractures rarely may be the cause of the rotary displacement. Rotary displacement of C1 on C2 usually occurs within the normal range

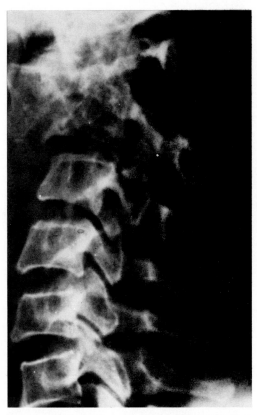

FIG. 15-28. Lateral roentgenographic projection showing the wedge-shaped lateral mass of C1 lying anteriorly where the oval arch of the atlas normally lies. This demonstrates marked rotation of C1 on C2 (may be normal).

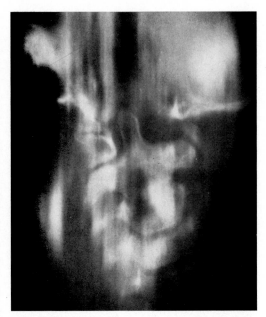

FIG. 15-29. This anteroposterior tomogram erroneously suggests the absence of one atlanto-axial mass which has rotated to a different plane (may be normal). (From Fielding, J. W.: Selected observations on the cervical spine in the child. *In* Ahstrom, J. P., Jr. (ed.): Current Practice in Orthopaedic Surgery, vol. 5. St. Louis, C. V. Mosby, 1973.)

of motion, and for some still unknown reason C1 fixes on C2 and the patient cannot return his head to the neutral position. The etiology of this type of displacement is still theoretical, since sufficient anatomical and autopsy evidence is unavailable. There are many theories.[114, 121, 124, 128, 146, 152] The obstruction is probably capsular and synovial interposition that produces pain in the initial stages with resultant muscle spasm. In most cases this resolves in a few days, representing the common rotary subluxation of childhood. However, it may persist, resulting in fixed contractures—rotary fixation.

The roentgenographic features of rotary displacement are sometimes difficult to demonstrate, partly because of difficulty in positioning due to associated pain and partly because of the occasional difficulty in roentgenographic interpretation. Indeed, assessment of normal upper neck roentgenograms is sometimes difficult due to malalignment of the head or the x-ray beam, along with the congenital anomalies which may occur in this area.[117, 118, 137, 144, 145] Tomographic techniques are often helpful for clarification.

Cineradiography has been invaluable to help elucidate the problems.[116, 117, 129, 133] This technique may be of little help in the acute stages of rotary displacement if pain precludes the motion necessary for cineradiographic study. If the pain has subsided and the deformity remains fixed, then cineradiography is helpful to confirm the diagnosis of a fixed rotary displacement by demonstrating the atlas and axis moving as a unit with rotation. This is seen best on the lateral projection.

With rotary displacement or torticollis from muscular and other causes or even

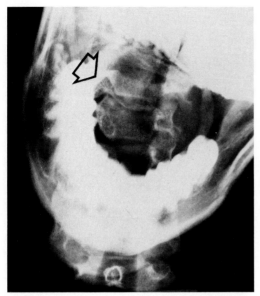

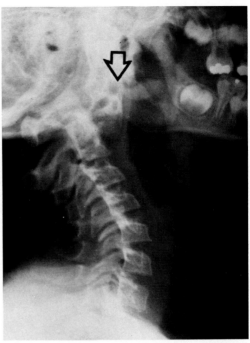

FIG. 15-30. The spine on the axis *(arrow)* and the chin are on the same side of the midline, demonstrating rotation of C2 (may be normal). (From Fielding, J. W.: Selected observations on the cervical spine in the child. *In* Ahstrom, J. P., Jr. (ed.): Current Practice in Orthopaedic Surgery, vol. 5. St. Louis, C. V. Mosby, 1973.)

FIG. 15-31. Lateral projection shows marked anterior displacement of the atlas on the axis with an atlantal-dens interval measuring 10 mm. (From Fielding, J. W., and Hawkins, R. J.: Roentgenographic diagnosis of the injured neck. *In* AAOS Instructional Course Lectures, vol. 25. St. Louis, C. V. Mosby, 1976.)

from normal tilt and rotation, the following radiologic features will be present in the open-mouth anteroposterior and lateral projections. The lateral mass of C1 that has rotated forward appears wider and closer to the midline (medial offset), while the opposite lateral mass is narrower and away from the midline (lateral offset). One of the facet joints may be obscured due to apparent overlapping.

On the lateral projection, the wedge-shaped lateral mass of the atlas lies anteriorly where the oval arch of the atlas normally lies (Fig. 15-28). The posterior arches of the atlas failed to superimpose due to head tilt. This may suggest assimilation of the atlas to the skull because, with tilt, the skull may obscure C1. Tomography in the anteroposterior projection may show the lateral masses of the atlas in different coronal planes and may erroneously suggest the absence of one atlantal mass which has rotated to a different plane (Fig. 15-29).

In most individuals, the spine of C2 is not deviated from the midline (indicating rota-

tion of C2) until greater than 50 per cent of head rotation has occurred (i.e., to the left with right rotation). With lateral flexion (tilt), even minimally, concomitant rotation below C1 causes the spine of C2 to be deviated from the midline much more than with rotation (i.e., to the right with left tilt). Therefore, with tilt in one direction and rotation in the opposite direction as occurs in torticollis from any cause, the spine of the axis and the chin would be on the same side of the midline, since rotation of C2 with head tilt is much more than in simple head rotation (Fig. 15-30).

Flexion-extension stress films are suggested to rule out the possible anterior displacement of the atlas on the axis occasionally seen with rotary displacement (Fig. 15-31).

Rotary displacement can be classified as follows (Fig. 15-32): *Type 1* is simple rotary displacement without anterior shift

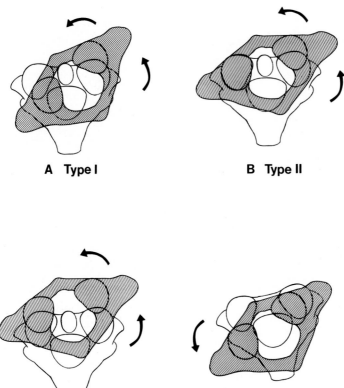

A Type I

B Type II

C Type III

D Type IV

Fig. 15-32. Classification of rotary displacement. *(A)* Type I, simple rotary displacement without anterior shift; *(B)* Type II, rotary displacement with anterior shift of 5 mm, or less; *(C)* Type III, rotary displacement with anterior shift greater than 5 mm.; *(D)* Type IV, rotary displacement with posterior shift. (From Fielding, J. W., and Hawkins, R. J.: Atlanto-axial rotary fixation, J. Bone Joint Surg., *59A*:37, 1977.)

of C1; *type 2* is rotary displacement with an anterior shift of 5 mm. or less. (Anterior displacement of greater than 3 mm. in older children and adults and greater than 4 mm. in younger children is considered pathologic.[119, 125, 131, 134, 138, 142, 145] *Type 3* is rotary displacement with an anterior shift greater than 5 mm.; and *type 4* is rotary displacement with a posterior shift.

Type 1 rotary displacement is by far the commonest seen in the pediatric age group. It is a much more benign lesion and may be approached with an expectant attitude. The type 2 deformity, however, does occur and is potentially more dangerous and must be carefully managed. Types 3 and 4 deformities are rare, but because of the problem of neurologic involvement or even instant death they must be very carefully managed.

In the acute stages, the diagnosis primarily is dependent upon history and clinical findings, because the roentgenographic features on plain films are not diagnostic and can be found in torticollis from other causes. Cineradiography, which would confirm the diagnosis, is precluded at this stage by the associated pain. However, if anterior displacement is demonstrated, the area of pathology is identified and the diagnosis is confirmed.

Clinical Findings. Atlantoaxial rotary displacement is predominantly a lesion of childhood. It may occur occasionally in adulthood. The onset is spontaneous, following an upper respiratory tract infection, following minor trauma or, very rarely, following major trauma.

The torticollis position is typically likened to a robin listening for a worm or the "cock-robin" position (Fig. 15-33). The head is tilted to one side and rotated to the opposite side with slight flexion. When it is acute, the child resists attempts to move the head, complaining of marked pain with any passive attempts to do so. Associated muscle spasm, unlike muscular torticollis, is predominantly in the side of the long sternocleidomastoid, since this muscle is attempting to correct the deformity. If the deformity becomes fixed the pain will subside, but the torticollis deformity may persist associated with a diminished range of motion. In long-standing cases, particularly in younger children, facial flattening may develop on the side of the tilt.

Rarely neurologic findings are present, indicating compromise to the atlantoaxial complex and neural structures.

Treatment. Many cases of atlantoaxial rotary displacement probably do not reach medical attention. A stiff neck and slightly twisted head often resolve over the ensuing days. The typical history and related clinical findings lead to the suspicion that the atlas is locked in position on the axis.

If the complaints are mild, use of a simple collar and analgesia suffices. Halter traction, muscle relaxants, and analgesia may be required in the more advanced cases, and usually they need to be continued for only a few days. If no anterior displacement is demonstrated, support need only be continued until symptoms have subsided. If the atlas is displaced anteriorly on the axis, immobilization should be continued for 6 weeks to allow ligamentous healing to occur. Careful follow-up is necessary in these patients because of potentially permanent atlantoaxial instability.

Rarely, these deformities become fixed. Atlantoaxial stability, particularly with anterior C1 displacement, is compromised and further insult could be catastrophic. Based on our experience with 17 such cases, we believe a C1–C2 fusion should be undertaken for stability and to maintain correction: (1) with neurological involvement, (2) with anterior displacement, (3) with failure to achieve and maintain correction if the deformity has been present for longer than 3 months, (4) with recurrence of the deformity following an adequate trial of conservative management, which should consist of at least 6 weeks of immobilization.

Torticollis Due to Rheumatoid Arthritis

Acute wryneck in childhood may be the first sign of rheumatoid disease. This may

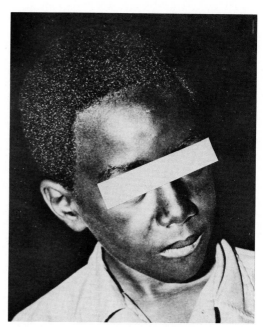

Fɪɢ. 15-33. Typical torticollis position of rotary displacement—the "cock-robin" position. The head is tilted to one side and rotated to the opposite side with slight flexion.

progress to become a fixed bony torticollis. Involvement with destruction of any of the lateral occipital-cervical joints may produce this wryneck. If present, it is usually associated with restriction of neck motion.[145]

Roentgenographic findings reveal evidence of rotation at C1 on C2 with plain films. Flexion films may reveal anterior displacement of the atlas on the axis, which may be fixed or mobile. The associated signs of rheumatoid arthritis are soon superimposed, if not already present. The treatment is directed primarily to the underlying disease; however, atlantoaxial instability, if significant or associated with neurologic involvement or persistent neck complaints, may require atlantoaxial arthrodesis.

REFERENCES

Basilar Impression

1. Bachs, A., Barraquer-Bordas, L., Barraquer-Ferre, L., Canadell, J. M., and Modolell, A.: Delayed myelopathy following atlanto-axial disloca-

tions by separated odontoid process. Brain, 78:537-553, 1955.

2. Bernini, F., Elefante, R., Smaltino, F., and Tedeschi, G.: Angiographic study on the vertebral artery in cases of deformities of the occipito-cervical joint. Am. J. Roentgenol. Radium Ther. Nucl. Med., 107:526-529, 1969.

3. Chamberlain, W. E.: Basilar impression (platybasia); a bizarre developmental anomaly of the occipital bone and upper cervical spine with striking and misleading neurologic manifestations. Yale J. Biol. Med., 11:487-496, 1939.

4. DeBarros, M. C., Farias, W., Ataide, L., and Lins, S.: Basilar impression and Arnold-Chiari malformation; a study of 66 cases. J. Neurol. Neurosurg. Psychiatr., 31:596-605, 1968.

5. Epstein, B. S., and Epstein, J. A.: The association of cerebellar tonsillar herniation with basilar impression incident to Paget's disease. Am. J. Roentgenol. Radium Ther. Nucl. Med., 107:535-542, 1969.

6. Fischgold, H., and Metzger, J.: Etude radiotomographique de l'impression basilaire. Rev. Rhum. Mal. Osteoartic., 19:261-264, 1952.

7. Fromm, G. H., and Pitner, S. E.: Late progressive quadriparesis due to odontoid agenesis. Arch. Neurol., 9:291-296, 1963.

8. Gunderson, C. H., Greenspan, R. H., Glaser, G. H., and Lubs, H. A.: Klippel-Feil syndrome: genetic and clinical re-evaluation of cervical fusion.

9. Hinck, V. C., Hopkins, C. E., and Savara, B. S.: Diagnostic criteria of basilar impression. Radiology, 76:572-585, 1961.

10. McGregor, M.: The significance of certain measurements of the skull in the diagnosis of basilar impression. Br. J. Radiol., 21:171-181, 1948.

11. Michie, I., and Clark, M.: Neurological syndromes associated with cervical and craniocervical anomalies. Arch. Neurol., 18:241-247, 1968.

11a. Whitesides, T. E., Jr., and Pendleton, E. B.: Lateral approach to the upper cervical spine for treatment of upper cervical-occipital-cervical disorders. J. Bone Joint Surg., 57A:1025, 1975.

Klippel-Feil Syndrome

12. Avery, L. W., and Rentfro, C. C.: The Klippel-Feil syndrome; a pathologic report. Arch. Neurol. Psychiatr. 36:1068-1076, 1936.

13. Baga, N., Chusid, E. L., and Miller, A.: Pulmonary disability in the Klippel-Feil syndrome. Clin. Orthop., 67:105-110, 1969.

14. Baird, P. A., Robinson, G. C., and Buckler, W. St. J.: Klippel-Feil syndrome. Am. J. Dis. Child., 113:546-551, 1967.

15. Bauman, G. I.: Absence of the cervical spine; Klippel-Feil syndrome. J.A.M.A., 98:129-132, 1932.

16. Bonola, A.: Surgical treatment of the Klippel-Feil syndrome. J. Bone Joint Surg., 38B:440-449, 1956.

17. Cattell, H. S., and Filtzer, D. L.: Pseudosubluxation and other normal variations in the cervical

spine in children. J. Bone Joint Surg., 47A:1295-1309, 1965.

18. Epstein, J. A., Carras, R., Epstein, B. S., and Levine, L. S.: Myelopathy in cervical spondylosis with vertebral subluxation and hyperlordosis. J. Neurosurg., 32:421-426, 1970.

19. Erskine, C. A.: An analysis of the Klippel-Feil syndrome. Arch. Pathol., 41:269-281, 1946.

20. Feil, A.: L'absence et la diminution des vertebres cervicales (etude clinique et pathogenique): le syndrome de reduction numerique cervicale. Theses de Paris, 1919.

21. Forney, W. R., Robinson, S. J., and Pascoe, D. J.: Congenital heart disease, deafness, and skeletal malformations: a new syndrome? J. Pediatr., 68:14-26, 1966.

22. Frawley, J. M.: Congenital webbing. Am. J. Dis. Child., 29:799-805, 1925.

23. Gray, S. W., Romaine, C. B., and Skandalakis, J. E.: Congenital fusion of the cervical vertebrae. Surg. Gynecol. Obstet., 118:373-385, 1964.

24. Gunderson, C. H., Greenspan, R. H., Glaser, G. H., and Lubs, H. A.: Klippel-Feil syndrome: genetic and clinical re-evaluation of cervical fusion. Medicine, 46:491-512, 1967.

25. Gunderson, C. H., and Solitare, G. B.: Mirror movements in patients with the Klippel-Feil syndrome; neuropathologic observations. Arch. Neurol., 18:675-679, 1968.

26. Hensinger, R. N., Lang, J. R., and MacEwen, G. D.: The Klippel-Feil syndrome: a constellation of related anomalies. J. Bone Joint Surg., 56A:1246-1253, 1974.

27. Illingworth, R. S.: Attacks of unconsciousness in association with fused cervical vertebrae. Arch. Dis. Child., 31:8-11, 1956.

28. Jalladeau, J.: Malformations congenitales Associessau syndrome de Klippel-Feil. These de Paris, 1936.

29. Kirkham, T. H.: Cervico-oculo-acusticus syndrome with pseudopapilloedema. Arch. Dis. Child., 44:504-508, 1969.

30. Klippel, M., and Feil, A.: Un cas d'absence des vertebres cervicales avec cage throacique remontant jusqu'a la base du crane. Nouv. Icon. Salpetriere, 25:223-250, 1912.

31. Krieger, A. J., Rosomoff, H. L., Kuperman, A. S., and Zingesser, L. H.: Occult respiratory dysfunction in a craniovertebral anomaly. J. Neurosurg., 31:15-20, 1969.

32. McElfresh, E., and Winter, R.: Klippel-Feil syndrome. Minn. Med., 56:353-357, 1973.

33. McLay, K., and Maran, A. G.: Deafness and the Klippel-Feil syndrome. J. Laryngol. Otol., 83:175-184, 1969.

34. MacRae, D. L.: Bony abnormalities in the region of the foramen magnum: correction of the anatomic and neurologic findings. Acta Radiol., 40:335-354, 1953.

35. Michie, I., and Clark, M.: Neurological syndromes associated with cervical and craniocervical anomalies. Arch. Neurol., 18:241-247, 1968.

36. Morrison, S. G., Perry, L. W., and Scott, L. P.: Congenital brevicollis (Klippel-Feil syndrome) and cardiovascular anomalies. Am. J. Dis. Child., 115:614-620, 1968.

37. Moseley, J. E., and Bonforte, R. J.: Spondylothoracic dysplasia—a syndrome with congenital heart disease. Am. J. Dis. Child., *102:*858-864, 1961.

38. Naik, D. R.: Cervical spinal canal in normal infants. Clin. Radiol., *21:*323-326, 1970.

39. Nora, J. J., Cohen, M., and Maxwell, G. M.: Klippel-Feil syndrome with congenital heart disease. Am. J. Dis. Child., *102:*858-864, 1961.

40. Notermans, S. L. H., Go, K. G., and Boonstra, S.: EMG studies of associated movements in a patient with Klippel-Feil syndrome. Psychiatr. Neurol. Neurochir., *73:*257-266, 1970.

41. Palant, D. I., and Carter, B. L.: Klippel-Feil syndrome and deafness. Am. J. Dis. Child., *123:*218-221, 1972.

42. Ramsey, J., and Bliznak, J.: Klippel-Feil syndrome with renal agenesis and other anomalies. Am. J. Roentgenol. Radium Ther. Nucl. Med., *113:*460-463, 1971.

43. Shoul, M. I., and Ritvo, M.: Clinical and roentgenological manifestations of the Klippel-Feil syndrome (congenital fusion of the cervical vertebrae, brevicollis); report of eight additional cases and review of the literature. Am. J. Roentgenol. Radium Ther. Nucl. Med., *68:*369-385, 1952.

44. Stark, E. W., and Borton, T. E.: Hearing loss and the Klippel-Feil syndrome. Am. J. Dis. Child., *123:*233-235, 1972.

45. Sullivan, R. C., Bruwer, A. J., and Harris, L.: Hypermobility of the cervical spine in children: a pitfall in the diagnosis of cervical dislocation. Am. J. Surg., *95:*636-640, 1958.

Congenital Anomalies of the Odontoid

46. Ahlback, I., and Collert, S.: Destruction of the odontoid process due to axial pyogenic spondylitis. Acta Radiol. [Diagn.] (Stockh.), *10:*394-400, 1970.

47. Bailey, D. K.: The normal cervical spine in infants and children. Radiology, *59:*712-719, 1962.

48. Bassett, F. H., and Goldner, J. L.: Aplasia of the odontoid process. Proc. A.A.O.S., *50A:*833-834, 1968.

49. Caffey, J.: Paediatric X-ray Diagnosis. Chicago, Year Book Medical Publishers, 1967.

50. Cattell, J. S., and Filtzer, D. L.: Pseudosubluxation and other normal variations in the cervical spine in children. J. Bone Joint Surg., *47A:*1295-1309, 1965.

51. Curtis, B. H., Blank, S., and Fisher, R. L.: Atlanto-axial dislocation in Down's syndrome. J.A.M.A., *205:*464, 1968.

52. Dzenitio, A. J.: Spontaneous atlantoaxial dislocation in mongoloid child with spinal cord compression; case report. J. Neurosurg., *25:*458-460, 1966.

53. Evarts, C. M., and Lonsdale, D.: Ossiculum terminale—an anomaly of the odontoid process; report of a case of atlantoaxial dislocation with cord compression. Cleve. Clin. Q., *37:*73-76, 1970.

54. Fielding, J. W.: Disappearance of the central portion of the odontoid process. J. Bone Joint Surg., *47A:*1228-1230, 1965.

55. ———: The cervical spine in the child. Curr. Pract. Orthop. Surg., *5:*31-55, 1973.

56. Fielding, J. W., and Griffin, P. P.: Os odontoideum: an acquired lesion. J. Bone Joint Surg., *56A:*187-197, 1974.

57. Fielding, J. W., and Hawkins, R. J.: Atlanto-axial rotary fixation. Unpublished, 1975.

58. Fielding, J. W., Hawkins, R. J., and Ratzan, S.: Fusion for atlanto-axial instability (A review of 57 cases). Unpublished, 1975.

59. Ford, F. K.: Syncope, vertigo and disturbances of vision resulting from intermittent obstruction of the vertebral arteries due to a defect in the odontoid process and excessive mobility of the axis. Bull. Johns Hopkins Hosp., *91:*168-175, 1952.

60. Freiberger, R. H., Wilson, P. D., Jr., and Nicholas, J. A.: Acquired absence of the odontoid process. J. Bone Joint Surg., *47A:*1231-1236, 1965.

61. Garber, J. N.: Abnormalities of the atlas and axis vertebrae. J. Bone Joint Surg., *46A:*1782-1791, 1964.

62. Giannestras, J. J., Mayfield, F. H., Provencio, F. P., and Maurer, J.: Congenital absence of the odontoid process. J. Bone Joint Surg., *46A:*839-843, 1964.

63. Gillman, C. L.: Congenital absence of the odontoid process of the axis; report of a case. J. Bone Joint Surg. *41A:*340-348, 1959.

64. Greenberg, A. D.: Atlanto-axial dislocations. Brain, *91:*655-684, 1968.

65. Greenberg, A. D., Scovillo, W. B., and Davey, L. M.: Transoral decompression of atlanto-axial dislocation due to odontoid hypoplasia; report of two cases. J. Neurosurg., *28:*266-269, 1968.

66. Gwinn, J. L., and Smith, J. L.: Acquired and congenital absence of the odontoid process. Am. J. Roentgenol. Radium Ther. Nucl. Med., *88:*424-431, 1962.

67. Hensinger, R. N., Lang, J. R., and MacEwen, G. D.: The Klippel-Feil syndrome: a constellation of related anomalies. J. Bone Joint Surg., *56A:*1246-1253, 1974.

68. Macalister, A.: Notes on the development and variations of the atlas. J. Anat. Physiol., *27:*519, 1892.

69. McKeever, F. M.: Atlanto-axial instability. Surg. Clin. North Am., *48:*1375-1390, 1968.

70. McRae, D. L.: Bony abnormalities in the region of the foramen magnum; correlation of the anatomic and neurologic findings. Acta Radiol., *40:*335-354, 1953.

71. ———: The significance of abnormalities of the cervical spine. Am. J. Roentgenol. Radium Ther. Nucl. Med., *84:*3-25, 1960.

72. Martel, W., and Fishler, J. M.: Observation on the spine in mongoloidism. Am. J. Roentgenol. Radium Ther. Nucl. Med., *97:*630-638, 1966.

73. Michaels, L., Prevost, M. J., and Crong, D. F.: Pathological changes in a case of os odontoideum (separate odontoid process). J. Bone Joint Surg., *51A:*965-972, 1969.

74. Minderhoud, J. M., Braakman, R., and Penning, L.: Os odontoideum; clinical, radiological, and therapeutic aspects. J. Neurol. Sci., *8:*521-544, 1969.

75. Nicholson, J. S., and Sherk, H. H.: Anomalies of the occipitocervical articulation. J. Bone Joint Surg., *50A:*295-304, 1968.
76. Rothman, R. H., and Simeone, F. A.: The Spine. Philadelphia, W. B. Saunders, 1975.
77. Rowland, L. P., Shapiro, J. H., and Jacobson, H. G.: Neurological syndromes associated with congenital absence of the odontoid process. Arch. Neurol. Psychiatr., *80:*286-291, 1958.
78. Schiller, F., and Nieda, I.: Malformations of the odontoid process. Report of a case and clinical survey. Calif. Med., *86:*394-398, 1957.
79. Shapiro, R., Youngsberg, A. S., and Rothman, S. L. G.: The differential diagnosis of traumatic lesions of the occipito-atlanto-axial segment. Radiol. Clin. North Am., *3:*505-526, 1971.
80. Shepard, C. N.: Familial hypoplasia of the odontoid process. J. Bone Joint Surg., *48A:*1224, 1966.
81. Sherk, H. H., and Nicholson, J. L.: Ossiculum terminale and mongolism. J. Bone Joint Surg., *51A:*957-964, 1969.
82. Spitzer, R., Rabinowitch, J. Y., and Wybar, K. C.: Study of the abnormalities of the skull, teeth and lenses in mongolism. Can. Med. Assoc. J., *84:*567-572, 1961.
83. Stratford, J.: Myelopathy caused by atlanto-axial dislocation. J. Neurosurg., *14:*97-104, 1957.
84. von Torklus, D., and Gehle, W.: The Upper Cervical Spine. New York, Grune & Stratton, 1972.
85. Wadia, N. H.: Myelopathy complicating congenital atlanto-axial dislocation (A study of 28 cases). Brain, *90:*449-472, 1967.
86. Wollin, D. G.: The os odontoideum; separate odontoid process. J. Bone Joint Surg., *45A:*1459-1471, 1963.

Occipitocervical Synostosis

87. Bailey, D. K.: The normal cervical spine in infants and children. Radiology, *59:*712-719, 1962.
88. Bharucha, E. P., and Dastur, H. M.: Craniovertebral anomalies (a report on 40 cases). Brain, *87:*469-480, 1964.
89. Caffey, J.: Paediatric X-ray Diagnosis, Chicago, Year Book Medical Publishers 1967.
90. Fielding, J. W.: The cervical spine in the child. Curr. Prac. Orthop. Surg., *5:*31-55, 1973.
91. Greenberg, A. D.: Atlanto-axial dislocations. Brain, *91:*655-684, 1968.
92. Hadley, L. A.: The Spine. Springfield, Charles C Thomas, 1956.
93. Macalister, A.: Notes on the development and variations of the atlas. J. Anat. Physiol., *27:*519, 1893.
94. McRae, D. L.: Bony abnormalities in the region of the foramen magnum: correlation of the anatomic and neurologic findings. Acta Radiol., *40:*335-354, 1953.
95. McRae, D. L.: The significance of abnormalities of the cervical spine. Am. J. Roentgenol. Radium Ther. Nucl. Med. *84:*3-25, 1960.
96. McRae, D. L., and Barnum, A. S.: Occipitalization of the atlas. Am. J. Roentgenol. Radium Ther. Nucl. Med., *70:*23-46, 1953.
97. Nicholson, J. S., and Sherk, H. H.: Anomalies of the occipito-cervical articulation. J. Bone Joint Surg., *50A:*295-304, 1968.
98. Rothman, R. H., and Simeone, F. A.: The Spine. Philadelphia, W. B. Saunders, 1975.
99. Sinto, G., and Pandya, S. K.: Treatment of congenital atlanto-axial dislocations. Proc. Aust. Assoc. Neurol., *5:*507-514, 1968.
100. Spillane, J. D., Pallis, C., and Jones, A. M.: Developmental abnormalities in the region of the foramen magnum. Brain, *80:*11-48, 1957.
101. von Torklus, D., and Gehle, W.: The Upper Cervical Spine. New York, Grune & Stratton, 1972.
102. Wadia, N. H.: Myelopathy complicating congenital atlanto-axial dislocation. Brain, *90:*449-472, 1967.
103. Wilkinson, M.: Cervical Spondylosis. Philadelphia, W. B. Saunders, 1971.

Congenital Muscular Torticollis

104. Brackbill, Y, Douthitt, T. C., and West H.: Psychophysiologic effects in the neonate of prone versus supine placement. J. Pediatr., *82:*82-84, 1973.
105. Brooks, B.: Pathologic changes in muscle as a result of disturbances of circulation. Arch. Surg., *5:*188-216, 1922.
106. Coventry, M. B., and Harris, L. E.: Congenital muscular torticollis in infancy; some observations regarding treatment. J. Bone Joint Surg., *41A:*815-822, 1959.
107. Hummer, D. C., Jr., and MacEwen, G. D.: The coexistence of torticollis and congenital dysplasia of the hip. J. Bone Joint Surg., *54A:*1255-1256, 1972.
108. Kaplan, E. B.: Anatomic pitfalls in the surgical treatment of torticollis. Bull. Hosp. Joint Dis., *15:*154-162, 1954.
109. Ling, C. M., and Low, Y. S.: Sternomastoid tumor and muscular torticollis. Clin. Orthop., *86:*144-150, 1972.
110. MacDonald, C.: Sternomastoid tumor and muscular torticollis. J. Bone Joint Surg., *51B:*432-443, 1969.
111. Staheli, L. T.: Muscular torticollis: late results of operative treatment. Surgery, *69:*469-473, 1971.

Torticollis Due to Bony Anomalies

112. Chandler, F. A.: Muscular torticollis. J. Bone Joint Surg., *30A:*556-569, 1948.
113. Corner, E. S.: Rotary dislocations of the atlas. Ann. Surg., *45:*9-26, 1907.
114. Coutts, M. B.: Atlanto-epistropheal subluxations. Arch. Surg., *29:*297-311, 1934.
115. DeBarros, M. C., Farias, W., Atoide, L., and Lins, S.: Basilar impression and Arnold-Chiari malformation; a study of 66 cases. J. Neurol. Neurosurg. Psychiatr., *31:*596-605, 1968.
116. Fielding, J. W.: Cineroentgenography of the normal cervical spine. J. Bone Joint Surg., *39A:*1280-1288, 1957.
117. ———: Normal and selected abnormal motion of the cervical spine from the second cervical

vertebra to the seventh cervical vertebra based on cineroentgenography. J. Bone Joint Surg., *46A:*1779-1781, 1964.

118. ———: The cervical spine in the child. Curr. Prac. Orthop. Surg., *5:*31-55, 1973.

119. Fielding, J. W., Cochran, G. V. B., Lawsing, J. F., III, and Hohl, M.: Tears of the transverse ligament of the atlas; a clinical and biomechanical study. J. Bone Joint Surg., *56A:*1683-1691, 1974.

120. Fielding, J. W., Kumar, R., and Poppolardo, P.: Fixed atlanto-axial rotatory subluxation. [*In* Proceedings of The American ·Academy of Orthopaedic Surgeons.] J. Bone Joint Surg., *53A:*1031-1032, 1971.

121. Fiorani-Gallotta, G., and Luzzatti, G.: Sublussazione Laterale e Sublussazione Rotatoria Dell-Atlanta. Arch. Ortop., *70:*467-484, 1957.

122. Gray, S. W., Romaine, C. B., and Shandalakis, J. E.: Congenital fusion of the cervical vertebrae. Surg. Gynecol. Obstet., *118:*373-385, 1964.

123. Greeley, P. W.: Bilateral (90 degrees) rotatory dislocation of the atlas upon the axis. J. Bone Joint Surg., *12:*958-962, 1930.

124. Grisel, P.: Enucleation de L'Atlas at Torticollis Naso Pharyngian. Presse Med. *38:*50-53, 1930.

125. Grogono, B. J. S.: Injuries of the atlas and axis. J. Bone Joint Surg., *36B:*397-410, 1954.

126. Gyorgyi, G.: Les Changements Morphologiques de la Region Occipitocervicale Associes au Torticolis. J. Radiol. Electrol. Med. Nucl., *45:*797-810, 1965.

127. Hensinger, R. N., Long, J. R., and MacEwen, G. D.: The Klippel-Feil syndrome: a constellation of related anomalies. J. Bone Joint Surg., *56A:*1246-1253, 1974.

128. Hess, J. H., Abelson, S. M., and Bronstein, I. P.: Atlanto-axial dislocation unassociated with trauma and secondary to inflammatory foci of the neck. Am. J. Dis. Child., *49:*1137-1145, 1935.

129. Hohl, M., and Baker, H. R.: The atlanto-axial joint. Roentgenographic and anatomical study of the normal and abnormal motion. J. Bone Joint Surg., *46A:*1739-1752, 1964.

130. Hunter, G. A.: Non-traumatic displacement of the atlanto-axial joint. J. Bone Joint Surg., *50B:*44-51, 1968.

131. Jackson, H.: Diagnosis of minimal atlanto-axial subluxation. Br. J. Radiol., *23:*672-674, 1950.

132. Jacobson, G., and Adler, D. C.: Examination of the atlanto-axial joint following injury with particular emphasis on rotational subluxation. Am. J. Roentgenol., Radium Ther. Nucl. Med. *76:*1081-1094, 1956.

133. Jones, M. D.: Cineradiographic studies of the normal cervical spine. Calif. Med., *93:*293-296, 1960.

134. Martel, W.: The occipito-atlanto-axial joints in rheumatoid arthritis and ankylosing spondylitis. Am. J. Roentgenol. Radium Ther. Nucl. Med., *86:*223-240, 1961.

135. McRae, D. L.: Bony abnormalities in the region of

the foramen magnum: correlation of the anatomic and neurologic findings. Acta Radiol. [Stockh.], *40:*335-354, 1953.

136. McRae, D. L.: The significance of abnormalities of the cervical spine. Am. J. Roentgenol. Radium Ther. Nucl. Med., *84:*3-25, 1960.

137. Paul, L. W., and Moir, W. W.: Non pathologic variations in relationship of the upper cervical vertebrae. Am. J. Roentgenol. Radium Ther. Nucl. Med., *62:*519-524, 1949.

138. Roy-Camille, R., De La Caffinière, J. Y., and Saillant, G.: Traumatisines du Rochis Cervical Supérieur C_1-C_2. Masson et Cie, Paris, 1973.

139. Schneider, R. C., and Schemm, G. W.: Vertebral artery insufficiency in acute and chronic spinal trauma. J. Neurosurg., *18:*348-360, 1961.

140. Shapiro, R., Youngsberg, A. S., and Rothman, S. L. G.: The differential diagnosis of traumatic lesions of the occipito-atlanto-axial segment. Radiol. Clin. North Am., *3:*505-526, 1971.

141. Sherk, H. H., and Nicholson, J. T.: Rotary atlanto-axial dislocation associated with ossiculum terminale and mongolism. J. Bone Joint Surg., *51A:*957-964, 1969.

142. Steele, H. H.: Anatomical and mechanical considerations of the atlanto-axial articulations. [*In* Proceedings of the Am. Orthop. Assoc.], J. Bone Joint Surg., *50A:*1481-1482, 1968.

143. Sullivan, Albert, W.: Subluxation of the atlanto-axial joint: sequel to inflammatory processes of the neck. J. Pediatr., *35:*451-464, 1949.

144. Sullivan, C. R., Brewer, A. J., and Harris, L. E.: Hypermobility of the cervical spine in children: a pitfall in the diagnosis of cervical dislocation. Am. J. Surg., *95:*636-640, 1958.

145. von Torklus, D., and Gehle, W.: The Upper Cervical Spine. New York, Grune & Stratton, 1972.

146. Watson-Jones, R.: Spontaneous hyperamic dislocation of the atlas. Proc. R. Soc. Med., *25:*586-590, 1932.

147. Webb, F. W. S., Hickman, J. A., and Brew, D. St. J.: Death from vertebral artery thrombosis in rheumatoid arthritis. Br. Med. J., *2:*537-538, 1968.

148. Werne, S.: Spontaneous atlas dislocation. Acta Orthop. Scand., *25:*32-43, 1955.

149. ———: Studies in spontaneous atlas dislocations. Acta Orthop. Scand. [Suppl.], *23:* 1-150, 1957.

150. Wilkinson, M.: Cervical Spondylosis. Its Early Diagnosis and Treatment. Philadelphia, W. B. Saunders, 1971.

151. Wilson, M. J., Michele, A., and Jacobson, E.: Spontaneous dislocation of the atlanto-axial articulation including a report of a case with quadraplegia. J. Bone Joint Surg., *22:*698-707, 1940.

152. Wortzman, G., and Dewar, F. P.: Rotary fixation of the atlanto-axial joint: rotational atlantoaxial subluxation. Radiology, *90:*479-487, 1968.

16 *The Spine*

Robert B. Winter, M.D.

INTRODUCTION

Deformity of the spine was probably the most neglected area of orthopaedics during the first half of this century. The past 25 years, however, have brought tremendous progress to this field. New approaches and devices have made possible better operative correction of advanced deformities and better nonoperative treatment of the lesser deformities. Despite all of these new advances, the basic fundamentals remain much the same. The care of the patient with a spinal deformity must be approached with thoughtfulness and attention to small details. There is no easy "cookbook" solution.

CLASSIFICATION OF SPINAL DEFORMITIES

The following classification is that which has been endorsed by the Scoliosis Research Society.[32] It is a "fluid" classification, (i.e., one which is constantly undergoing revision and alteration according to new advancements in the basic sciences).

Structural Scoliosis

Idiopathic
  Infantile
    Resolving
    Progressive
  Juvenile
  Adolescent
Neuromuscular
  Neuropathic
    Upper motor neuron
      Cerebral palsy

Spinocerebellar degeneration
    Friedreich's
    Charcot-Marie-Tooth
    Roussy-Lévy
   Syringomyelia
   Spinal cord tumor
   Spinal cord trauma
   Other
  Lower motor neuron
   Poliomyelitis
   Other viral myelitides
   Traumatic
   Spinal muscular atrophy
    Werdnig-Hoffmann
    Kugelberg-Welander
   Myelomeningocoele (paralytic)
  Dysautonomia (Riley-Day)
  Other
  Myopathic
   Arthrogryposis
   Muscular dystrophy
    Duchenne (pseudohypertrophic)
    Limb-girdle
    Facioscapulohumeral
   Fiber-type disproportion
   Congenital hypotonia
   Myotonia dystrophica
   Other
Congenital
  Failure of formation
   Wedge vertebra
   Hemivertebra
  Failure of segmentation
   Unilateral (unsegmented bar)
   Bilateral
  Mixed
Neurofibromatosis
Mesenchymal disorders
  Marfan's
  Ehlers-Danlos
  Others

Rheumatoid disease
Trauma
  Fracture
  Surgical
    Postlaminectomy
    Postthoracoplasty
  Irradiation
Extraspinal contractures
  Postempyema
  Post burns
Osteochondrodystrophies
  Diastrophic dwarfism
  Mucopolysaccharidoses (e.g., Morquio's)
  Spondyloepiphyseal dysplasia
  Multiple epiphyseal dysplasia
  Other
Infection of bone
  Acute
  Chronic
Metabolic disorders
  Rickets
  Osteogenesis imperfecta
  Homocystinuria
  Others
Related to lumbosacral joint
  Spondylolysis and spondylolisthesis
  Congenital anomalies of lumbosacral region
Tumors
  Vertebral column
    Osteoid osteoma
    Histiocytosis X
    Other
  Spinal cord (see Neuromuscular, below)

Nonstructural Scoliosis

Postural scoliosis
Hysterical scoliosis
Nerve root irritation
  Herniation of nucleus pulposis
  Tumors
Inflammatory (e.g., appendicitis)
Related to leg length discrepancy
Related to contractures about the hip

Kyphosis

Postural
Scheuermann's disease
Congenital
  Defect of formation
  Defect of segmentation
  Mixed
Neuromuscular
Myelomeningocoele
  Developmental (late paralytic)
  Congenital (present at birth)
Inflammatory
  Due to bone and/or ligament damage without
    cord injury
  Due to bone and/or ligament damage with cord
    injury
Postsurgical
  Postlaminectomy
  Post excision of vertebral body
Postirradiation
Metabolic
  Osteoporosis
    Senile
    Juvenile
  Osteomalacia
  Osteogenesis imperfecta
  Other
Skeletal dysplasias
  Achondroplasia
  Mucopolysaccharidoses
  Neurofibromatosis
  Other
Collagen disease
  Marie-Strümpell
  Other
Tumor
  Benign
  Malignant
    Primary
    Metastatic

Lordosis

Postural
Congenital
Neuromuscular
Postlaminectomy
Secondary to hip flexion contracture
Other

TERMINOLOGY

A glossary of terms has been developed by the Scoliosis Research Society in order to have a working set of words which are understood by all.[32] In the past there was much confusion between the terms "major," "primary," "secondary," "compensatory," "structural," "nonstructural," "postural," and "functional." The reader is referred to p. 681 for a full glossary of terms used in this chapter.

EVALUATION OF THE PATIENT

HISTORY TAKING

As in all fields of medicine, the taking of an adequate history is important. Quite frequently this seems to be ignored in the field of scoliosis and other spinal deformities.

Important clues for both diagnosis and treatment can be derived from the taking of a good history.

The following questions are important: When did the deformity first appear? In what manner did it come to attention (pain, elevated shoulder, prominent hip, etc.)? Is the deformity progressive? Is there pain? Is there fatigue? Is there any family history of spinal deformity? Is there any weakness, numbness, a tingling sensation, or awkwardness of gait? Is there any family history of neurologic disease? Have there been any past illnesses? Is there any shortness of breath, either with or without exertion?

One of the most important aspects of spinal problems is growth. It is of the utmost importance to determine the status of growth. Therefore we ask: Is there still active growth? Have the menses begun? When? Has pubic hair development begun? Has breast development begun? In boys one asks about onset of pubic hair development and change of voice.

It is also important to ask about other observations or treatment. Has the patient seen another doctor? What was that opinion? Was treatment given? Was a roentgenogram taken? Were chiropractic treatments given? Was a brace applied? What kind of brace? Was surgery done? What kind of surgery? Has the patient had surgery elsewhere than on the spine? Was a cast applied? What type? For how long? Were there any complications?

PHYSICAL EXAMINATION

Physical examination of the patient with spinal deformity involves far more than the spine alone. The patient who presents with a scoliosis and who has, on further examination, dislocation of the lenses of the eyes, a heart murmur, and long thin fingers has Marfan's syndrome *with* scoliosis, not just scoliosis alone.

Therefore, it must always be remembered that scoliosis, kyphosis, and lordosis are only *symptoms* of an underlying disease process. It is unfortunate that the etiology of the most common type of scoliosis (idiopathic) remains unknown. It is easy to fall into the habit of calling all scolioses "idiopathic," but one must be careful not to miss a spinal cord tumor or a syringomyelia, or a Friedreich's ataxia, or any number of conditions which may present first with a scoliosis.

Examination of the Spine

Physical examination of the spine includes noting the area of the curve (e.g., right thoracic, or double right thoracic and left lumbar), the magnitude of the curve, the amount of deviation of the spine from a plumb line (measured in centimeters) from the occiput or from C7, and the presence or absence of shoulder elevation (also measured in centimeters). The presence or absence of the flank crease is noted. The prominence of one hip should be noted, if present. Are the hips (iliac crests) level? Any deviation should be measured.

On forward bending *toward* the observer, the presence or absence of rib hump should be noted. A high left thoracic curve may show a slight hump on forward bending, but the curve usually can be seen more easily by noting prominence in the trapezius area at the base of the neck. The typical thoracic rib hump may be very mild or very severe. The quantity of rib hump should be measured in centimeters. A level is placed at the point of maximal deformity. A vertical ruler is placed on the concave side at a point an equal distance from the midline as is the point of maximal rib hump from the midline on the convex side (Fig 16-1). This quantitates the rib hump deformity (it really measures the amount of "hump" plus the amount of "valley").

Anteriorly one should note the presence or absence of rib flare on one side, asymmetry of breast development, the presence or absence of pectus excavatum or carinatum, and the state of breast development in the female.

It should be noted whether there is pure scoliosis, pure kyphosis, pure lordosis, or a combination of the above. The term "kyphoscoliosis" must be preserved for those patients with *both* kyphosis and scoliosis. A rib hump due solely to rotation should never be called kyphoscoliosis. Most

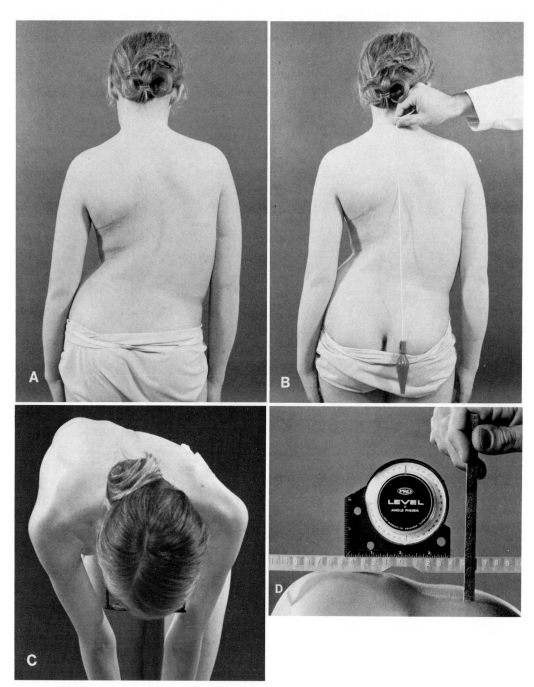

FIG. 16-1. Physical examination. *(A)* Back view of a patient. *(B)* Back view of a patient with a plumb line. *(C)* Forward bending view from the head to show the thoracic rotation. *(D)* The thoracic bending as measured by a standardized technique. The center of the level is placed over the midline spinus processes. The level is placed at the zero mark. The maximal prominence is noted to be at 5 cm. lateral to the midline, and therefore 5 cm. to the opposite side. A ruler is dropped and the distance is measured. This technique measures both the hump and the valley, as a single figure. In this case, it is 2.4 cm.

patients with adolescent idiopathic scoliosis have *lordosis* of the thoracic spine, not kyphosis.

Examination of Other Areas

The skin should be examined for the presence or absence of abnormal defects in the spinal area, such as lipomas, dermal sinuses, hairy patches, hemangiomas, or nevi. Then one should look for generalized skin abnormalities, especially café-au-lait spots (more than six of which, when 1 cm. or larger, is a sign of neurofibromatosis). Hyperelasticity of the skin suggests Ehlers-Danlos syndrome.

The ears should be examined for congenital abnormalities, such as preauricular skin tags, which are signs of Goldenhar's syndrome (oculoauriculovertebral dysplasia).

The palate should be examined. A high-arched palate is suggestive of Marfan's syndrome. A cleft palate suggests a congenital deformity.

The hands should be examined for congenital anomalies, for joint hyperelasticity (Ehlers-Danlos and Marfan's syndromes), and muscle weakness (e.g., clawing of the fingers in syringomyelia).

The hips should be examined for range of motion and especially for contractures. In paralytic disorders, look for tightness of the extensors, flexors, aductors, abductors, and the iliotibial bands. (See the section on neuromuscular spinal deformity, page 661).

The feet can reveal much, especially in the diagnosis of neuromuscular problems. High arches suggest Friedreich's ataxia. Clubfeet, vertical tali, or heel varus suggests spinal dysrhaphism. The presence of both a foot deformity and a spinal deformity in the same patient suggests either a generalized neurological disorder or spinal dysrhaphism (diastematomyelia, intraspinal lipoma, filum terminale, etc.).

Neurologic examination should include biceps, triceps, patellar- and Achilles-tendon reflexes. The Babinski's reflexes should be tested in all patients. A basic motor and sensory examination of the extremities is important. A Romberg test and finger-to-nose examination should be done for any existent or suspected neuromuscular problem.

ROENTGENOGRAPHIC EVALUATION

Measurement of Curvature

One of the greatest advancements in the field of scoliosis and other spinal deformities was the development of techniques for accurate measurement of the quantity of deformity. All techniques suffer from certain inadequacies, particularly in that most spinal deformities are three-dimensional and the measurement techniques are only two-dimensional. Nevertheless, by measuring both the anteroposterior and lateral projections, the physician can document well the quantity and pattern of deformity. Several techniques for measurement have been developed, but the most widely accepted, and the one officially recommended by the Scoliosis Research Society, is the *Cobb technique*.

This technique must be learned well and applied precisely, otherwise major errors in treatment will result. Whether or not a curve is progressive may be absolutely critical. Only precise measurement can give the answer. It is impossible to compare two roentgenograms accurately without measurement.

In the Cobb technique, first select the end vertebrae of the curve. *The end vertebrae are those vertebrae which are the most tilted from the horizontal.* By convention, the upright roentgenogram is used for this determination (usually with the patient standing, but with the patient sitting for those with leg paralysis). A line is drawn along the upper end-plate of the upper end vertebra and along the lower end-plate of the lower end vertebra. Perpendiculars are erected from these two lines. The angle of intersection of these perpendiculars is the angle of the curvature.

If there is difficulty in determining which is the end vertebra, lines can be drawn along the end-plate of *every* vertebra and projected out to the edge of the roentgenogram. It then will be noted that those lines from the vertebrae in the curve will converge in the concavity of the curve. Those vertebrae outside the curve being measured will diverge.

When there is a double curvature, both curves should be measured. There is one

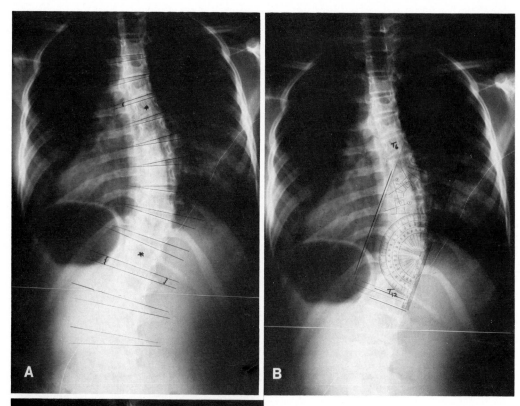

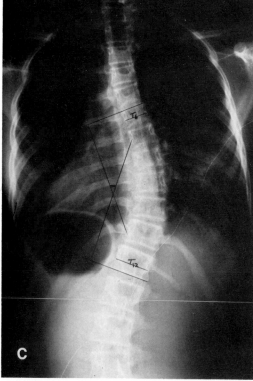

Fig. 16-2. Measurement of roentgenograms for scoliosis. *(A)* On an upright anteroposterior roentgenogram, lines have been drawn along the end-plates of each vertebra. One can see that between T6 and T12 all of the lines converge to the left. Above T6 and below T12 these lines are divergent. In addition, the disc spaces are wedged open to the right between T6 and T12, and wedged open to the left above T6 and T12, T6 and T12 are the vertebrae most tipped from the horizontal. All these factors identify T6 and T12 as the end vertebrae of this curve. *(B)* To measure the curve, a straight line is drawn along the lower end-plate of T12 and a perpendicular is erected to that line. *(C)* A second line is drawn along the end-plate of T6, and a second perpendicular is erected to intersect the first. The angled intersection measures the angle of the curve. This is the Cobb-Lippman technique for curve measurement. It is the officially recognized system of the Scoliosis Research Society. *(Continued on facing page.)*

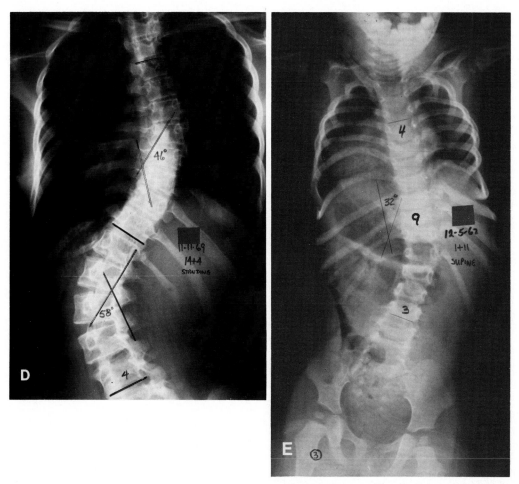

FIG. 16-2 *(Continued)*. *(D)* A double structural curve, right thoracic, left lumbar is illustrated. T11 is the lower end vertebra of the upper curve and is simultaneously the upper vertebra of the lower curve. T11 is thus the "transitional" vertebra. T4, T11, and L4 are the maximally tipped vertebrae, and are thus the end vertebrae of the two curves. *(E)* This patient exhibits a single curve with indistinct ends. There are multiple parallel vertebrae. The patient shows a lack of compensatory curves. In such circumstances, one should select as the end vertebra those vertebra parallel and farthest from the apex. The lack of compensatory curves is an indication of the extensive involvement of the spine by the disease process.

vertebra which will be the upper end vertebra for the lower curve and the lower end vertebra for the upper curve. This is called the *transitional* vertebra. It is necessary to place only one line on this vertebra, since usually the upper and lower end-plates are parallel.

Once these end vertebrae have been established, measurement should always be from the same vertebrae. The supine roentgenogram and the bending roentgeno-gram should also be measured from the *same* end vertebrae as chosen on the erect film, even though they may not be the maximally tilted vertebrae on these other films.

Occasionally, one will see a curve in which the end vertebra is difficult to determine because two or more vertebrae are parallel. In such a case, select the parallel vertebra *farthest* from the apex of the curve.

Usually the end-plates are clearly seen and the line along the end-plate can be

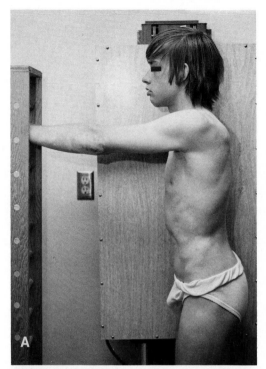

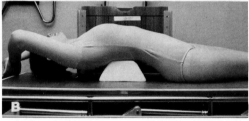

Fig. 16-3. Positioning for lateral roentgenograms. *(A)* The proper position for obtaining a lateral standing roentgenogram. Note that the patient's arms are resting on a ladder at 90° to the torso. The patient is looking straight ahead. The patient is standing in a neutral posture (i.e., neither attempting to stand slouched or "super" straight). *(B)* To obtain a hyperextension roentgenogram to test the flexibility of a kyphosis, the patient is hyperextended over a firm plastic block placed at the apex of the kyphosis. A cross-table lateral roentgenogram is then obtained.

at its maximum deformity (i.e., with gravity acting on the spine). The bending films show the spine without gravity and with the flexibility, or correctability, of the curves. Comparison of all the films shows which curves are structural versus nonstructural, and for structural curves, how rigid or flexible they are. The upright films are best taken on 14- by 36-inch films (36 by 91 cm.).

For patients unable to stand, or able to stand only with crutch support, sitting rather than standing films should be obtained. Sitting films will show the spine with gravity acting on it, but without the effect of uneven leg length or contractures about the hips.

For patients unable to actively bend the torso (paralytic disorders), bending films must be done by passive bending. Correctability can also be determined by a traction film, either in suspension or longitudinal traction.

In dealing with problems of kyphosis or lordosis, a different "routine" is used. The upright anteroposterior and lateral views are included. A supine lateral view is taken, and a "correction" view is taken. For kyphosis, the patient is placed supine with the apex of the kyphosis on a rigid plastic block. A cross-table lateral view is then taken. For lordosis, the patient lies on the side, with the knees drawn tightly to the chest, while a lateral view is taken (Fig. 16-3A, B).

drawn with great precision. Independent observers should be able to measure the same roentgenogram within 1 or 2 degrees. On some occasions the end-plate cannot be clearly defined (especially in congenital scoliosis), in which case it is permissible to use a line drawn along the lower border of each pedicle. The same points of reference should be used on subsequent films (Fig. 16-2).

Most scoliosis clinics have a "scoliosis routine" series of roentgenograms for the average patient coming to the clinic for the first time. What is "routine" varies from clinic to clinic, but almost all clinics include: (1) standing anteroposterior and lateral view and (2) supine bending films to the right and left. The standing films show the spine

Measurement of Rotation

It is important to be able to recognize rotation on the roentgenogram, because the length of the fusion is partly determined by the appreciation of rotation. The quantity or

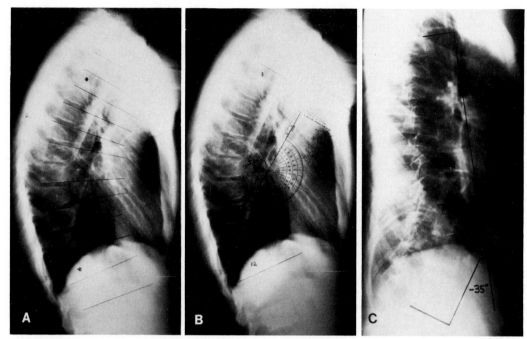

FIG. 16-4. Measurement of roentgenograms for kyphosis and lordosis. *(A)* A standing lateral roentgenogram with lines drawn along the end-plate of all the vertebrae. Note that T3 and T12 are the vertebrae most tipped from the horizontal, and are thus the end vertebrae. *(B)* By the same technique as is used for scoliosis, perpendiculars are erected from the lines along the end-plates, and the angle of intersection defines the angle of the curvature. In this case the patient exhibits a 54° T3 to T12 thoracic kyphosis. *(C)* This patient exhibits thoracic lordosis. The same technique of measurement is used. Any lordotic measurement less than 0° is recorded as a negative number, in this case −35°.

amount of rotation can be measured and graded, but at the present time, this technique seems to be of little practical value.[68]

This technique is based on a comparison of position of the pedicle relative to the lateral border of the vertebral body. Techniques based on the spinous process are very inaccurate due to the warping of the spinous process by the deformity or paralysis, the absence of the spinous process in spina bifida, and the surgical absence of the spinous processes after fusion.

Measurement of Kyphosis and Lordosis

The measurement of the lateral roentgenogram has largely been ignored, but is just as important as the anteroposterior roentgenogram. The Cobb technique can be readily applied to the measurement of both kyphosis and lordosis. The same basic principles ap-

ply, namely, the selection of end vertebrae based on the maximally tilted vertebrae as seen on a lateral upright roentgenogram, preferably with the patient standing (Fig. 16-4).

Special Roentgenographic Techniques

Laminograms are useful for special problems. The most common use is in the better definition of congenital anomalies. It may be difficult to determine the exact nature of a jumbled mass of abnormal bones on a routine film, but the laminogram can distinguish the exact anomaly. Laminograms are also useful in the detection of an osteoid osteoma, which, if present in the spine, usually produces scoliosis.

Myelography is also useful in certain complex problems. A myelogram is always indicated if there is *any suspicion* of a spinal cord tumor, *any suspicion* of a spinal dysrhaphism (see p. 627), or any neurologic problems secondary to the curvature. Myelography, if done, should always examine the entire spinal canal, never just the lower spine. If there is a kyphosis problem, the patient will require either a high-volume myelogram or supine positioning in order to adequately visualize the cord at the apex of the curve.

Radioactive technetium bone scans have become useful adjuncts in spinal roentgenography, especially for the detection of infections and tumors. In the scoliosis field, they are especially useful for the detection of osteoid osteomas.

Optional views are: (1) a hand film for bone age, (2) spot lateral and oblique views of the L5-S1 area to detect spondylolysis and spondylolisthesis, (3) oblique view of the curve area to demonstrate the curve in its maximal projection (Stagnara *"plan d' election"* view), and (4) the "Ferguson" view, an anteroposterior view of the L5-S1 area with the tube directed 30° cephalad.

PULMONARY FUNCTION TESTING

The major reason for treating scoliosis, especially thoracic scoliosis, is preservation of lung capacity. Thus, it can be quite important to know whether or not pulmonary function has been affected by the curve. In the patient with significant deformity, it is important to know how much damage has been done, as this can materially affect the risks of surgery, and thus the technique of surgical management.

In borderline situations when a decision must be made as to whether or not the patient should have surgery, pulmonary function testing should be utilized to assist in the decision. If there is a decrease in the lung function, surgery should be done. If the lung function is normal, perhaps surgery is not needed.

When pulmonary function tests are performed in scoliotic patients, serious errors can occur if the patient's *actual* height is used for calculation. The scoliosis causes loss of height, and a falsely high value will be obtained. Always correct for true height. We use arm span with a conversion factor to eliminate this problem.[42]

Both volume analysis, including flow rates and blood gases are necessary for the evaluation. The blood gases are more reliable than the volumes, since they are independent of true height and independent of voluntary action.

Beware of patients with thoracic lordosis. These patients have a far greater loss of pulmonary function than one would expect from their anteroposterior roentgenograms. The presence of thoracic lordosis significantly alters the indications for surgery.[92]

THE ADULT SEQUELAE OF UNTREATED SPINAL DEFORMITY

What happens to the patient with scoliosis who receives no treatment during the growing years? How do they function as adults? Do they have problems related to their spine? These are all very pertinent questions and must be answered before undertaking the active treatment of the growing child. Indeed, if there were no problems in the scoliotic adult, we would be hard pressed to justify the stresses, anxieties, and problems which are encountered in treating the child.

One way to answer these questions would be to document the actual natural history of a group of untreated patients who have gone many years into adulthood. Such documentation is available in three studies. The best is by Nilsonne and Lundgren,[70] in which 113 patients with idiopathic scoliosis were reviewed an average of 50 years after being seen at a scoliosis clinic from 1913 to 1918. Ninety per cent of the patients were located. Forty-five per cent of the patients were dead, twice the expected mortality rate for the age. Most of the deaths were from cardiac or pulmonary diseases. There was a noticeable increase in mortality after age 45. Seventy-six per cent of the females had never married. No one was engaged in heavy labor, and 47 per cent of patients were on disability pensions, 30 per cent specifically because of their spinal deformities. Ninety per cent had back symptoms.

In a similar article in the same journal issue, Nachemson[66] reviewed 130 patients with various types of scoliosis. Again, 90 per cent were located for follow-up an average of 35 years later. Again the mortality rate for the group as a whole was twice that of the

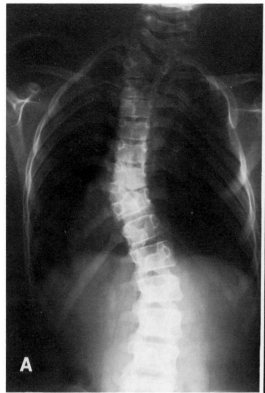

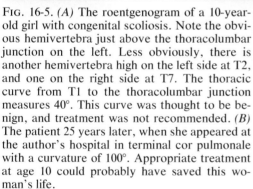

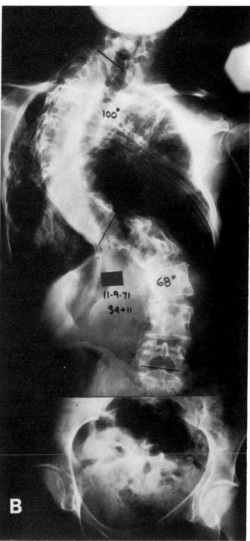

FIG. 16-5. *(A)* The roentgenogram of a 10-year-old girl with congenital scoliosis. Note the obvious hemivertebra just above the thoracolumbar junction on the left. Less obviously, there is another hemivertebra high on the left side at T2, and one on the right side at T7. The thoracic curve from T1 to the thoracolumbar junction measures 40°. This curve was thought to be benign, and treatment was not recommended. *(B)* The patient 25 years later, when she appeared at the author's hospital in terminal cor pulmonale with a curvature of 100°. Appropriate treatment at age 10 could probably have saved this woman's life.

population in general. If only thoracic curves were considered, the mortality rate was four times that of the general population. The mortality rate was higher in those patients with paralytic and congenital curves. Forty per cent of the patients noted backache, 30 per cent were disabled (expected rate of disability—1%). No one was employed in heavy labor.

The third paper on the long-term results of untreated idiopathic scoliosis is by Collis and Ponseti.[13] They attempted to locate the 353 patients reviewed in 1950 by Ponseti and Friedmann.[73] They located and personally examined 105 patients, while another 100 were reviewed only by questionnaire. The average follow-up was 24 years. Most curves increased after skeletal maturity. Thoracic curves of 60° to 80° progressed the most, an average of 28°. Thoracic curves less than 60° showed an average 9° progression. Lumbar curves of more than 30° pro-

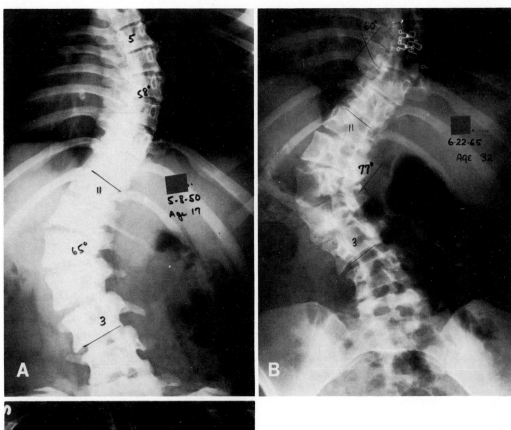

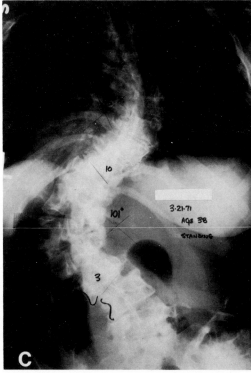

FIG. 16-6. *(A)* A double structural idiopathic scoliosis in a 17-year-old girl with a Risser sign of 4+. The thoracic curve measures 58°, and the lumbar curve 65°. She was told at this time that she had "nicely balanced curves which should give her no problem in the future."*(B)* The patient at age 32. The curves now measuring 60° in the thoracic spine and 77° in the lumbar spine. She had been having low backache for about 2 years at this time. *(C)* The patient at age 48. Now exhibiting a 75° degree right-thoracic and 101° left-lumbar curve. Note the lateral subluxation of L3 on L4. A this time she was having severe low back pain and left leg sciatica. Progression of curves during adult life is common, particularly lumbar curves over 60°.

gressed an average of 18°, while those less than 30° did not progress.

The mortality rate was less than that seen in the two Swedish series noted above, but the length of follow-up was shorter. Decreased vital capacity was noted in all thoracic curves over 60°. Dyspnea was noted in 40 per cent of patients, usually in those with thoracic curves of 85° or more. Although 54 per cent of patients had backache complaints, the authors did not feel that this incidence was higher than the population as a whole. Only eight of the 205 patients had been hospitalized for back pain. It is unfortunate that 148 (42%) of patients in the original series could not be located.

The great lesson of these papers is that scolioses are not static once growth ceases. They do progress, especially thoracic curves of 60° or more, and they do cause decreased pulmonary function and a significant likelihood of premature death due to respiratory failure. The question of lumbar curves is less obvious. Undoubtedly, lumbar curves over 30° do tend to progress, but whether there is a statistically higher incidence of back pain is unknown.

Another way to determine the presence or absence of adult problems in the patient with scoliosis is to examine the files of those physicians who might have contact with the scoliosis patient in adult life. If no adults came to these physicians, then one could safely say that adults do not have significant problems. However, that is not the case. Many patients come to internists and pulmonary physicians because of respiratory failure, with or without secondary right heart failure. The pathodynamics of "scoliotic heart failure" were well outlined by Bergovsky and his colleagues in 1959.[3]

Similarly, the orthopaedic surgeon interested in scoliosis sees many adult scoliosis patients for a variety of problems. Some are young ladies who are concerned about the cosmetic disfigurement of their "humps." Others come because of pain. Pain seems to be more common in the lumbar curves, but may also occur in thoracic curves. The most common complaint is pain, especially in lumbar curves. Some come to the orthopaedic surgeon because of dyspnea. They are hopeful that the curve can be straightened and their breathing improved. Finally, there is a small group of patients who come because of paralysis due to the spinal deformity. They are more likely to be patients with severe kyphosis.

Thus, it can be said with certainty that scoliosis is not always a benign condition. Premature death from respiratory failure is likely in patients with thoracic curves over 60°, if they are left untreated. Lumbar curves, especially those over 50°, are likely to progress in adult life. These patients have a high likelihood of degenerative disc disease and pain. Therefore, even if cosmetic and emotional factors are not taken into account (and they may be of considerable importance), aggressive treatment of the child with a spinal deformity is justified (Figs. 16-5, 16-6, 16-7).

NONSTRUCTURAL SCOLIOSIS

POSTURAL SCOLIOSIS

Although the normal spine is straight in the frontal plane, there are certain children who do not voluntarily stand straight. This usually results in increased thoracic kyphosis and increased lumbar lordosis, but there also may be a scoliosis of mild degree as well. It usually is easy to detect the difference between postural and structural scoliosis by careful physical and roentgenographic examination. Postural scoliosis is not associated with a rib hump on forward bending. It disappears in the prone position and when the child is asked to stand in a very straight position. On the roentgenogram, the curves are different than those in structural scoliosis. There is a long curve, usually extending from one end of the spine to the other, that is not associated with rotation. The supine roentgenogram is usually straight, and bending films show no areas of contracture. Such curves neither progress nor become structural.

LEG LENGTH DISCREPANCY

A difference in the length of the legs will result in a curvature of the spine in the standing position. This is a functional or nonstructural curvature. When the patient is sitting

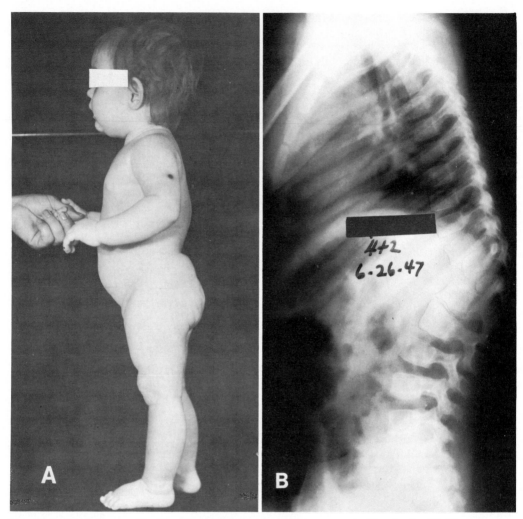

Fig. 16-7. *(A)* A 1-year-old girl with a slight thoracolumbar congenital kyphosis. *(B)* The patient at age 4 has a congenital kyphosis, with a defect of formation of two vertebral bodies. No treatment was given at that time. *(Legend continued on facing page.)*

or lying down, the curve disappears. When the difference in leg length is corrected, the curve disappears. One is frequently asked whether the presence of a leg length discrepancy for a long period of time will result in a functional curve becoming structural. This is highly doubtful, since we spend so little of our time standing on our feet with even weight. When we walk, we shift weight from one leg to the other. When we sit, the discrepancy disappears. We usually spend a great deal of time lying down. Thus, the inequality of leg length does not act on the spine more than a small percentage of each

day. People with leg length discrepancies over a long period of time, such as those with hemihypertrophy or hemiatrophy, usually do not have any fixed scoliosis. However, neuromuscular conditions which may result in leg length discrepancy (e.g., poliomyelitis) can also cause a structural scoliosis, so that the two may coexist because of the common etiology (Fig. 16-8).

HYSTERICAL SCOLIOSIS

Hysterical scoliosis has been reported to occur in some emotionally disturbed teenag-

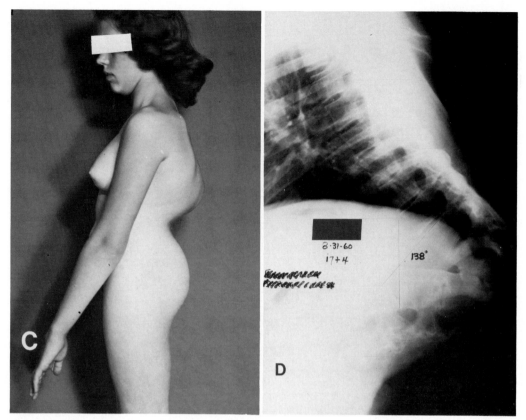

FIG. 16-7 *(Continued)*. *(C)* At age 12, the patient has marked increase in her kyphosis. *(D)* The patient at age 17 has an extremely severe kyphosis. She was showing early signs of spinal cord compression at this time.

ers. The curvature is constant in the upright position, is usually constant in the sitting position, and may or may not be present in the prone or supine position. It is always absent while sleeping and disappears under an anesthetic. It is characterized by curvatures which have a long, sweeping, bizarre pattern not associated with rotation on the roentgenogram or a true rib hump on forward bending. There may be considerable contortions of the torso during the examination, which may confuse the examiner as to the presence of thoracic deformity. Roentgenograms taken in the supine or prone position may demonstrate the absence of any fixed curve. If necessary, roentgenograms can be obtained under heavy sedation or even under an anesthetic. Before labeling a child as a hysteric, one must be absolutely sure that there is no spi-

nal cord tumor or other neurologic pathology present. Consultation is strongly recommended. Hysterical scoliosis should not be treated by orthopaedic methods (e.g., exercises, braces, or casts), and certainly never by surgery. This is a psychiatric problem and should be dealt with promptly by specialists in this field. Continued orthopaedic treatment will only lead to a greater degree of fixation of the hysteria (Fig. 16-9).

IDIOPATHIC SCOLIOSIS

Idiopathic scoliosis is the most common form of scoliosis. The child is usually healthy, has a normal spine at birth, and develops a curvature at some time during growth, usually around ages 10 to 12. Idiopathic scoliosis is slightly more common

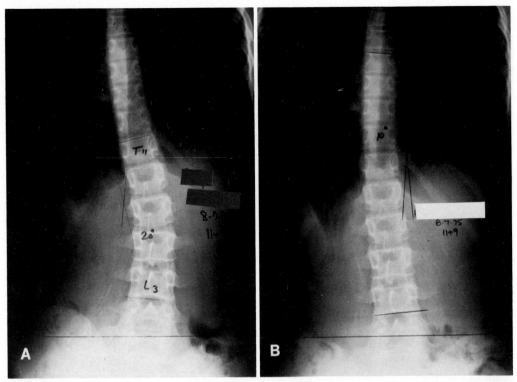

FIG. 16-8. *(A)* This 11-year-old girl was seen with a complaint of scoliosis. She exhibits a 20° T11 to L3 lumbar curve without rotation. A standing roentgenogram demonstrates significant leg length discrepancy. *(B)* The same patient, the same day, in a second roentgenogram, with the patient standing on a 2.5 cm. lift. Note that the lumbar curve has disappeared. She was treated by epiphysiodesis of the longer leg.

in females, and the female has a far greater tendency to progression of the curve to the point where treatment is required. There certainly is a genetic pattern, but the exact nature of the genetic mechanism is unknown at this time. Cowell and his associates[14] feel that it is an autosomal dominant trait, but Wynn-Davies[95] feels that it is a multifactorial trait.

INFANTILE IDIOPATHIC SCOLIOSIS

Infantile idiopathic scoliosis is a definite entity, most commonly seen in Great Britain, but also seen to a lesser extent in other parts of Europe. In this condition, the scoliosis appears some time between birth and 3 years.

Infantile idiopathic scoliosis is more common in the male than in the female. It usually produces a curve to the left; the curve is thoracolumbar. Fortunately, approximately 85 per cent of the time, the curve spontaneously disappears without treatment.[40, 49, 82]

The other 15 per cent of curves are progressive, and lead to very severe deformities. Thus, it is important to note whether or not an infantile idiopathic scoliosis is progressive. This can only be determined by careful serial examinations and serial roentgenograms. Mehta[58] has developed a method for measurement of the difference in the angle at which the rib meets the spine at the apex of the curve. This measurement is called the "rib-vertebral angle difference." If the angle is greater than 20°, it is likely that the child will have a progressive infantile idiopathic scoliosis. This has proven help-

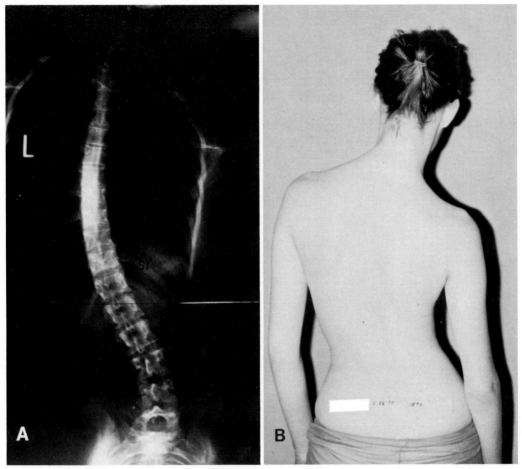

FIG. 16-9. *(A)* A long, sweeping nonrotated scoliosis. This particular pattern of curvature does not resemble any of the usual types of scoliosis. *(B)* A photograph of the patient, taken at the same time as the roentgenogram, demonstrates the clinical appearance. This patient had a purely hysterical scoliosis. The curve eventually disappeared after 3 years of psychiatric treatment.

ful, but not absolutely reliable, in determining the prognosis.

Treatment

No treatment is necessary for the non-progressive type, but progressive infantile idiopathic scoliosis must be treated vigorously. Patients with curvatures of 35° or more, or a rib-vertebral angle difference of 20° or more, must be treated (Fig. 16-10).

The treatment of choice for the progressive curve is a Milwaukee brace. It is difficult to make a good brace for a 1-year-old child, but with care it can be done. The model for the pelvic section of the brace should be obtained under an anesthetic. A lateral holding pad should be applied. The brace should be maintained on a full-time schedule and should be removed only for bathing purposes. Usually the brace will successfully manage the curve for many years. Most patients will eventually require spinal fusion.

Milwaukee brace treatment must continue until the curve is maximally corrected and is stable. The curve must never be allowed to go beyond 60°. If in spite of satisfactory Milwaukee brace treatment, the curve progresses, application of a Risser

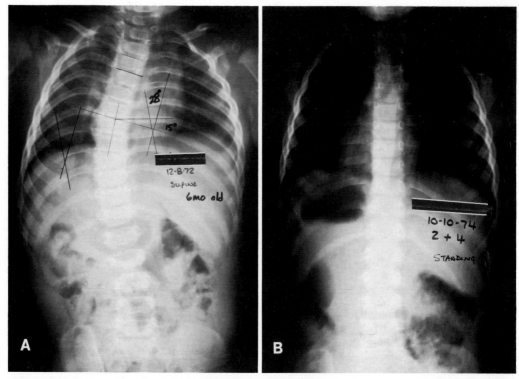

FIG. 16-10. *(A)* This 6-month-old child exhibits a 28° left thoracic scoliosis. No congenital anomalies are visible. The rib-vertebral angle difference is 15°. *(B)* The patient at age 2 years and 4 months. The curve has totally disappeared without treatment.

localizer cast will often improve the curvature. If the curve progresses despite all nonoperative measures, fusion is necessary, *regardless of age*. James has recommended fusion at 10 years of age, regardless of the situation of the curve at that time. We feel that this is arbitrary, and each case should be determined individually. Even after fusion, Milwaukee bracing must be continued to prevent lengthening of the curve and bending of the fused area (Fig. 16-11).

JUVENILE IDIOPATHIC SCOLIOSIS

By definition, juvenile idiopathic scoliosis is that type of idiopathic scoliosis occuring after the age of 3, but before the onset of puberty. The age difference between late onset of juvenile idiopathic scoliosis and early onset of adolescent idiopathic scoliosis is not precise. Nevertheless, there is a sig-

nificant difference between a deformity appearing at age 6 or 7 and one beginning at age 10 or 11. Juvenile idiopathic scoliosis is quite different from the infantile type, in that the curvatures do not resolve spontaneously. The curvature usually progresses steadily for many years, producing an extremely severe deformity. A few curves may remain relatively small and rather static for several years, and then later progress. Thus, any patient with juvenile idiopathic scoliosis and a progressive curve must be treated. Any patient with a curve of 20° or more should be treated, since the likelihood of progression is so high. It is not wise to watch curves greater than 20° without treatment. A golden opportunity to achieve permanent correction of the curve will have been lost.

The best treatment for curves of less than 60° is the Milwaukee brace. In the juvenile years, the spine is more flexible and correctable than later. The results of Milwaukee

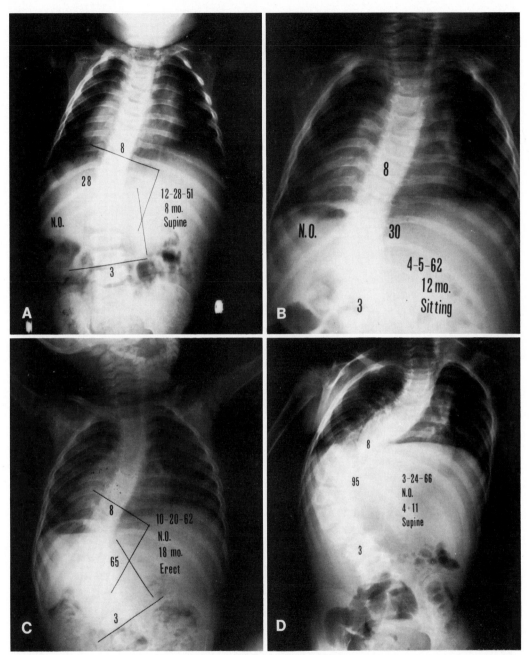

Fig. 16-11. *(A)* An 8-month-old girl with a 28° left thoracolumbar infantile idiopathic scoliosis. *(B)* The patient, sitting, at age 12 months. The curve measures 30°. *(C)* The patient at age 18 months. In a sitting roentgenogram, the curve now measures 65°, indicating a rapidly progressive curvature. The curve should not have been allowed to deteriorate to this degree without treatment. *(D)* The patient at age 4 years 11 months. A supine roentgenogram shows the curve to have increased to 95°. This progression represents a tragic delay in treatment. Photographs kindly donated by Dr. John A. Moe.

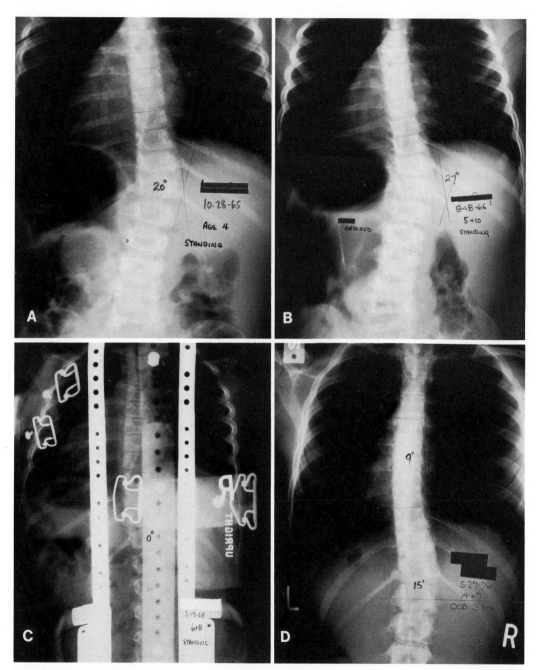

FIG. 16-12. *(A)* This 4-year-old girl shows a 20° right thoracolumbar curve from T9 to L2. No treatment was given at this time. *(B)* The patient 10 months later, the curve having increased to 27°. Note the increased rotation, as well as increased lateral curvature. A Milwaukee brace was fitted at this time. *(C)* The patient 2 years later, in her Milwaukee brace. The curve has been corrected to 0°. *(D)* The patient, who is now 14 years 7 months old, in the process of being weaned out of her Milwaukee brace. The original curve measures 15°, and a 9° left thoracic compensatory curve has developed. Although the patient has spent many years in a Milwaukee brace, it has not harmed her in any way, psychologically or otherwise.

brace treatment are excellent, even though many years of brace treatment are necessary. Quite often, one can achieve such a stable correction that part-time wearing is possible, even though the patient is still growing. A minimum of 2 years of full-time use is necessary. The brace should never be completely discontinued while the child is still growing (Fig. 16-12).

Juvenile idiopathic scoliosis that is progressive despite brace or cast treatment mandates fusion. Curves should not be allowed to progress beyond 60°, and fusion should be carried out regardless of age. Milwaukee brace treatment is necessary following fusion to prevent lengthening of the curve and bending of the fusion area (Fig. 16-13).

ADOLESCENT IDIOPATHIC SCOLIOSIS

Adolescent idiopathic scoliosis is the most common cause of spinal deformity seen on the North American continent. By definition, the onset is at or just after puberty. In actual practice, the age of onset is very difficult to determine. Several curve patterns may occur, the most common being a right thoracic curve. The second most common are right thoracic and left lumbar curves. The third most common is thoracolumbar, the fourth most common is double thoracic (left thoracic-right thoracic), and the least common is an isolated left lumbar curve. On rare occasions, one sees a right lumbar curve or a right thoracic and left thoracolumbar double pattern (Fig. 16-14).

The etiology is unknown. There is a strong genetic tendency, and females are more likely to have the progressive curve requiring treatment. Most series of spine operations for idiopathic scoliosis show a female-to-male ratio of 5 to 1, but school screening surveys show a female-to-male ratio of 1.5 to 1.0.[10, 50]

The curves usually begin early, at age 10 or 11. At this point they are very small and not easily detected. At the time of puberty, the influence of hormonal changes is associated with an increase in the curvature in certain patients. Thus, we see during the growth spurt the appearance of a number of patients with significant curvatures. Careful history and physical examination must be carried out to be sure that other conditions which may mimic idiopathic scoliosis are not overlooked. Syringomyelia is probably the most likely diagnosis to be missed, since it quite often produces a curve that precisely mimics idiopathic scoliosis. Neurologic changes early in the course of syringomyelia are quite subtle. Spinal cord tumors may also closely simulate idiopathic scoliosis.

The natural history of adolescent idiopathic scoliosis is quite varied. Some patients never progress at all. They may have a 10° curve at age 10, which remains constant, disappears, or progresses. At the present time, there is no way to distinguish in the 10-year-old child whether or not the curve is going to progress, resolve, or remain static. Thus, the physician is obligated to observe this situation carefully and to note whether or not progression occurs. Progression indicates the need for treatment (Figs. 16-15, 16-16).

Treatment

The treatment for adolescent idiopathic scoliosis is either bracing or surgery. There are no other available methods which have been proven to be successful. Exercises do not influence the curves unless combined with bracing. Exercises have not been demonstrated to even stop the progression of curves, much less improve them. Exercises have been tried on thousands of patients. No series of patients has ever been reported to have been improved by exercises.

The Milwaukee brace is the standard orthosis for the treatment of adolescent idiopathic scoliosis. This brace was developed in 1945 by Drs. Blount and Schmidt and has subsequently been further refined.[4] The basic Milwaukee brace must have a well-formed pelvic girdle, deeply indented above the iliac crests to maintain a solid foundation. This is the most critical part of the brace. There are two posterior uprights and a single anterior upright. There is a neck ring at the upper end, with a throat mold anteriorly and two occipital pads posteriorly. For a right thoracic curve, an L-shaped thoracic pad is positioned on those ribs lead-

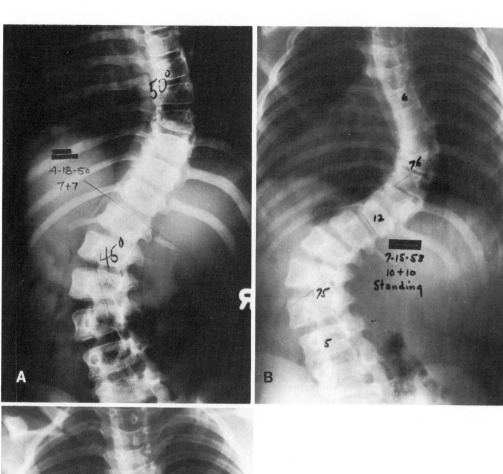

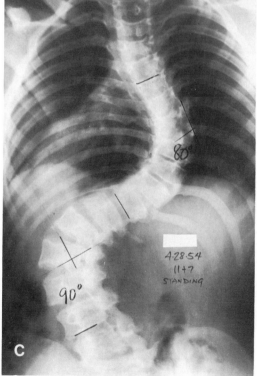

Fig. 16-13. *(A)* Juvenile idiopathic scoliosis, a double structural, right thoracic, left lumbar curve. When first seen at age 7, this boy exhibited a 50° right thoracic curve and a 45° left lumbar curve. No treatment was given at that time. *(B)* The patient at age 10 years and 10 months. The curves had increased to 76° in the thoracic spine and 75° in the lumbar spine. Again no treatment was given. *(C)* At age 11 years and 7 months, his curves had increased to 80° in the thoracic spine and 90° in the lumbar spine. Still no treatment was given. *(Legend continued on facing page.)*

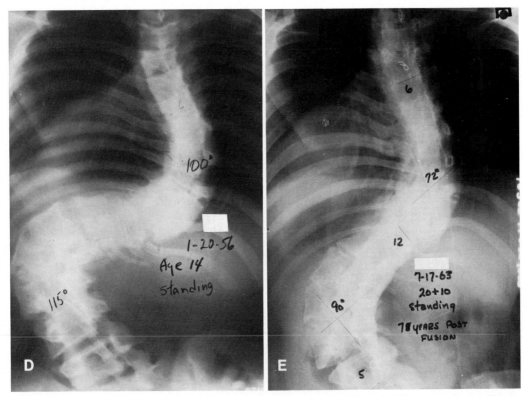

FIG. 16-13 *(Continued)*. *(D)* By age 14 the curves had reached 100° and 115°, respectively. Finally treatment was rendered, but much too late. In 1956 the only thing that could be offered was Risser casting and fusion, which was done at this time. *(E)* At age 20 years and 10 months, 7 years after fusion, the curves were noted to be 72° in the thoracic spine and 90° in the lumbar spine. He appears to have a pseudarthrosis between L4 and L5 in the lumbar curve. Progression has been stopped, although minimal correction has been obtained.

ing to the apex of the curve. For a lumbar curve, a lumbar pad is applied to the transverse process area above the iliac crest and below the most caudad ribs. It is best to fit this pad to the inside of the pelvic girdle with Velcro. For right-thoracic, left-lumbar double structural curves, both pads are used. For high curves involving the upper thoracic area, a shoulder ring is used. The pelvic section is usually made of plastic material, which is heated and then shaped from a model of the patient's waist and hip line. Sometimes prefabricated pelvic sections can be utilized if the patient's shape fits a standard model. Some orthotists prefer to use leather for the pelvic section, with metal bands in the iliac crest area. It is not important whether the brace is made of plastic or leather, but it is important that the girdle fits precisely (Fig. 16-17).

For more details of Milwaukee brace treatment, the reader is referred to the classic text by Blount and Moe.[5]

Indications. The Milwaukee brace is effective for mild to moderate curves. It is not a device which can effectively correct or even control severe curves. The optimal area for the use of the brace is for curves of between 20° and 40°. Below 20°, many curves are nonprogressive or even spontaneously resolving, and thus brace treatment is unnecessary. On the other hand, curves above 40° tend to respond poorly to the brace, particularly if the child has reached the later stages of puberty. Therefore, if the brace treatment is to be effective,

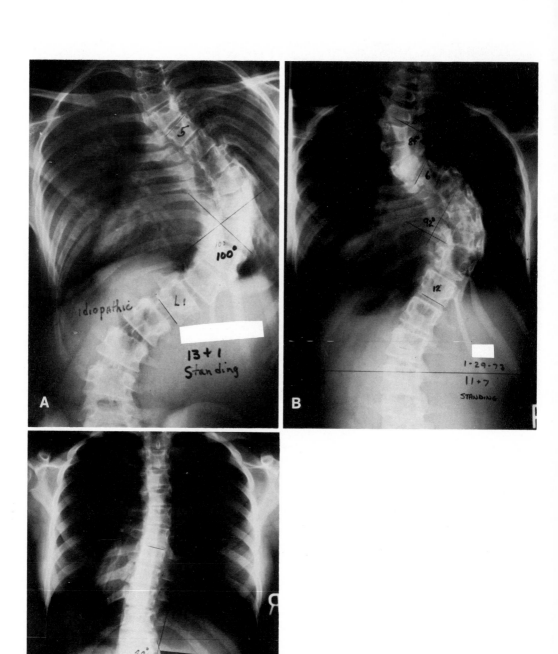

FIG. 16-14. Adolescent idiopathic scoliosis curve pattern. (A) Patient with a classic right thoracic curve, T5 to L1. (B) A patient with a double structural thoracic idiopathic curve, high left thoracic and low right thoracic. (C) A true idiopathic thoracolumbar curve. The apex is at T12. (Legend continued on facing page.)

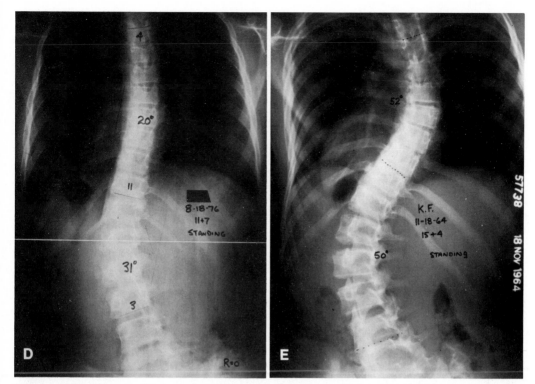

Fig. 16-14 *(Continued)*. *(D)* A single left lumbar idiopathic scoliosis. *(E)* A double structural, right thoracic, left lumbar adolescent idiopathic scoliosis.

it is important that the brace be applied when the curve is small and flexible. Thus, from a practical point of view, *the Milwaukee brace is ideal for growing children with curves of between 20° and 40°*. The brace is primarily a device to prevent small curves from becoming large curves, not to transform large curves into small curves.

Some patients with curves of less than 20° should be braced. These are usually patients with juvenile idiopathic scoliosis of between 15° and 20° for whom it is important to begin treatment early. There are also curves between 15° and 20° which are known to be progressive because of previously documentation of a smaller curve (e.g., a 12° curve that has increased to 18°). Under these circumstances, it is wise to start the bracing, even though the curve has not yet reached 20°. It is the presence of a *progressive* curve that is important.

Curves above 40° can be treated in a Milwaukee brace, but the results are poor, and the physician should warn the family and the patient that results are unpredictable. Thus, it should be attempted only on a trial basis. If an adequate correction is not obtained, surgery should be considered without delay.

Management of the patient in a Milwaukee brace is not easy. The patient should be seen as frequently as necessary to maintain a quality fitting of the brace and quality maintenance of the brace and control of the patient. We find in our own clinics that every 3 to 4 months seems appropriate. More frequent visits are necessary early in the course of management and less frequent visits are necessary later when growth is slower and the patient is more accustomed to the brace.

At the time the brace treatment is started, the brace should be checked by the responsible physician to be sure it fits well. The brace should be started on a full-time basis. The patient should *not* be "weaned" into the brace. Under a full-time program, there

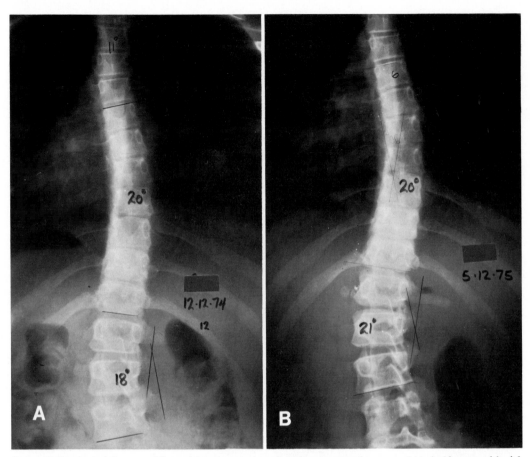

FIG. 16-15. An adolescent idiopathic progressive double structural curve. *(A)* A 12-year-old girl with a 20° right thoracic curve and an 18° left lumbar curve. *(B)* The patient 5 months later. The curves are 20° thoracic and 21° lumbar. *(Legend continued on facing page.)*

is usually a period of approximately 1 week where the child will not be very happy, will often cry, and will not sleep well the first night or two. Nevertheless, this period of adjustment passes, and a happy and outgoing patient soon emerges. A slow weaning into the brace only prolongs the period of adjustment. After the patient has worn the brace for 2 or 3 weeks, he or she should be seen for further adjustments of the brace, as it may need to be lengthened due to correction of the curve. At this point, there will be many questions about activities in the brace; the patient will need verbal support. Roentgenograms should be obtained to check the response of the curve to the brace.

After this, the patient can usually be seen at intervals of 3 months. A roentgenogram should be obtained either every visit or every other visit, and it must be carefully measured.

It is very important to recognize whether or not correction is being maintained. The patient who progressively loses correction while wearing the brace is either not wearing the brace regularly, has a brace that does not fit well, or has a curve that is simply beyond the ability of the brace to manage. Provided there is a good brace and it is being worn full-time, a loss of correction usually means a difficult curve problem. A patient with a curve progressing beyond 40° should have

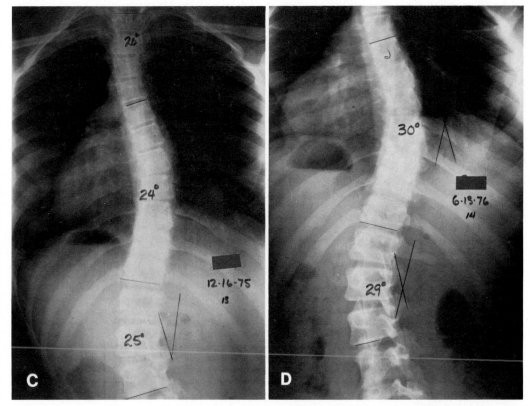

Fig. 16-15 *(Continued). (C)* The patient 7 months later. The curves are 24° right thoracic and 25° left lumbar. *(D)* The patient at age 14, 1½ years after the original roentgenogram was taken. The curves now measure 30° and 29°. No treatment had been given.

correction and spinal fusion. As long as the curve can be maintained under 35°, surgery is not necessary.

Techniques of Brace Fitting. For the typical right thoracic curve, the main lateral holding pad is the contoured thoracic pad. This is customarily situated posterolaterally, with the anterior strap fixed to the anterior outrigger. The posterior strap is attached to the ipsilateral posterior upright. If the patient has a kyphotic component to the curve, the posterior margin of the pad should be placed underneath the posterior upright; thus, the pad is primarily posterior and slightly lateral. If the patient has no kyphosis, and especially if the patient has a flat or slightly lordotic thoracic spine, the pad must be placed purely laterally. It is

very important not to promote an increase of thoracic lordosis. Patients with idiopathic thoracic scoliosis quite often have a tendency to thoracic lordosis.

Particularly when beginning the brace, it is customary to apply a left axillary sling to counteract some of the lateral forces of the right lateral thoracic holding pad. The axillary sling is designed to allow the patient to maintain the neck in the center of the neck ring, otherwise the right thoracic holding pad will push the patient against the left side of the neck ring, producing discomfort and irritation along the side of the neck. With the axillary sling, the patient can maintain a neutral and nonirritated position in the neck ring. The axillary sling is not a device that corrects a curve. It is not intended to elevate

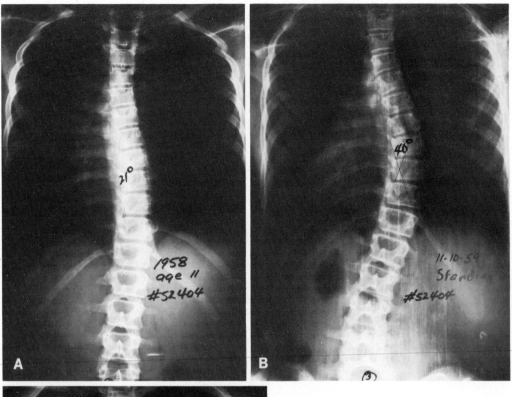

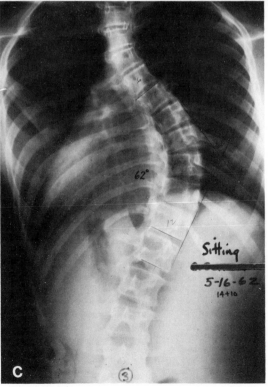

Fig. 16-16. Adolescent idiopathic scoliosis, with progression of a single curve. *(A)* An 11-year-old girl with a 21° right thoracic curve. *(B)* The patient 1 year later, showing an increase to 40°. No treatment was given. *(C)* The patient 2½ years later. The curve has increased to 62°. Note the persistence of rotation into the lumbar spine. L4 is the first neutrally rotated vertebra, although the end vertebra is either T12 or L1.

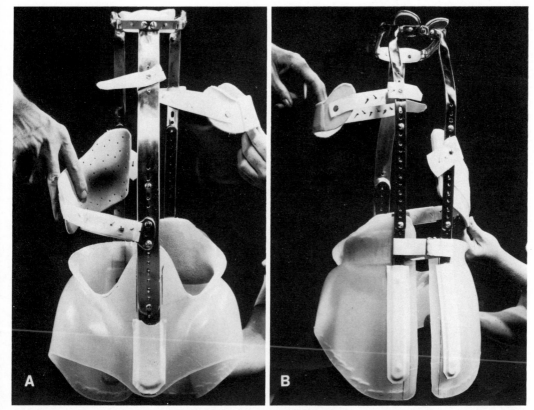

FIG. 16-17. The general design of the idiopathic scoliosis Milwaukee brace. *(A)* A modern Milwaukee brace. The pelvic section is made of polypropylene, and the brace is fitted with a left lumbar pad, a right thoracic pad, and a left axillary sling. *(B)* The brace viewed posteriorly. Note how the brace is carried low, posteriorly, and cut high, anteriorly, in the pelvic section.

the left shoulder. Correction of the elevated right shoulder is accomplished by correcting the right thoracic scoliosis.

Quite often the axillary sling can be discontinued after 3 or 4 months of brace wearing. By this time, the patient will have learned through voluntary muscle control to maintain a central position in the neck ring (Fig. 16-18).

If structural lumbar curve is also present, it is treated with a left lumbar pad. A large number of techniques has been attempted to position and hold this pad. After hundreds of patients and dozens of techniques, we have settled upon the use of a lumbar pad which is held to the inside of the pelvic girdle by means of Velcro. By this attachment technique, the pad can be moved slightly in several directions, thus affording immediate alterations of pad position. The thickness of the pad varies with the anatomic variations of the patient, and it must maintain the most lateral correcting force possible. It should not be a force that presses purely forward. If properly applied, the lumbar pad produces redness of the skin, but no blisters or ulcerations. The pad must exert pressure against the transverse process area, and it must lie above the iliac crest and below the ribs (Fig. 16-19).

For the statistical results of Milwaukee brace treatment, the reader is referred to the classic article by Moe and Kettleson.[65]

Lumbar and Thoracolumbar Braces in Idiopathic Scoliosis. There recently has been enthusiasm for treatment of lumbar and thoracolumbar idiopathic scoliosis with underarm braces. The advent of thermoplastic

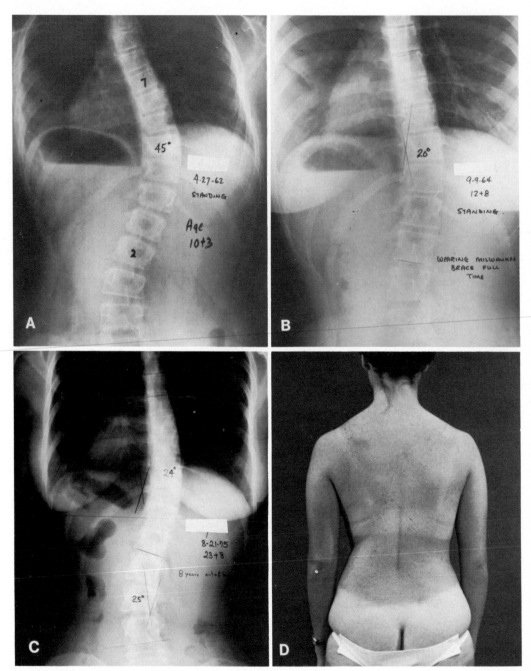

FIG. 16-18. Milwaukee brace treatment of idiopathic scoliosis with a right thoracic curve. (A) This girl, 10 years and 3 months old, was seen for a 45° T7 to L2 progressive curvature. The mother had a severe and painful thoracic scoliosis. Milwaukee brace treatment was started at this time. (B) At age 12 years and 8 months, a standing roentgenogram out of the brace shows correction of the curve to 20°. She was wearing the brace full-time at this point. (C) The patient at age 23, 8 years after coming out of the brace. She has lost only 3°, since the time when the brace was removed. (D) A photograph of the patient at age 23. This is obviously an excellent result from brace treatment.

materials has stimulated this reactivation of an old idea.

The lumbar brace is effective only for flexible curves of less than 40°. It is effective only in curves with the apex at T12 or lower (Fig. 16-20). It is *neither designed nor intended* for thoracic curves.

The brace should be made from a cast of the patient taken in the corrected position. Lumbar lordosis must be eliminated. The brace must be worn for 23 of each 24 hours, and removed on the same schedule as is a Milwaukee brace (Fig. 16-21).

Sometimes it is advantageous to prescribe the "TLSO" (thoracic lumbar sacral orthosis) in the daytime and the Milwaukee brace at night for stubborn teenagers who refuse to wear the Milwaukee brace in the daytime (Fig. 16-22).

Weaning From the Brace. Total nonoperative treatment with a brace demands that the treatment continue until growth ceases. Otherwise, relapse occurs. There is considerable controversy concerning the completion of growth and the time when the brace should be discontinued. To obtain optimal results, the brace should be maintained on a full-time schedule until: (1) full vertical height has been achieved, as determined by serial height measurement, and (2) the Risser sign shows full capping (Risser IV). In girls, these factors usually coincide, but in boys, there is customarily another 2 cm. of vertical growth after full capping of the iliac epiphysis.[1]

Once vertical growth has ceased and full capping has occurred, weaning can *begin*. Weaning progresses slowly; time in the brace usually decreases about 1 hour each day per month. Thus, it requires 1 year to go from full-time use to "nights only" use. The patient must wear the brace only at night for at least 1 year.

SURGICAL TREATMENT OF IDIOPATHIC SCOLIOSIS

With modern techniques, the surgical approach to idiopathic scoliosis has become a safe and reliable procedure. It should not be viewed as a "last-ditch" measure, and it should not be avoided when it is clear that the patient would benefit by such a procedure.

At the same time, it is a surgical procedure of significant magnitude that never should be entered into lightly. There are several basic components to the surgical program: (1) selection of the patient for surgery; (2) selection of the exact area to be fused; (3) the actual fusion procedure itself; (4) the instrumentation procedure; (5) the immediate postoperative management; and (6) the postoperative immobilization.

Selection of the Patient for Surgery

The indication for surgery is based upon the magnitude of the curvature and the problems that it has caused or may cause in the future. Over the years, a solid, rational basis has evolved for the selection of the patient for surgery. Based upon the Cobb measurement system, adolescent curves beyond 50° are best treated by surgery. This is true, regardless of the curve pattern. The reason for the use of 50° as a baseline for making this decision comes from long-term studies of untreated patients. As was noted in the section on natural history (p. 582), patients with curves of greater than 50° at the end of growth usually have progression of their curves during adult life, and subsequently they have curves of 75° to 80° 20 to 30 years later. With curves of this magnitude, symptomatology is so apparent that it is obviously better to take care of the situation in childhood rather than allowing the adult to deteriorate to a point of malfunction. Thus, the recommendation for surgery is based on the predictability of complications in adult life.

The most important indication for fusion is the *prevention* of respiratory insufficiency. Thoracic curvatures above 60° are associated with a progressive decline in pulmonary function with age and with increase in curvature. Correction of curvatures in adults seldom gives significant improvement of respiratory function. Therefore, it is best to prevent a patient from having a respiratory insufficiency, rather than waiting for insufficiency to develop and then trying to correct it.

The use of the 50° baseline is not a magic

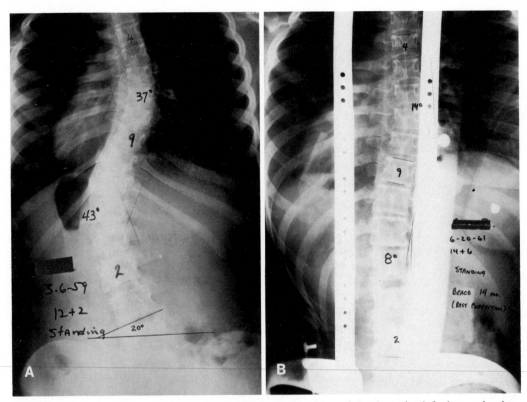

FIG. 16-19. *(A)* A double structural idiopathic scoliosis with a right thoracic, left thoracolumbar, double curve pattern. The patient was 12 years old, and was placed in a Milwaukee brace at this time. *(B)* The patient after 14 months in a Milwaukee brace. The curves have been corrected to 14° and 8° in the brace. *(Legend continued on facing page.)*

figure below which surgery must never be done and above which surgery must always be done. It is merely intended as a guideline. It must always be remembered that scoliosis is a three-dimensional deformity and that the anteroposterior roentgenogram is only a two-plane evaluation. The prudent physician must look at the lateral roentgenogram and especially must look at the patient, putting all factors together to make a determination. Some patients with 40° curves require surgery. These are patients who have a considerable structural deformity of the thorax, particularly if they have thoracic lordosis or a larger-than-average rib hump. Other patients with 40° curves may require fusion because of pain. Some patients with 55° curves have virtually no deformity at all, and on testing of pulmonary function they are entirely normal. These patients do not require surgery, but they should be periodically observed for progression of the curve.

Selection of the Fusion Area

Improper selection of the fusion area leads to many tragedies. It is wrong to fuse either too much or not enough of the spine. The question of exactly what area to fuse is a constant problem. One should fuse the structural (major) curve, and generally, one should avoid fusing the compensatory or secondary curves. The determination of whether a curve is structural or secondary is based upon analysis of bending and traction films. It is also determined upon examination of the patient, since the absence of rotation is usually a sign of a secondary curve.

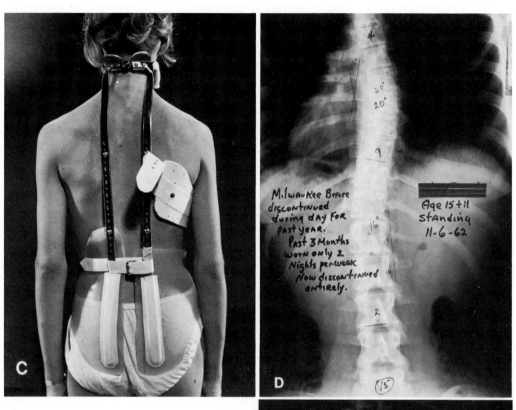

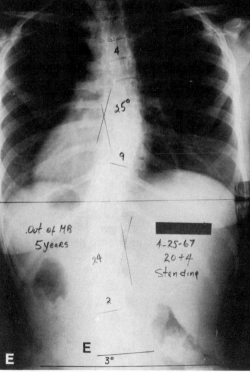

FIG. 16-19 *(Continued)*. *(C)* A patient with similar curve patterns in a modern Milwaukee brace with right thoracic and left lumbar pads. *(D)* The patient at the time the brace was discontinued. A standing roentgenogram shows a 20° thoracic curve and a 16° lumbar curve. *(E)* The patient at age 20, 5 years after removing the brace. The thoracic curve is 25° and the lumbar curve is 24°; essentially no loss has occurred since discontinuing the brace. She is married and has had two children by this time. (Photographs kindly donated by Dr. John H. Moe.)

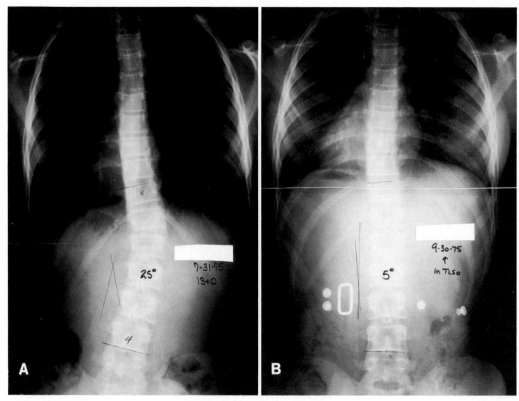

FIG. 16-20. *(A)* A 13-year-old girl with a progressive 25° right lumbar idiopathic scoliosis. A TLSO was prescribed at this time. *(B)* The patient standing in the TLSO, the curve measuring 5°. Results like this are typical of this brace. The authors do not have any long-term follow-up at the time of this writing.

The presence of significant degrees of rotation indicates a structural curve.

One must never fuse less than the measured curve. Thus, if the curve is T5 to T12, the fusion must never be less than T5 to T12. Usually this is not enough, and one vertebra above and one vertebra below the measured area should be included. Thus, the rule that *"one above and one below the measured curve is the area for fusion"* is a practical one which is used by many surgeons.

Even this rule is not totally adequate. There are certain curves in which the fusion will still be too short. The curve will lengthen after the cast is removed. Careful analysis of these complications has led to the use of vertebral rotation as a guideline for selection of the fusion area. With this rule, one should include in the fusion area *all of the vertebrae rotated in the same direction as the vertebra at the apex of the curve, and the fusion should extend to the first vertebra that is not rotated.* Thus, if the end of the measured curve is L1, but L2 and L3 are both rotated in the same direction as the apical vertebra, and L4 is the first neutral vertebra in terms of rotation, then the fusion should extend to L4. The fusion may stop at L3 if on the supine roentgenogram L3, rather than L4, would be the neutral vertebra on rotation. If the child still has more than a year of growth remaining, it is better to select the more distal vertebra rather than the more proximal one. If, however, the patient has completed growth, lengthening of the curve is less likely and the slightly shorter fusion area can be chosen (Fig. 16-23).

If the patient has a double structural curve pattern, both curves must be fused. It is useless to fuse only one curve, since the

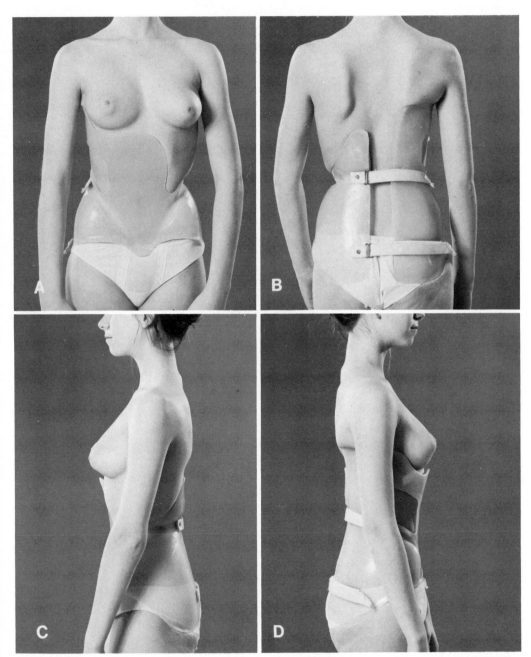

Fig. 16-21. (A) A thoracolumbar sacral orthosis for the treatment of a lumbar idiopathic curvature, front view. (B) The same brace, as viewed posteriorly. She has a left lumbar curve. (C) The patient as viewed from the left side. (D) The patient as viewed from the right side. Note that the brace is cut high in the front for sitting, kept low in the back to control lumbar lordosis, and is kept below the breast area to avoid compression.

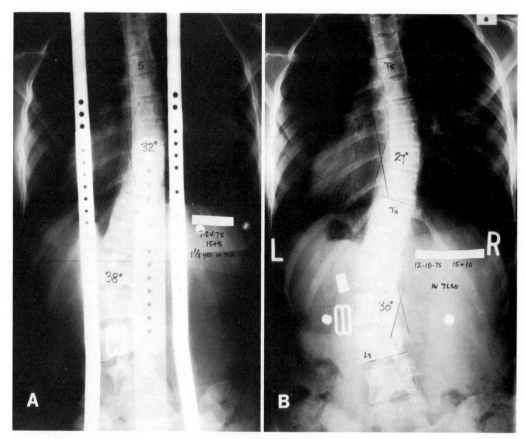

FIG. 16-22. *(A)* This 15-year-old girl spent 1¹/₂ years in a Milwaukee brace. The curve in the brace measures 32°. Unfortunately, she developed "rebellion syndrome" and now refuses to wear her Milwaukee brace in public. A compromise was reached, and she wears the Milwaukee brace at night and a TLSO in the daytime. *(B)* The same patient in a TLSO showing curves to measure 27° and 30°. This shows that the TLSO can, in her particular case, manage the curves as well as the Milwaukee brace.

second curve will progress and a second fusion will be necessary at some other time. Fusion of two curves is a larger procedure than a single curve, but with care it is quite possible to accomplish both at one time. If there is any concern about this being excessive surgery, it is perfectly reasonable to fuse one curve, wait 2 weeks, and then fuse the other curve.

There are conflicting ideas about the proper level for fusion of lumbar curves. The rule that the fusion must extend to the first neutrally rotated vertebra does not hold when that vertebra is L5. In most lumbar curves, the fusion should stop at L4, even if L4 is still rotated in the same direction as the apical vertebra.

There are certain occasions when it may be necessary to fuse to L5. This is particularly true when there is a great deal of rotational shift between L4 and L5. *It is never necessary to fuse the spine of a child with idiopathic scoliosis to the sacrum, unless there is a coincident and symptomatic spondylolisthesis.*

Patients undergoing fusion to L4 or L5 must have a careful physical examination and roentgenographic evaluation of the lumbosacral area to be sure that there is no spondylolysis or spondylolisthesis. It is safe to extend a fusion to L4 if there is an asymptomatic and nondisplaced spondy-lolysis at L5.

Patients with idiopathic scoliosis do not have curves that extend into the cervical spine. Thus, the uppermost vertebra that should be included in the fusion area for idiopathic scoliosis is T1. Any curve extend-ing into the cervical spine must be suspected of being a condition other than idiopathic scoliosis.

One of the common mistakes has been the failure to fuse the high left thoracic curve in the double structural thoracic curve pattern. It is sometimes difficult to decide whether this upper curve needs fusion.

If, on erect films, the upper curve has the same magnitude at the right thoracic curve, if on bending films it has the same quantity of rigidity, and if, on upright films, the upper-most ribs on the left side are higher than the uppermost ribs on the right side, then this upper curve must be included in the fusion area (Fig. 16-24).

One of the most difficult problems in all of scoliosis is the question of whether to fuse the lumbar curve in patients with double structural, right thoracic, left lumbar curve patterns in which the lumbar curve is not as structural as the thoracic curve. These pa-tients have curves which are usually of equal magnitude on the standing film, but on the supine and bending films, the lumbar curve is of less magnitude and is more flexible than the thoracic curve. Here the decision-making becomes quite difficult. As stated before, if the two curves are of equal mag-nitude on the standing film, of equal mag-nitude on the supine film, and of equal struc-tural quality on the bending films, then both curves *must* be fused. If, however, the lum-bar curve is considerably more flexible than the thoracic curve, and if the lumbar curve on voluntary supine side-bending corrects to a degree which is equal to or better than the *expected* correction of the thoracic curve, then it is satisfactory to fuse only the thoracic curve and not the lumbar curve. The lumbar curve must be carefully fol-lowed, and if it progresses beyond the curva-ture in the fused thoracic spine, it also must be fused at a later time.

It is a nuisance to the patient to have a second fusion at a later time, but this is sometimes preferable to a single procedure in which a lumbar curve is fused unnecessar-ily (Fig. 16-25, 16-26).

Surgical Technique

The reader is referred to standard texts and references on fusion technique, as it is beyond the scope of this chapter to give de-tails on surgical technique. The author stresses the importance of: (1) complete facet joint excision on both sides (concave and convex); (2) replacement of the facet joint area by a plug of iliac, cancellous, au-togenous bone; (3) complete decortication of all exposed laminae and transverse pro-cesses; and (4) the routine addition of fresh, autogenous, iliac bone. When these components are religiously applied to each and every case, consistently good results are obtained. Surgeons who try to "get by" without excising the facet joints or using extra bone have much poorer results than those surgeons who use the preferred proce-dure.[18, 29, 31, 60, 63]

Surgical technique must be learned in the operating room from a skilled surgeon. It is simply not possible to review a textbook, slides, or movie and then perform this type of procedure.

Harrington instrumentation has become almost standard throughout the world for the surgical treatment of idiopathic scolio-sis. It must be remembered that the Har-rington instruments are an *adjunct* to the fusion technique and never replace fusion.[35] Therefore, the instrumentation is only a de-vice that gives internal correction and inter-nal stabilization to the fused area. There was a tendency at one time for surgeons to de-pend too much upon instrumentation and to not perform an adequate fusion. This has been proven over and over again to lead to bad results. Scoliosis surgery was done for many years prior to the invention of the Har-rington instruments; very good results were obtained and are still obtained in cases with-out instrumentation. There are many situa-tions in which Harrington instruments should not be used, as a better result can be obtained without them.

There is also considerable controversy as

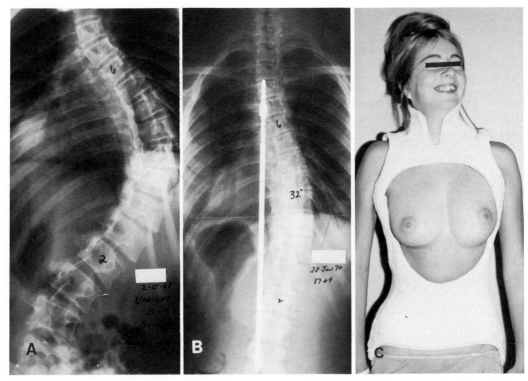

FIG. 16-23. *(A)* A 15-year-old girl with a T6 to L12 right thoracic adolescent idiopathic scoliosis. Note the marked rotation of the vertebra and note also the continuation of rotation beyond the end vertebra, L2. She also exhibits "thoracic overhang," with deviation of the torso to the right. In such cases it is important to have lowermost end of the fusion mass directly above the sacrum; therefore, for both reasons, the fusion was carried down to L4. *(B)* The patient 2 years later. The curve has been corrected to 32° and maintained at that point. The thorax has been totally and completely corrected, in terms of its alignment over the pelvis. It is important that the fusion mass be vertical in its orientation, and it should be centered over the center of the sacrum *(Legend continued on facing page.)*

to whether the only distraction rod should be used in most cases of idiopathic scoliosis, or whether the contracting rod assembly should also be used in addition to the distraction rod. It is the author's opinion that the contracting assembly adds little to the procedure except time and inconvenience, and it should be used only in those cases with a kyphotic component to the curve. Other prominent surgeons, such as Harrington, Dickson, and Hall, feel strongly that the compression assembly should always be used. Good results are obtained by surgeons using both techniques, so this discrepancy of opinion is not important. Certainly, if there is an existent thoracic lordosis, the

compression rod *must* be avoided (Fig. 16-27).

It is important that the patient with true kyphoscoliosis have a compression assembly applied to the convex side *before* insertion of the distraction rod on the concave side.

Bending of the distraction rod is frequently necessary; it should not be avoided when the indication arises. This is usually necessary to fit a distraction rod to the normal roundness of the thoracic spine, particularly when dealing with double thoracic curves. Some patients with right thoracic, left lumbar double curves also have a slight kyphosis at the junction of the two curves,

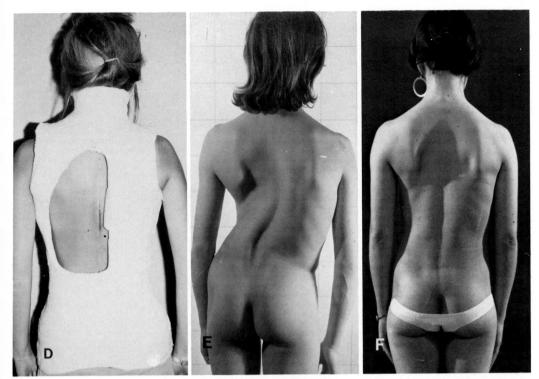

Fig. 16-23 *(Continued)*. *(C)* An anterior view of the Risser-Cotrel cast for postoperative management of a patient with thoracic idiopathic scoliosis. On the anterior view, note the large anterior thoracic window, which provides maximal opportunity for inspiration, expiration, and rib movement. Care is taken that there is no compression of the breasts. Note that the abdomen is kept firmly held in to promote thoracic breathing. The slot in front of the neck is to eliminate any pressure against the trachea. The cast is cut sufficiently high in front to permit 100° of hip flexion for comfortable sitting. *(D)* The same cast as viewed from behind. The cast comes low on the buttocks, and has a large window cut out of the concavity of the thoracic curve. Firm pressure is maintained over the rib hump area on the right, and the patient is encouraged to deeply breathe and thus bring out the "rib valley" holding in the rib hump. *(E)* A preoperative photograph of the patient. *(F)* A postoperative photograph a few years later. She demonstrated an increase in vital capacity of 500 ml.

and the rod should be slightly bent to accommodate this at the time of insertion. Failure to bend the rod in these circumstances may result in hook dislocation. The rod should be bent only in the nonratcheted portion.

The Harrington distraction system is customarily inserted into the facet joint at the upper end, using a No. 1262 hook. The lower insertion is underneath the lamina of the most caudad vertebra to be included in the fusion area. A small window is made in the ligamentum flavum; a blunt dissector is placed between the dura and the lamina, and a No. 1254 hook is placed in this area. All of the facet joint fusion and decortication fusion on the concave side should be done prior to the insertion of the rod. The rod is distracted to the comfortable limit. The amount of force used can only be learned in the operating room. It cannot be verbally described. Certainly it is possible to overstretch the tissues. Overstretching can cause fractures of the lamina and can produce paraplegia.[54]

After insertion of the rods to the desired limit, it is our custom to awaken the patient to a lighter level of anesthesia and command the patient to move the hands and then the feet. When the patient has demonstrated the

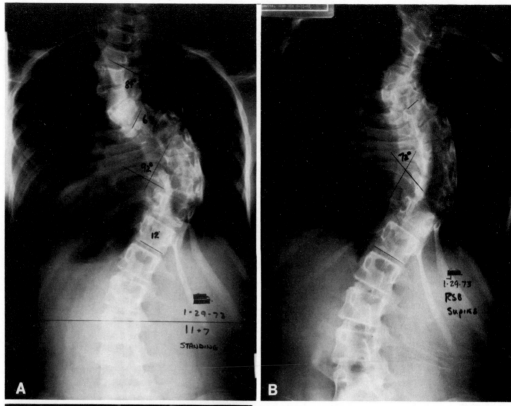

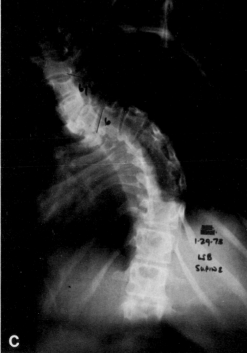

FIG. 16-24. *(A)* This patient exhibits a double thoracic idiopathic scoliosis. Note the elevation of the first rib on the left, as compared to the right, and clinically the patient showed a higher left shoulder than right shoulder. Correction and fusion of the T6 to T12 curve alone would produce a disastrous worsening of the patient's appearance, due to increase of the elevation of the left shoulder. This high left thoracic curve is one reason that it is important to have long roentgenograms in analyzing the scoliosis patient. *(B)* A supine voluntary right side-bending roentgenogram of the patient, showing correction of the right thoracic curve to 72°. *(C)* A supine voluntary left side-bending roentgenogram of the high thoracic curve, showing correction to 67°. Both curves are thus highly structural and of equal structural character. This readily defines this condition as a double-major or double-primary or double-structural idiopathic thoracic scoliosis. *(Legend continued on facing page.)*

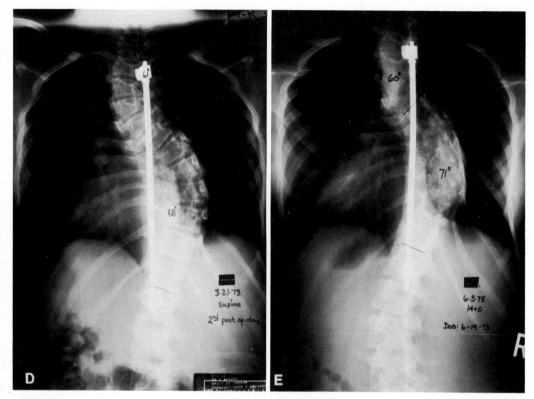

Fɪɢ. 16-24 *(Continued). (D)* The same patient on the second postoperative day, showing the instrumentation from T1 to L1 with a single Harrington distraction rod. The rod has been turned upside down so that the smaller #1254 hook could be inserted in the smaller T1, T2 facet joint. This also permits bending of the rod in the thoracic area to accommodate the normal thoracic kyphosis. It also prevents any prominence of the ratcheted end of the rod at the base of the neck. The patient was managed in a standard Risser cast, as shown in Fig. 16-23. *(E)* A roentgenogram of the patient 2 years after fusion showing minimal loss of correction, none in the high thoracic curve, and only 3° in the lower curve. This patient was ambulatory throughout the entire course of treatment.

ability to move the feet *voluntarily,* he is placed back to the deeper level of anesthesia. With good anesthetic control, this is easy to perform and provides a simple and immediate evaluation of the neurologic status. This test was designed by Stagnara and his associates, of Lyon, France. It has been our experience that patients do not remember this episode.

After surgery, the patient is nursed in a regular bed and turned with a careful log-rolling technique. If the rod is well inserted and if the nurses use good care, dislocation of the rod is most unusual. Patients with osteoporotic bone should be protected in a cast

or placed on a turning frame. At the end of a week, the wound is usually sufficiently healed to apply the postoperative cast. We apply a Risser-Cotrel cast with a small amount of padding around the hips and no padding elsewhere, except two layers of stockinette. The cast is applied with traction, and a localizer force is created by a Cotrel derotation lateral-flexion strap.

After the cast has dried for 2 or 3 hours, the patient can be started on ambulation and should be fully ambulatory by the time of discharge from the hospital.

This early ambulation program is possible, provided there has been proper inser-

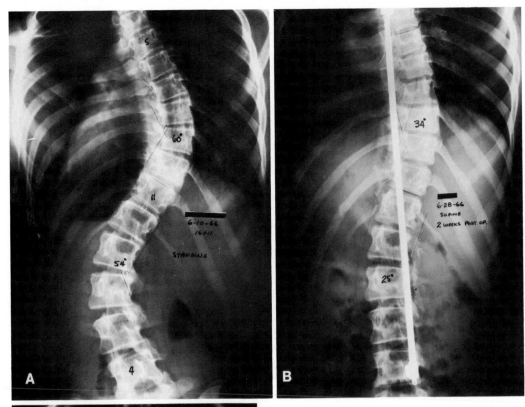

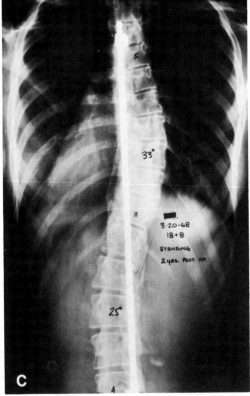

FIG. 16-25. (A) An idiopathic double curve, right thoracic and left lumbar, in a 16-year-old boy. Due to the equal structural characteristics, it was felt necessary that both curves be fused. (B) The same patient, supine, 2 weeks postoperatively, showing correction of the upper curve to 34° and the lower to 25°. The fusion area is T4 to L4. (C) The patient 2 years postoperatively, showing maintenance of the correction at 33° in the thoracic spine and 25° in the lumbar spine. There had been no loss of correction, despite ambulation, since the second week postoperatively. The cast was worn a total of 9 months. (*Legend continued on facing page.*)

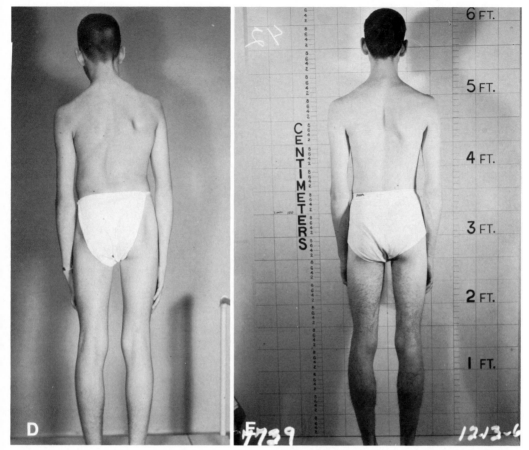

FIG. 16-25 *(Continued)*. *(D)* Preoperative photograph of the patient. *(E)* A photograph of the patient 2 years postoperatively.

tion of the Harrington rod and proper application of the Risser-Cotrel cast. Provided these conditions are met, a loss of correction by early ambulation can be limited to no more than 5° or 6°.[47, 59]

The duration of casting varies from center to center and from surgeon to surgeon. But like all other bone healing processes, it should be individualized according to the patient's healing capacity. Generally, most scoliosis fusions require 8 to 9 months of cast time to become sufficiently solid, with good vertical trabeculation of the fusion mass. Some surgeons remove the cast in as short a time as 6 months, but this is the bare minimum. The most important thing is that good quality roentgenograms demonstrate a solid fusion. In our experience, this seldom is present at 6 months and is usually present at 8 to 9 months in the usual patient with idiopathic scoliosis. In the patient with *adolescent* idiopathic scoliosis, no further support is needed after cast removal.

Some surgeons prefer to use a Milwaukee brace postoperatively, rather than a cast. Provided it is a well-made brace, and provided the patient can be trusted not to remove the brace, this a useful method.

Pseudarthrosis is a recognized problem in the surgical treatment of any type of scoliosis, including idiopathic scoliosis. The incidence of pseudarthrosis has decreased steadily as better surgical and cast immobilization techniques have developed.

If, at the time of cast removal, a definite *(Text continues on page 619.)*

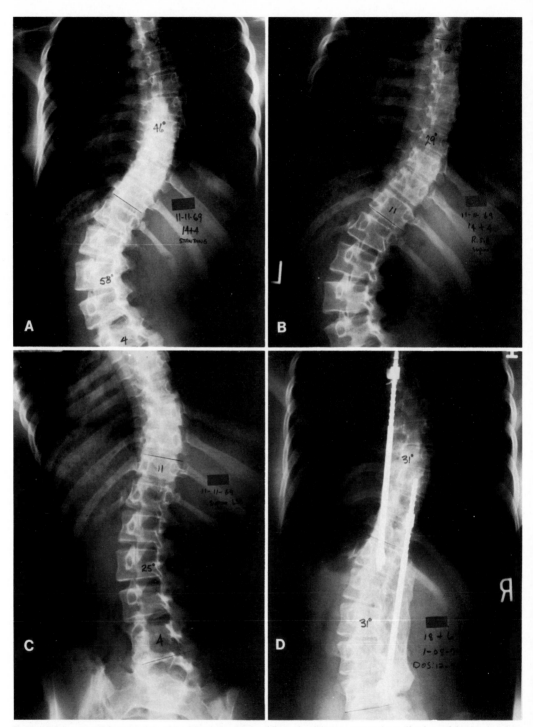

FIG. 16-26. *(A)* This 14-year-old girl presented with a double structural scoliosis, with the lumbar curve being the larger of the two curves. Both curves were clinically apparent. *(B)* Supine right side-bending for the thoracic curve, showing correction to 29°. *(C)* Supine left side-bending, showing correction of the lumbar curve to 25°. Both curves are thus equally structural, and both require fusion. *(D)* Standing roentgenogram 4 years postoperatively. In this case, two distraction rods were used, one for each curve, with a two-segment overlap of the rods. It is the author's preference to use a single rod for this type of curve situation at the present time. Note on this film the massive transverse process fusion on the concavity of the lumbar curve. The fusion mass extends in a straight linear fashion from T4 to L4.

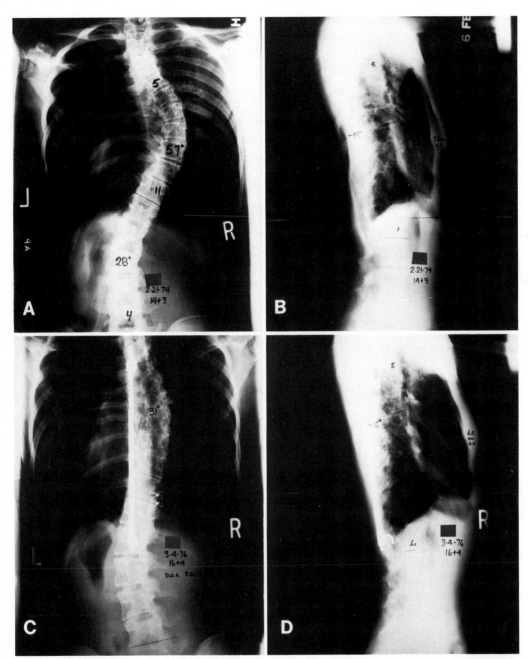

Fig. 16-27. (A) This 14-year-old girl demonstrates a T5 to T11 57° right thoracic scoliosis. (B) This lateral standing roentgenogram demonstrates a serious degree of thoracic lordosis, measuring − 19°. Since the lower limit of normal thoracic kyphosis is 20°, this patient has 39° of lordotic deformity. The distance from the front of her spine to the back of the sternum is 3.8 cm. (C) The patient 2 years postoperatively showing a solid fusion. Correction of the curve was to 31°. Note that the rods in the lower end of the fusion mass are centered over the midsacrum. (D) A standing lateral roentgenogram taken 2 years postoperatively, showing correction of lordosis from −39° to −6°. There is now 6.5 cm. between the front of the spine and the back of the sternum. Her vital capacity was increased by 1050 ml.

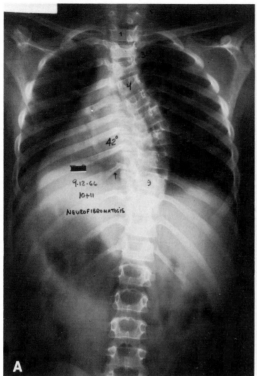

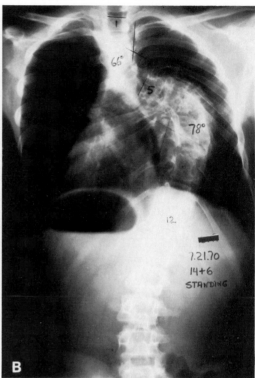

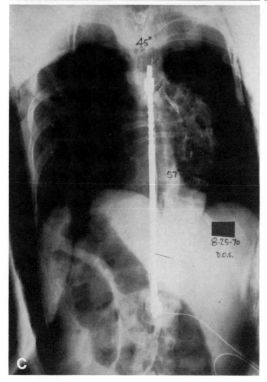

FIG. 16-28. (A) This 10-year-old boy presented elsewhere with a 42° right thoracic scoliosis. He had a multiple café-au-lait spots on the skin, and his mother also demonstrated café-au-lait spots and multiple subcutaneous tumors, typical of neurofibromatosis. On this roentgenogram, note the scalloping of the vertebral body borders on the convexity of the curve, the warping of the necks and heads of the ribs and transverse processes, and the concavity of the curve. Note also the 35° T1 to T4 high left thoracic curve. This patient was placed in a Milwaukee brace, which he wore faithfully for 4 years. Such curves should not be placed in a Milwaukee brace, but should be fused immediately. (B) The patient at age 14, after 4 consecutive years in the Milwaukee brace. His right thoracic curve has increased to 78° and the high left curve to 66°. (C) Surgical correction was performed, with a fusion extending from T1 to L2 and the Harrington rod from T4 to L2. Note that the lower end of the rod and the fusion is centered over the midsacrum, and the uppermost ribs are level. (*Legend continued on facing page.*)

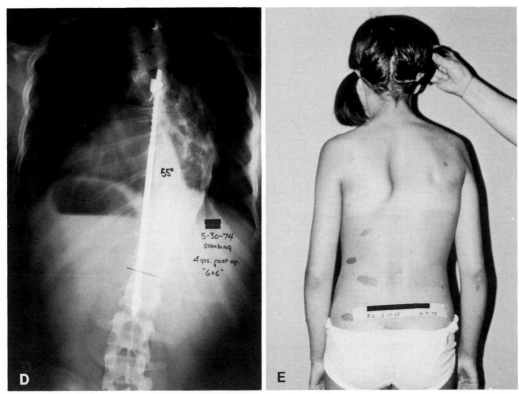

Fig. 16-28 *(Continued)*. *(D)* The patient 4 years later. His correction has been completely maintained with no loss of correction, whatsoever. Six months after the original fusion the wound was reopened, the bone graft lightly decorticated and the other iliac crest added as a further thickening bone graft. Note the massive strong fusion. *(E)* A patient with multiple café-au-lait spots and right thoracic scoliosis secondary to neurofibromatosis.

pseudarthrosis is noted, the patient should be scheduled for pseudarthrosis repair without further delay. It is unwise to "observe" the pseudarthrosis and allow any loss of correction to take place. Harrington rods do not ordinarily break, but they can break with the repeated stresses of a pseudarthrosis.

NEUROFIBROMATOSIS SPINAL DEFORMITY

CLINICAL AND ROENTGENOGRAPHIC FEATURES

Neurofibromatosis is a special problem in scoliosis. Bone lesions are common in this disorder, and of the many bone lesions, scoliosis is the most common. The classic type of scoliosis described in neurofibromatosis is a very short and sharply angulated curve with marked distortion of the vertebrae in the curve and spindling of the ribs leading to the apex of the curve. This curve is most frequently thoracic and may be to the right or the left. This classic form appears to be quite different from idiopathic or paralytic scoliosis. The astute physician should be able to recognize from the roentgenogram that a curve is probably due to neurofibromatosis. Clinical examination of the patient demonstrating the presence of a multitude of café-au-lait spots or skin nodules, or a positive family history of neurofibromatosis will clinch the diagnosis. Not all curvatures have this classic pattern. Included among other patterns are long sweeping curves, curves in the cervical spine, and curves which are totally like an idiopathic scoliosis and may merely represent the coexistence of idiopathic scoliosis in a patient with neurofibromatosis.[12, 16, 81] The special problem about neurofibromatosis is that it may produce extremely severe spinal deformities, even to the point of paraplegia. In addition, it is very difficult to treat. As stated previously, the classic curve is a very special problem. If the classic curve is neglected, it usually progresses rapidly, and it may become extraordinarily severe. When there is a kyphotic component to the curve, paraplegia may result. Neurofibromatosis is the second most common cause of paraplegia due to untreated spinal deformity, congenital kyphosis being first.[52, 86] Thus, there is a compelling indication to fuse these curves before they become severe.

TREATMENT

Brace treatment is of no benefit to patients with the classic neurofibromatosis curve. Fusion is the procedure of choice and should be performed immediately, regardless of the age of the child. The fusion must encompass all of the curve, plus two vertebrae above and below. In patients with dystrophic bone, at the end of 6 months the incision should be reopened, the fusion mass explored and lightly decorticated, and additional autogenous iliac bone should be added to reinforce the graft, *regardless of how good the fusion mass looks at that time*. A cast should then be reapplied and the patient continued in cast treatment for an additional 6 months, giving a total of 1 year in the cast. The reason for the long cast time and the extra surgical procedure is the notorious tendency of these patients to have pseudarthrosis. These patients cannot be treated as those with simple idiopathic scoliosis. After the cast is removed, the patient must be monitored very carefully for pseudarthrosis, and further fusion must be performed, if necessary (Fig. 16-28).

Anterior interbody fusion is necessary for all patients with neurofibromatosis kyphosis. Posterior fusion alone will not suffice for the kyphotic type of curvature. Anterior fusion should be done through the *concave* side of the scoliosis, even though this is the more difficult approach. Anterior fusion should encompass the entire kyphotic area. Posterior arthrodesis with Harrington instruments should also be done in addition to the anterior arthrodesis. Halo-femoral traction is highly effective for preoperative correction (Fig. 16-29).

Patients who develop paralysis with neurofibromatosis have one of two problems. They may have the spinal cord pressed upon by deformity of the spine; this only occurs with the kyphotic types of patients. The other cause for paralysis may be an intraspinal tumor, particularly a neurofibroma in the spinal canal. This may occur in the presence of a curve, leading to a considerable dilemma in diagnosis.

Myelography should always be carried out in these patients. If the patient has a kyphosis, the myelogram must be done in the supine position so that the dye can pool in the area of the maximum deformity. The usual prone myelogram is virtually useless unless it is done by the high-volume technique. If the patient has an intraspinal tumor, neurosurgical excision of the tumor should be performed, removing as little bone as possible. Following removal of the tumor, a fusion *must* be performed either at the same time or within a month. The patient must never be allowed out of immobilization until this fusion is solid. Laminectomy performed in the region of a curve for neurofibromatosis will result in extraordinarily rapid decompensation of the curve, and paralysis becomes a very real possibility.

Patients without a curvature who are subjected to laminectomy because of a tumor must also have a fusion performed before a curve develops. If the curve is allowed to develop, it becomes very difficult to fuse, since the lamina are absent due to the laminectomy. Under such circumstances, anterior interbody fusion is an absolute necessity.

For severe deformities in which there is diminished respiratory function, curvatures should be first corrected by halo-femoral traction. When the maximal correction has been obtained, usually in 2 to 3 weeks, fusion should be performed, with both anterior and posterior fusions done 2 weeks apart. If satisfactory correction has been obtained by the traction, either the anterior or the posterior fusion may be done first. It is sometimes helpful to do the posterior fusion with Harrington instrumentation first, to provide the best possible correction and a stable fixation. Two weeks later the anterior fusion is done. Since the spine is already fixed in the maximally corrected position, the bone graft can be inserted with greater ease and security. Again, cast immobilization for 1 year is recommended.

The essence of treatment of neurofibromatosis scoliosis is to never allow the deformities to become severe. Fusion must be done early, regardless of the age of the child or the severity of the curve.

CONGENITAL SPINAL DEFORMITY

Congenital spinal deformities arise from anomalous development of the vertebrae. A curve in a very young child without congenital anomalies is usually an infantile idiopathic scoliosis and should not be called congenital. Because these anomalies are present at birth, children with congenital scoliosis tend to have a curvature either at birth or much earlier in life than the typical patient with idiopathic scoliosis or paralysis. Adequate bracing is difficult for a very small child. Fusion is frequently necessary, but it is difficult for the surgeon to bring himself to perform fusions on very young children because of the fear of stunting growth.

All of these problems have resulted in a tendency for the young child with a congenital scoliosis to receive less than optimal care. The curves are all too frequently allowed to progress to a serious degree. Congenital curves tend to be rigid and resistant to correction. Thus, these curves must not be allowed to progress. Early fusion is necessary in a large number of cases. Early fusion is far preferable to allowing severe curves to develop. Usually early fusion will not stunt growth, since the area of the anomalies and the area which needs to be fused cannot grow in a normal vertical manner due to the undeveloped growth plates.

There are many different types of congenital spinal deformities (Fig. 16-30). They are customarily classified first as to whether they are scoliotic, kyphotic, lordotic or a combination thereof. Secondly, one should establish the type of congenital anomaly present. This quite often gives very useful clues as to the prognosis of the deformity.

CONGENITAL SCOLIOSIS

Classification of Congenital Scoliosis
Failure of Formation
   Partial unilateral failure of formation (wedge)
   Complete unilateral failure (hemivertebra)
Failure of Segmentation
   Unilateral failure of segmentation (unilateral unsegmented bar)
   Bilateral failure of segmentation (bloc vertebrae)
Miscellaneous
Mixed

Although one theoretically would like to associate a certain prognosis with a certain anomaly, this is not always possible. It is best to consider the curve in its general character and to see what problem it produces and whether it is progressive or not, regardless of the specific type of anomaly. Thus, careful documentation of the curve by high-quality roentgenograms and photographs is necessary on the first examination. Subsequently, serial photography and serial roentgenography are important. Children should be followed at 6-month intervals and must be followed until they stop growing. Many patients have mild curves which are very stable for many years and then suddenly become severe at the time of the adolescent growth spurt.

Some patients' curves never progress at all. These patients, of course, do not need any treatment, and it is foolish to apply a brace or perform a fusion for a condition which is not progressive and not disabling (Fig. 16-31).

Statistically, about 25 per cent of patients in the average clinic with congenital scoliosis do not show any progression and do not need any treatment. Conversely, about 75 per cent show some progression, and approximately 50 per cent progress significantly and require treatment. Thoracic curves are almost always progressive.[90]

Certain anomalies are associated consis-

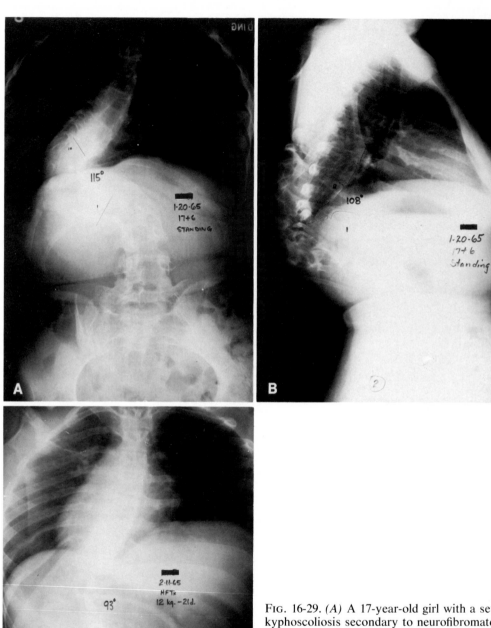

FIG. 16-29. *(A)* A 17-year-old girl with a severe kyphoscoliosis secondary to neurofibromatosis. The anteroposterior standing roentgenogram shows the sharply angular 115° curve. *(B)* The lateral standing roentgenogram shows a sharply angular 108° kyphosis. Surprisingly, the neurologic examination was normal. *(C)* The patient in halo-femoral traction, showing correction of the scoliosis to 93°. There is a mild degree of spindling of the ribs leading into the concavity at the apex of the curve. The scalloping of the convex border of the apical vertebral body can also be seen. *(Legend continued on facing page.)*

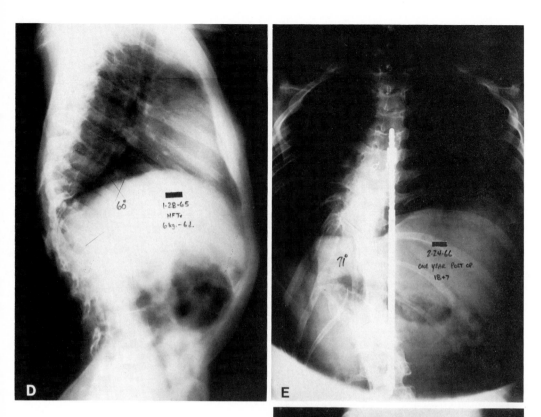

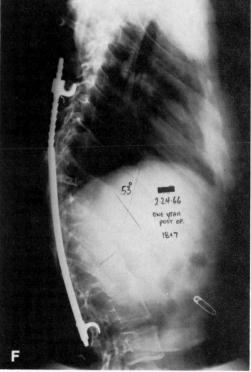

Fig. 16-29 *(Continued).* *(D)* A lateral roentgenogram of the patient in halo-femoral traction with correction to 60°. This film was taken after only 6 days in traction, with 6 kg. of traction on the head and 3 kg. on each femur. Note the marked improvement, showing the easily obtained correction of the kyphotic component of the curvature. Posterior fusion with Harrington instrumentation was performed after 3 weeks of traction. *(E)* The patient, 1 year postoperatively, at age 18. Scoliosis has been maintained at 71°. On this film the fusion mass along the concavity of the curve appears to be excellent. *(F)* A lateral roentgenogram, taken at the same time, showing the Harrington rod to be in good position and also showing the bending of the rod necessary to conform to the residual kyphosis. At this point the correction was thought to be satisfactory, and casting was discontinued. This was incorrect judgment. A patient with this degree of kyphosis always requires anterior fusion in order to obtain a solid and stable graft. *(Legend continued on overleaf.)*

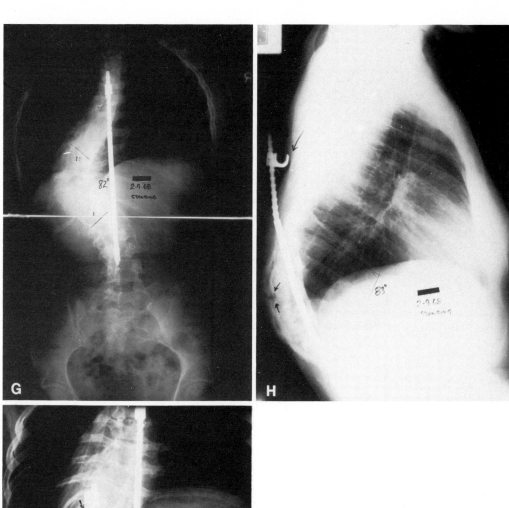

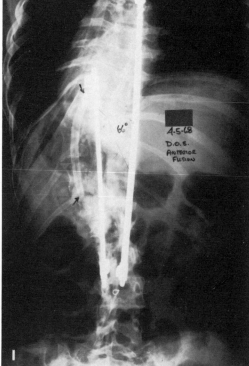

FIG. 16-29 *(Continued)*. *(G)* One year later, the patient shows loss of scoliosis correction to 82°. *(H)* The lateral roentgenogram shows the obvious pseudarthrosis at the apex of the kyphosis and complete dislocation of the upper Harrington hook. The patient was replaced in halofemoral traction to once again correct the deformity. *(I)* The lateral roentgenogram, following reoperation, showing the contraction rod and the longer and slightly bent distraction rod. *(Legend continued on facing page.)*

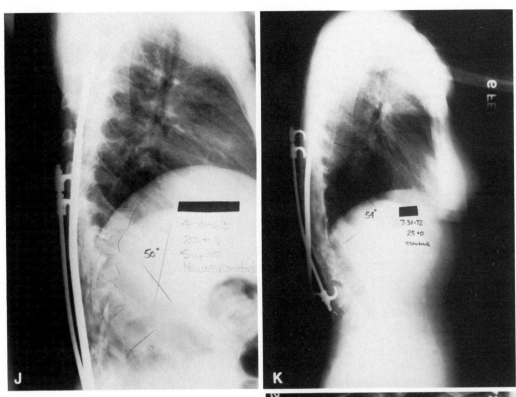

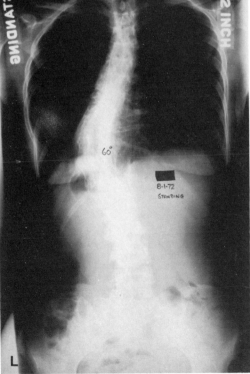

FIG. 16-29 *(Continued). (J)* The patient after two operative procedures. The original Harrington rod was removed and the pseudarthrosis repaired. Two weeks later an anterior interbody fusion was performed, using an autogenous iliac bone graft. The arrows show the ends of the anterior rib graft. *(K)* A lateral standing roentgenogram taken 4 years later. There had been no loss of correction. The fusion mass is solid, both anteriorly and posteriorly, and the kyphosis measurement is 54°. She was having difficulty with bursitis over the lower Harrington hooks, so the rods were removed. The fusion was found to be solid. *(L)* An anteroposterior standing roentgenogram after rod removal, showing solid fusion and permanent correction of the curve to 60°. (Photographs kindly donated by Dr. John H. Moe.)

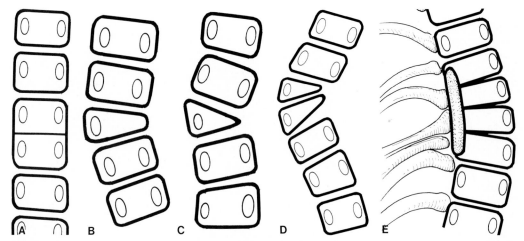

FIG. 16-30. *(A)* A symmetrical defect in segmentation or "block" vertebra. *(B)* A partial lateral vertebral hypoplasia or "wedge" vertebra. *(C)* A lateral defect of formation or "hemivertebra." *(D)* A double lateral defect of formation or "double hemivertebra." *(E)* A unilateral defect of segmentation or "unilateral unsegmented bar."

tently with progression, especially the unilateral unsegmented bar. This problem is so reliably malicious that the patient should have a fusion immediately and not wait for progression. The unilateral unsegmented bar causes a total lack of growth on the concave side of the curve. If growth continues on the convex side, the patient grows into severe deformity. Naturally, this deformity is extremely rigid and virtually impossible to correct, except by extraordinary and difficult surgery. Therefore, it is far better to prevent an increase in the deformity than to correct it once it has become severe (Fig. 16-32).

Hemivertebrae may be single or multiple, balanced or unbalanced. Balanced hemivertebrae often may not progress and may not require treatment. Contralateral hemivertebrae, when separated by several segments, quite often produce a double curve; both curves may progress. In such cases, both curves require fusion. A single hemivertebra may or may not cause deformity; this is difficult to predict. The patient must be followed carefully, and if deformity occurs, fusion should be performed. A single hemivertebra at the lumbosacral level produces a significant decompensation of the patient, because there is no room below the

hemivertebra for natural compensation to occur. These patients develop a severe list to one side which is progressive with growth. This produces a rigid deformity which is extraordinarily difficult to correct. These patients should have very early correction and fusion of the most caudad segments of the lumbar spine.

Evaluation of the Patient With Congenital Scoliosis

Patients with congenital anomalies of the spine quite frequently have congenital anomalies involving regions other than the spine. It is extremely important that these patients receive a complete evaluation.

The most frequently associated congenital anomaly is found in the genitourinary tract. Studies of patients with congenital scoliosis by MacEwen, Winter and Hardy[56] revealed an incidence of 20 per cent having anomalies of the urinary tract on routine intravenous pyelography. Many of the anomalies noted are not demanding of urologic treatment—for example, a unilateral kidney with good function or a crossed-fused ectopia with good function. However, in the study by MacEwen and colleagues, 6 per cent of the patients were noted to have

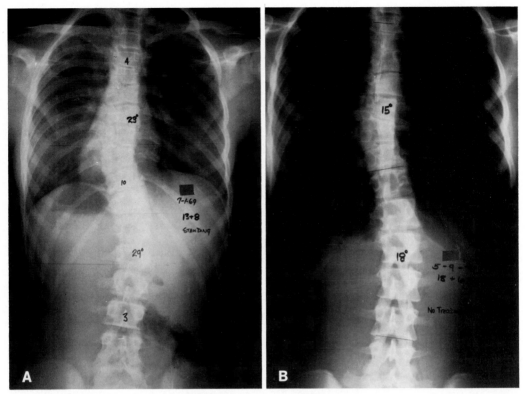

FIG. 16-31. *(A)* This 13-year-old girl was seen with congenital spinal deformity. She has many abnormal vertebrae, the most obvious being a hemivertebra on the left at T9. She exhibited a left thoracic T4 to T10 curve of 23° and a T10 to L3 curve of 29°. External clinical examination revealed no curve at all, and there was no rotation associated with the thoracic curve and only 5 mm. of rotational prominance in the lumbar curve. It was elected not to treat her at this time, but to watch her carefully. *(B)* The patient 5 years later. The thoracic curve measures 15°, the lumbar curve 18°. The curve never progressed, she never had any treatment of any kind, and she was seen twice a year during this period of time. No exercises were given; had exercises been used, they would have mistakenly been given the credit for this spontaneous stabilization.

a life-threatening urologic problem, usually obstructive uropathy. If such obstructive uropathy is detected during screening of the scoliotic patient, appropriate urologic procedures should be carried out before instituting orthopaedic treatment of the scoliosis (Fig. 16-33).

A second area of great concern is cardiac anomalies. As many as 10 to 15 per cent of patients with congenital scoliosis have been noted to have congenital heart defects. These may have been previously undetected. It is tempting to blame murmurs on distortion of the thorax due to the scoliosis, but in actuality, scoliosis alone does not produce murmurs. Therefore, any murmur must be considered as intrinsic in the heart until proven otherwise.

Examination of the back and extremities for any evidence of a hidden neurologic disorder is very important. There is a fairly high frequency of spinal dysrhaphism in patients with congenital scoliosis.[91] These are frequently associated with hair patches on the back, dimples, hemangiomata and various abnormalities on the lower extremities. These abnormalities include such things as flat feet, cavus feet, vertical tali, clubfeet, and more subtle signs, such as slight atrophy of one calf, a slightly smaller foot on one

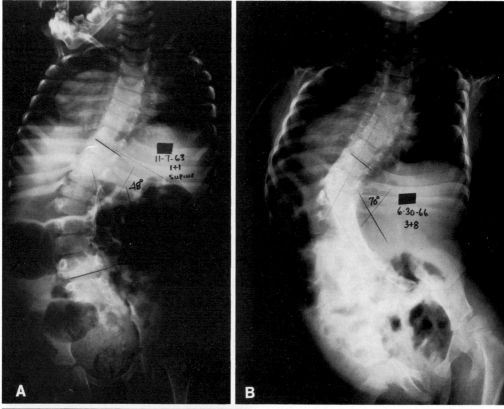

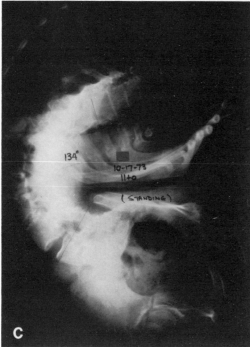

Fig. 16-32. (A) This 1-year-old child was seen because of the obvious spinal deformity at an early age. There is a 48° left lumbar scoliosis with fixed pelvic obliquity. A very obvious unilateral unsegmented bar can be seen extending from T11 to L3. In the thoracic spine, the interpedicular space is noted to be wider than normal, and the disc spaces are narrower than normal. She was neurologically intact and there was no hair patch or other evidence of spinal dysrhaphism. She was seen elsewhere at this time, and no treatment was given. (B) The patient at age 3 years. Her curvature has already progressed to 70°. The unilateral unsegmented bar is clearly visible. The increasing pelvic obliquity is obvious, as is the narrowing of the disc spaces in the thoracic spine. (C) The patient at age 11 was now showing a 134° completely rigid scoliosis. Pelvic obliquity has reached such a severe proportion that her rib cage is abutting against the lateral wall of the pelvis. This case represents the usual and customary malignant progression of the unilateral unsegmented bar. To allow such a curve to progress in this manner is indefensible. Salvage at this point is extraordinarily difficult.

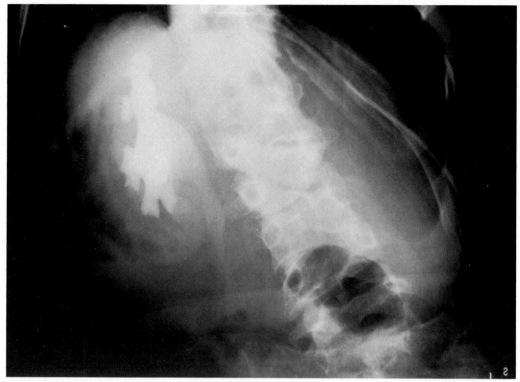

FIG. 16-33. Complete evaluation of a patient with congenital spine anomaly includes the taking of an intravenous pyleogram. This patient exhibits a unilateral kidney with mild dilation of the upper urinary tract.

side, and asymmetry of the reflexes. It is possible to have a patient with a diastematomyelia who has none of these associated findings. The physician must be very astute to evaluate the roentgenograms for interpedicular widening or midline bony spicules (Fig. 16-34).

Milwaukee Brace Treatment

Because the primary deformity in congenital scoliosis is in the bones rather than in the soft tissues, the curves tend to be rigid, and thus they are not as amenable to brace treatment as are idiopathic and paralytic curves. Nevertheless, there are definite indications for the brace treatment of congenital spinal deformities.[94]

Certain patients do well in the Milwaukee brace for many years, and a few can even be treated permanently in a brace and surgery can be avoided. Patients with congenital scoliosis who do well have very flexible curves. These patients have the curvature primarily in nonanomalous vertebrae. On the other hand, short rigid curves do poorly in braces.

There is need for the Milwaukee brace following a fusion in many patients with congenital curves. There is a tendency for fused areas to bend and for curves to lengthen into areas of the spine that formerly were without curves. These additional curve problems are significantly helped by the Milwaukee brace, since these other curves tend to develop in nonanomalous vertebrae.

It is important that the physician recognize that the brace must accomplish its goal. That is, it must maintain the curve in an improved and acceptable condition. The pa-

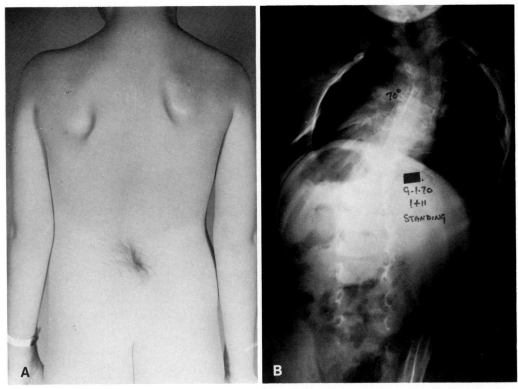

FIG. 16-34. *(A)* This patient presented with thoracic scoliosis (no prominence of the right scapula) and a hairy patch in the low back. One foot was smaller than the other, and there was an absence of the ankle reflex on the side of the smaller foot. *(B)* The patient exhibits a 70° right thoracic scoliosis with a unilateral unsegmented bar in the thoracic spine, and marked interpediculate widening in the lumbar spine. *(Legend continued on facing page.)*

tient with a 90° curve is done no service when brace treatment is attempted. The main indication for bracing in congenital scoliosis is to delay surgery until a more suitable age. This is particularly true of a long curve in which a long fusion at a very early age would be less desirable than at a later age. This delay in fusion can be accomplished with a Milwaukee brace in some patients. If the patient's curve progresses despite the brace, fusion must be done without further delay. It is only when the brace successfully holds the curve that it can be continued.

Certain special brace adaptations are necessary for the patient with congenital scoliosis. Very young children (as young as 6 months of age) can be fitted with a Milwaukee brace, if necessary. Under these circumstances, a padded neck ring is used instead of the conventional chin pad or throat mold. For cervicothoracic curves, a shoulder ring is mandatory to bring the shoulder down and the curve inward. When there is a congenital scoliosis extending into the cervical spine, the head is often tilted to one side. A lateral extension up the side of the head helps to hold the head in a neutral position, or, with serial correction, a lateral extension actually helps correct a fixed head tilt.

The two most common errors seen in the treatment of congenital scoliosis by a Milwaukee brace are the attempt to treat with the brace a curve that requires surgery and the failure to recognize that the brace is not adequately controlling the curve. It is imperative that the physician carefully monitor

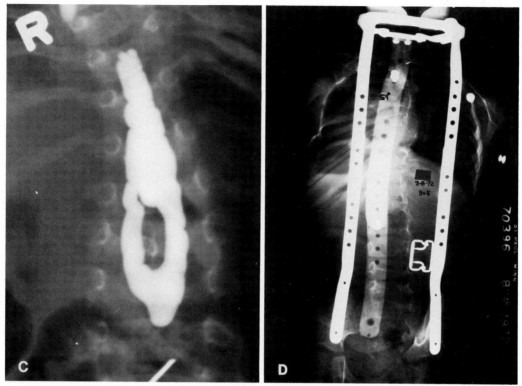

FIG. 16-34 *(Continued)*. *(C)* A myelogram demonstrating a classic diastematomyelia. *(D)* The patient underwent excision of the spur of the diastematomyelia, followed 2 weeks later by fusion of the thoracic spine from C7 to T10, for treatment of the progressive thoracic congenital scoliosis. Here, the patient at age 3 years and 5 months, 1¹/₂ years after surgery, shows correction of the thoracic curve to 59°, solid fusion and maintenance of the overall spinal contours with a Milwaukee brace. Such early fusion for such severe problems requires long-term bracing to prevent bending of the fusion mass and extension of the curves.

the progress of the patient in the brace; he must not delegate this responsibility to anyone else, and he must be prepared to admit that it is not working and to proceed to a fusion (Fig. 16-35).

Surgical Treatment

The indications for surgical treatment of congenital scoliosis are: the presence of any curve over 50° and any curve that is progressive despite adequate nonoperative treatment. The age of the patient should not be a deterrent to fusion if these criteria are met.

At the least, the fusion area must always include *all vertebrae in the measured curve*. Usually, one must also include at least one above and one below this area. As in idiopathic scoliosis, all vertebrae rotated in the same direction as the apical vertebra must be included.

What is the best method of correction of congenital scoliosis? This question is frequently asked, but is difficult to answer exactly. Harrington instruments are dangerous in the *correction* of congenital scoliosis, due to the high incidence of paraplegia.[54] Harrington rods should be used primarily to *maintain* correction which has been *obtained* by other methods, either cast or traction correction.

By far the best results have been obtained by the early recognition of congenital curves, careful monitoring of the curve, and prompt cast correction and fusion when progression is determined. This method of

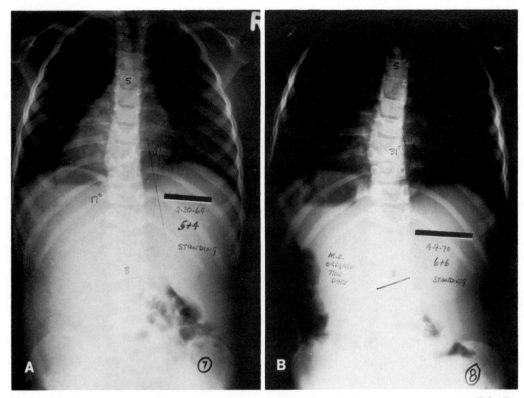

FIG. 16-35. *(A)* This 5-year-old girl was seen for a congenital scoliosis. It was not apparent clinically, but had been detected on a chest roentgenogram taken for other reasons. She exhibits a 17° long left curve from T5 to L3. In her situation, there are two anomalous areas separated by two or three normal vertebrae. Such anomalous situations are difficult to predict, and it is best for the surgeon to observe these carefully and let nature give the answer.) *(B)* At age 6 years and 6 months the curve showed a sudden increase to 31°, and the Milwaukee brace was ordered at this time. *(Legend continued on facing page.)*

treatment is reliable, well tested, free of dangerous complications, and has produced the best results[90] (Fig. 16-36).

For more advanced and serious deformities not previously detected, slow and gradual correction by halo-femoral traction over a period of 2 weeks is best. This is followed by spinal fusion with or without instrumentation (Fig. 16-37).

Patients with a unilateral unsegmented bar are best recognized early and fused before severe deformity exists. Unfortunately, some patients are seen by an orthopaedist only after a severe deformity has developed. In such cases, the bar can often be excised or divided, correction can be obtained by halo-femoral traction, and fusion of the entire curve can be carried out.

Most patients with hemivertebrae are best managed by early detection and early fusion of the curve, before severe deformity develops. Only rarely is hemivertebra excision indicated. The most common indication for hemivertebra excision is the low lumbar hemivertebra. In this area, there is no compensatory curve below the hemivertebra, and severe decompensation results. The compensatory curve develops structural qualities, and, therefore, early prompt treatment of the lumbosacral hemivertebra is needed. If detected *very* early, simple correction and fusion of L3 to S1 is all that is needed. If L3 cannot be corrected to a horizontal alignment over S1 on bending films, excision of the hemivertebra is needed. Hemivertebra excision is best performed by

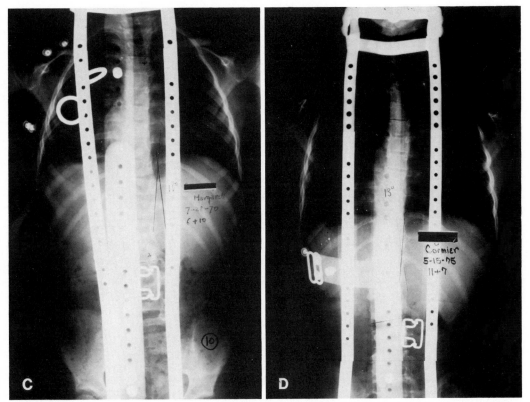

FIG. 16-35 *(Continued)*. *(C)* After application of the brace, the curve was corrected to 11°. *(D)* Five years later, after 5 years of continuous brace use, the curve is well maintained at 13°. This patient may possibly avoid surgery altogether, or may require fusion if the curve goes out of control during the adolescent growth spurt. The goal of the brace has already been obtained, that is, allowing adequate spine growth while controlling the curve.

the two stage technique of Leatherman[46] (Fig. 16-38).

If associated with a diastematomyelia, the midline bony septum should be removed before correcting and fusing the scoliosis. Such spurs should be removed early in life, since any neurologic damage which might result from neglect will usually be permanent.[33]

CONGENITAL KYPHOSIS

Congenital kyphosis is a kyphotic deformity due to congenitally anomalous vertebrae. There are two basic types. The first (Type I) is caused by a congenital failure of formation of all or part of the vertebral body (Fig. 16-39). This may range from the absence of two or even three vertebral bodies, with the preservation of the posterior element in which a severe deformity is produced, to only a partial absence of a vertebral body with a less severe deformity. The second (Type II) is due to congenital failure of segmentation of the vertebral body anteriorly, producing an "anterior unsegmented bar" (Fig. 16-40). In both situations, progressive deformity occurs as a result of no growth anteriorly and persistent growth posteriorly.

The more severe deformities may be manifest at birth and may progress steadily thereafter. The less obvious deformities may not appear until years later, and the deformity is accentuated at the time of the adolescent growth spurt.

Once progression begins, it does not cease spontaneously, but continues until full

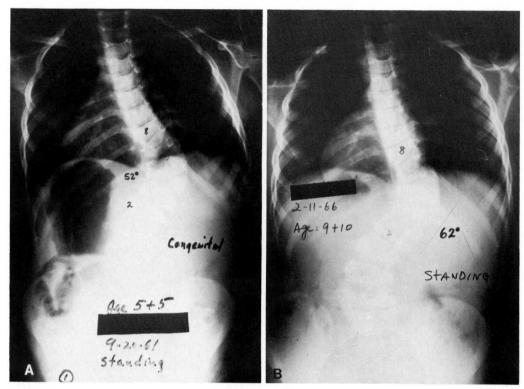

FIG. 16-36. *(A)* A 5-year-old girl with a 52° right thoracolumbar curve due to two hemivertebrae on the right side, one at T11, the other at L1. An attempt was made to treat this girl with a Milwaukee brace, which she wore from age 5 to age 9. *(B)* At age 9, the patient exhibits a 62° curve, thus indicating the failure of the brace to control this curve. Surgical corrective fusion was felt necessary at this time. *(Legend continued on facing page.)*

growth is reached. The more severe types of kyphotic problems may progress even after growth is complete.

Progression takes place not only due to growth differential, but also because of actual erosion of the vertebral body from mechanical pressure related to the disturbance of biomechanics of the kyphosis. Studies of the natural history of progression revealed very severe deformity to occur, particularly with congenital failure of formation of one or more vertebral bodies (Fig. 16-41).[94]

Paraplegia can result from a progressive kyphotic deformity, particularly when the kyphosis is in the thoracic spine. Paraplegia is associated with Type I deformities, but it has not been described in Type II deformities. Partial paralysis can be present even at birth, or the onset of paralysis may not

occur until adulthood. Congenital kyphosis is the most common noninfectious spinal deformity that causes paraplegia.

Treatment

The ideal treatment for congenital kyphosis is early detection and early posterior fusion. The best results obtained are in those patients who have posterior fusion prior to the age of 3 years. Fusion can be done as early as 6 months of age, if necessary. A posterior fusion stops the posterior growth and appears to allow growth to take place anteriorly where there are viable growth plates (Fig. 16-42).

Posterior fusion is often inadequate to stabilize the spine in the patient with significant kyphosis. The posterior fusion mass is under a distraction force and does not develop strongly. The pseudarthrosis rate is

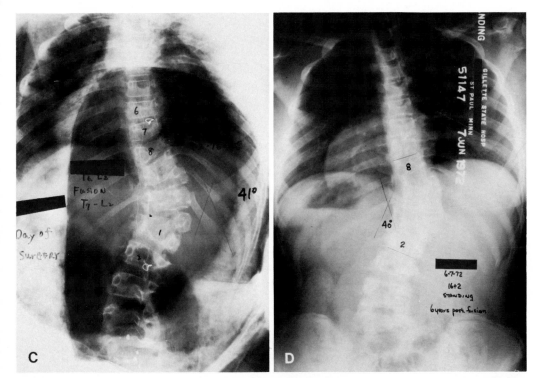

Fɪɢ. 16-36 *(Continued)*. *(C)* A roentgenogram taken shortly after fusion. Correction was obtained by a Risser localizer cast applied before surgery, and the surgery was performed through a window in the cast. The two hemivertebra are more obvious on this film. The curve was corrected to 41°. *(D)* The patient 6 years after fusion. The curve has lost nothing, and now measures 40°. This case is a good example of the ability of a well-performed spinal fusion to stabilize a curve due to a hemivertebra. It is not necessary to excise such hemivertebra to obtain some correction or to obtain stabilization of the curve.

extremely high, and beyond a certain point a solid posterior arthrodesis cannot be accomplished. Thus, if posterior fusion is to be attempted for these problems, the fusion mass must be thickened at the apex. The best way to achieve thickening is by concentrating the bone-graft material in this area on the first operation. Six months later, the incision is intentionally reopened, and the fusion mass is stimulated by "feathering" the graft and adding additional autogenous bone. The fusion mass takes a long time to develop vertical trabeculation sufficiently strong to withstand gravity and flexion forces. Therefore, a period in the cast of at least 1 year is necessary. Protection in a brace for 1 or more years thereafter is strongly recommended.

Anterior fusion has become the treatment of choice for the more severe congenital kyphosis problems. Patients with kyphosis of greater than 50° who are 5 years of age or older require anterior interbody fusion. If anterior fusion is performed, posterior fusion is done also, usually one more level above and below the anterior fusion. This allows the fusion mass to develop some degree of lordosis with time.

The surgical treatment of a well-established and severe kyphosis is one of the greatest challenges to the orthopaedic surgeon. In our clinic, the best results for *thoracolumbar* kyphosis have been obtained by very cautious and carefully monitored halo-femoral traction. After 2 weeks, the patient is taken to the operating room where an anterior transthoracic exposure is made, the anterior longitudinal ligament is

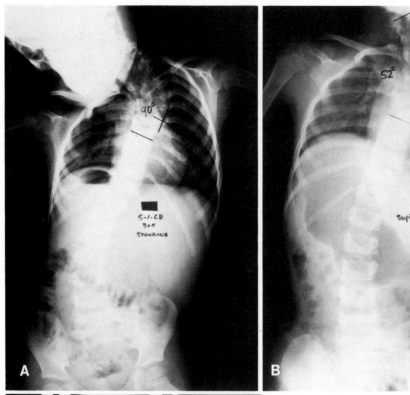

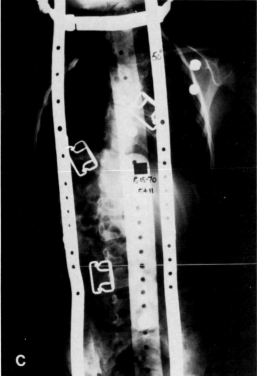

FIG. 16-37. (A) This girl, 3 years and 11 months old, was seen for the first time, presenting with this severe 90° cervicothoracic congenital scoliosis and severe head tilt due to the curve. (B) The same patient, showing a correction of the curve with Cotrel passive traction. Note, on the concavity of the curve, the areas in which there is no bone visible, the so-called "empty space." Such empty spaces usually are areas into which the spine will collapse, and they do not represent cartilage which subsequently ossify. After partial correction of the curve with traction, the patient was placed in a Milwaukee brace. (C) Two years later, after 2 years of Milwaukee brace treatment, the curve is being maintained at 50° in the brace, with the head in neutral alignment. (Legend continued on facing page.)

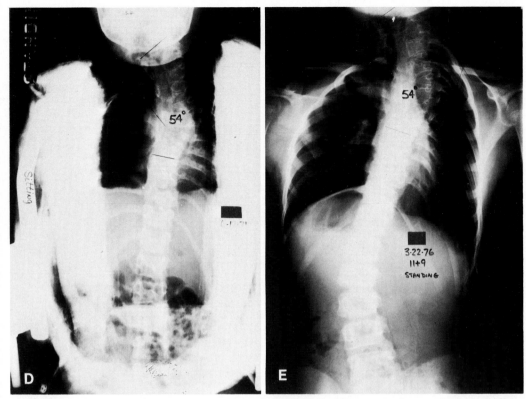

Fig. 16-37 *(Continued). (D)* Surgical fusion was deemed necessary for the curve, in preference to full-time bracing until the end of growth. Due to the severe segmentation defects, fusion at this age does not produce any stunting of growth that would not already have been caused by nature. Therefore fusion was done without instrumentation, utilizing iliac autogenous bone. The correction was maintained in a halo cast. *(E)* The patient, 5 years later, showing maintenance of correction at 54°. A compensatory left lumbar curve has developed to balance the high right curve. The plumb line is in the center and the head is directly over the pelvis.

excised, several discs are removed, and a strong anterior strut-graft operation is performed, using rib or fibular bone and additional rib or iliac bone. During the operative procedure, the traction weights are reduced to 50 per cent of the weight used prior to surgery. For the first 48 hours afterwards, the traction is maintained at this lower level. Once the edema phase of surgery has subsided, the traction weights are gradually restored to their previous levels. Under no circumstances should traction exceed 10 kilograms on the head or 5 kilograms on each leg. At the slightest suggestion of any neurologic deficit, the weights should be markedly reduced or discontinued.

Approximately 2 weeks following the initial procedure, the patient is returned to the operating room, where once again, under reduced traction weights and in a hyperextended prone position, a posterior fusion of adequate length is performed, supplemented by Harrington instrumentation (if the patient is 10 years or older). One week following the second operation, a snug cast is applied, utilizing either a halo cast or Risser-Cotrel type of hyperextension cast. The patient can be ambulated if there is adequate interal fixation, or a period of 6 months of bedrest may *(Text continued on page 640.)*

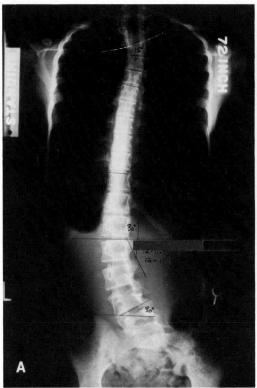

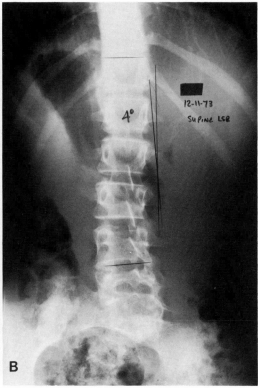

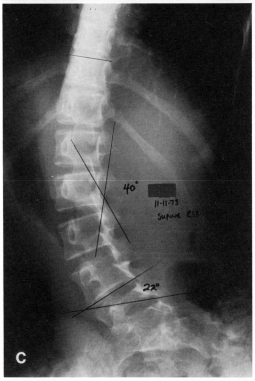

FIG. 16-38. *(A)* This girl, 12 years and 11 months old, was seen for a peculiar curvature of the spine. It was particularly evident as an offset of the plumb line. There was a 30° left lumbar curve at T11 to L4, and a 30° angle between L4 and the sacrum. *(B)* A voluntary maximal, supine left side-bending film demonstrated complete correction of the left lumbar curve. Note the derotation of these vertebrae as they correct. *(C)* A maximal, voluntary, right side-bending film showed the lumbosacral curve (i.e., that curve between L4 and S1 is quite rigid, and L4 remains in its tilted and deviated position relative to the sacrum). These bending films demonstrate the primary curve to be lumbosacral, and the T11 to L4 curve is a compensatory curve. *(Legend continued on facing page.)*

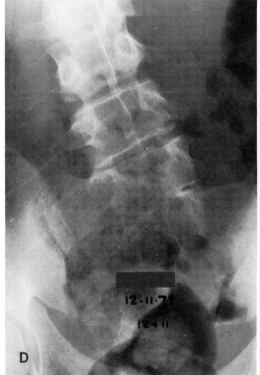

D

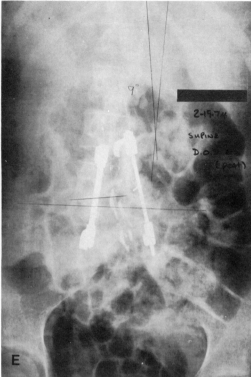

E

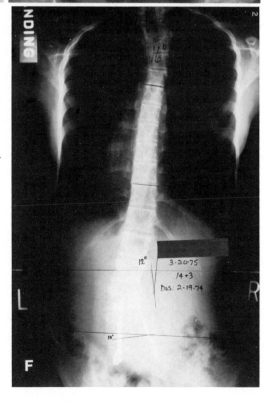

F

FIG. 16-38 *(Continued)*. *(D)* A Ferguson view revealed the true nature of the pathology. There is a hemivertebra between L5 and the sacrum, which is fused with the sacrum. There was no alternative but for the spine to start out in a deviated manner and to attempt to achieve compensation through compensatory mechanisms. It was felt appropriate to treat the primary curve by wedge excision of the low lumbar spine. *(E)* The patient first had an anterior wedge excision of the lower half of L5. The hemivertebra was so low that it was tucked behind the bifurcation of the aorta and the innominate vein and was very difficult to remove, so a wedge was taken out in the vertebra above the hemivertebra. Two weeks later, through a posterior approach, the posterior wedge of the same dimension was removed, a contracting rod inserted to pull the wedge closed, and a short distracting rod added to lift and deviate L4 toward the midline. This roentgenogram was taken in the operating room on the day of the second surgery. *(F)* The patient is shown 1 year after the osteotomy and fusion. Her body alignment is now normal. She has a 16° high thoracic curve due to a congenital anomaly in this area. The patient's postoperative management consisted of bedrest and a double-pantaloon underarm cast for 4 months, followed by 3 more months in a short body cast, which allowed her to be ambulatory. *(Legend continued on overleaf.)*

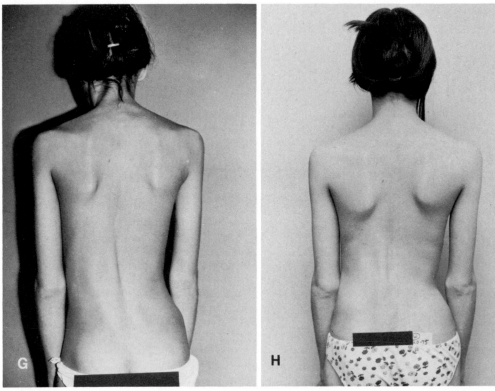

FIG. 16-38 *(Continued)*. *(G)* A preoperative posterior photograph of the patient, demonstrating the left lumbar curve and the deviation of the torso to the left in relation to the pelvis. *(H)* Photograph 1 year postoperatively, showing restoration of the plumb line to a central location.

be necessary if there is any question about the ability to control the deformity in the upright position. A period of 1 year in this type of cast is necessary to achieve total and complete healing (Fig. 16-43).

The patient with a severe angular kyphosis in the thoracic area, with the apex in the T3 to T8 area, is in great jeopardy of paraplegia, both with and without treatment. Traction should be avoided. Anterior fusion without traction is the procedure of choice. Posterior fusion without instrumentation should follow 2 weeks later.

For severe Type II deformities, anterior osteotomy of the unsegmented bar, disc excision, anterior bone grafting followed by halo-femoral traction, and posterior fusion with Harrington rods are recommended. It is obvious that a correction cannot be obtained unless the anterior osteotomy is performed first. It is desirable to detect these problems early and to perform a simple posterior fusion, obviating the need for such radical surgery (Fig. 16-44).

MARFAN'S SCOLIOSIS

Scoliosis is a common manifestation in the patient with Marfan's syndrome. The reported incidence of scoliosis in this condition ranges from 30 per cent to 70 per cent.[77] Patients with Marfan's syndrome have a defect of the connective soft tissues. Therefore, it is not surprising that deformity of the spine should occur. Scoliosis may appear at a young age, or it may occur in the adolescent period, particularly in its less obvious forms.

Clinical Features

The scoliosis in Marfan's syndrome has some typical characteristics. The curvatures

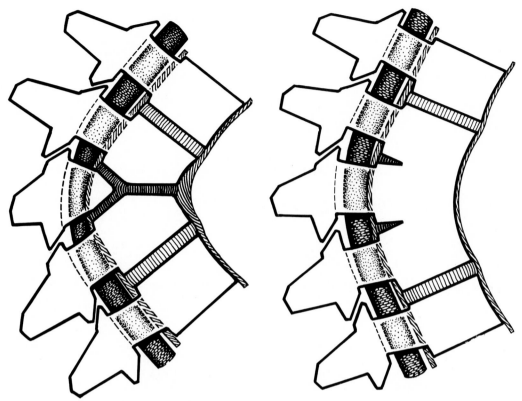

FIG. 16-39. Congenital kyphosis, Type I (anterior failure of formation of the vertebral body.)

FIG. 16-40. Congenital kyphosis, Type II (anterior failure of segmentation).

are usually those same patterns as seen in idiopathic scoliosis. Pelvic obliquity, commonly noted in neuromuscular diseases, is not seen. Patients usually have double structural right thoracic and left lumbar curves, or right thoracic curves, or thoracolumbar curves, all of which are roentgenographically similar to idiopathic scoliosis. Double curve patterns are seen more frequently in Marfan's syndrome, whereas single curve patterns are more common in idiopathic-scoliosis.

The quantity of curvature varies from very mild to extremely severe. In view of the high incidence of scoliosis in patients with Marfan's syndrome, all patients with this syndrome should have regular spinal examinations. Scoliosis must be looked for in these patients, as should the more classic manifestations of the disease, such as dislocation of the lens of the eye, heart murmurs and arachnodactyly.

Treatment

The treatment of the scoliosis of Marfan's syndrome is very similar to that for most all structural scolioses. Very mild curves of 15° or less need no treatment, but the patient must be very carefully followed to be sure that the curves do not progress.

Brace treatment is appropriate for moderate curves of less than 40°, particularly in the younger child. Brace treatment has not been as effective in the patient with Marfan's syndrome as it has been in the patient with idiopathic scoliosis, apparently due to the inability of the soft tissues to "stabilize." Because of the great flexibility of the curve in Marfan's syndrome, particularly early in the course of the disease, excellent correction can be obtained with the brace. However, despite 2 or more years of full-time brace wearing, it is not unusual to see a patient relapse to the original deformity or

(Text continues on page 644.)

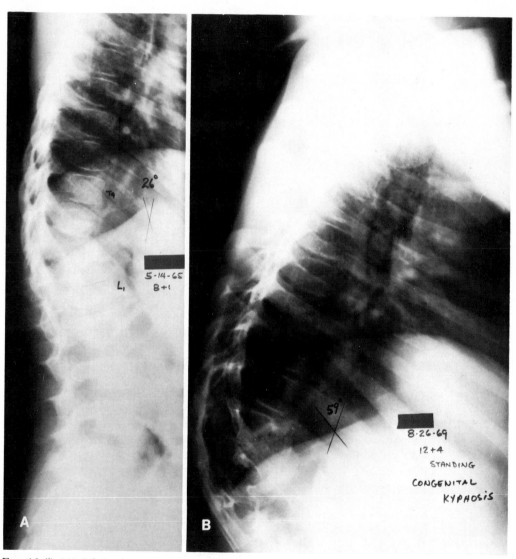

Fig. 16-41. *(A)* A lateral roentgenogram of an 8-year-old boy with a 26° congenital kyphosis at T11, with partial absence of the body of T11. No treatment was given at this time. The ideal treatment would have been a fusion of five segments posteriorly, at this time. *(B)* The patient at age 12. His kyphosis has progressed to 59°, and he has mild bladder symptoms. *(Legend continued on facing page.)*

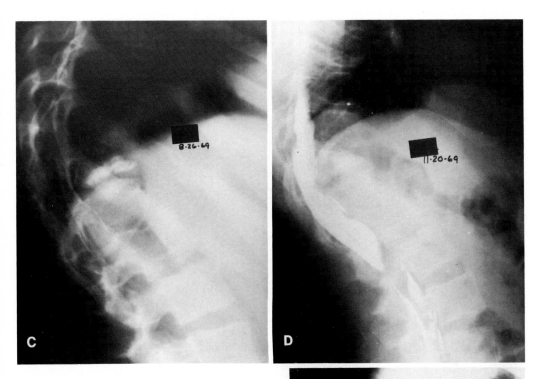

C

D

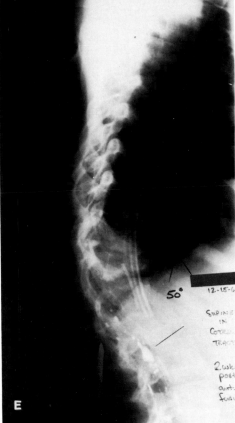

Fig. 16-41 *(Continued).* (C) A detailed view to show how the body of T10 has rubbed against and compressed the body of T12, producing sclerosis and an erosive reaction. This is indicative of the very high pressure forces existent in such a lesion. *(D)* The same patient, demonstrating myelographic findings. In the prone position, the myelogram shows a complete block. By turning the patient to a supine position, the dye easily flows around the apex of the kyphosis. Protrusion of the anulus and disc material posteriorly can be seen on the myelogram. This was felt to be secondary to the compressive effect anteriorly. *(E)* The patient was placed in Cotrel traction, and then an anterior interbody fusion was performed, using autogenous rib strut grafts, as shown in the roentgenogram. The discs were removed, as was the anterior longitudinal ligament. No attempt was made to expose the spinal cord. It was felt that simply correcting and fusing the area would alleviate the pathology. *(Legend continued on overleaf.)*

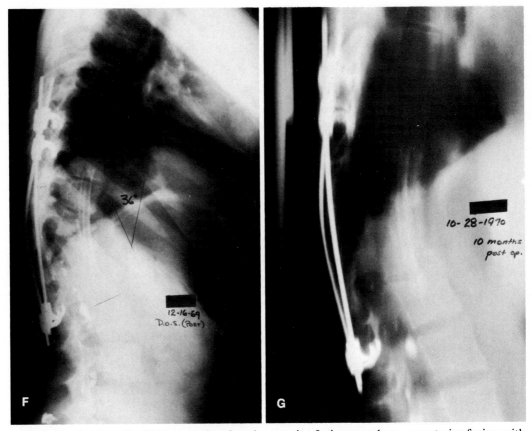

FIG. 16-41 *(Continued)*. *(F)* Two weeks after the anterior fusion was done, a posterior fusion with Harrington compression rods was performed. No attempt was made to explore the spinal canal. Autogenous iliac bone was added. The patient was kept on bedrest for 6 months in a Risser cast, and was ambulatory for 6 further months in a Risser cast. *(G)* The lateral laminogram 10 months following the fusion shows incorporation of the anterior bone graft. Note the disappearance of the angulation at the apex of the kyphosis and the conversion to a smooth posterior contour of the vertebral bodies. Lateral laminography is extremely helpful in evaluating the quality of an anterior arthrodesis. *(Legend continued on facing page.)*

worse after removal of the brace. A few patients have been successfully managed with the brace, but the incidence of relapse is certainly much higher than it is in idiopathic scoliosis.

Surgical Treatment. Most patients with Marfan's scoliosis of moderate to severe degree should be considered as surgical candidates. The only confraindications to surgery are known cardiac decompensation or aortic aneurysm. Because of the high incidence of cardiac and aortic defects in this disease, all patients considered for scoliosis surgery must have a very thorough cardiovascular

evaluation. Aortic insufficiency and mitral insufficiency are also common.

The moderately advanced curve (40° to 70°) can usually be corrected by direct surgical instrumentation and fusion. Patients with more severe curves, particularly those with curves of 90° or more, should have preliminary correction by halo-femoral traction, followed by instrumentation and fusion. The fusion area encompasses the same limits as for idiopathic scoliosis; the reader is referred to that section for selection of the fusion area.

The healing time appears to be normal in

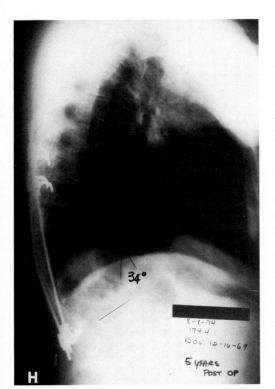

(H) Fig. 16-41 *(Continued).* The patient 5 years after surgery. There has been no loss of correction. Fusion is solid. He has no symptoms of back pain or neurologic defects. All of the extensive surgery could have been prevented by performing a simple posterior fusion when the child was 8 years old.

these patients, and usually 9 to 10 months of cast immobilization is sufficient. With good internal fixation by Harrington instruments and good cast fixation externally, early ambulation is possible. Prolonged bedrest is not necessary.

Surgical treatment is often withheld from the patient with Marfan's syndrome, because of the fear of creating an aortic aneurysm or the expectation of early death. To the author's knowledge, no patient has ever had aortic rupture due to scoliosis treatment.

The average life expectancy in patients with Marfan's syndrome is 45 years. Any patient who does not have a cardiac defect at the time of the surgical consideration for scoliosis has a good life expectancy and should not be denied adequate orthopaedic care (Fig. 16-45).

POSTLAMINECTOMY KYPHOSIS

In the thoracic and thoracolumbar spine, the forces of gravity have a natural tendency to produce kyphosis. In the normal spine these gravity forces are counteracted by the posterior ligament complex, including the interspinous ligament, the ligamentum flavum, and the facet joint ligaments. A radical laminectomy, regardless of the indication, results in the removal of some or all of these supporting structures. In the growing child, when the laminectomy is sufficiently extensive to result in bilateral removal of facet joints, a kyphotic deformity inevitably occurs. The more radical the laminectomy and the younger the child at the time of laminectomy, the more severe is the deformity likely to become.

Dubousset and his associates,[21] in an excellent review of children subjected to laminectomy, showed that 80 per cent of children who have had bilateral facet removal have developed a significant spinal deformity. Other studies by Lonstein and his associates[51] have also demonstrated a very high incidence of severe deformity in patients having this type of surgery.

In most situations, laminectomy is absolutely necessary because of the original diagnosis, usually a spinal cord tumor. Facetectomy is not always necessary, except in the case of dumbbell neurofibromas or neuroblastomas. When the ligaments and facets have been removed, a deformity develops if the child survives the tumor. Therefore, it is pertinent that the deformity potential be recognized, that the child be followed on a regular basis by an orthopaedic surgeon familiar with spinal problems, and that early bracing be instituted if a deformity develops. Most postlaminectomy spinal deformities do not respond well to bracing, and fusion may be necessary. The fusion should utilize an anterior interbody technique, since there are no laminae or bony structures posteriorly to support a posterior fusion. In some circumstances, it may be wise to perform a prophylactic anterior spinal fusion following a laminectomy, if the general prognosis is known to be good.

Certainly, if a child develops a progressing deformity, the necessary steps to correct and stabilize the spine should be under-

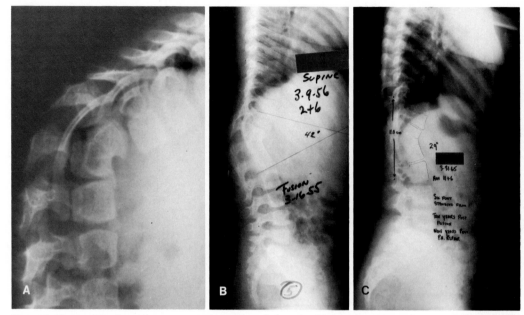

FIG. 16-42. *(A)* The lateral roentgenogram of an 8-month-old boy demonstrating a peculiar type of congenital kyphosis. At the apex there is a defect in segmentation of two vertebral bodies, and posteriorly there is no contact of the facets with one another. At the level just below the apex there is an anterior bridge with posterior disc material remaining. Just above the apex of the kyphosis there is a partial spondylolisthesis. The physical examination was neurologically normal and there were no other findings. The patient was placed in a plaster cast and maintained in the cast until age 16 months. At 16 months, he underwent a posterior spinal fusion. *(B)* In a roentgenogram taken 1 year after the posterior spinal fusion, a pseudarthrosis is evident at the apex of the curve in the region where the T11 and T12 facets do not contact one another. Note the reduction of the spondylolisthesis of T10 on T11 by the cast and posterior fusion. Note the increased ossification anteriorly, between T12 and L1. The kyphosis angle measures 42°. The pseudarthrosis repair was done at this time. *(C)* The patient at age 11, 9 years after the pseudarthrosis repair. His posterior fusion is now solid. Due to lack of posterior growth and some continued anterior growth, there has been a spontaneous correction to 29°. The patient was not in any cast or brace after the age of four. *(Legend continued on facing page.)*

taken without delay. It is tragic to see a child deteriorate profoundly without the institution of adequate spinal surgery.

Many times there is a lack of understanding of the basic nature of the original tumor process. All too often, the physicians feel that the child has a doomed prognosis from the spinal cord tumor and will die at a young age. Thus, the spinal deformity is ignored. However, the child may live for many years or may even have a normal lifespan, despite the original diagnosis, and a valuable opportunity to correct and stabilize the spine will have been lost.

Neurosurgeons must learn that these de-formities can develop and that the amount of bone removed should be minimized, if at all possible. Especially important is the preservation of the facet joint complex (Fig. 16-46).

POSTIRRADIATION SPINAL DEFORMITY

Irradiation of the young child can produce deformity of the spine due to the effect of the irradiation on the growth plates of the vertebrae and the soft tissues. The usual conditions requiring irradiation of young children are Wilms' tumor and neuroblastoma. With

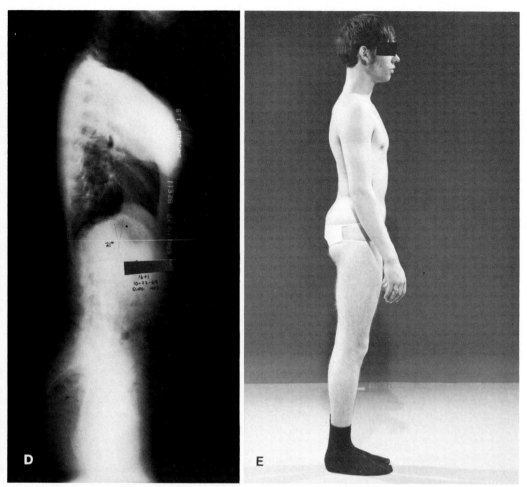

Fig. 16-42 *(Continued).* *(D)* A lateral roentgenogram at age 16 showing complete correction of the external deformity. The kyphosis measures only 21°, and his body alignment is now normal. He remains neurologically normal. *(E)* A lateral photograph of the patient at age 16. Note the normal body contour. Note the normal relationship of trunk height to leg length. The early fusion of this low number of segments has not materially altered his total body height or torso-leg ratio. He is an active athletic boy, participating in all activities.

the increased survival rate of patients with these tumors under modern medical treatment, there is probably an increased number of patients at risk for spinal deformity.

Quite often the scoliosis does not manifest itself until many years after the irradiation. Therefore, it is mandatory that these children be followed until they are grown, if the radiation has been given at a young age.

Treatment of the irradiation deformity may be either bracing, if the curve is mild, or surgery, for more severe curves. Recently, we have seen cases with kyphosis following symmetrical anterior irradiation of the vertebral bodies and following irradiation of the anterior abdominal wall, producing shortening in the rectus abdominus and its fascia.

Healing following surgery may be delayed due to the irradiation effect. The patient should be warned that the cast will probably have to remain on for a longer period than would be expected for a patient with a nonir-

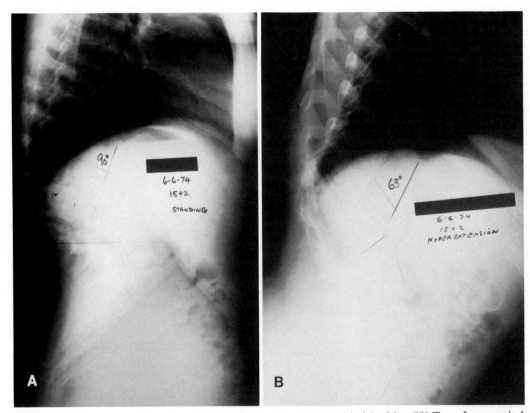

FIG. 16-43. *(A)* A lateral standing roentgenogram of a 15-year-old girl with a 90° Type I congenital kyphosis. There is total absence of the body at T11 and wedging of the body at T12. The anterior interior corner of the body of T10 is touching the superior anterior corner of the body of L1. This patient had been under "observation" for several years, the orthopaedic surgeon waiting for the patient "to finish her growth before the fusion." *(B)* A hyperextension supine lateral roentgenogram, showing correction of the rigid portion of the curve to 63°. *(Legend continued on facing page.)*

radiated condition. Anterior and posterior fusion is necessary if there is kyphosis greater than 50° (Fig. 16-47).

SCHEUERMANN'S DISEASE

Scheuermann's disease is a common problem affecting the spine of the adolescent child. In our experience, females with this disease outnumber males 2 to 1. Second to idiopathic scoliosis, it is the most common cause of patients' coming to spinal deformity clinics.[8]

ETIOLOGY

The cause of Scheuermann's disease is unknown. In the past it has been called an "epiphysitis," but there is no evidence of any inflammatory changes. Histologic examination of disc and end-plate material removed at surgery has revealed only marked irregularity of the end-plates and frequent perforations of nuclear material into the vertebral body.

Scheuermann's disease is a hereditary condition, but the hereditary patterns are not clearly defined. It is quite common to see several children in one family with the condition, as well as one or both parents.

DIAGNOSIS

The typical patient is between the ages of 12 and 15 years, with a round-shouldered

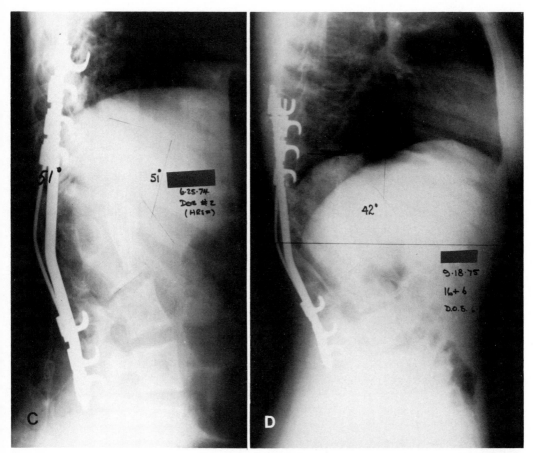

FIG. 16-43 *(Continued)*. *(C)* The patient underwent an anterior exposure resection of the anterior longitudinal ligament, and a resection of all discs over five levels, including the abnormal cartilage tissue at the apex of the curve. With a laminar spreader, the bones were opened up and strong autogenous rib strut grafts were added. Two weeks later, a posterior spinal fusion was performed, using a compression rod and a bent distraction rod because of a slight scoliosis in this area. One week later, the patient was placed in an ambulatory Risser localizer cast, which she wore for 9 months. She was fully ambulatory during the entire course of her treatment after discharge from the hospital. *(D)* A lateral standing roentgenogram taken 15 months after the fusion, demonstrating a solid anterior and posterior fusion with no loss of correction.

appearance; the patient may or may not have pain of the thoracic spine.

The differential diagnosis is usually a problem of distinguishing Scheuermann's disease from postural roundback, although other conditions causing kyphosis, such as idiopathic juvenile osteoporosis, congenital kyphosis, and infectious disorders of the spine, may cause diagnostic confusion.

Scheuermann's disease can usually be readily distinguished from postural kyphosis by a basic physical examination and roentgenographic examination. Patients with true postural roundback can readily assume a very straight spinal position if they are correctly encouraged. The patient with Scheuermann's disease and a fixed spinal deformity cannot truly correct the kyphosis, either in the standing or in the prone hyperextended position. When viewed from the side while bending forward, the back of

(Text continued on page 652.)

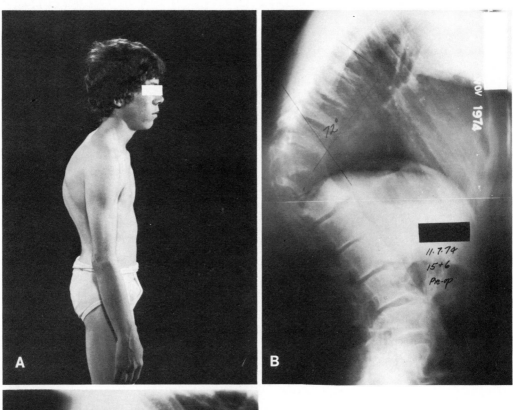

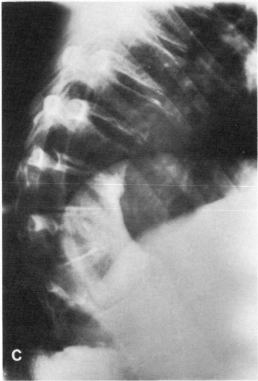

FIG. 16-44. (A) A lateral view of a boy with the clinical appearance of Scheuermann's disease. The curve was quite rigid to clinical examination. (B) A lateral standing roentgenogram of the patient taken at the same time as the photograph, demonstrating a Type II congenital kyphosis with anterior failure of segmentation at the thoracolumbar junction with a secondary kyphosis. In the lumbar spine there is anterior defective segmentation without deformity. (C) A lateral laminogram, showing the bony anterior bridge in greater detail. Proximally, one can see the normal vertebrae with the open ring apophyses. Because of the progressive nature of this deformity, it was felt that surgical correction and fusion were indicated. Bracing has no effect upon such rigid anterior unsegmented bars. (Legend continued on facing page.)

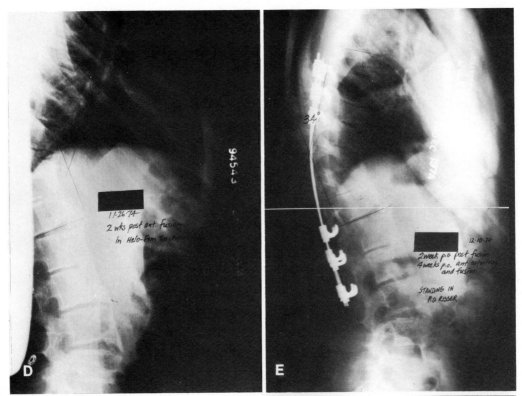

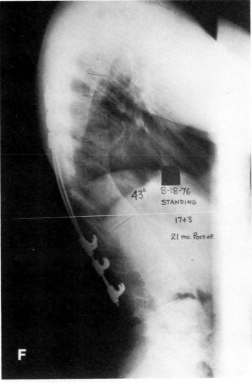

Fig. 16-44 *(Continued)*. *(D)* The patient underwent anterior osteotomy of the unsegmented bar
at two levels, T9 and T10, and T11 and T12. In
addition, the anterior longitudinal ligament and
semiosseous material between T12 and L1 was
removed. The discs were also removed proximal
to the anomalous area. The anterior longitudinal
ligament was cut proximal to the anomalous
area. Halo-femoral traction was applied during
this anesthesia. Postoperatively, he was kept for
2 weeks in halo-femoral traction with a minimal
amount of weight and with hyperextension in
bed. *(E)* Two weeks after the anterior fusion was
done, posterior fusion with Harrington compression rods placed bilaterally was performed. His
kyphosis, which had been corrected to 44° in
traction, was corrected to 34° following the posterior fusion and instrumentation. The patient
was placed in an ambulatory Risser cast 1 week
following the posterior procedure. He was discharged from the hospital 2 weeks following this
procedure. He remained in the Risser cast for 8
months, fully ambulatory during the entire time.
(F) A lateral standing roentgenogram, when the
patient was 17 years old, 21 solid anterior and
posterior fusion with a kyphosis permanently
corrected at 43°.

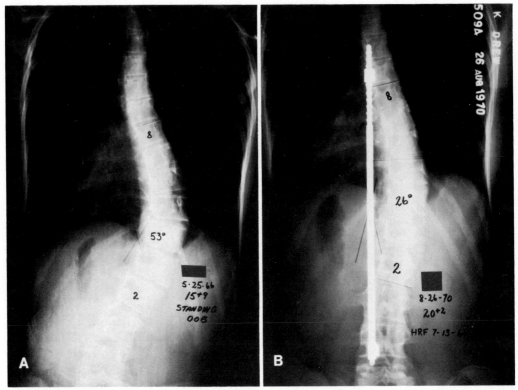

FIG. 16-45. *(A)* This girl, 15 years and 9 months old, with Marfan's syndrome presented with a T8 to L2 53° right thoracolumbar curve. She had spent 3 years in a Milwaukee brace with good correction in the brace, but had a total loss of correction on coming out of the brace. *(B)* An anteroposterior standing roentgenogram of the patient 4 years after surgical correction by Harrington instrumentation and spinal fusion. The patient with Marfan's syndrome can be readily managed by techniques identical to those used for idiopathic scoliosis.

the patient with Scheuermann's disease shows an area with acute angulation, usually at about T7. The patient with postural roundback shows a smooth, symmetrical contour. Most patients with Scheuermann's disease have a fixed or relatively fixed kyphosis. These two simple clinical tests usually distinguish structural kyphosis from postural roundback (Fig. 16-48).

Roentgenographic examination will provide the final diagnosis. The classic findings include narrowing of the disc spaces, increased anteroposterior diameter of the apical thoracic vertebrae, loss of normal height of the involved vertebrae, irregularity of the end-plates, and there may or may not be Schmorl's nodes. On the spinal hyperextension roentgenogram, loss of the normal

flexibility of the spine can be noted. In addition, there is usually wedging of one or more apical vertebrae.

Sorensen[85] believes that one cannot diagnose Scheuermann's disease without there being three consecutive vertebrae with at least 5° of wedging. The author does not feel that this wedging is necessary for diagnosis, and the presence of other signs, particularly the presence of a relatively fixed deformity, is sufficient to make the diagnosis.

NATURAL HISTORY

Scheuermann's disease may exist in the spine without causing either pain or defor-

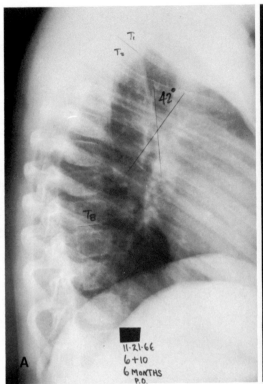

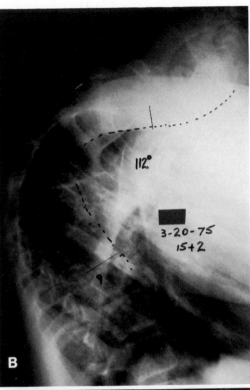

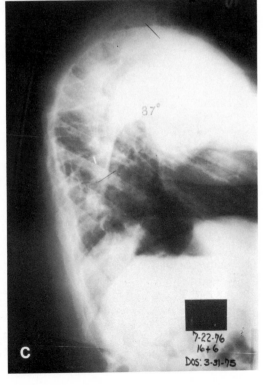

FIG. 16-46. *(A)* This 6-year and 10-month-old boy had a neuroblastoma requiring a laminectomy, thoracotomy and irradiation. This lateral roentgenogram taken 6 months following the tumor surgery shows a T2 to T8 kyphosis of 42°. *(B)* The patient, as seen 9 years later, with a rapidly progressive 112° upper kyphosis. Progression will continue unless surgical stabilization is performed. The development of paraplegia from the kyphosis is a distinct possibility. *(C)* The same patient at age 16 years and 6 months, 1 year and 4 months following anterior spinal fusion from T1 to T10, with multiple strut grafts and interbody fusion, after correction with halo-femoral traction. The curve is permanently stabilized at 87°. Fusion should have been performed much earlier, before the deformity reached this degree of severity.

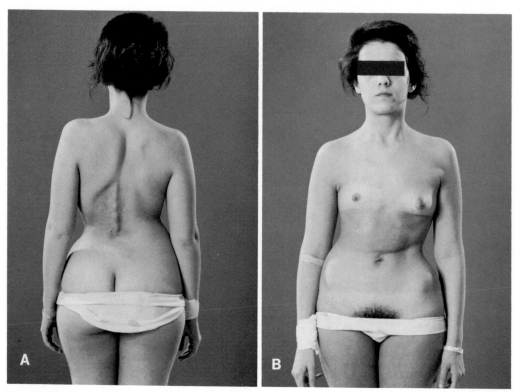

FIG. 16-47. *(A)* Posterior view of a 16-year-old girl with changes in the skin and spine secondary to irradiation treatment of a Wilms' tumor when she was 3 years old. She exhibits a slight left lumbar scoliosis, atrophy of the paravertebral muscles and irradiation changes of the skin. *(B)* Anterior view of the patient showing the scar of the nephrectomy, and also showing the irradiation changes in the skin, anteriorly. She had some mild tightness of the rectus fascia. *(Legend continued on facing page.)*

mity. Thus, it can run its natural course without creating any clinical problem. More often, however, it creates either pain or deformity or both. A slight scoliosis is quite common, but the main problem is kyphosis, usually in the midthoracic spine. There is one variety of Scheuermann's disease involving the thoracolumbar area in which the kyphosis is less prominent, but pain is more prominent and more lasting.

Most adolescents outgrow the pain at the conclusion of growth and are left only with the fixed deformity. Only a few have chronic pain in adult life. These are usually the patients with the more marked kyphoses. The cosmetic aspect of kyphosis considerably bothers some adults, others it does not.

TREATMENT

The question then arises as to whether treatment is appropriate, and if treatment is to be instituted, what is the best treatment.

Exercises

Postural exercises have been tried for many years, but they have never been demonstrated to cause any significant improvement in any documented series of patients with *structural* kyphoses. Exercises are important, in conjunction with brace or cast treatment.

Nonoperative Treatment

There are only two documented methods of nonoperative treatment which have

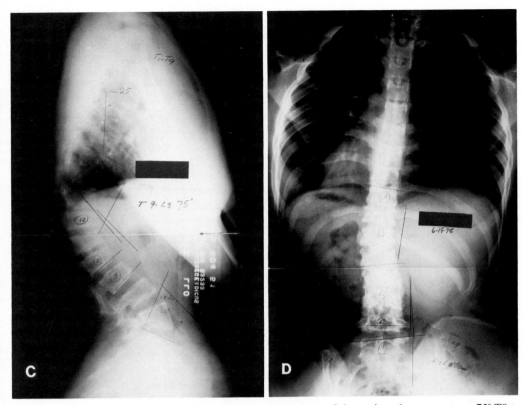

FIG. 16-47 *(Continued)*. *(C)* A lateral standing roentgenogram of the patient demonstrates a 75° T9 to L3 kyphosis. The vertebral bodies show loss of height and irregularity of the growth plates, secondary to the irradiation effect. Milwaukee bracing had already been attempted in this patient, but failed to effect correction. *(D)* This anteroposterior roentgenogram demonstrates only a slight degree of scoliosis. The patient underwent excision of the anterior longitudinal ligament and excision of all intervertebral discs throughout the kyphosis area, autogenous strut grafting and intersegmental autogenous chip grafting. Two weeks later she had a posterior fusion with Harrington compression instrumentation. The patient is still in a cast at the time of this writing.

proven beneficial—corrective plaster casts and the Milwaukee brace. Plaster casts are used, and if they are maintained for at least 1 year and are followed by an exercise program, they do, in most patients, effect and maintain a satisfactory correction. A few patients (15 to 20%) may relapse and require a second period of casting. The author prefers to use a Milwaukee brace, which is usually less objectionable to the patient than the plaster cast. The brace is certainly cooler, and it can be removed daily for bathing and other activities. A patient can be "weaned" from a brace, but a cast is an "all-or-nothing" device. Braces other than the Milwaukee brace have not been demonstrated to be successful. Some of the thoracolumbar types of roundback can be managed in hyperextension underarm braces, but the majority of patients with Scheuermann's disease have the apex at about T7 and T8. At this level, only the Milwaukee brace has been demonstrated to be beneficial. Most patients with Scheuermann's disease have a forward-jutting head, and only the Milwaukee brace will hold the head back on the same plane as the hips (Fig. 16-49).

A good Milwaukee brace for the patient with Scheuermann's disease maintains pelvic tilt to eliminate lumbar lordosis. It has two posterior kyphosis pads and a neck ring that is centered above the thorax. The most

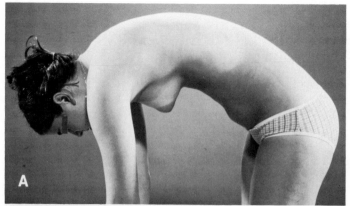
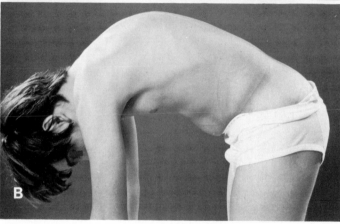

Fig. 16-48. *(A)* A lateral view of a normal spinal contour on forward bending. This patient *does not* have Scheuermann's disease. *(B)* A lateral forward-bending view to demonstrate a "break" in the contour of the spine, as viewed from the side on forward bending. This patient *does* have Scheuermann's disease.

frequent mistake is to have the neck ring in a forward position, perpetuating the forward jutting of the head, and thus perpetuating the kyphosis.

The patient who is placed in a Milwaukee brace and on an exercise program typically experiences a 1- to 2-week period of adjustment, after which the pain disappears and significant height is gained, requiring adjustment of the brace. Usually within 4 to 6 weeks, the flexible type of deformity has been corrected. After this, it is only a problem of maintaining the correction and allowing the soft tissues and the vertebrae to readjust and to grow more normally. The patient typically requires a year of full-time brace wearing (23 out of 24 hours), coupled with a supervised physical therapy program, to maintain and improve thoracic extensors and to eliminate the lumbar lordosis. At the end of 1 year, if the deformity has remained fully corrected, weaning can be instituted gradually, even though full growth may not have been reached. Patients with Scheuermann's disease usually require less intensive Milwaukee brace treatment than patients with idiopathic scoliosis. For weaning, usually a minimum period of 1 year is necessary. If there is loss of correction at any time during the weaning process, a return to full-time brace wearing is necessary, with weaning being resumed 6 to 12 months later.

Some patients, particularly those with the structural types of Scheuermann's disease with marked wedging, cannot achieve correction with this brace program. These patients require full and intensive brace treatment, including exercises, until growth is complete. Weaning is to be done only after

Fig. 16-49. (A) Diagrams of lateral views, illustrating both the deformity of the Scheuermann's disease and its correction by the multiple forces of a Milwaukee brace. (From Blount, W. P., and Moe, J. H.: The Milwaukee Brace. Baltimore, Williams & Wilkins, 1973.) (B) A patient fitted with a Milwaukee brace for kyphosis. The posterior uprights are kept close to the body, the occipital pads are below the occiput, and the throat mold is kept fairly high under the chin to encourage posterior displacement of the head. The anterior upright is sufficiently far from the chest to permit full and complete inspiration, along with correction of the curve. The patient's ear is directly above the shoulder and the hip line, showing satisfactory total body alignment. (C) A posterior view of the patient, showing the brace for Scheuermann's kyphosis. In this illustration the pads are too large and they encroach upon the scapular wing. To be properly applied, the pad should be quite narrow and should not extend lateral to the posterior upright.

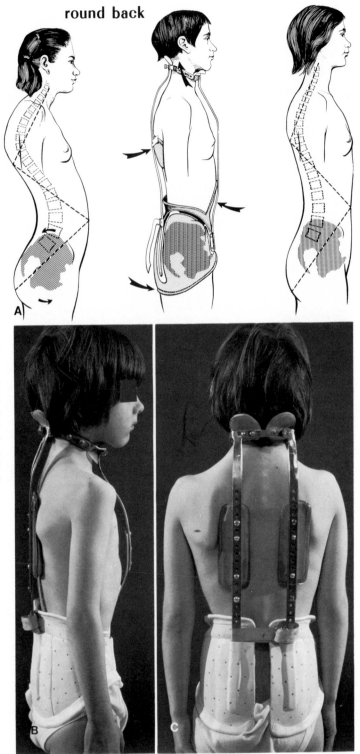

round back

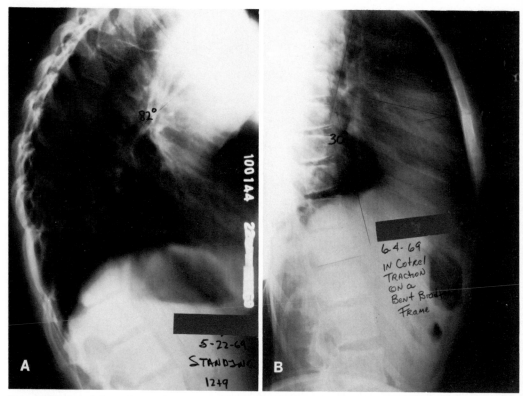

Fig. 16-50. *(A)* A lateral standing roentgenogram of a girl with classic Scheuremann's disease; the curve measures 82°. Details cannot be seen on this film. *(B)* A lateral roentgenogram in traction and hyperextension demonstrates correctability of the curve to 30° and shows, with unusual clarity, the wedging of the apical vertebra. This girl exhibits relatively little end-plate irregularity. The obviously viable and normal ring apophyses and the lack of end-plate irregularity give this girl an excellent prognosis, provided a brace can relieve the stresses of the kyphotic deformity. *(Legend continued on facing page.)*

there has been closure of the ring apophyses of the involved vertebral bodies.

The age at which treatment can be started with the brace depends on the maturity of the vertebrae in the area of the disease. Bone age, as determined by the hand film and the status of the iliac epiphyses, is of less importance than the degree of growth in the area of the disease. Growth is delayed in many patients. The author has seen successful brace treatment in patients started as late as 17 years in males and 15 years in females.

The results of brace treatment are usually excellent. In a series of 75 patients who had completed Milwaukee brace treatment, Bradford and his colleagues demonstrated that good correction was obtained in most patients. The average correction of the kyphosis was 40 per cent, and the average correction of the vertebral wedging was 41 per cent. Patients with more severe and rigid deformities, especially those whose growth was nearly complete, had the least improvement, but all groups had some improvement (Fig. 16-50).[8]

Surgical Treatment

Surgical treatment in Scheuermann's disease is rarely necessary. It is indicated only for those patients who have completed growth, who have a significant deformity (greater than 60°), and who have chronic pain in the curve area. Thus, out of several hundred patients seen with Scheuermann's

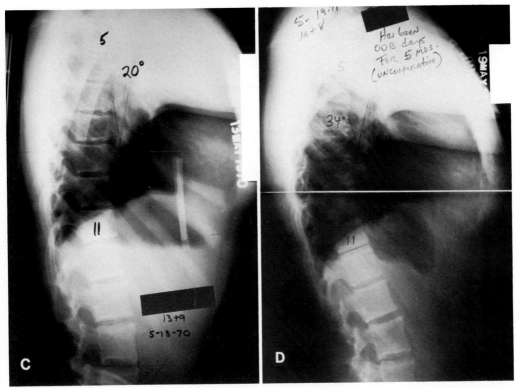

FIG. 16-50 *(Continued)*. *(C)* The patient 1 year later in the Milwaukee brace. Not only is her curve maintained at 20°, but the vertebral bodies have rapidly returned to a more normal contour. *(D)* One year later, the kyphosis measures 34°, with the patient standing without the brace. The patient has been wearing her brace only at night for the past 5 months. The brace was discontinued at this time.

disease, the authors have found it necessary to operate upon only a few.

Initially, the authors were pleased with the correction obtained by posterior Harrington instrumentation and spinal fusion. Satisfactory correction was obtained, and the patients were relieved of their discomfort. Unfortunately, many of these patients subsequently lost their correction, particularly those with curves greater than 70°.[9]

At the present time, we feel that if a patient with Scheuermann's disease requires fusion (as stated above, this situation is rare), both anterior and posterior arthrodeses should be done. The patient with kyphosis of this degree cannot obtain a posterior fusion sufficiently solid to withstand the tension forces placed upon it. It is only by anterior interbody fusion that permanent maintenance of correction is achieved for patients with the more severe deformities. The patient is first placed in halo traction. Then an anterior approach is performed, usually through a left thoracotomy. The five apical discs are removed, and the anterior longitudinal ligament is either excised or incised transversely at each disc level. The anterior longitudinal ligament has been found to be quite thickened and hypertrophied in these patients, and certainly it has been responsible for limiting correction. Thus, the release of the anterior longitudinal ligament is quite important. The discs are removed back to the posterior longitudinal ligament, leaving the posterior anulus and posterior longitudinal ligament intact. The end-plates are perforated into cancellous bone. The rib removed during the thoractomy is broken up into tiny pieces, and the disc spaces are packed with fragments of this autogenous

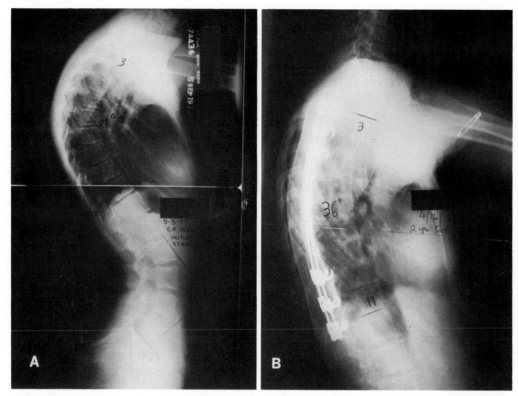

FIG. 16-51. *(A)* A lateral standing roentgenogram of a 15-year-old skeletally mature girl with a painful 79° Scheuermann's kyphosis. This curve is extremely rigid on attempted hyperextension. She underwent anterior longitudinal ligament release, anterior disc excision, and anterior bone grafting of the disc spaces, followed by two weeks of halo Cotrel traction and hyperextension, and posterior spinal fusion with Harrington compression instrumentation. She was kept in a Risser ambulatory hyperextension cast for 9 months. *(B)* A lateral standing roentgenogram of the patient taken 2 years after surgical correction and fusion.

bone. If there is not enough bone obtained from the single rib, iliac bone should be obtained. On rare occasions, a strut graft has been used, but the segmental small grafts have been quite satisfactory for most cases of Scheuermann's disease. They appear to heal more rapidly.

The patient is continued in halo traction with thoracic extension for 2 weeks, to obtain further correction. Then a posterior arthrodesis is performed, encompassing the entire kyphotic curve. Harrington instrumentation (usually two compression instruments) should be used. On occasion, one distraction rod and one compression rod can be used when there is some scoliosis.

Approximately 1 week following the second procedure, a Risser type of cast is applied, with a hyperextension strap placed underneath the apex of the kyphosis. The patient is then allowed to ambulate but remains in the cast for approximately 9 months. We have not been impressed with attempting this type of surgery without a full Risser cast, since it is very important to maintain the head in an extended position and to prevent its falling forward, anterior to the gravity line. A Milwaukee brace can be used postoperatively just as well as a Risser cast, provided that the patient is completely reliable and the brace is maintained at all times (Fig. 16-51).

NEUROMUSCULAR SPINAL DEFORMITY

As noted in the classification of spinal deformity (p. 573), there is a large number of neurologic conditions which may result in a spinal deformity. It is simplest to remember that *any* neuromuscular condition in a growing child may cause a spinal deformity. Formerly, most such spinal deformities were caused by poliomyelitis, but now, at least in the United States and Canada, poliomyelitis is rare. However, other neuromuscular problems still confront the physician, particularly myelomeningocele, cerebral palsy, posttraumatic paralysis and spinal muscular atrophy. Myelomeningocele spinal deformity is covered in Chapter 10. The spinal-cord-injured child is discussed in Chapter 14.

GENERAL PRINCIPLES

Neuromuscular spinal deformities are quite different from idiopathic scoliosis, and the management is quite different. Many errors have occurred when surgeons have used the principles of treating idiopathic scoliosis in the treatment of paralytic problems.

The curve patterns are different. Most paralytic curves are long, and they may lack the compensatory curves seen in idiopathic scoliosis. The curves may extend up into the cervical spine and down to the sacrum, neither of which ever occur in idiopathic scoliosis.

The patient has problems other than the spinal deformity. The primary condition may cause respiratory problems due to intercostal paralysis, contractures around the hips, deformities of the legs, problems in ambulation, problems in cerebration, and sometimes anesthetic skin in the trunk, hips and legs.

Neuromuscular curvatures tend to respond poorly to bracing, and they require arthrodesis in a high percentage of patients. The arthrodesis is more difficult to accomplish due to the longer curve, softer bone, less abundant amount of iliac bone, and greater problems of immobilization postoperatively. Thus, a higher rate of pseudarthrosis is to be expected, and pseudarthrosis repair should be anticipated and carried out without hesitation.

EVALUATION

In addition to the general examination mentioned earlier in this chapter, attention must be directed to the extent and pattern of muscle weakness in the torso, paying particular attention to the intercostal, abdominal, quadratus lumborum and erector spinae muscles. The hip area must be examined for range of motion, muscle strength and contractures. If there is pelvic obliquity, is it due to contractures between the spine and pelvis only, contractures of both? Is there leg length inequality? The reader is referred to Chapter 18 for further details regarding paralytic problems about the hips.

Special attention must be directed toward lung function, since the paralytic patient often has intercostal paralysis. Vital capacity may be significantly reduced, even with a small curvature. Curvatures must never be allowed to progress to the point of further embarrassment of already compromised lung function. Special management may be needed at the time of spinal fusion.

POLIOMYELITIS

Most of the general principles in the treatment of neuromuscular spinal problems were developed in treating the large numbers of poliomyelitis victims between 1940 and 1960. Although poliomyelitis is no longer seen in highly developed countries, it is still found in many areas of the world. Many adults with untreated curvatures are still coming to my attention. All of these patients should have had spinal fusions years ago.

Brace treatment of poliomyelitis curves is possible, even though the goal of bracing is to delay surgery until a greater degree of spinal growth has occurred. For thoracic curves, the Milwaukee brace is ideal. Pad placement is similar to that with idiopathic scoliosis. For lumbar curves, the new molded lumbar braces work well. No brace should inhibit pulmonary function. The thorax must never be constricted (Fig. 16-52).

(Text continues on page 664.)

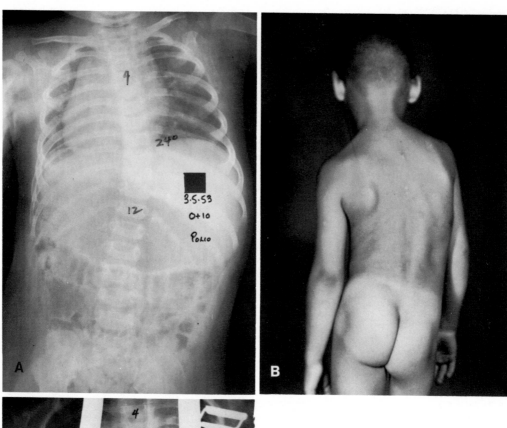

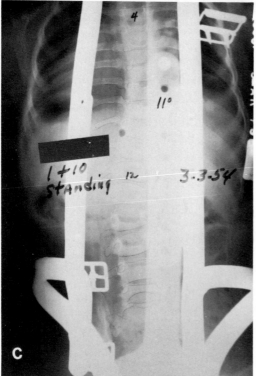

Fig. 16-52. *(A)* A 10-month-old boy who had severe poliomyelitis at the age of 2 months. At the age of 10 months, he already exhibits a 24° right thoracic scoliosis of T4 to T12. The prognosis for such a curve is extremely poor. *(B)* The patient a few years later, showing the very structural right thoracic scoliosis. He also has a severe leg length discrepancy, due to the involvement of the right leg. *(C)* A standing roentgenogram of the patient, at age 1 year and 10 months, in a Milwaukee brace. The curve measures 11° and is well controlled at this time. *(Legend continued on facing page.)*

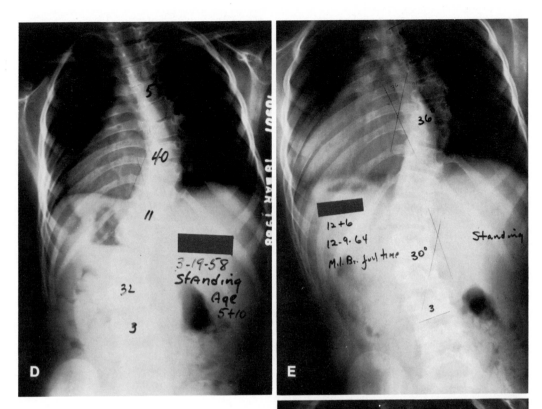

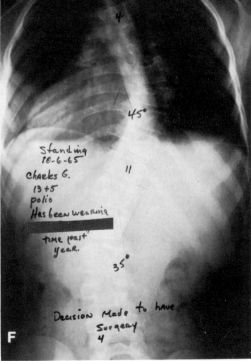

FIG. 16-52 *(Continued)*. *(D)* A standing roentgenogram taken when the patient was 5 years and 10 months old, showing the curve to measure 40°. However, he had not been wearing the brace full-time, due to incorrect instructions by the physicians. Full-time Milwaukee brace treatment was instituted at this time. *(E)* At 12 years and 6 months of age, this patient's spine has been kept well under control, with the thoracic curve measuring 36°. There now exists a 30° left lumbar compensatory curve. He is still wearing the Milwaukee brace full-time. He has now been in the Milwaukee brace for 11 years. *(F)* One year later the patient's curve is showing deterioration, despite continued full-time brace use. He is now 13½ years of age. It was felt this was the optimal time for surgery, that further bracing would not be likely to be productive, and for psychologic reasons it would be beneficial to remove him from the brace at this time. The lumbar curve remains completely flexible, so it was necessary to fuse only the thoracic curve. *(Legend continued on overleaf.)*

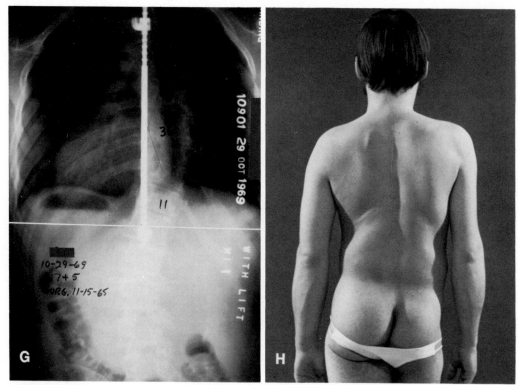

FIG. 16-52 *(Continued).* *(G)* This roentgenogram was taken 4 years after the posterior spinal fusion with Harrington instrumentation of T2 to T12. The curve was corrected to 30° and has remained stable at 36°. The leg length discrepancy has been managed by appropriate epiphysiodesis. *(H)* A posterior view of the patient at age 17 showing the well-controlled spine. This combination of brace treatment for many years, to obtain adequate growth and to keep the curve under control, followed by spinal fusion at an appropriate age has given the best possible results for this boy's very difficult, potentially catastrophic curvature problem.

Surgical arthrodesis is the mainstay of treatment in poliomyelitis scoliosis. The fusion must never be delayed until the child is fully grown. If a curve can be maintained at 50° or less by bracing, then bracing should be continued, but if a curve progresses beyond 50° in the brace, fusion should be done regardless of age.

The fusion area is longer than for idiopathic scoliosis. Should there be pelvic obliquity due to contractures *above* the hips, fusion to the sacrum is mandatory. If the patient has a "collapsing" type of spinal deformity, fusion to the sacrum is mandatory. Patients with thoracic scoliosis and no pelvic obliquity do *not* require fusion to the sacrum. It was once thought that fusion to the sacrum inhibited ambulatory ability; it does not. Cervicothoracic curves require fusion up into the cervical spine. In such cases, a halo cast or halo brace is essential (Fig. 16-53).

Harrington instrumentation should be used if at all possible. It is desirable to have maximal internal fixation to lessen the dependence on external cast or brace forces that may interfere with respiration. Rapid return to the upright position is also highly desirable, for the same reason.

Patients with severe lumbar scoliosis and pelvic obliquity are best managed by the combined anterior and posterior approach.[72] Halo-femoral traction for 2 weeks is followed by a Dwyer anterior instrumentation and fusion.[24] Two weeks later, a long posterior fusion and Harrington instrumentation is done from the upper thoracic spine to the sacrum. The patient is immobilized in a halo cast, a Risser localizer cast or a brace and returned to the upright position in 1 to 2 weeks. The legs and hips are *not* immobilized. The *minimal* period of time in the cast or brace is 1 year.

The most common errors of treatment in poliomyelitis are: (1) failure to brace soon enough, (2) failure to fuse soon enough, (3) failure to fuse an adequate length, and (4) failure to recognize and repair pseudarthroses.

CEREBRAL PALSY

Spinal deformity in cerebral palsy has been a long-neglected topic. A few series of patients have been analyzed to find the incidence of scoliosis, which seems to be about 25 per cent in the average patient with cerebral palsy who is ambulatory.[2, 78, 79] The more extensively involved patient has a higher incidence of scoliosis, and the scoliotic curves are more severe.[80] Studies of the results of treatment have not been done, except for reports by MacEwen[53] and Bonnett and his associates.[6]

Bracing for spinal problems of cerebral palsy has been felt by many to be futile. Such is not always the case. The Milwaukee brace has successfully delayed surgery for thoracic curvatures, and the molded plastic lumbar braces and underarm braces have done well for lumbar and thoracolumbar curves. In no case has bracing alone permanently solved a curve problem. As stated for poliomyelitis and other conditions, no curve should be allowed to progress beyond 50° without fusion (Fig. 16-54).

As in poliomyelitis, the patient with cerebral palsy requires an extensive area of fusion, usually from high in the thoracic spine down to the sacrum. Many patients with spastic quadriplegia have lumbar or thoracolumbar curves. These must *always* be fused to the sacrum, or pelvic obliquity will rapidly recur. It is tempting to stop the fusion at T9 or T10, proximally, since that is often the upper end of the curve. Unfortunately, the spastic abdominal muscles pull the thoracic spine forward into kyphosis. Therefore, it is best to always extend the fusion proximally to the upper thoracic spine (T2). The combined approach of halo-femoral traction, Dwyer procedure, and long posterior fusion with Harrington instrumentation has shown the best results in our hands for the severe lumbar or thoracolumbar curve. The Dwyer procedure alone is insufficient. For the less common thoracic curve, halo-femoral traction and posterior fusion with Harrington instrumentation has been best. Postoperative immobilization in well-padded Risser or halo casts has given the best results. The cast extends only to the pelvis, even though the fusion extends to the sacrum. Rapid return to the upright position is routinely done (Fig. 16-55).

When the technical aspects of correcting and fusing the spine in cerebral palsy have been solved, the chief problem is in deciding whether or not to fuse the spine of retarded patients. One can choose one of three paths: (1) fuse no retarded child on the premise that "nothing of benefit is being accomplished," or "the child has no appreciation of having a straighter spine;" (2) fuse all children with spinal deformity, regardless of mental status, on the premise that "no child should be denied treatment just because of retardation;" or (3) take a middle path, treating those in whom there is disability, malfunction, or pain because of the curve. Those in whom the curve is causing no problems are not treated, regardless of the magnitude of the curve.

At the present time, the authors feel that the "middle path" is preferable. Pain, loss of sitting balance, and painful hip subluxation are our more frequent indications for treating a retarded patient. The patient with cerebral palsy who is not retarded should be given every possible opportunity for improved quality of life. (Fig. 16-56).

SPINAL MUSCLE ATROPHY

This group of disorders is characterized by degeneration of the anterior horn cells; the etiology is unknown. (See Chapter 8.) Various names have been applied to spinal muscle atrophy, such as Werdnig-Hoffmann disease, Kugelberg-Welander disease, and

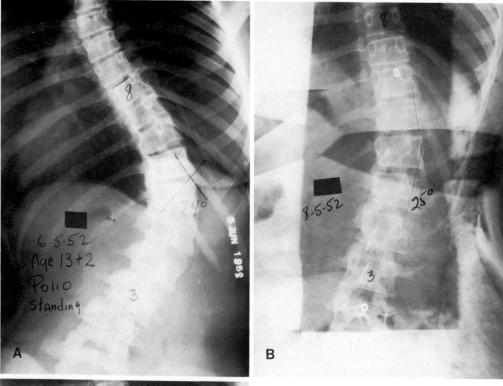

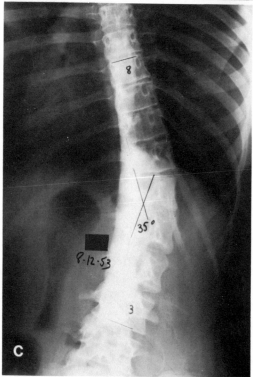

FIG. 16-53. (A) This 13-year-old girl was first seen at Gillette Hospital in 1952 by Dr. Moe, exhibiting this 74° T8 to L3 right thoracolumbar curve secondary to poliomyelitis. The treatment of choice was surgical correction and fusion. In 1952 Harrington instrumentation was still 8 years away. The traditional method at that time was cast correction and posterior fusion. These were performed. (B) A supine roentgenogram taken in the corrective Risser cast, showing improvement of the curvature from 74° to 25°. (C) One year postoperatively, after 6 months in bed in a cast and 6 months ambulatory in a cast, the patient's curve measured 35°, and the fusion was apparently solid. The cast was discontinued at that time. (Legend continued on facing page.)

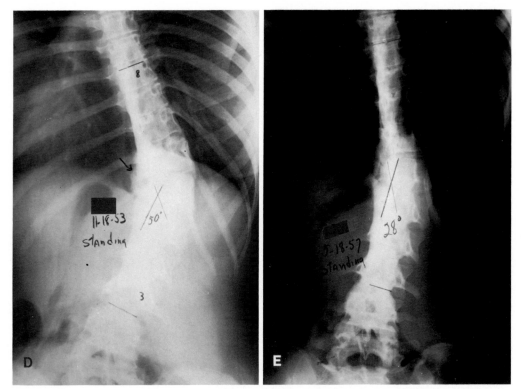

FIG. 16-53 *(Continued)*. *(D)* Three months later the patient returned for routine follow-up. Her curve had shown a loss of correction to 50° and pseudarthrosis was quite evident at T11 to T12 region. The patient was taken back to the operating room, where the pseudarthrosis was excised and bone-grafted, and the curve was corrected once again by cast technique. *(E)* A standing roentgenogram taken 4 years after pseudarthrosis repair and 5 years after fusion. The correction has been maintained at 28°, and the fusion is now solid. This demonstrates that successful correction and fusion can be obtained without instrumentation. It must always be remembered that instrumentation, either Harrington or Dwyer, is always an adjunct. A positive result from spinal arthrodesis always depends upon maintaining a high quality of fusion technique, coupled with meticulous postoperative external immobilization.

amyotonia congenita. Many children born with this condition go rapidly downhill and die before the age of 6 years. However, some do not, and they seem to stabilize neurologically. These patients, however, are extensively paralyzed and usually do not ambulate. This group of survivors always develops severe spinal deformities.

A second group (those with the Kugelberg-Welander form) develops the disease later in age, and they are ambulators up until about 12 to 15 years. This group usually develops scoliosis, but it occurs when growth is advanced, and it is not as severe as the other types.

Bracing may be quite effective if begun early, but as in all paralytic problems, bracing seldom is adequate without fusion. Spinal fusion is best done at 10 to 12 years of age. If, however, the patient is still ambulatory, fusion should be delayed until ambulation is no longer possible (Figs. 16-57. 16-58).

SPONDYLOLISTHESIS

"Spondyl-" means spine and "-olisthesis" means slipping; thus, spondylolisthesis means a slipping of the spine. There are several types of spondylolisthesis, as outlined

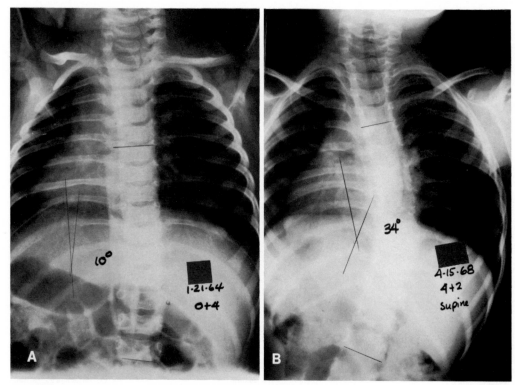

FIG. 16-54. *(A)* This 4-month-old child has cerebral palsy with spastic quadriplegia. A chest roentgenogram taken at 4 months demonstrates an apparently innocuous 10° low right thoracic scoliosis. *(B)* A supine roentgenogram taken at age 4 demonstrates an increase of curvature to 34°. This curve has now become structural. Without treatment, this curve will inevitably progress to well beyond 100°. It was therefore elected to treat the patient, despite her spastic quadriplegia and mental retardation. *(Legend continued on facing page.)*

by Wiltse.[89] They are: congenital, isthmic, traumatic, pathologic and degenerative.

In this section, we are not concerned with the degenerative spondylolisthesis (a problem of the elderly patient), the pathologic defects due to tumors and infections, or the traumatic type, but we are concerned with the congenital and the isthmic types.

PATHOLOGY

In the congenital type, the defect is present at birth. There is a specific congenital anomaly of development. There are the more extreme congenital types appearing at birth, and there is a less obvious type that shows progressive slipping during growth.

This quite often leaves a long "stretched out" pars interarticularis, but there apparently is no lytic defect. This type has a high incidence of associated congenital anomalies, such as spina bifida occulta and maldeveloped facet joints.

The most common type, the lytic (or "isthmic") type, has a defect in the pars interarticularis, usually bilaterally, and a defect at L5 in 85 to 90 per cent of patients. In a small percentage of cases, there may be involvement of the L4, and in rarer cases, L3 or more than one vertebrae are involved.

The presence of a defect in the pars interarticularis is referred to as "spondylolysis," and a defect with a slip is known as

(Text continues on page 675.)

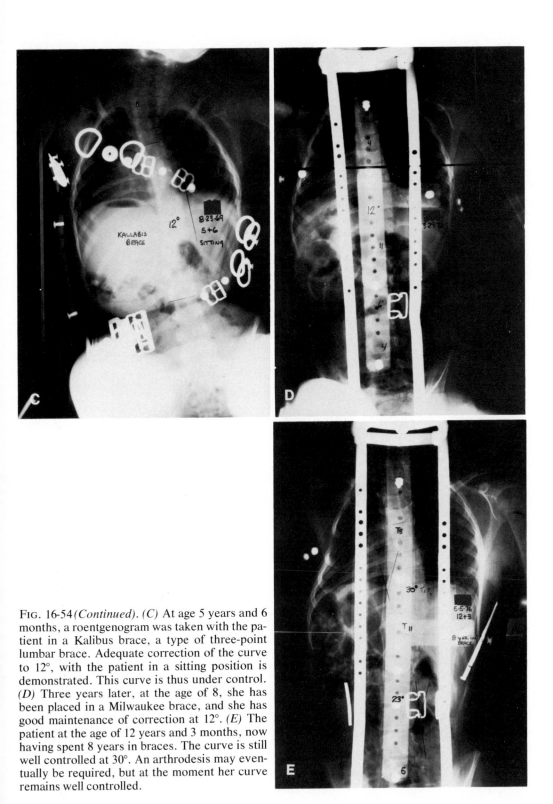

FIG. 16-54 (Continued). (C) At age 5 years and 6 months, a roentgenogram was taken with the patient in a Kalibus brace, a type of three-point lumbar brace. Adequate correction of the curve to 12°, with the patient in a sitting position is demonstrated. This curve is thus under control. (D) Three years later, at the age of 8, she has been placed in a Milwaukee brace, and she has good maintenance of correction at 12°. (E) The patient at the age of 12 years and 3 months, now having spent 8 years in braces. The curve is still well controlled at 30°. An arthrodesis may eventually be required, but at the moment her curve remains well controlled.

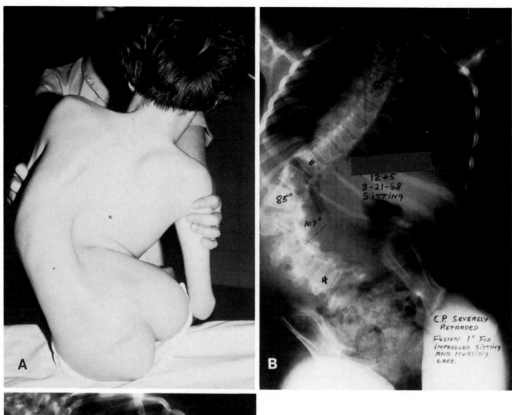

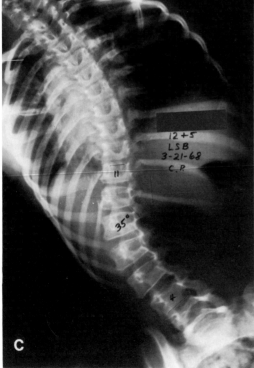

FIG. 16-55. *(A)* A 12½ year-old girl with total loss of sitting balance due to spastic quadriplegic cerebral palsy. She is mentally retarded and lives at home with her family. She had previously been able to sit, but within the past year had lost all sitting ability. *(B)* An anteroposterior roentgenogram taken with the patient in a sitting position demonstrates a 107° left lumbar scoliosis, with severe pelvic obliquity. *(C)* A forced left side-bending film demonstrates significant correctability of her curve to 35°. Note that the thorax can be placed in appropriate position over a level pelvis. This roentgenogram demonstrates that she has sufficient correctability, and it is only a matter of surgical technology to stabilize her curve in this corrected position. Such a patient does not require preliminary traction. *(Legend continued on facing page.)*

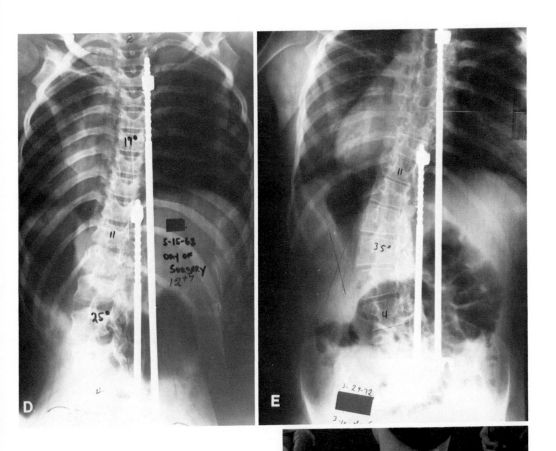

FIG. 16-55 (Continued). (D) The patient underwent posterior spinal fusion of T4 to the sacrum with two Harrington distraction rods and abundant autogenous bone graft. The pelvis was deliberately slightly overcorrected, in expectation of some settling. It is always necessary to stabilize these curves high into the thoracic spine. A lower fusion results in bending of the spine over the top of the fusion area. (E) An anteroposterior roentgenographic view of the patient taken 3 years after the posterior spinal fusion. The curve is solidly stabilized at 35°. The pelvis is perfectly level. The thorax is well centered over the pelvis. (F) A posterior view of the patient at that time, showing reconstitution of sitting balance.

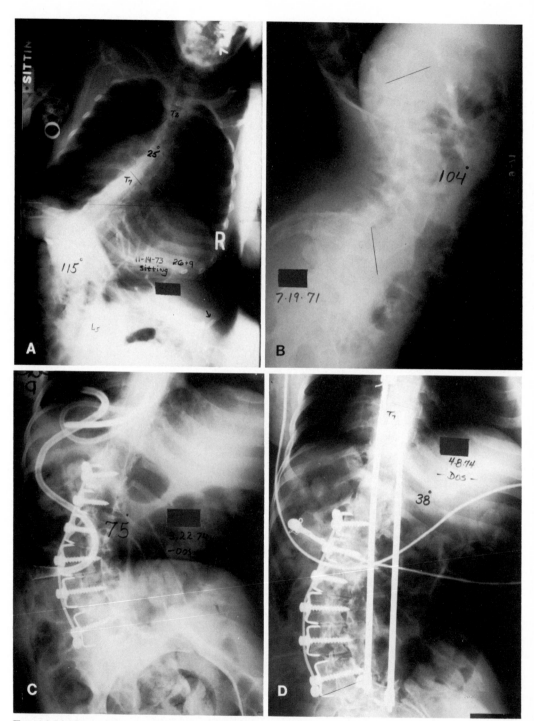

FIG. 16-56. (A) A sitting roentgenogram of a patient with spastic quadriplegic cerebral palsy, who presented with spinal pain and pain in the right hip due to partial subluxation. She is 26 years old at this time. The pain severely limited her ability to sit for an extended period. (B) A lateral standing roentgenogram taken at this time, showing a severe increase in lumbar lordosis, which measured 104°. (C) An anterior view of the patient, showing Dwyer instrumentation, during 2 weeks of halo- and right-legged femoral traction. (D) An anterior view following Harrington instrumentation and spinal fusion of T5 total sacrum. Note the marked correction of the pelvic obliquity. (*Legend continued on facing page.*)

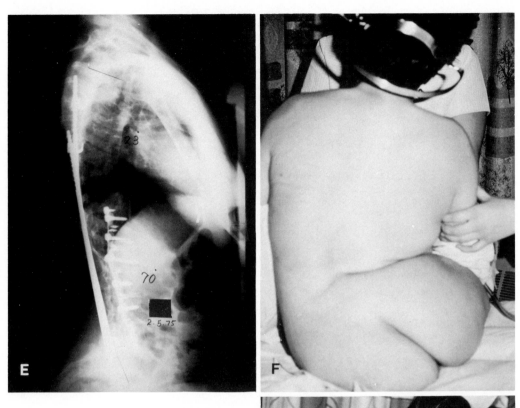

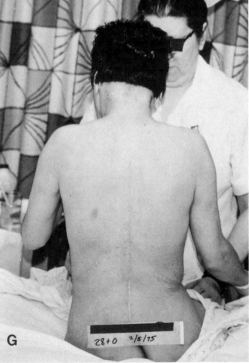

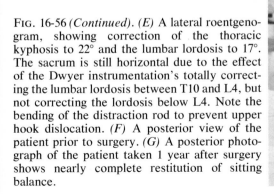

E

F

G   28+0 2/5/75

FIG. 16-56 (Continued). (E) A lateral roentgenogram, showing correction of the thoracic
kyphosis to 22° and the lumbar lordosis to 17°.
The sacrum is still horizontal due to the effect
of the Dwyer instrumentation's totally correcting the lumbar lordosis between T10 and L4, but
not correcting the lordosis below L4. Note the
bending of the distraction rod to prevent upper
hook dislocation. (F) A posterior view of the
patient prior to surgery. (G) A posterior photograph of the patient taken 1 year after surgery
shows nearly complete restitution of sitting
balance.

673

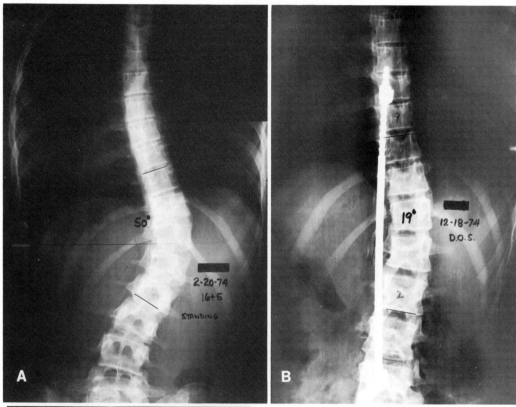

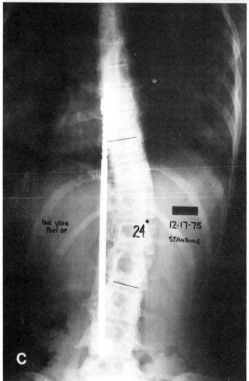

FIG. 16-57. (A) A roentgenogram of a 16-year-old girl with a 50° thoracolumbar curve of the late onset type of spinal muscle atrophy. She was still ambulatory at this time. (B) A film taken on the day of surgery, following Harrington instrumentation and spinal fusion. She was placed in a lightweight plaster cast and placed back in the sitting position the day after surgery. One week after surgery she was placed in a bivalved polypropylene body jacket. (C) A standing roentgenogram taken 1 year following surgery, showing solid fusion and correction maintained at 24°. She was kept fully ambulatory the entire time. The use of the plastic body jacket permitted ambulation, since the weight of plaster was too much for her weak legs.

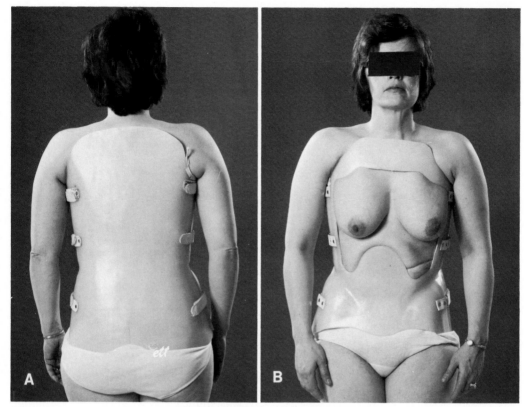

Fig. 16-58. *(A)* A patient in a bivalved polypropylene body jacket, posterior view. *(B)* An anterior view of the same patient. Note the large anterior window to avoid breast compression and to allow for lung expansion. This brace must be made after correction of the patient's deformity.

"spondylolisthesis." Spondylolysis is present in about 5 per cent of North Americans after the age of 5 years (Figs. 16-59, 15-60).

Low back pain is the most common complaint bringing these patients to the physician. Other complaints may be lordosis, scoliosis, peculiar gait, tight hamstrings, or even a neurologic deficit, such as bladder weakness or drop foot.

PHYSICAL FINDINGS

Depending on the reason for the patient's coming to the physician, various physical findings may be elicited. In a mild case without a gross slip but with pain, the most common physical finding is localized tenderness at the lumbosacral level. Careful examination shows a palpable forward displacement of the L4 spinous process relative to the L5 spinous process. There may be tightness of the hamstrings. This may assume severe proportions, with even total absence of straight-leg- raising ability.

The gait may be peculiar due to tight hamstrings and the inability to bring one leg ahead of the other without bending the knees. This gait is not seen in any other condition. The neurologic examination should be carefully done, testing particularly the reflexes and motor and sensory components in the lower extremities. Severe degrees of slip of L5 on S1 may impair the L5 nerve root, producing hyperesthesia of the medial border of the foot, weakness of toe dorsiflexion, weakness of ankle dorsiflexion and diminution of the ankle reflex. The presenting problem may be a scoliosis due to muscle spasm and related to pain or slipping of a vertebra.

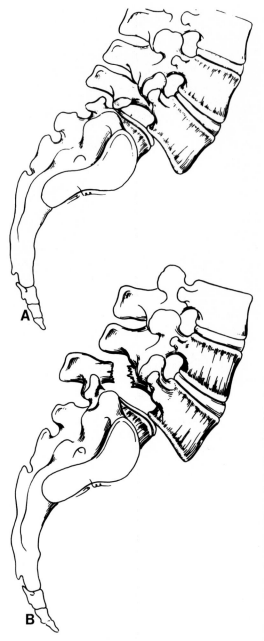

A

B

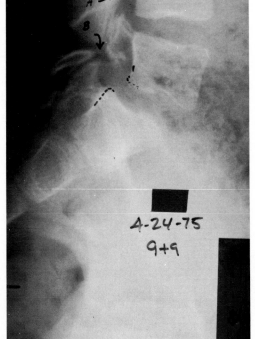

Fig. 16-59. *(A)* Congenital lumbosacral subluxation. This drawing demonstrates the congenital type of spondylolisthesis in which slipping occurred without a defect in the pars interarticularis. This may occur by slipping at the facet joint of L5 to S1, or may occur with a gradual elongation of the pars interarticularis of L5. Neurologic symptomatology is more likely when there is the facet dislocation type. *(B)* A diagram of the more common type of isthmic spondylolisthesis, in which there is forward slipping. There is a defect in the pars articularis of L5. (From Hensinger, R. N., Lang, J. R., and MacEwen, G. D.: Surgical management of spondylolisthesis in children and adolescents. Spine, *1:*207, 1976.)

the focus of the roentgenograms, rather than the lumbar spine, since roentgen beams directed at L2 will not produce a proper view at L5 to S1. It is important that the spot lateral roentgenogram be taken with the patient

Fig. 16-60. A lateral standing roentgenogram of a 9-year-old boy with a Grade I spondylolisthesis. Arrow *A* points to the intact pars interarticularis of L4. Arrow *B* points to the defect in the pars interarticularis of L5.

ROENTGENOGRAPHIC FINDINGS

When spondylolysis or spondylolisthesis is suspected, the patient should have a lateral, standing, detailed roentgenographic view of the lumbosacral level. In addition, one should obtain anteroposterior and oblique views of the lumbosacral area. It is important that the lumbosacral region be

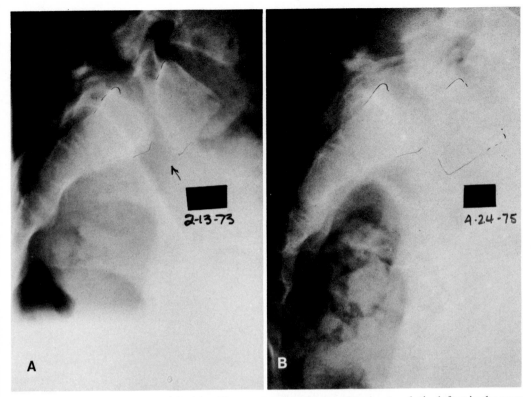

Fig. 16-61. *(A)* A 13-year-old girl with a 30 per cent slip of L5 on S1, due to a lytic defect in the pars interarticularis of L5. A 30 per cent slip would classify this as a Grade II spondylolisthesis, under the Myerding classification. She had no symptoms of any kind at this time. She had no tightness of the hamstrings. She was observed. *(B)* The patient 2 years later. She had progressed to a 60 per cent slip (now a Meyerding Grade III). She still had no symptoms whatsoever. She could easily bend forward and put her hands flat on the floor with her knees straight. Despite the lack of symptoms it was felt necessary to surgically fuse her spine to prevent complete slipping. The rounding of the upper border of the sacrum and the trapezoidal shape of L5 carry a poor prognosis for further slipping.

standing to maximize the quantity of slip. If there is any scoliosis associated with the spondylolisthesis, which there may be, full-length anteroposterior roentgenograms and sometimes full-length lateral roentgenograms are appropriate for evaluation of associated spinal deformity. With severe degrees of slip, the body of L5 is displaced anterior to S1, and there will be an overlapping shadow in this area on the anteroposterior view known as the "Napoleon's hat." On the oblique views, the defect in the pars interarticularis can be seen. Usually it is not possible to see this defect on any other view. One looks for the defect in the "scotty dog neck."[69] The lateral view of the lumbosacral level should be examined for displacement of L5 relative to S1. There may be reactive

changes anterior to the body of S1, which are physiologic remodelings that help support the body of L5. Thus, the anterior border of S1 may be indistinct. It is easier to look at the posterior aspect of S1 relative to the posterior aspect of L5 to see the proper alignment relationship. The traditional system developed by Myerding[88] indicated that a Grade I slip involves up to 25 per cent of the vertebral body; Grade II, 25 to 50 per cent; Grade III, 50 to 75 per cent; and Grade IV, 75 per cent or greater (Fig. 16-61).

TREATMENT

Treatment depends on the symptomatology and the quantity of displacement. The growing child who presents with an occa-

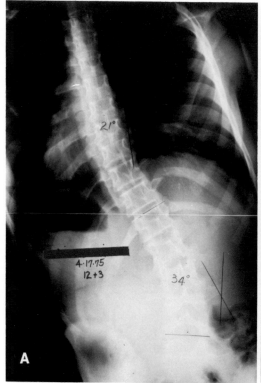

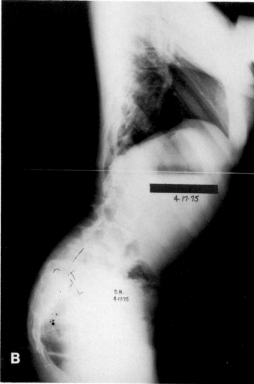

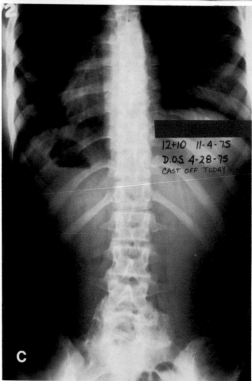

FIG. 16-62. *(A)* This 12-year-old girl presented with severe muscle spasm in her lower back and a minimal amount of low back pain. *(B)* A lateral, standing full-length roentgenogram of the patient shows the 65 per cent (Grade III) slip of L5 on S1. Note the flexion relationship of L5 to S1; the long sweeping lordosis is thus a secondary curve in order to maintain the head over the thighs. The sacrum becomes more vertical as the slip progresses. Such a patient must have surgical stabilization. In the absence of objective neurologic findings, such as motor weakness, sensory deficit, or reflex changes, it is not necessary to excise the lamina of L5. It is important to perform a thorough transverse process fusion from L4 to the sacrum. The patient should be maintained postoperatively in a double-pantaloon underarm cast, with the lumbar spine in tolerable hyperextension, in order to maintain L5 in the most extended relationship to S1 possible. Further slipping can occur in the child with this type of spondylolisthesis, even in a cast, if the patient is allowed to be ambulatory. *(C)* An anteroposterior standing roentgenogram taken 7 months following fusion. She spent 4 months supine in a double-pantaloon cast and 3 months ambulatory in a short body cast. The fusion appears solid on this anteroposterior view, and the scoliosis has disappeared. *(Legend continued on facing page.)*

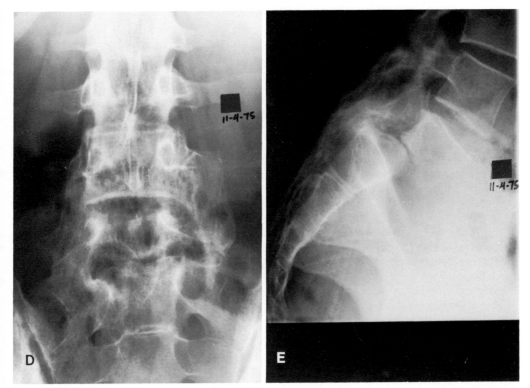

FIG. 16-62 *(Continued). (D)* A Ferguson view of the same patient on the same day. This shows the fusion mass between the transverse processes of L4 and L5 and the ala of the sacrum in much better perspective than does the ordinary anteroposterior view. Oblique views of the fusion mass should also be obtained in this Ferguson projection. *(E)* A lateral roentgenogram taken at time of cast removal, 7 months following fusion. Note the solid fusion and the partial improvement of the alignment of L5 in relation to the sacrum. The percentage of slip has not been appreciably changed, but the tilting of L5 in relation to S1 has been significantly altered. The sacrum is now considerably less vertical.

sional backache and a Grade I slip requires no treatment other than careful periodic observation to make sure that the slip is not progressing. Follow-up should be at 6-month intervals, with a lateral standing roentgenogram of the L5 to S1 area on each visit.

A child who presents with acute low back pain and little or no slipping requires treatment of back pain by conservative measures, such as bedrest, casting and Williams' exercises. Fusion is not necessary unless pain is persistent. Braces may be of temporary benefit during periods of low back pain.

A patient who has presented with a more significant slip of Grade III or IV, or one who has been followed periodically and shows progressive slipping from Grade I to Grade II or more, should have fusion, regardless of the presence or absence of symptoms at that time. Certainly, the patient with a Grade II slip or better who presents with pain or tight hamstrings or neurologic deficit must have fusion.

Fusion is usually performed from L4 to S1, using the transverse process fusion procedure. The author prefers to perform this through a vertical midline incision. Theoretically, it is only necessary to fuse L5 to S1, but because the lamina of L5 is floating free and there is no pars interarticularis, the only part of L5 that can be utilized for fusion is the transverse process. This is quite often small, atrophic and displaced forward, and it is very difficult to adequately expose. Thus, for practical reasons, most patients with significant spondylolisthesis have arthrodesis of L4 to S1.

Removal of the loose lamina is not necessary in most patients. It should be removed in those who have neurologic deficits. The L5 nerve root is the one involved, and it is compressed by the fibrocartilaginous reactive material at the region of the pars interarticularis defect. Roots that go over the prominence of the sacrum are not involved, so removing this does not appear to be of any benefit, except in circumstances when there is bladder paralysis. Adequate decompression of the L5 nerve root can be performed by removing this fibrocartilaginous material in the region of the pars defect. Fusion is done lateral to the decompression site, in the transverse process area. Removal of the loose lamina without fusion (Gill procedure) is *never* indicated in the growing child.

The author has always utilized the transverse process fusion and has had no failures with this technique. Midline posterior fusion is not adequate. Anterior interbody arthrodesis, commonly advocated overseas, has not been found to be necessary in our hands, but there is certainly nothing wrong with doing this procedure in the female if the surgeon is skillful with this type of surgery. A double-pantaloon underarm cast, with the hips hyperextended, and bedrest should be used for 4 months, and a lumbosacral brace should be used for the 4 subsequent months (Fig. 16-62).[37]

Reduction of severe slips by instrumentation has been attempted by several authors,[15] but in the author's experience, better results have been obtained by the hyperextension cast.

DISC CALCIFICATION IN CHILDREN

Disc space calcification is a distinct clinical syndrome of uncertain etiology occasionally seen in the cervical spine in children. Boys are more commonly affected than girls, and it occurs usually between the ages of 6 and 12 years. The child presents with pain and stiffness in the neck, usually with local tenderness and torticollis due to localized muscle spasm. There may be mildly elevated temperature, increased sedimentation rate, and mildly increased white blood count, suggesting an infectious etiology. Roentgenograms may be normal early in the course, but 1 to 2 weeks later they may begin to show fluffy calcific densities centrally in the nucleus of one of the discs in the lower cervical spine or, on occasion, in the thoracic spine. Treatment is symptomatic, including neck support, traction, analgesics, and muscle relaxants. The condition runs a self-limiting course, with a consistently good prognosis. Most patients are symptom-free after 3 or 4 weeks. They may have intermittent neck discomfort for 1 to 2 years. Calcification usually regresses and disappears with time, but may stay permanently. The etiology is unknown.

LUMBAR DISC HERNIATION IN CHILDREN

Lumbar disc herniation in children is relatively uncommon. Approximately 1 to 2 per cent of all patients having surgery for herniated lumbar discs are under the age of 20 years. Herniated discs have been reported in patients as young as 10 years, with the incidence slightly higher with advancing years.

The complaints are usually low back pain with or without pain radiating into one or both legs. The patient may present with stiffness in the lower back, a sciatic scoliosis, a deviation to one side on forward bending, and positive straight-leg-raising tests. Objective neurologic findings, such as sensory defects, motor defects, and reflex changes, are much less common in children than adults. This is presumably due to the more resilient nerve roots in the child, which are able to tolerate more pressure without showing objective evidence of nerve deficit.

The differential diagnosis should include spondylolisthesis, disc space infection, osteomyelitis, sacroiliac joint disorder, bone tumor, and instraspinal tumor. Bone scans are appropriate to rule out inflammatory diseases and active bone tumors whereas myelography is indicated to rule out intraspinal neoplasms such as meningioma or spinal cord tumor. Myelography should be routinely performed prior to any surgery.

Virtually all disc lesions in children are at L5-S1 or at L4-L5. Conservative treatment should consist of at least 2 weeks of bedrest with the patient maintaining the contour position and receiving heat and analgesics to relax the muscle spasm. If, at the end of this time, the abnormal findings are still apparent, particularly the positive straight-leg-raising test, myelography should be performed. Even in the presence of a negative myelogram, if the physical findings are consistently positive, surgical exploration should be carried out. False-negative myelograms are consistently found in 5 to 10 per cent of the cases.

At surgery, a hemilaminectomy should be performed with removal of the offending disc. Care should be taken to preserve the facet complex to maintain normal lumbar stability. Fusion is not indicated.

Results are quite good. Contrary to the case of adults, where the recurrence rate is fairly high and persistent symptoms common, the child usually obtains a good or excellent result with a very small likelihood of recurrence.

GLOSSARY

Adolescent Scoliosis. Spinal curvature developing after the onset of puberty and before maturity.

Adult Scoliosis. Spinal curvature existing after skeletal maturity.

Apical Vertebra. The most rotated vertebra in a curve (not necessarily structural); the most deviated from the vertical axis of the patient.

Cervical Curve. Spinal curvature which has its apex from C1 to C6.

Cervicothoracic Curve. Spinal curvature which has its apex at C7 or T1.

Compensation. Accurate alignment of the skull over the sacrum, or the shoulders over the hips.

Compensatory Curve. A curve (which can be structural), above or below a major curve, that tends to maintain normal body alignment.

Congenital Scoliosis. Scoliosis due to congenitally anomalous vertebral development.

Double Structural Curve (Scoliosis). Two structural curves in the same spine.

Double Thoracic Curve (Scoliosis). A scoliosis with two structural thoracic curves and a relatively nonstructural lumbar curve.

End Vertebra. The most cephalad vertebra of a curve whose superior surface, or the most caudad one whose inferior surface,

tilts maximally toward the concavity of the curve.

Gibbus. A sharply angular kyphos.

Fractional Curve. A compensatory curve that is incomplete because it returns to the erect. Its only horizontal vertebra is its caudad or cephalad one.

Full Curve. A curve in which the only horizontal vertebra is at the apex.

Infantile Scoliosis. Spinal curvature developing during the first 3 years of life.

Juvenile Scoliosis. Spinal curvature developing between the skeletal age of 4 years and the onset of puberty.

Kyphos. A change in the alignment of a segment of the spine in the sagittal plane, which increases the apex's posterior angulation.

Kyphoscoliosis. Lateral curvature of the spine, associated with either increased posterior or decreased anterior angulation in the sagittal plane in excess of the accepted normal for that area. In the thoracic region, 20° to 40° of dorsal rounding is considered normal.

Lordoscoliosis. Lateral curvature of the spine, associated with either an increase in anterior curvature or a decrease in posterior angulation in the sagittal plane in excess of normal for that area. In a thoracic spine, where posterior angulation is not normally present, less than 20° of curvature would constitute lordoscoliosis.

Lumbar Curve. Spinal curvature which has its apex from L1 to L4.

Lumbosacral Curve. Spinal curvature which has its apex at L5 or below.

Pelvic Obliquity. Deviation of the pelvis from the horizontal in the frontal plane.

Nonstructural Scoliosis. Spinal curvature without structural characteristics. (See structural curve.)

Primary Curve. The first or earliest of several curves to appear. Usually, but not necessarily, it is the most structural curve.

Structural Curve. The segment of the spine with a fixed lateral curvature. It is not necessarily the largest curve. Roentgenographically it is identified in supine lateral side-bending films by the failure to fully correct.

Thoracic Curve (Scoliosis). Curve with the apex between T1 and T12. There may be upper (T2 to T6) and lower (T7 to T11) thoracic curves. (See double thoracic scoliosis)

Thoracolumbar Curve. Spinal curvature which has its apex at T12 or L1 or at the interspace between these.

REFERENCES

1. Anderson, M., Hwang, S. C., and Green, W. T.: Growth of the normal trunk in boys and girls during the second decade of life. J. Bone Joint Surg., *47A:*1554, 1965.
2. Balmer, G. A., and MacEwen, G. D.: The incidence and treatment of scoliosis in cerebral palsy. J. Bone Joint Surg., *52B:*134, 1970.
3. Bergofsky, E. H., Turino, G. M., and Fishman, A. P.: Cardiorespiratory failure in kyphoscoliosis. Medicine, *38:*263, 1959.
4. Blount, W. P. Use of the Milwaukee brace. Orthop. Clin. North Am., *3:*3, 1972.
5. Blount, W. P., and Moe, J. H.: The Milwaukee Brace. Baltimore, Williams & Wilkins, 1973.
6. Bonnett, C., Brown, J., and Grow, T.: Thoracolumbar scoliosis in cerebral palsy. Results of surgical treatment. J. Bone Joint Surg., *58A:*328, 1976.
7. Bonnett, C., Brown, K. C., Perry, J., Nickel, V. L., Walinski, T., *et al.:* Evolution of treatment of paralytic scoliosis at Rancho Los Amigos Hospital. J. Bone Joint Surg., *57A:*206, 1975.
8. Bradford, D. S., Moe, J. H., Montalvo, F. J., and Winter, R. B.: Scheuermann's kyphosis and roundback deformity—results of Milwaukee brace treatment. J. of Bone and Joint Surgery *56A:*740-758, 1974.
9. ———: Scheuermann's kyphosis—results of surgical treatment by posterior spine arthrodesis in twenty-two patients. J. Bone Joint Surg., *57A:*439, 1975.
10. Brooks, H. L., Azen, S. P., Gerberg, E., Brooks, R., and Chan, L.: Scoliosis: A prospective epidemiologic study. J. Bone Joint Surg., *57A:*968, 1975.
11. Bunch, W. H.: The Milwaukee brace in paralytic scoliosis. Clin. Orthop. *110:*63, 1975.
12. Chaglassian, J. H., Riseborough, E. J., and Hall, J. E.: Neurofibromatosis scoliosis. Natural history and results of treatment in thirty-seven cases. J. Bone Joint Surg., *58A:*695, 1976.
13. Collis, D. K., and Ponseti, I. V.: Long term follow-up of patients with idiopathic scoliosis not treated surgically. J. Bone Joint Surg., *51A:*425, 1969.
14. Cowell, H. R., Hall, J. N., and MacEwen, G. D.: Genetic aspects of idiopathic scoliosis. Clin. Orthop., *86:*121, 1972.
15. Dandy, D. J., and Shannon, M. J.: Lumbosacral subluxation (group I spondylolisthesis). J. Bone Joint Surg., *53B:*578, 1971.
16. Dawson, E., Moe, J. H., and Pedras, C. V.: Spinal deformity in neurofibromatosis—natural history, classification and treatment. (Proc. AAOS.) J. Bone Joint Surg., *55A:*1321, 1973.
17. dePeloux, J., Fauchet, R., Faucon, B., and Stagnara, P.: Le plan d'election pour l'examen radiologigue des cypho-scolioses Rev. de chir. orthop. e repar. de l Appareil Motor *51:*517, 1965.
18. Dickson, J. H., and Harrington, P. R.: The evolution of the Harrington instrumentation technique in scoliosis. J. Bone Joint Surg., *55A:*993, 1973.
19. Dommissee, G. F.: The blood supply of the spinal cord, a critical vascular zone in spinal surgery. J. Bone Joint Surg., *56B:*225, 1974.
20. Drummond, D.: Untreated scoliosis in the adult. Scoliosis Research Society, 1975.
21. Dubousset, J., Guillaumat, M., and Méchen, J. F.: Retentissement rachidjen des laminectomies, les compressions medullaires non-traumatiques de l'enfant. J. Rougerie, Mason et Cie, Chapitre XI, Paris, 1973.
22. Duval-Beaupere, G.: Pathogenic relationship between scoliosis and growth. *In* Zorab, P. A. (ed.): Scoliosis and Growth. London, Churchill Livingstone, 1971.
23. Dwyer, A. F.: Experience of anterior correction of scoliosis. Clin. Orthop., *93:*191, 1973.
24. Dwyer, A. F., Newton, N. C., and Sherwood, A. A.: An anterior approach to scoliosis. A preliminary report. Clin. Orthop. *62:*192, 1969.
25. Dwyer, A. F., and Schafer, M. F.: Anterior approach to scoliosis, results of treatment in 51 cases. J. Bone Joint Surg., *56B:*218, 1974.
26. Ferriera, J. H., and James, J. I. P.: Progressive and resolving infantile iodiopathic scoliosis—differential diagnosis. J. Bone Joint Surg., *54B:*648, 1972.
27. Garrett, A. L., Perry, J., and Nickel, V.: Stabilization of the collapsing spine. J. Bone Joint Surg., *43A:*474, 1961.
28. Ghavamian, T.: The future of minor scoliotic curves of the spine. J. Bone Joint Surg., *57A:*134, 1975.
29. Goldstein, L. A.: Surgical management of scoliosis. J. Bone Joint Surg., *48A:*167, 1966.
30. ———: Treatment of idiopathic scoliosis by Harrington instrumentation and fusion with fresh autogenous iliac bone grafts. J. Bone Joint Surg., *51A:*209, 1969.
31. ———: The surgical treatment of idiopathic scoliosis. Clin. Orthop., *93:*131, 1973.
32. Goldstein, L. A., and Waugh, T. R.: Classification and terminology of scoliosis. Clin. Orthop., *93:*10, 1973.
33. Guthkelch, A. N.: Diastematomyelia with median septum. Brain, *97:*729, 1974.
34. Hall, J. E.: The anterior approach to spinal deformities. Orthop. Clin. North Am., *3:*81, 1972.
35. Harrington, P. R.: Treatment of scoliosis—correction and internal fixation by spine instrumentation. J. Bone Joint Surg., *44A:*591, 1962.
36. ———: Technical details in relation to the successful use of instrumentation in scoliosis. Orthop. Clin. North Am. *3:*49, 1972.
37. Hensinger, R. N., Lang, J. R., and MacEwen, G. D.: Surgical management of spondylolisthesis in children and adolescents. Spine, *1:*207, 1976.
38. James, J. I. P.: Idiopathic scoliosis, the prognosis, diagnosis, and operative indications related to

curve patterns and the age of onset. J. Bone Joint Surg., *36B:*36, 1954.

39. ———: Kyphoscoliosis. J. Bone Joint Surg., *37B:*414, 1955.

40. ———: Infantile idiopathic scoliosis. Clin. Orthop., *77:*57, 1971.

41. ———: The management of infants with scoliosis. J. Bone Joint Surg., *57B:*422, 1975.

42. Johnson, B. E., and Westgate, H. D.: Methods of predicting vital capacity in patients with thoracic scoliosis. J. Bone Joint Surg., *52A:*1433, 1970.

43. Keim, H. A., and Reina, E. G.: Osteoid-osteoma as a cause of scoliosis. J. Bone Joint Surg., *57A:*159, 1975.

44. Kuhns, J. G., and Hormel, R. S.: Management of congenital scoliosis. Arch. Surg., *65:*250, 1952.

45. Laurent, L. E., and Einola, S.: Spondylolisthesis in children and adolescents. Acta Orthop. Scand., *31:*45, 1961.

46. Leatherman, K. D.: The management of rigid spinal curves. Clin. Orthop., *93:*215, 1973.

47. Leider, L. L., Moe, J. H., and Winter, R. B.: Early ambulation after the surgical treatment of idiopathic scoliosis. J. Bone Joint Surg., *54A:*1792, 1972.

48. Lindh, M., and Bjure, J.: Lung volumes in scoliosis before and after correction by the Harrington instrumentation method. Acta Orthop. Scand., *46:*934, 1975.

49. Lloyd-Roberts, G. C., and Pilcher, M. F.: Structural idiopathic scoliosis in infancy—a study of the natural history of 100 patients. J. Bone Joint Surg., *47B:*520, 1965.

50. Lonstein, J. E., Winter, R. B., Moe, J. H., Bianco, A. J., Campbell, R. G.: School screening for the early detection of spinal deformities—progress and pitfalls. Minn. Med., *59:*51, 1976.

51. Lonstein, J. E., Winter, R. B., Moe, J. H., Bradford, D. S., and Bianco, A.: Post laminectomy spine deformity. New Orleans, AAOS, 1976.

52. Lonstein, J. E., Winter, R. B., Moe, J. H., Chou, S., and Pinto, W. C.: Spinal cord compression due to spine deformity. Paper presented to the Scoliosis Research Society, Gothenberg, Sweden, 1973.

53. MacEwen, G. D.: Operative treatment of scoliosis in cerebral palsy. Reconstr. Surg. Traumatol., *13:*58, 1972.

54. MacEwen, G. D., Bunnell, W. P., and Sriram, K.: Acute neurologic complications in the treatment of scoliosis. (A report of the Scoliosis Research Society). J. Bone Joint Surg., *57A:*404, 1975.

55. MacEwen, G. D., Conway, J. J., and Miller, W. T.: Congenital scoliosis with a unilateral bar. Radiology, *90:*711, 1968.

56. MacEwen, G. D., Winter, R. B., and Hardy, J. H.: Evaluation of kidney anomalies in congenital scoliosis. J. Bone Joint Surg., *54A:*1451, 1972.

57. McKee, B. W., Alexander, W. J., and Dunbar, J. S.: Spondylolysis and spondylolisthesis in children, a review. J. Can. Assoc. Radiol., *22:*100, 1971.

58. Mehta, M. H.: The rib-vertebra angle in the early diagnosis between resolving and progressive infantile scoliosis. J. Bone Joint Surg., *54B:*230, 1973.

59. Mir, S. R., Cole, J. R., Lardone, J., and Levine,

D. B.: Early ambulation following spine fusion and Harrington instrumentation in idiopathic scoliosis. Clin. Orthop, *110:*54, 1975.

60. Moe, J. H.: A critical analysis of methods of fusion for scoliosis. An evaluation in 266 patients. J. Bone Joint Surg., *40A:*529, 1958.

61. ———: Complications of scoliosis treatment. Clin. Orthop., *53:*21, 1967.

62. ———: The Milwaukee brace in the treatment of scoliosis. Clin. Orthop., *77:*18, 1971.

63. ———: Methods of correction and surgical techniques in scoliosis. Orthop. Clin. North Am., *3:*17, 1972.

64. ———: Indications for Milwaukee brace nonoperative treatment in idiopathic scoliosis. Clin. Orthop., *93:*38, 1973.

65. Moe, J. H., and Kettleson, D. N.: Idiopathic scoliosis—analysis of curve patterns and the preliminary results of Milwaukee brace treatment in 196 patients. J. Bone Joint Surg., *52A:*1509, 1970.

66. Nachemson, A.: A long-term follow-up study of nontreated scoliosis. Acta Orthop. Scand., *39:*466, 1968.

67. Nasca, R. J., Stelling, F. H., and Steel. H. H.: Progression of congenital scoliosis due to hemivertebrae and hemivertebrae with bars. J. Bone Joint Surg., *57A:*456, 1975.

68. Nash, C. L., and Moe. J. H.: A study of vertebral rotation. J. Bone Joint Surg., *51A:*223, 1969.

69. Newman, P. H.: The etiology of spondylolisthesis. J. Bone Joint Surg., *45B:*39, 1963.

70. Nilsonne, U., and Lundgren, K. D.: Long-term prognosis in idiopathic scoliosis. Acta Orthop. Scand., *39:*456, 1968.

71. Nordwall, A.: Studies in idiopathic scoliosis—relevant to etiology, conservative and operative treatment. Acta Orthop. Scand. [Suppl.], *150,* 1973.

72. O'Brien J. P., and Yau, A. C.: Anterior and posterior correction and fusion for paralytic scoliosis. Clin. Orthop., *86:*151, 1972.

73. Ponseti, I. V., and Friedman, B.: Prognosis in idiopathic scoliosis. J. Bone Joint Surg., *32A:*381, 1950.

74. Reckles, L. N., Peterson, H. A., Bianco, A. J., and Weidman, W. H.: The association of scoliosis and congenital heart defects. J. Bone Joint Surg., *57A:*449, 1975.

75. Riseborough, E. J.: The anterior approach to the spine for the correction of deformities of the axial skeleton. Clin. Orthop., *93:*207, 1973.

76. Riseborough, E. J., and Wynn-Davies, R.: A genetic survey of idiopathic scoliosis in Boston, Mass. J. Bone Joint Surg., *55A:*974, 1973.

77. Robins, P. R., Moe, J. H., and Winter, R. B.: Scoliosis in Marfan's syndrome. Its characteristics and results of treatment in 35 patients. J. Bone Joint Surg., *57A:*358, 1975.

78. Robson, P.: The prevalence of scoliosis in adolescents and young adults with cerebral palsy. Dev. Med. Child Neurol., *10:*447, 1968.

79. Rosenthal, R. K., Levine, D. B., and McCarver, C. L.: The occurrence of scoliosis in cerebral palsy. Dev. Med. and Child Neurol., *16:*664, 1974.

80. Samilson, R., and Bechard, R.: Scoliosis in cere-

bral palsy: incidence, distribution of curve patterns, natural history and thoughts on etiology. Curr. Pract. Orthop. Surg., *5:*183, 1973.

81. Scott, J. C.: Scoliosis and neurofibromatosis. J. Bone Joint Surg., *47B:*240, 1965.

82. Scott, J. C., and Morgan, T. H.: Natural history and prognosis of infantile idiopathic scoliosis. J. Bone Joint Surg., *37B:*400, 1955.

83. Shannon, D. C., Riseborough, E. J., Valenca, L. M., and Kazeuri, H.: The distribution of abnormal lung function in kyphoscoliosis. J. Bone Joint Surg., *52A:*131, 1970.

84. Sommer, J.: Congenital functional scoliosis. Acta Orthop. Scand., *39:*447, 1968.

85. Sörenson, K. H.: Scheuermann's Juvenile Kyphosis. Copenhagen, Munksgaard, 1964.

86. Stagnara, P., Fauchet, R., Boulliat, G., dePeloux, J., Mazoyer, D., *et al.:* A propos de 17 observations de paraplegies par deformations vertebrales traites par redressment partiel. Rev. d. Chir Orto e Repar. Appar. Moteur *54:*623, 1968.

87. Tachdjian, M. O., and Matson, D. D.: Orthopaedic aspects of intraspinal tumors in infants and children. J. Bone Joint Surg., *47A:*223, 1965.

88. Turner, R. H., and Bianco, A. J.: Spondylolysis and spondylolisthesis in teenagers and children. J. Bone Joint Surg. *53A:* 1298, 1971.

89. Wiltse, L. L., Widell, E. H., and Jackson, D. W.: Fatigue fracture: the basic lesion in isthmic spondylolisthesis. J. Bone Joint Surg., *57A:*17, 1975.

90. Winter, R. B., Moe, J. H., and Eilers, V. E.: Congenital scoliosis—a study of 234 patients treated and untreated. J. Bone Joint Surg., *50A:*1, 1968.

91. Winter, R. B., Haven, J. J., Moe, J. H., and Lagaard, S. M.: Diastematomyelia and congenital spine deformities. J. Bone Joint Surg., *56A:*27, 1974.

92. Winter, R. B., Lovell, W. W., and Moe, J. H.: Excessive thoracic lordosis and loss of pulmonary function in patients with idiopathic scoliosis. J. Bone Joint Surg., *57A:*972, 1975.

93. Winter, R. B., MacEwen, G. D., Moe, J. H., and Peon, H.: Milwaukee brace in congenital scoliosis. Spine, *1:*85, 1976.

94. Winter, R. B., Moe, J. H., and Wang, J. F.: Congenital kyphosis. Its natural history and treatment as observed in a study of 130 patients. J. Bone Joint Surg., *55A:*223, 1973.

95. Wynn-Davies, R.: Familial (idiopathic) scoliosis —a family survey. J. Bone Joint Surg., *50B:*24, 1968.

17 *The Upper Limb*

Daniel C. Riordan, M.D.

SPRENGEL'S DEFORMITY (CONGENITAL ELEVATION OF THE SCAPULA)

Clinical Features

This condition was described by Eulenberg[1] in 1863. It is an uncommon congenital anomaly characterized by elevation and medial rotation of the inferior pole of the scapula. The elevation may vary from 2 to 10 centimeters. The deformity is usually unilateral, but may be bilateral. It is frequently associated with other deformities of the cervical and thoracic spine, such as hemivertebrae[3] and fusion or absence of the ribs.

The affected scapula is usually small, with a decreased vertical length and anterior bending of the upper portion. There may be a bony, cartilaginous or fibrous connection to the cervical or upper thoracic spine.[4] The connection may be to the lamina, to the transverse process or the spinous process of the vertebrae, and may be single or multiple. Occasionally the connection is by bone, and if so, this bone is known as the omovertebral bone.[2]

Diagnosis

Roentgenograms are necessary to determine the degree of development of the scapula, the degree of angular deformity, the presence or absence of a connection to the cervical or thoracic spine and the presence or absence of an omovertebral bone (Fig. 17-1).

The clinical examination shows the amount of elevation and the presence or absence of an associated torticollis,[5] with or without muscle contraction. The limitation of abduction of the shoulder is generally proportional to the severity of angulation and elevation of the scapula (Fig. 17-2). For differential diagnosis, the muscle examination should rule out paralysis of the serratus anterior muscle and obstetrical or birth paralyses. The degee of fixation of the scapula should be determined, as well as the quantity of malrotation and malposition. The muscles about the shoulder should be tested as thoroughly as possible, which may be quite difficult with the fixed position of the scapula.

Treatment

The treatment of choice is surgery. The deformity does not progress, but it does not spontaneously improve without surgery. Conservative treatment does not result in any improvement. Physical therapy also is not helpful.

Numerous surgical treatments have been described. The basic goal of surgery is to lower the scapula to a more normal position and to decrease its fixation or, conversely, to increase its mobility. The Schrock procedure[4] was used in the past, but it involved only excision of the upper portion of the scapula; it neither lowered the body of the scapula nor increased mobility. This procedure is not recommended.

The two procedures which have had the best results are the Green[2] and Woodward[5] procedures. The Green procedure consists of an extra-periosteal dissection of the mus-

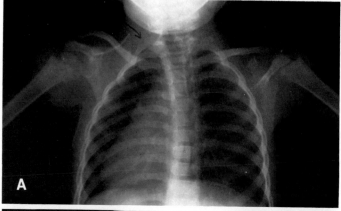

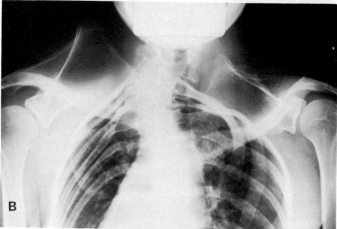

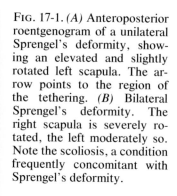

FIG. 17-1. *(A)* Anteroposterior roentgenogram of a unilateral Sprengel's deformity, showing an elevated and slightly rotated left scapula. The arrow points to the region of the tethering. *(B)* Bilateral Sprengel's deformity. The right scapula is severely rotated, the left moderately so. Note the scoliosis, a condition frequently concomitant with Sprengel's deformity.

cles from the scapula, resection of the upper corner of the scapula, which is affixed over the upper aspect of the first rib, insertion of a pull-out wire to pull the scapula down, resuturing of the scapula at a lower level, and reattachment of the muscles in a more anatomic position. This is followed by a period of traction, in which the scapula is gradually pulled down by rubberband traction attached to the wire. The rubberband is attached to a hip spica.

The Woodward procedure uses a somewhat different approach. A midline incision is made, rather than the scapular incision of the Green procedure. Basically, in the Woodward procedure the muscles are dissected at the point of their origin along the spine, rather than at the point of their insertion along the scapula. The trapezius, leva-

tor scapulae and rhomboids must all be detached from the scapula. Any fibrous, cartilaginous or bony bridge must be excised, as must any attachment of the upper corner of the scapula over the first rib. The scapula is then brought down to a more nearly normal anatomic position, and the muscles are reattached, also to approximate a normal anatomic position. Great care must be taken to protect the eleventh cranial nerve.

This procedure can be supplemented by a small incision over the midportion of the clavicle, and, with a rongeur, a small segment of the scapula can be osteotomized, thus giving more mobility to the shoulder girdle and protecting the great vessels and brachial plexus from the clavicle's exerting excessive pressure against the first rib.

In general, this combined procedure of

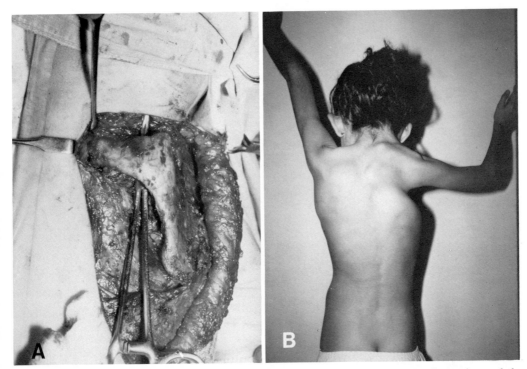

FIG. 17-2. *(A)* In this patient there is an omovertebral bone connecting the cervical spine and the scapula. *(B)* Posterior view of a patient with a right Sprengel's deformity, showing the typical loss of shoulder abduction and elevation.

clavicular osteotomy, coupled with the Woodward procedure, has given consistently good results, in terms of the cosmetic appearance of the scapula, as well as providing improved motion, particularly in elevation. Only those patients with severe deficits of motor muscle function to the shoulder girdle have not benefited functionally from this operation. The ideal age for surgery is between 4 and 7 years, but it has been done for both younger and older children.

CONGENITAL DISLOCATION OF THE SHOULDER

Clinical Features

Congenital dislocation of the shoulder is usually seen only when there are other associated deformities of the upper extremity. It is seen in general underdevelopment of the upper extremity, in absence of the radius, and in arthrogryposis in varying degrees. The shoulders are small in appearance, and the humerus is unstable in all directions, but its instability does not produce pain. The deltoid, pectorals and other periscapular muscles are deficient or absent. The proximal, central, or distal humerus may be deficient, or it may be totally absent. Roentgenograms show a small scapula in normal position, an undeveloped glenoid, and a small or absent one-third of the humerus. If the condition is associated with arthyrogryposis, the biceps or triceps, or both, may be absent or markedly underdeveloped.[6]

Diagnosis

Diagnosis is made by observation of a small shoulder and an unstable shoulder

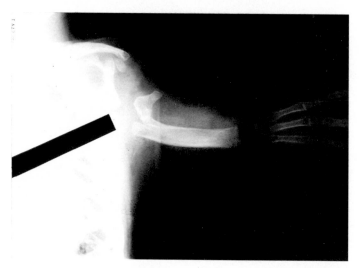

FIG. 17-3. Anteroposterior roentgenogram of congenital dislocation of shoulder due to incomplete formation of the scapula and humerous.

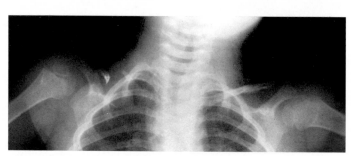

FIG. 17-4. Anteroposterior roentgenogram of pseudarthrosis of right clavicle, the central portion being defective.

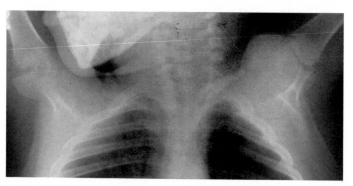

FIG. 17-5. Anteroposterior roentgenogram of congenital absence of the lateral half of both clavicles.

joint, and the diagnosis is confirmed by roentgenograms. The physical examination shows a more or less unstable, paralyzed shoulder, as seen in poliomyelitis. Motion is attained by contortions of other body parts and gravity.

Treatment

No satisfactory surgical treatment is available at this time. In rare instances, shoulder fusion may offer some functional improvement, if there is sufficient bone present to achieve fusion and sufficient muscular support of the scapula to achieve control (Fig. 17-3).[7]

CONGENITAL PSEUDARTHROSIS OF THE CLAVICLE

Clinical Features

The term "congenital pseudarthrosis of the clavicle"[8] implies the presence of a proximal and distal clavicle, with an absent central section. This is more common than total absence of the clavicle. A partial absence of the clavicle may be seen. This may be an absence of the lateral half of the clavicle, and may be unilateral or bilateral.

In true pseudarthrosis of the clavicle, there is usually a deficient central one-third of the clavicle (Fig. 17-4), or absence of lateral half (Fig. 17-5). Occasionally it is present at birth, but is overlooked. It may also exist as a thinned, central portion of the clavicle, which may be fractured by lifting the infant or child, or by the child's falling. When this occurs, the area is painful when the shoulder is moved. Consequently, this type is often diagnosed by the presence of pain and shoulder instability, and the diagnosis is confirmed by roentgenogram. Lack of callus and failure to heal means that surgery is necessary.

Treatment

The best treatment is early operation, at age 3 to 6 years (Fig. 17-6). Internal fixation is achieved with an intramedullary pin, the type being dependent on the size of the child. Multiple bone grafts are taken from the ilium, the bone grafts are fixated to the site by sutures placed like bands around barrel staves. The graft should be long enough to bridge the defect between the proximal and distal fragments and to fill the intervening spaces in the medullary canal with cancellous bone. If good technique is used, adequate fixation is obtained, and an adequate amount of bone is used, union should result. The symptoms of pain and instability disappear. Fixation of grafts with screws, such as on a double onlay graft, is not recommended because of the proximity of the brachial artery and plexus.

Cleidocranial Dysostosis

Absence of the clavicle associated with cranial deformation is known as cleidocranial dysostosis.[9] In this condition, there may be a total absence of the entire clavicle, absence of all but a small bony remnant of the distal or proximal ends, or both (Fig. 17-7A). The skull is broad, with an increased transverse diameter and widely opened fontanelles due to the delayed or absent ossification of the skull (Fig. 17-7B). The clinical appearance of the absence of the clavicle is that of drooping shoulders (Fig. 17-7C). This is usually bilateral, and the neck is quite wide at its base, giving the appearance of a web between the neck and shoulders. With the total absence of the clavicles, the patient usually has the ability to bring the shoulders together anteriorly (Fig. 17-7D). The muscles attaching to the clavicle are anomalous or absent. The patient usually has no symptoms, except that the adult may occasionally have difficulty carrying heavy weights due to the traction on the brachial plexus. Treatment for this condition is not indicated. There are few or no symptoms.

OSTEOCHONDRITIS DISSECANS OF THE ELBOW

Clinical features

Osteochondritis dissecans of the elbow (Fig. 17-8) is probably not a congenital lesion, but it is seen predominently in adolescent males.[10,11] Although trauma is frequently blamed, it has not been definitely linked to this condition. Clinically, the onset is insidious and may be manifested by a dull aching pain and slight limitation of motion. Occa-

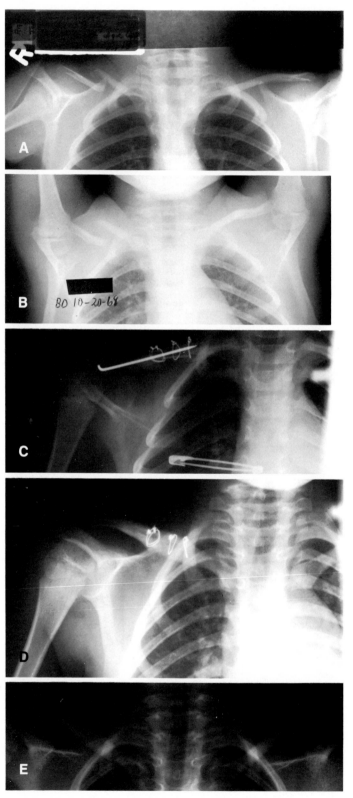

Fig. 17-6. *(A)* Anteroposterior roentgenogram of congenital pseudoarthrosis of the right clavicle, which was painful. *(B)* Roentgenogram of the same patient with the arms elevated, showing motion at the pseudoarthrosis. *(C)* Roentgenogram of the patient 2 months later after iliac segmental grafting. Barrel-stave grafts were fixed with an intrameduallary .062 Kirschner wire and wire loops. *(D)* Roentgenogram of the patient 5 months after grafting and after removal of the intramedullary pin. *(E)* A roentgenogram of the patient taken 1 year postoperatively.

FIG. 17-7. (A) This roentgenogram, although marred, shows a 25-year-old adult with cleidocranial dystosis, showing absence of proximal third of both clavicles and pseudarthrosis of both clavicles. (B) Lateral view of the skull, showing open suture lines and frontal bossing. (C) A child with cleidocranial dystosis, showing drooping shoulders. (D) The same child, showing the left shoulder swinging anteriorly.

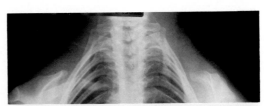

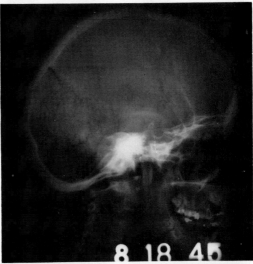

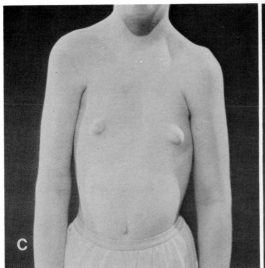

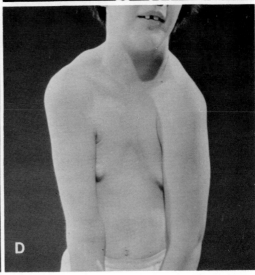

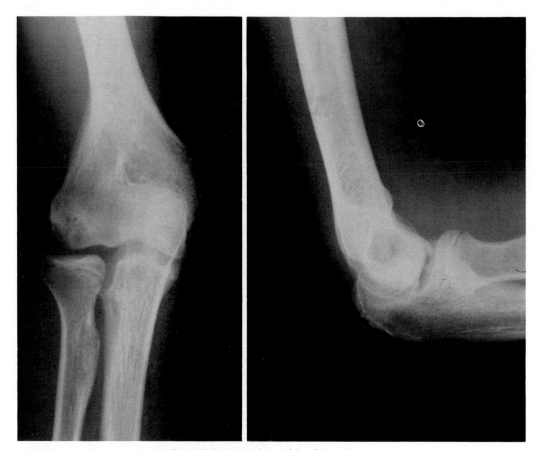

Fig. 17-8. Osteochondritis of the elbow.

sionally a loose body may separate and cause locking of the elbow, followed by pain and effusion. It may be a silent lesion, which is discovered only accidentally on a roentgenogram taken for another condition. The radial head may become enlarged clinically, and this is confirmed by roentgenogram. The early roentgenographic changes are rarefaction of a small area in the capitellum and, later, separation of a small fragment, leaving a small punched-out cavity. This usually results in a loose body that locks the elbow.

Treatment

Treatment should not be surgical, unless locking occurs or the presence of loose body can be proven by roentgenogram. Conservative treatment, consisting of rest and limited activities, including the use of a sling or posterior splint, if necessary, can result in healing of the bone lesion if treatment is undertaken before separation of the fragment occurs. The radial head should not be resected in children for this condition.[12] Resection should be reserved for adults, but only after marked degenerative changes and limitation of motion has resulted.

CONGENITAL RADIOULNAR SYNOSTOSIS

Congenital radioulnar synostosis is present at birth, and may be bilateral. It occurs in the proximal one-third of the forearm (Fig. 17-9). The lack of rotation may be the only finding in a newborn or very young infant, as roentgenograms of children this young do

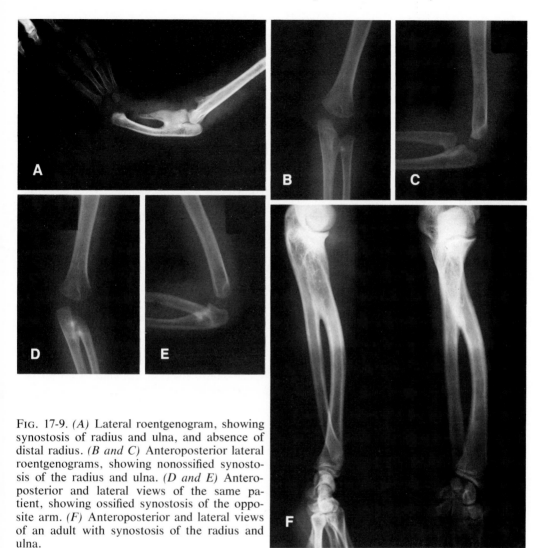

FIG. 17-9. *(A)* Lateral roentgenogram, showing synostosis of radius and ulna, and absence of distal radius. *(B and C)* Anteroposterior lateral roentgenograms, showing nonossified synostosis of the radius and ulna. *(D and E)* Anteroposterior and lateral views of the same patient, showing ossified synostosis of the opposite arm. *(F)* Anteroposterior and lateral views of an adult with synostosis of the radius and ulna.

not show the synchondrosis, which later becomes the osseous bridge between the radius and ulna. The joining of the marrow cavities of the radius and ulna may not be evident on roentgenograms at birth, and only appears after the age of 1 year, when more ossification has occurred. In some cases, the elbow may be dislocated anteriorly or posteriorly. Because of the lack of rotation, there is usually an absence of the supinator brevis muscle and underdevelopment or absence of the pronator teres and pronator quadratus. The forearm is usually in pronation, and occasionally may be so pronated that derota-

tional osteotomy is indicated on one arm, if the condition is bilateral. Other surgical procedures, such as resection of the synostosis or resection of the radial head and arthroplasty of the synostosis by insertion of a swivel type of joint, have been uniformly unsuccessful, and these procedures are not recommended. Generally this condition produces no symptoms, except for the inability to supinate. This loss of function is usually not too much of a handicap, except if it is bilateral, in which case the person usually is unable to supinate the forearm and cup the palm, as for receiving change.

If osteotomy for derotation of the forearm is contemplated, it is usually felt that it should be done on the minor arm rather than on the major arm, since the position of the function is usually considered to be in mild to moderate pronation, the usual position of most cases of synostosis.

CONGENITAL RADIOHUMERAL SYNOSTOSIS

Clinical Features

Congenital radiohumeral synostosis is rarely seen, except in association with other deformities of the forearm and hand. The most commonly associated deformity is partial or complete absence of the ulna. In this condition (Fig. 17-10A), there is failure of segmentation of an elbow joint during development, so that the distal humeral epiphysis and proximal radial epiphysis are not formed, and there is fusion of those two bones. There may be partial or complete absence of the ulna. Most commonly, the absence is in the distal half of the ulna, with only a small cartilaginous anlage present at the elbow region. This results in considerable shortening of the upper extremity, since growth attributable to the distal humeral epiphysis and the proximal radius and ulna is absent (Fig. 17-10B). There is usually deformity of the forearm, with the radius being markedly bowed, and frequently the hand points toward the posterior aspect of the body, rather than the anterior aspect. This is further discussed on page 714.

Treatment

Surgical treatment of the elbow joint is not recommended, unless the forearm is pointed posteriorly. The absence of the elbow joint is usually accompanied by absence or deficiency of the muscles associated with flexion of the elbow or rotation of the forearm. Surgical attempts to provide motion of the elbow joint are not recommended, since the deformity results in severe shortening of the forearm. It is felt that if osteotomy is done to correct the posterior angulation of the arm, the anterior angulation accomplished by the osteotomy should be not more than 25° of flexion. This puts the

hand into a range of function, avoiding its being so acutely flexed that the person is unable to take care of normal toilet needs because of the shortness of the extremity. Arthroplasty performed in an attempt to establish motion is not advised.

CONGENITAL DISLOCATION OF THE RADIAL HEAD

Clinical Features

Congenital dislocation of the radial head (Fig. 17-11A) may occur as an isolated deformity with no other deformity of the extremity. It is probably due to a malformed capitellum, which leads to a dome-shaped rather than a cup-shaped radial head, thus resulting in instability. The radial head may be dislocated at birth, or dislocation may occur shortly after birth. The head may dislocate anteriorly, posteriorly or posterolaterally. The anterior dislocation is not obvious clinically at birth and may not be diagnosed early. The posterior or posterolateral dislocation causes a prominence at the elbow and is usually more easily recognized. Therefore, it may be diagnosed at birth or shortly thereafter. The anterior dislocation may not be evident for some months until it is noticed that the patient is unable to fully flex the elbow. Roentgenograms of both elbows taken shortly after birth reveal the dislocation of the radius, even though there is not full ossification of the proximal end of this bone at birth. There may be some limitation of flexion or extension, depending on the direction of the dislocation of the radius. There is usually loss of rotation, with supination usually being the motion lost.

Treatment

There are usually few symptoms associated with the congenital form of this condition, and the need for surgical correction is not usually great. Traumatic anterior dislocation of the head of the radius from traction on the forearm may be difficult to differentiate from congenital dislocation, although this condition is usually seen in a child of 2 years or older, as it is usually as-

FIG. 17-10. *(A)* Anteroposterior roentgenogram, showing synostosis of humerus and radius, with partial absence of distal ulna, and ulnar defects of the hand and wrist. *(B)* Anteroposterior and lateral views of synostosis of the humerus and radius in a straight line, with the ulna appearing as a supracondylar bone.

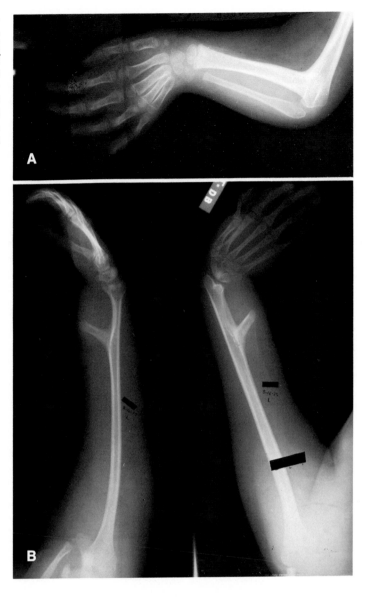

sociated with a child who is walking. The radial head is cup-shaped, not dome-shaped (Fig. 17-11B).

If the dislocation of the radius is diagnosed at or shortly after birth, it may be possible in some cases to reduce the dislocation, but it is usually quite difficult to maintain the reduction. Even if an open surgical procedure should be done to accomplish the reduction and reconstruct the ligaments around the radial head and the capitellum, the success rate of maintaining the reduction is usually not very high. The capitellum is usually deformed and rather flat, and the radial head is dome-shaped, so that the dislocation frequently recurs within a short period of time. Resection of the radial head is not advised on growing children, as it usually produces considerable disturbance of the distal radioulnar articulation and results in proximal migration of the radius, increasing the shortening of the forearm. Late complications usually can be expected at the distal articulation if the radial head is resected in a

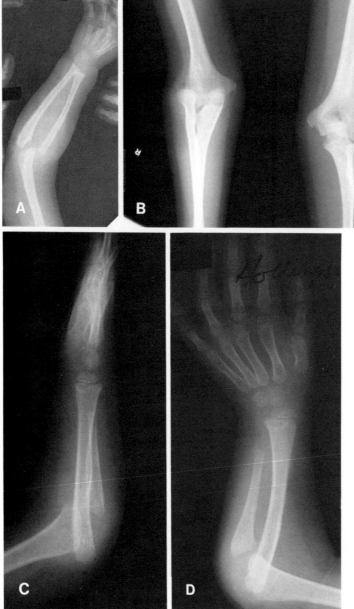

Fig. 17-11. *(A)* Anteroposterior roentgenogram, showing dislocation of radial head at elbow. *(B)* Anteroposterior views of both elbows of a 10-year-old child, showing a dislocated radial head on the right and a dome-shaped radial head. *(C and D)* Anteroposterior and lateral views, showing dislocation of the radial head in association with partial absence of distal ulna.

FIG. 17-12. Anteroposterior and lateral views of a dislocated elbow.

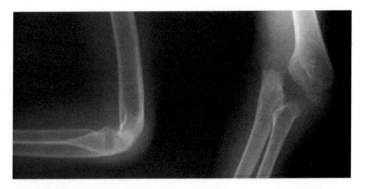

growing child. This approach to the treatment of the condition is not recommended.

Congenital dislocation of the radial head can also be seen in association with partial or complete absence of the ulna (Fig. 17-10C and D), and this will be discussed in that section. Resection of the radial head can be done after growth is complete if the problem is symptomatic.

CONGENITAL DISLOCATION OF THE ELBOW

Clinical Features

Congenital dislocation of the elbow is a rare condition as an isolated deformity. If the dislocation is posterior, there is limitation of flexion. Most commonly, deformity of the forearm bones is the cause for the dislocation of the elbow. It is either incomplete formation of the distal humerus or incomplete formation of the proximal ulna that results in an unstable or dislocated elbow. In contrast to a traumatic dislocation of the elbow, the congenitally dislocated elbow is usually not painful (Fig. 17-12).

Treatment

The dislocation is usually obvious at birth, and if treated then, a reduction can usually be obtained, and should be immobilized in plaster. The treatment should be similar to the type of treatment used for a congenital clubfoot, with frequent cast changes to obtain the reduction and maintain the reduction, gradually bringing the elbow into flexion in a normally articulated position between the humerus and ulna. In the rare case

in which an open reduction of the elbow may be necessary, it is usually difficult to maintain the reduction. Short-term pinning with Kirschner wires is recommended to maintain the reduction until ligament reconstruction is given a chance to heal. Immobilization should probably not exceed 2 months, and efforts should be made to establish motion early, so that the motion will help in the formation of a proximal ulna and distal humerus.

CONGENITAL ABSENCE OF THE THUMB

Clinical Features

Congenital absence of the thumb may involve a total absence, partial absence or perhaps only a slight underdevelopment of the thumb (Fig. 17-13). Total absence of the thumb is usually associated with other deformities of the hand or forearm. The deformity may be unilateral or bilateral. In some cases the remainder of the hand and forearm may be practically normal, except for some mild shortening of the radius. There may be incomplete development of the proximal part of the first metacarpal, so that there is instability of the thumb at the carpometacarpal joint. There may be a partial or total absence of the first metacarpal, which leaves the proximal and distal phalanx with only flail motion. Partial absence of the thumb is frequently associated with defects of the radius, ranging from a partial absence or total absence of the radius. On rare occasions, the absence of the thumb is

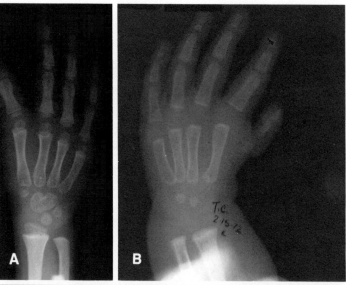

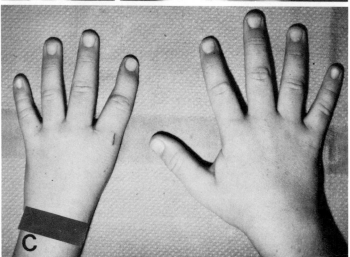

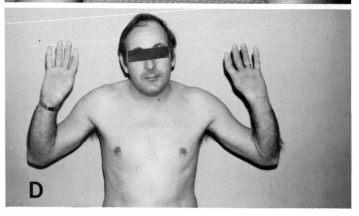

FIG. 17-13. (A) Anteroposterior roentgenogram, showing total absence of the thumb with a delta middle phalanx of the index finger and fusion of capitate and hamate. (B) Partial absence of the first metacarpal. (C) An absent thumb with a normal hand; no other deformities are present. (D) Bilateral absence of the thumbs in an adult.

FIG. 17-14. *(A)* Preoperative view of a hand with absence of the thumb. *(B)* The thumb as it appears 1 year after pollicization.

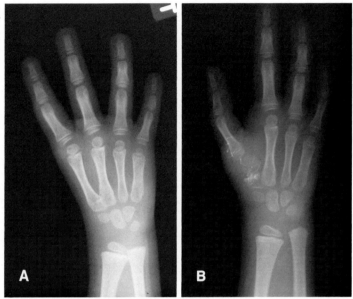

associated with partial or complete absence of the ulna and its attendant deformities.

Treatment

Reconstruction of the thumb depends upon the type of deformity present. The thumb that has only slight underdevelopment of the proximal end of the first metacarpal may be stabilized by reconstructing ligaments, giving some stability between the greater trapezium and the loose base of the first metacarpal. If this is done in a young patient, it should be remembered that the growth center for the first metacarpal is the proximal end, and no drilling of the bone should be done at this point. The cartilaginous part of this first metacarpal may be sutured, but no holes should be drilled in this bone until the child is old enough so that the epiphysis is visualized on roentgenogram. If there is absence of the proximal half of the first metacarpal with a distal metacarpal and thumb of reasonable size with tendons, it may be possible to do a proximal reconstruction of this bone by transplanting the distal one-third of the fourth metacarpal. In this case, the entire joint surface is taken with the attendant collateral ligaments, so that stability can be obtained when grafting this part of the bone. As is usual with the

transplant of epiphyses on growing children, this graft should not be expected to grow. Unless the first metacarpal has an anomalous distal epiphysis, the thumb at full maturation will be a very short digit. Some authors have recommended repeated bone grafting to lengthen these thumbs.[16] In some conditions this is warranted. If the entire first metacarpal is absent, it is recommended that an early amputation of the floating thumb be done. If the condition is unilateral, it is not recommended that pollicization of the thumb be carried out. If the condition is bilateral, it is recommended that reconstruction of the thumb by pollicization of the index finger be done bilaterally. If reconstruction of the thumb is carried out by pollicization of the index finger, it is recommended that the principles outlined by Littler[15] and Buck-Gramcko[13] be used. The technical details of this procedure can be obtained from the original articles. The preferred age for pollicization, as recommended by Buck-Gramcko, is at least 4 years.[14] This author performs pollicization on patients between the ages of 6 and 12 months, and finds that satisfactory development of the thumb can be achieved even when the procedure is done at this early age. It is recommended that if pollicization

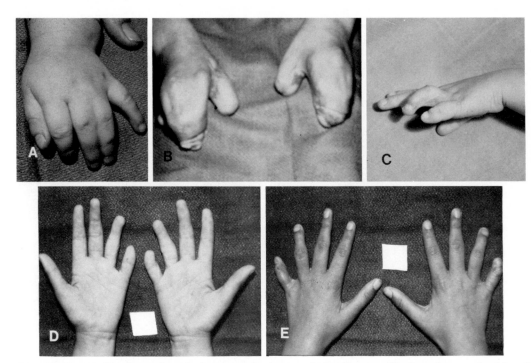

FIG. 17-15. *(A)* Simple syndactyly between the long and ring fingers. *(B)* Complex syndactyly of Apert's syndrome, with partially separated thumbs. *(C)* Lateral view of a hand 4 years after separation and grafting of the ring and little fingers, showing residual curvature of ring finger. *(D)* The hands of the patient in *C,* 13 years after operation for separation of both ring and little fingers. *(E)* Dorsal view of the hands of the same patient.

is carried out, the techniques of utilizing the second metacarpal head and its ligaments as the greater trapezium and advancing the interossei to the middle joint of the index finger establish a much better functioning thumb and a better appearing thumb (Fig. 17-14).

SYNDACTYLY

Clinical Features

Syndactyly is one of the most common hand anomalies, and is seen most often between the long and ring fingers. The next most common area is between the ring and little fingers. It occurs slightly more often in males than in females. It is frequently accompanied by syndactyly of the feet. It is also associated with a number of syndromes with multiple anomalies, such as Apert's syndrome (acrocephalosyndactyly). Different degress of webbing may occur. The simplest is for the fingers to be joined only by a skin bridge, each finger having its own tendons, nerves and bone structures, which are essentially normal.

Treatment

Treatment requires reconstruction of the skin web and skin grafting at the bases of the adjoining fingers and, in varying amounts on the contiguous sides of the involved fingers (Fig. 17-15). The distal phalanges may be joined by fusion, and they usually have a common nail. If the fingers are of equal lengths, the need for surgical separation is not urgent. If the fingers are of different lengths, the fingers should be separated in the period betwen 6 months and 1 year, or the shorter finger causes curved growth of the longer finger.[17] Treatment in these cases requires web reconstruction and skin grafting of the contiguous sides, including grafting directly on the bone laid bare by the separation of the fused distal phalanges. In

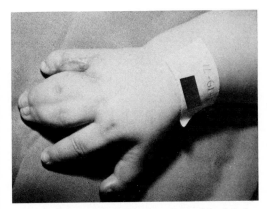

FIG. 17-16. In this hand, separation of the border fingers was the first operation.

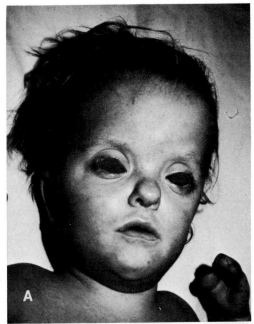

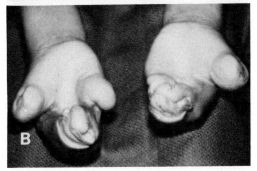

FIG. 17-17. (A) A child with Apert's syndrome, showing the typical facies. (B) The fused nails and distal phalanges of Apert's syndrome.

some cases the bones are fused the full length of the fingers, which requires splitting of the bone of all three phalanges. Skin grafting is necessary to a greater degree. In this type of case, the flexor and extensor tendons may be Y-shaped, with a single tendon at the metacarpal head level, or the tendons may be broad and flat, necessitating the splitting of the tendons along the full length of the fingers. In this case, there are no collateral ligaments of the interphalangeal joints and no pulleys for the flexor tendon. Usually, however, the joint motion is so poor that a fibrous ankylosis usually results, and the fingers are best immobilized in the position of some flexion during the healing phase. There is some disagreement as to when separation of the fingers should be done. The best rule to follow is to separate the fingers early, between the ages of 6 and 12 months if the distal bones are fused, and certainly by age 1 or 2 years if only a skin bridge exists. If a web is properly constructed with a flap of skin and subcutaneous fat, the tissues usually remain where they are placed during growth. Occasionally they may have to be revised if they migrate distally during the rapid growth period of adolescence. When separating the skin of these fused fingers, surgical incisions should be zig-zagged or S-shaped to prevent longitudinal scars from contracting at a later time and leading to late deformities.

If more than two fingers are included in the syndactyly, it is not recommended that both sides of the finger be operated on at the

same time. If the index, long, ring and little fingers are all joined, it is best to separate the border fingers (the index and little) first, separating the central fingers after an interval of approximately 3 months (Fig. 17-16). Nerves can be split and made to go to individual fingers, but vessels cannot. It requires some care and demands proper spacing of procedures if all four fingers are to be separated safely.

Apert's Syndrome

Complicated syndactylies are seen in syndromes such as Apert's achrocephalo-syndactyly.[18] In this condition the facies

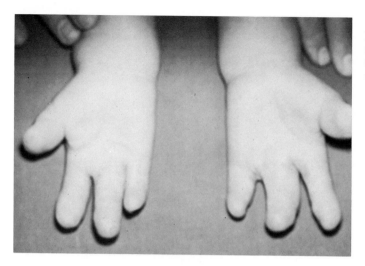

Fig. 17-18. Palmar view of the hands of a child with Apert's syndrome, after separation and construction of the thumb and three fingers.

is characterized by a high broad forehead, wide-set eyes with the outer canthus lower than the inner, a prominent lower jaw and a sunken, small maxilla (Fig. 17-17A). The teeth are crowded, the hard palate is high and arched and may be cleft posteriorly. The hand deformities are usually symmetrical, and there is complicated syndactyly of the long, ring and little fingers. There is little or no interphalangeal joint motion. The fingers are shorter than normal. The syndactyly is usually complete, with bone fusion of the distal phalanges of the central fingers (Fig. 17-17B). The fingernail may be a broad sheet covering all distal phalanges. The different finger lengths combined with the distal fusion results in a diamond-shaped configuration of the fingers and their metacarpals. The little finger is not usually fused at the distal phalanx. The thumb is usually separate and short and may have a single phalanx, although the thumb metacarpal is usually normal.

The finger metacarpals are short. The bases of the fourth and fifth metacarpals may be fused. If separation of the bony fusion of the distal phalanges of the index, long, ring and fifth fingers is not done early, the third and fourth metacarpals are forced to diverge because of differential growth and distal tethering. A roentgenographic appearance of diamond-shaped, longitudinally arranged fusions is a characteristic feature.

The surgical treatment of Apert's syndrome is difficult because of the complex syndactylies present. It is recommended that the separation of the border digits—the thumb and little finger—be done before the age of 1 year. Separation of the central fingers can be delayed until sufficient ossification has occurred to determine which bones belong to which fingers. Because of the complex syndactyly involving the bones, there is usually insufficient skin to provide adequate coverage for all four fingers, and it is wiser to produce a hand containing a thumb and three fingers (Fig. 17-18). Generally separation of the thumb and index fingers and the ring and little fingers is done before 1 year, and separation of the remaining fingers is usually best accomplished by amputation of the central or long finger, making two fingers out of the three. Because of the marked bony involvement, there is usually marked limitation of motion of the interphalangeal joints. When the fingers are separated, it is best to place the interphalangeal joints in some degree of flexion when doing the skin grafting. This is most easily accomplished by using Kirschner wires to maintain bone position during the healing phase of the skin graft. This may prevent a second operative procedure for fusion of the interphalangeal joints in flexion at a later date. Late surgery is frequently indicated in these unfortunate children because of the lack of interphalangeal joint motion and the need to place the fingers

FIG. 17-19. Dorsal view of gigantism of the index and long fingers.

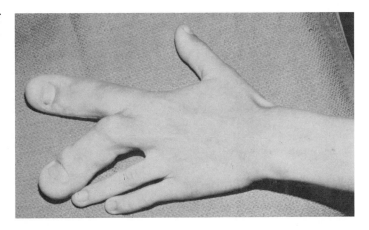

in a more curved position to allow better grasping of medium-sized objects.

GIGANTISM OF THE FINGERS

Clinical Features

Gigantism in fingers may also be termed "macrodactyly." It is characterized by an increased size of all structures of a finger, including the bony phalanges, tendons, nerves, blood vessels, fat, finger nails and skin. Macrodactyly must be distinguished from other causes of finger enlargement, such as neurofibroma, hemangioma, lymphangioma, arteriovenous fistula, fibrous dysplasia and lipoma.[19]

In true macrodactyly, there is usually no family history of the condition. It is more common in males than females. One type usually stops growing at puberty, while the second type continues to enlarge the soft tissues after bony growth ceases, resulting in a tremendously large finger. The most frequently involved single finger is the index finger, followed closely by the long finger (Fig. 17-19), and then the thumb and ring fingers, in decreasing occurrence. Some cases show multiple finger involvement, usually two fingers. The most common pair of involved fingers are the index and long fingers, while the thumb and index finger are almost as commonly involved. Slightly less frequently, the long and ring fingers are involved. The little finger seems to be strangely free of this type of involvement. Of the cases of gigantism with multiple digital involvement, about 10 per cent also have syndactyly of the fingers. Syndactyly involving the index and long fingers is probably the most common, followed closely by the syndactyly of the long and ring fingers.

About 5 per cent of the cases with macrodactyly have bilateral involvement. There may occasionally be pedal gigantism along with the hand involvement. Associated systemic anomalies are uncommon. The roentgenogram shows larger-than-normal bones of the involved finger or fingers. The metacarpals are moderately enlarged, but the phalanges are markedly enlarged. In some at the age of 7 or 8 years, the finger or fingers are already of adult size.

Treatment

If untreated, these hands acquire a cosmetically unsatisfactory appearance. At cessation of growth, the involved fingers are one and one-half to two times the normal circumference, and about one and one-half times as long as the other fingers. Cosmesis becomes an increasingly important factor as the child gets older. If seen early, no treatment is indicated. The child should be followed at regular intervals until age 7 or 8 years, and then, if the involved digit or digits are of a size comparable to that of the fingers of the parents, epiphysiodesis of the metacarpal and all three phalanges is performed. If the child is not treated until 9 or 10 or more years, the involved fingers will be too large for the other fingers to catch up to them. The affected fingers therefore require some sort of bone shortening, at one or more levels, and narrowing of the bone structure, defatting of the finger, and narrowing of the nail and the terminal phalanx. Cosmetically, the child treated late in childhood incurs poor results, while one treated at age 7 or 8 shows considerably less difference in finger size when fully grown.[20]

The treatment of gigantism due to neurofibroma requires the same bone treatment, but, in addition, defatting, partial nerve resection and carpal tunnel release are needed to allow for the usually marked enlargement of the median nerve. Gigantism due to hemangiomas or arteriovenous fistulas requires the appropriate treatment for these respective conditions, which is limited resection of the involved tissues. Occasionally, amputation is necessary in conditions where there is erosion of the skin and the life-endangering episodes of hemorrhage.

CAMPTODACTYLY

Clinical Features

This term means "bent finger." There is much confusion concerning the definition condition, but strictly speaking, it means a bent little finger. Primarily, the flexion contracture occurs at the middle joint or the proximal interphalangeal joint. It is usually hereditary, appearing in early childhood, and gradually increases in severity. When it first appears, it is correctable with passive extension, but with growth there is secondary shortening of the skin, tendons and joint, and the bend eventually becomes a fixed deformity that is not correctable by splinting.[21]

The early roentgenograms are normal, but roentgenograms taken at puberty or later show notching of the fossa at the neck of the proximal phalanx because of the acute flexion of the middle phalanx. The bone structure is otherwise normal.

Treatment

The treatment in the early stages is dynamic splinting in the daytime and fixed extension splinting at night. Fixed deformities may be prevented with prolonged diligent splinting. Splinting should begin as soon as the deformity is noticed. Fre-

quently, however, late fixed deformity does not respond well to splinting.[22]

The surgical treatment, therefore, requires correction of all the involved tissues. This means a shift of a lateral skin flap to cover the short volar skin surface and skin grafting of the donor area on the lateral and dorsal side of the finger. If the sublimis tendon is short, it may be lengthened at the wrist level, if surgery is performed when the patient is still quite young. If the extensor central slip is attenuated, sublimis slips may be used as an intrinsic central slip replacement. If the joint capsule is contracted, it usually requires capsulotomy. If these surgical procedures are carried out, prolonged follow-up treatment and splinting are necessary. Even with the best efforts at treatment, prolonged splinting and follow-up care, the results are usually incomplete correction. In late untreated cases with severe flexion deformities, arthrodesis of the middle joints in 30° to 35° of flexion is indicated.[23]

CONSTRICTING BANDS

Clinical Features

Much confusion exists as to the cause of this condition. Constriction by the umbilical cord or amniotic bands is frequently mentioned, and the common association of shortened or partially absent phalanges suggests that there must be a common cause. Recent experimental work tends to show that this may be due to an injury to the fetal extremity in early stages of gestation.

The constricting band may be a partially or completely encircling ring or band. There may be single or multiple bands involving single or multiple fingers. They may also be associated with similar bands involving the hand, forearm or upper arm and may be accompanied by similar bands around the toes, feet, lower leg or thigh. The abdomen and thorax are also occasionally encircled by constricting bands. The depth of the constricting bands varies, and they may be deep enough to result in circulatory embarassment and, occasionally, to late nerve involvement.

Some bands seem to slowly deepen with growth, which probably indicates lack of

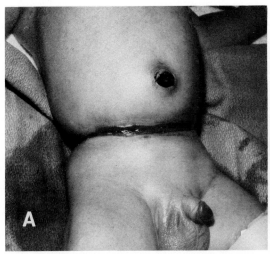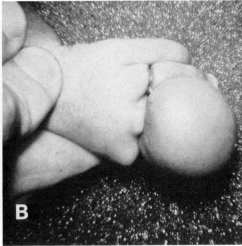

FIG. 17-20. *(A)* A newborn with a constricting band encircling the body at trunk level, with loss of skin and fat at the level of band. *(B)* Dorsal view of an edematous long finger from a constricting band on long finger. There is amputation of the index finger, and another band is present on the long finger.

growth at the area of the band, and therefore there is a slowly increasing tourniquet effect. Edema and a fluid-filled distal part may result. Gangrene may occur if release of the constriction is not done early. This type of involvement is usually seen in the newborn or very young and demands release of the constricting band, since the increasing edema tends to further constrict circulation to the finger.

The relation between constricting bands and ainhum is not clear, but they are probably different conditions. The latter condition is not present at birth and appears at a later time. Constricting bands are probably not inherited, although there are some reports of a recessive inheritance. The most severe form of constricting bands may be associated with the absence of a phalanx or phalanges, and the associated metacarpals may also be absent (Fig. 17-20).

Treatment

The surgical treatment is usually delayed until age 2 years or later, unless interference with circulation is noted. Multiple Z-plasties are necessary in most cases; at least two Z-plasties are needed for a completely encircling band. Constricting bands at the proximal phalanx, near the metacarpal head, are probably better treated with a

Y-V procedure. The Y-V procedure can also be combined with a Z-plasty, if necessary. The Y-V procedure on the dorsal surface over the metacarpal head or base of the proximal phalanx yields a less obvious scar than a Z-plasty at this level. If proper care is taken to preserve skin, nerves and vascular supply, a total of 360° of correction can be done at one operation. For the occasional operator, however, correction of one-half of the circumference at a time is recommended for safety.

TRIGGER THUMB

Clinical Features and Diagnosis

Congenital trigger thumb, sometimes called "clasped thumb," is easily misdiagnosed or unrecognized at birth, due to the clenched-fist attitude of the newborn hand. It can be easily diagnosed at birth if the obstetrician or pediatrician passively extends the fingers and thumb as a part of the initial physical examination.

Treatment

If the diagnosis is made at birth, and if the thumb can be passively extended, splinting in extension for 6 to 8 weeks may overcome the triggering; however, even some that are

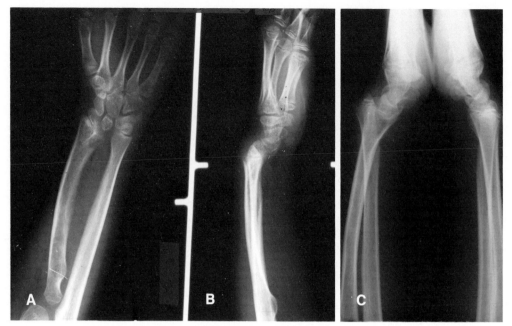

FIG. 17-21. *(A)* Anteroposterior roentgenogram of Madelung's deformity of the left wrist. *(B)* A year and 4 months later, there is a worsening of the deformity. *(C)* Lateral view showing overgrowth and prominence of the distal ulna as compared to the normal wrist *(right).*

diagnosed at birth do not allow passive extension, and splinting does not correct the condition. Occasionally, continuous splinting or casting, as for a clubfoot, gradually produces full extension of the thumb.[24]

Mechanically, the annular ligament at the metacarpal head is too tight or too small for the flexor pollicis longus. The distal swelling of the tendon may result in formation of a nodule or enlargement of the tendon. This can be palpated and causes the triggering. If this goes untreated, the fibrosis in the swollen area of the tendon progresses to a permanent nodule on the flexor tendon. If the trigger thumb cannot be extended by splinting with 6 or 8 weeks of treatment, surgical correction is recommended. It can be done under premedication and local anesthetia, but it is more commonly done under general anesthesia, if there are no contraindicating physical conditions of the newborn. If surgery is necessary, resection of the small pulley at the metacarpal head is recommended. The more distal cruciate or oblique ligament is preserved to prevent marked bowstringing of the flexor pollicis longus.[25]

MADELUNG'S DEFORMITY

Clincial Features and Diagnosis

This is probably not a true congenital deformity, in that it is not present at birth. It is, however, known to be inherited as an autosomal dominant condition. It is more common in females than in males (by four to one), and it is frequently bilateral (by two to one).

Roentgenograms reveal that the changes begin to appear at age 2 years. The ulnar and volar half of the distal radial epiphysis does not grow as rapidly as the radial half. This results in a radius whose ulnar half is shorter than the radial half, and there is a curving toward the ulnar side. The volar part of the ulnar half of the epiphysis is also involved in the delayed growth, so that the radius curves volarward and ulnarward, simultaneously. This results in dorsal prominence of the distal ulna and, subsequently, greater ulnar length (Fig. 17-21). The combination of these factors leads to limited dorsiflexion of the wrist, with resultant loss of supination. The proximal end of the radius is usually normal, but may occasionally be somewhat deformed. There are many other bony anomalies frequently associated with this condition, and there are many reports concerning their relationships. These include such anomalies as scoliosis, cervical ribs, defects of the humerus and many types of bony anomalies of the lower extremities. In recent years deformities of Hurler's and Morquio's syndromes, and the association of these with mucopolysaccharidosis, have been studied and compared with Madelung's deformity.

Treatment

Surgical treatment is not indicated early. After closure of the epiphyses, osteotomy of the radius to correct the volar and ulnar angulation can be done, as can a limited resection of the distal ulna. Resection of the extra length of the ulna must be accompanied by reconstruction of the ulnar carpal ligament and the ulnar radial ligaments, to prevent the distal radial ulnar instability so commonly seen when excessive bone is removed. There is rarely a great degree of loss of function of the fingers in this condition. Most of the lost function is in dorsiflexion of the wrist; there is usually good residual supination and finger function.

LOBSTER-CLAW HAND

Clinical Features

Unfortunately, this term is widely used to describe what is actually a clefting of the hand. This widely varying deformity is hereditary, is frequently bilateral, and may also involve the lower extremities.

The term "lobster claw" is used to describe the absence of the central ray of the hand. The index finger may also be absent, as may be the thumb. Many combinations have been described, with absence of the central ray or rays and preservation, either partial or complete, of the border rays being the most common. Roentgenograms show which bones are absent or which parts of the osseous structures are present. There may be a simple absence of a central ray, or there may be complex anomalies with transverse phalanges or metacarpals and absence of the central finger. There are many variations of

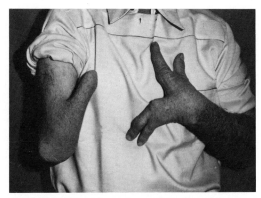

FIG. 17-22. In this patient, there is no hand on the right and a lobster-claw hand on the left.

the tendon, vessel and nerve involvement, and these are only identifiable at surgery (Fig. 17-22).

Treatment

The treatment of choice is surgery. Early treatment between the ages of 6 and 24 months is recommended. In the absence of the central metacarpal and long finger, surgery must provide skin cleft closure and web reconstruction between the index and ring fingers. Realignment of the second and fourth metacarpals to a parallel position is essential, and may require osteotomy of one or both metacarpals. This necessarily means construction of a transverse metacarpal ligament between the second and fourth metacarpal heads to prevent recurrence of the deformity. The excess skin resulting from the closure between the second and fourth metacarpals gives adequate skin for widening of the web between the thumb and index fingers, if this web is contracted. In this latter condition, the index finger must be shifted ulnarward to take the place of the third metacarpal, and the surrounding skin is shifted into the thumb web (Fig. 17-23).

In the more complicated cases with other deformities, metacarpal osteotomies are usually necessary to realign the fingers or the thumb in cases where there are transversely oriented phalanges. Closure of the central defect is essential in all cases, probably combined with osteotomies of the metacarpals or phalanges, if necessary.

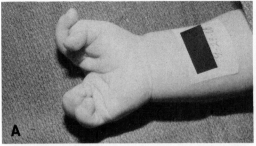
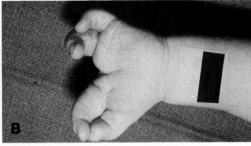
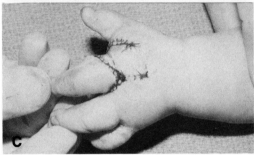

FIG. 17-23. *(A)* A 1-year-old male with a cleft hand and syndactyly of the ring and little fingers. *(B)* The hand as it appeared 2 months after separation of the ring and little fingers. *(C)* The hand as it appeared after completion of closure of the central cleft and reconstruction of the thumb web.

CONGENITAL ABSENCE OF THE RADIUS

Clinical Features

Congenital absence of the radius is characterized by radial deviation of the hand, marked shortening of the forearm, and general underdevelopment of the upper extremity. There are two types, one where there is total absence of the radius and one with only partial absence of the radius. The most common manifestation of this type is absence of the distal half of the radius. There may also be absence of only the central segment or absence of the proximal segment of the radius. Approximately 50 per cent of the reported cases are bilateral. There may or may not be associated anomalies, and there does not seem to be any pattern of these anomalies.

The lack of the support of the radius to the carpus results in radial deviation of the hand and carpus. This may vary from a mild radial deviation of the hand, if the radius is only mildly shortened, to more than 90° of deviation, if the radius is totally absent. The greater the radial deviation, the less effective are the forearm muscles, due to the greater relaxation and proportionate loss of strength (Fig 17-24 A,B,C).

In addition to the radial deviation of the hand, the forearm is shortened. The ulna is usually short, hypertrophied, and in most cases curved, with the concavity toward the radial side. In unilateral cases, the hand, forearm, upper arm and shoulder girdle are usually underdeveloped in comparison to the normal arm and shoulder. At maturity, the total length of the upper extremity is between one-half and two-thirds of the length of the normal extremity.

As is true in other congenital anomalies, there may be associated deformities. There is no set pattern of associated anomalies and no relationship to a partial or complete absence of the radius. The list of associated anomalies includes: hairlip, cleft palate, clubfoot, hydrocephalus, hernia, kyphosis, scoliosis, hemivertebrae, rib deformity including fusions, and aplasia or absence of a lung.

The skeletal changes that occur in this deformity may involve any bone of the upper extremity. The scapula is commonly reduced in size, and the clavicle may be shortened and more curved. The humerus is usually shorter than normal, and either end may be deformed. The carpal bones are rarely complete in number. The scaphoid is the bone most frequently absent, and occasionally it is fused to the lunate. The trapezium is the next most commonly absent. The capitate, hamate, triquetrum and pisiform bones are usually present. The first metacarpal may be absent, whether or not the thumb is present. Varying degress of floating thumb result, depending on whether all or only the first part of the metacarpal is absent.[26]

The muscles are frequently involved in the deformity. The pectoralis major may have an abnormal insertion, or either the clavicular or costal part may be absent. The pectoralis minor and deltoid are usually present, but may have abnormal insertions. The biceps may be absent. If it is present, it inserts into the lacertus fibrosis, or may be fused to the brachialis. The brachialis is usually present. The brachioradialis is usually present and may insert into the carpus, acting as a tether. The extensor carpi radialis longus and brevis are usually present, or may be fused together. The extensor digitorum communis is usually present, and is fairly normal. The supinator is usually absent, unless the proximal radius is present, as is the pronator. If the thumb is present and is fully developed, its extensor is usually normal, but the flexor pollicis longus may or may not be present, depending on whether the distal radius is present or absent. The interosseous, lumbrical and hypothenar muscles are usually present and normal.

The nerve supply of the brachial plexus and upper arm is usually normal. The radial nerve sensory branch may not extend below the elbow, and the median nerve then gives off a branch to the dorsal surface of the hand, and may unite with the dorsal branch of the ulnar nerve. If this is the case, the median nerve is the most superficial nerve found on the radial side of the forearm (Fig. 17-24D). It must be looked for in any surgical approach from the radial side. The ulnar nerve is usually normal and supplies its normal flexors of the ring and little fingers, the interosseous and hypothenar muscles.

Fanconi's syndrome, a hypoplastic anemia, should be sought in any child with this anomaly or multiple anomalies involving the bones. This syndrome is characterized by a severe, progressive, refractory, macrocytic anemia, with neutropenia and thrombopenia and hypoplastic bone marrow. This condition may be fatal, and the extent of the hypoplastic factors must be determined before any surgical reconstruction is undertaken.

Treatment

Casting. Treatment for congenital absence of the radius should be started as soon as possible after birth, if the condition of the child permits.[27] If seen shortly after birth, plaster cast correction of the deformity should be undertaken (Fig. 17-24E). Like a cast for a clubfoot, the cast should be put on in three parts, with only one part of the deformity being corrected with each section of the cast. A hand piece, leaving the fingers free, is applied first. The elbow is then flexed to 90°, allowing relaxation of the forearm muscles, and traction is applied to the hand to move the carpus as far distally as possible in relation to the distal end of the ulna. The plaster is then applied to the forearm and is joined to the hand section, with the hand in neutral rotation. The cast should be trimmed out over the anterior aspect of the elbow so that there is no pressure exerted anteriorly when the third part is applied. The third part of the cast is then applied, while the hand-forearm is held in neutral rotation and the elbow is flexed to 90°, and the upper section is joined to the forearm section. As with a clubfoot cast, unless this technique is followed every time, satisfactory correction is not obtained. If the cast is applied within the first few days of life, a great deal of correction can be obtained quickly. If not started until 2 years or later, casting does not achieve very much correction.[28]

Surgery. If there is no contraindication for surgery, such as Fanconi's syndrome or heart anomalies that preclude surgery, the surgical correction can be started as early as 2 or 3 months. Historically, the surgical treatment of this deformity has been by osteotomy of the ulna, leaving the hand and distal ulna alone, to bone grafting (tibial, fibular, ulnar, and epiphyseal graft), to centralization of the hand over the ulna by a number of methods (Fig. 17-24 F,G,H,I). In the past 75 years, treatment methods have made a full circle. The treatment recommended by most individuals actively engaged in managing this condition today is centralization of the hand over the distal end of the ulna, coupled with osteotomy of

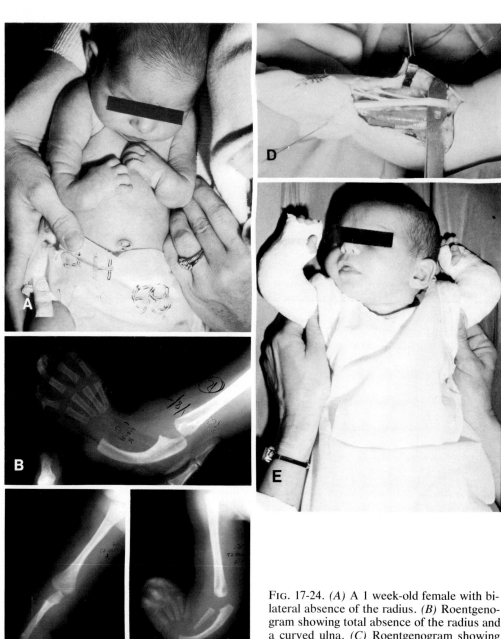

FIG. 17-24. (A) A 1 week-old female with bi-lateral absence of the radius. (B) Roentgeno-gram showing total absence of the radius and a curved ulna. (C) Roentgenogram showing partial absence of the radius, a curved ulna, and an absent thumb. (D) Operative view, showing branches of the median nerve supplying the dorsal side of the hand. (E) Plaster casts in place for correction of the deformity prior to surgery.
(Continued on facing page.)

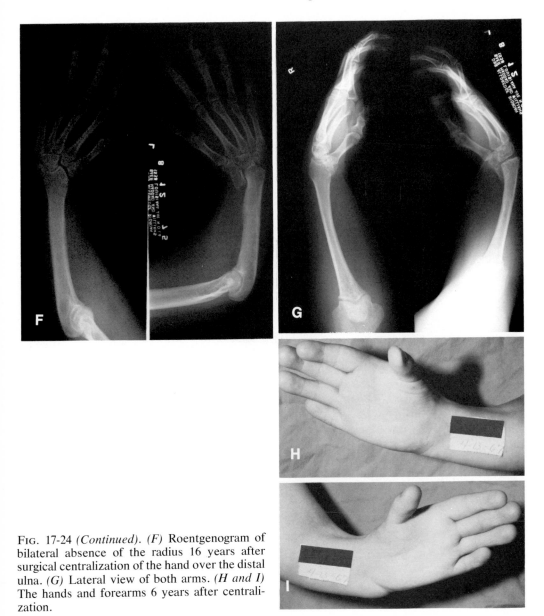

FIG. 17-24 *(Continued)*. *(F)* Roentgenogram of bilateral absence of the radius 16 years after surgical centralization of the hand over the distal ulna. *(G)* Lateral view of both arms. *(H and I)* The hands and forearms 6 years after centralization.

the ulna if it is curved. Internal fixation for 8 to 10 weeks with a pin no larger than a .062 Kirschner wire is recommended. The pin is then removed to prevent damage to the distal ulnar epiphysis. Short-arm splints are used to maintain correction and keep the hand over the distal ulna. The splints must be worn 24 hours a day until the child is 6 years old, removing them only for bath-ing. After school age is reached, the splints may be left off during the day and worn at night until full maturation is achieved. This allows the distal ulna full enlargement, with the hand centralized. The ulna frequently becomes almost as large as the distal radius would have been. Arthrodesis of the wrist is rarely necessary, except in a few cases, which are usually only those in whom treat-

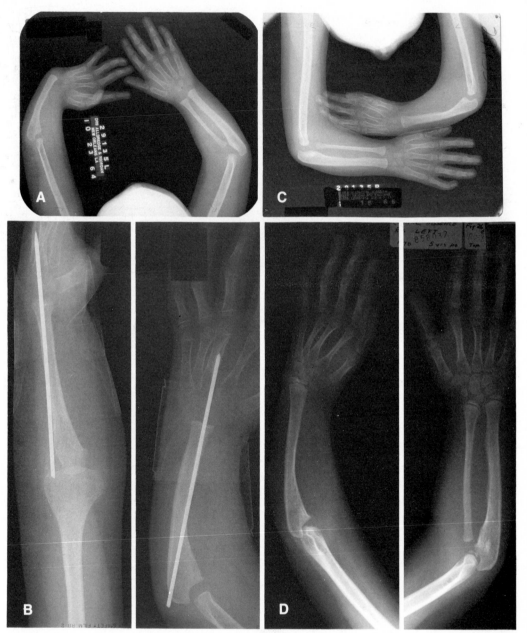

FIG. 17-25. *(A)* Roentgenogram of both arms of a 5-year-old male with an absent radius on the left, and a slightly small radius on the right. *(B)* Roentgenographic view 3 months after surgical centralization of the left hand. *(C)* Seventeen months after centralization. *(D)* Five years after centralization. *(Continued on facing page.)*

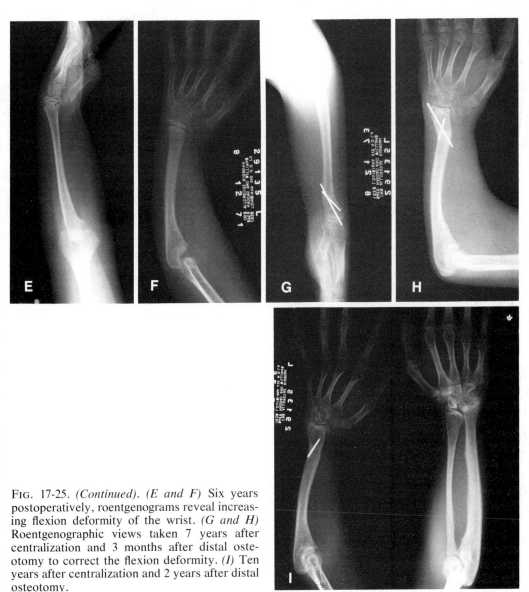

FIG. 17-25. *(Continued). (E and F)* Six years postoperatively, roentgenograms reveal increasing flexion deformity of the wrist. *(G and H)* Roentgenographic views taken 7 years after centralization and 3 months after distal osteotomy to correct the flexion deformity. *(I)* Ten years after centralization and 2 years after distal osteotomy.

ment was started after age 4, so that full development of the distal ulna could not take place.

The surgical approach varies from surgeon to surgeon. Some recommend an approach from the radial side, coupled with a Z-plasty, and an ulnar approach for the osteotomy, if necessary. This author prefers to use an ulnar approach, transversely oriented at the distal ulna, excising a football-shaped wedge of skin and fat, thus removing excess skin and fat that would give a cosmetically poor result if allowed to remain. The dorsal branch of the ulnar nerve is identified and protected. The extensor ulnaris and extensor digiti quinti are freed from their compartment and the distal ulna is then exposed. This bone should not be widely exposed, so as to preserve as much of the blood supply of the distal epiphysis as possible. Then, by increasing the deformity, the proximal end of the proximal row of carpal bones can be exposed, the capsule freed from the inner side of the ulna, and by flexing the elbow, the hand carpus can usually be brought over the distal end of the ulna to the centralized position. If the structures are still too tight on the radial side and there is not a need for a Z-plasty, the central carpal bone (lunate) can be partially or wholly removed.[30] This shortens the bone length without interfering with growth, and usually allows the hand to be centralized on the distal ulna. If successful, the hand is then moved out of the way, the distal ulna is exposed, and a Kirschner wire is drilled through the ulna and made to come out the forearm (if the ulna is bowed), or out of the olecranon process (if the ulna is not bowed). This does not interfere with growth. The drill is then placed on the proximal end of the wire and it is drilled into the carpus and third metacarpal, after recentralizing the hand over the distal ulna. The wire is not drilled across the metacarpal epiphysis, but is stopped short of it. Long-arm splints over adequate padding are used to assist the fixation. After 1 or 2 weeks, a long-arm cast can be applied for 8 to 10 weeks, followed by a short-arm plastic splint. This method has given good results, but it is dependent upon the complete cooperation of the parents, since the splints must be continuously worn if Wolff's law is to prevail and the distal end of the ulna is to enlarge sufficiently to support the hand.

If the treatment is started within the first year of life, the ulna develops into a bone large enough to support the hand by the time the child is 6 or 7 years old. At that time the splint may be left off during the day while the child is at school, but should be worn at night. It is essential that the splint be kept on until full development of the hand and forearm has occurred. If this is done, the hand remains corrected and a wrist stabilization procedure does not have to be done.

If splinting is discontinued and the deformity recurs, it is necessary to do another centralization procedure or, perhaps, an osteotomy at the distal end of the ulna. The distal ulna frequently has a curvature within the distal inch or so, and an osteotomy at this level, leaving the carpus in its relation with the distal end, repositions the hand and corrects the distal curve. After the osteotomy has healed, splinting can be resumed until growth is complete (Fig. 17-25).[31,32,33]

CONGENITAL ABSENCE OF THE ULNA

Clinical Features

Congenital absence of the ulna is characterized by ulnar deviation of the hand, radial bowing of the radius with concavity toward the ulna, and dislocation of the head of the radius, when present. This deformity is about one-third as common as congenital absence of the radius. It may be seen with other deformities, but usually only on the involved extremity. It may be unilateral or bilateral (Fig. 17-26).

There are three types of congenital absence of the ulna. The rarest type is that with complete and total absence of the ulna. The child has an unstable elbow, since there is no ulna present to give stability at the elbow. Since there is no distal cartilaginous ulnar anlage to tether the wrist, the radius is usually straight. In the second type there is absence of the distal or middle third of the ulna and the proximal third has an articulation with the humerus. The radial head may be articulating with the capitellum, or it may be dislocated laterally and displaced posteriorly. In the third type the radius is fused with the humerus in flexion or extension. Even though there is no elbow joint, there is usually a cartilaginous anlage. Since this cartilaginous anlage has no longitudinal growth, the distal radial epiphysis is compressed on its ulnar side, and the wedge-shaped epiphysis produces further ulnar deviation of the hand with growth. The longitudinal growth of the radius occurring while the distal radial epiphysis is tethered by the anlage results in a radial bowing of the radius. If the radial head is articulating with the humerus at birth, the combination of radial bowing and ulnar anlage tethering result in eventual dislocation of the radial head on the humerus. If the ulnar anlage tether is not released early by excision of the anlage, ulnar deviation of the hand increases with growth, and the radial head slides posteriorly past the humerus, thus wasting longitudinal growth.

In the third type, the proximal radius is fused with the distal humerus. Thus, there is

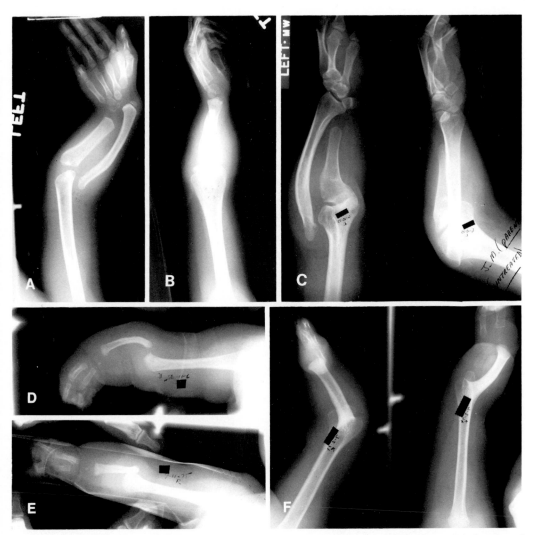

FIG. 17-26. *(A and B)* Anteroposterior and lateral roentgenograms of a child with partial absence of the distal ulna, showing the dislocation of the radial head and marked ulnar drift of the hand. *(C)* Roentgenogram showing the arms of the 34-year-old father of the child in *A*. The father was untreated. *(D and E)* Roentgenogram of a 3-month-old male with absence of the ulna and the fourth and fifth rays of the hand. *(F)* Roentgenogram of a 2-year-old male with synostosis of the humerus and radius, and partial absence of the ulna.

no distal humeral epiphysis, and there is no proximal radial epiphysis. Even though there is fusion of the radius and humerus, there is a proximal ulnar anlage which extends distally and attaches to the carpus. This fibrocartilage also tethers the distal radius and causes it to bow, and the distal radial epiphysis grows in a wedge shape. As with the other types, this anlage should be excised early to lessen the tendency for the radial bowing and to lessen the wedging of the distal radial epiphysis.

Treatment

If the anomaly is detected at birth, plaster casts should be used to prevent increasing deformity. If the child has no other congenital anomalies preventing surgery, the ulnar

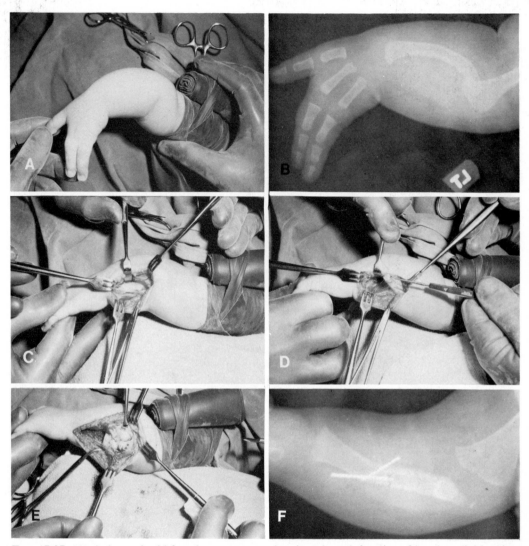

FIG. 17-27. *(A)* A 6-month-old female at surgery, showing ulnar deformity of hand, radial bowing, and absence of the fourth and fifth rays. *(B)* Roentgenogram of the arm at age 6 months. *(C)* View at surgery, with the ulnar anlage exposed. *(D)* The ulnar anlage is detached and is pulled upward by a hook. *(E)* The anlage is excised to the point just distal to the joint. The capsule is opened to show the capitellum of the humerus. *(F)* The postoperative roentgenogram, showing pins in the osteotomy site of the radius. Wire sutures were used to connect the cartilaginous ulna with the radius as close to the joint as possible. *(Continued on facing page.)*

anlage should be excised early, perhaps at 6 months. When there is marked radial bowing and dislocation of the radial head, an osteotomy of the radius and creation of a one-bone forearm can be done at the same time. With care, the osteotomy can be done from the ulnar side, after excision of the ulnar anlage. The removal of the anlage gives adequate exposure through the interosseous membrane to osteotomize the radius from the ulnar side. The radial osteotomy is done as close to the elbow as possible, and the distal radial shaft is brought into alignment with the remaining proximal

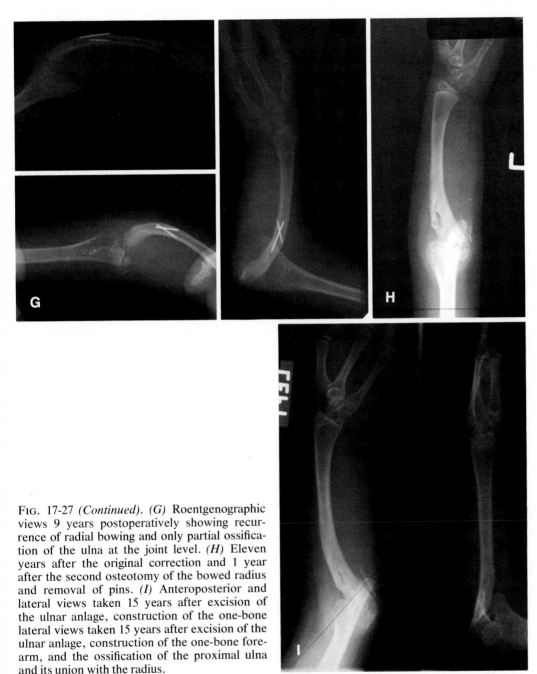

FIG. 17-27 *(Continued)*. *(G)* Roentgenographic views 9 years postoperatively showing recurrence of radial bowing and only partial ossification of the ulna at the joint level. *(H)* Eleven years after the original correction and 1 year after the second osteotomy of the bowed radius and removal of pins. *(I)* Anteroposterior and lateral views taken 15 years after excision of the ulnar anlage, construction of the one-bone lateral views taken 15 years after excision of the ulnar anlage, construction of the one-bone forearm, and the ossification of the proximal ulna and its union with the radius.

ulna. This can be done even if the ulna is still cartilaginous. Intrameduallary fixation with a .062 Kirschner wire is used to affix the radius to the ulna. The proximal part of the neck of the radius and radial head are left alone at this time, unless they are interfering with motion. It is safest to wait some months before removing the proximal radius, since the combined procedures are extensive. Occasionally, the radial bowing is so great that several osteotomies of the radius are necessary to straighten the curve, and the intramedullay pin is used to skewer the multiple fragments. Thus, the ulnar anlage can be excised, a one-bone forearm made, and the radius straightened at one operation.

As with absence of the radius, the initial immobilization is with a plaster cast, followed in 2 months by splints (usually short-arm splints), until school age is reached. This 24-hour wearing of the splint is continued until school age, and if conditions are satisfactory, the splint can be left off while the child is at school and worn the rest of the day and night. Once full growth has been achieved, splinting can be discontinued. The total length of this forearm will be about two thirds of the length of a normal arm on the same child (Fig. 17-27).

There are many different hand deformities associated with absence of the ulna. The most common deformity is presence of a thumb and an index and long finger, with the fourth and fifth rays being absent. However, there may be a normal five-ray hand present. The thumb and index ray may be absent, and the third, fourth and fifth rays present. The fingers may be webbed in varying combinations. The hand problems should be solved after the arm deformity has been corrected. If there is webbing and the bones are fused distally, this must be corrected as early as possible to prevent the shorter finger from causing a deformity of the longer finger. It must be emphasized that the earlier the deformity is corrected, the greater the growth potential of the arm.

REFERENCES

Sprengel's Deformity

1. Eulenberg, M.: Casuistis Mittheilungen aus dem Begiete der Orthopädie. Arch. Klin. Chir., *4:*301, 1863.
2. Green, W. T.: The surgical correction of congenital elevation of the scapula (Sprengel's deformity). [Proc. Am. Orthop. Assoc.] J. Bone Joint Surg., *39A:*149, 1957.
3. Horwitz, A. E.: Congenital deviation of the scapula—Sprengel's deformity. Am. J. Orthop. Surg., *6:*260, 1908.
4. Shrock, R. D.: Congenital abnormalities at the cervicothoracic level. AAOS Instruct. Course Lect.*6,* 1949.
5. Woodward, J. W.: Congenital elevation of the scapula. Correction by release and transplantation of muscle origins. J. Bone Joint Surg., *43A:*219, 1961.

Congenital Dislocation of the Shoulder

6. Cozen, L.: Congenital dislocation of the shoulder and other anomalies. Arch. Surg.,*35:*956, 1937.
7. Whitman, R.: The treatment of congenital and acquired luxations at the shoulder in childhood. Ann: Surg.,*42:*110, 1905.

Congenital Pseudarthrosis of the Clavicle

8. Alldred, A. J.: Congenital pseudarthrosis of the clavicle. J. Bone Joint Surg.,*45B:*312, 1963.
9. Fitzwilliams, D. C. L.: Hereditary craniocleidodysostosis. Lancet,*2:*1, 466, 1910.

Osteochondritis Dissecans of the Elbow

10. Heller, C. J., and Wiltse, L. D.: A vascular necrosis of the capitelum humeri (Panner's disease). J. Bone Joint Surg.,*42A:*513, 1960.
11. Panner, H. J.: An affection of the capitulum humeri, resembling Calvé-Perthes disease of the hip. Acta Radiol.,*8:*617, 1927.
12. Smith, M. G. H.: Osteochondritis of the humeral capitelum. J. Bone Joint Surg.,*46B:*50, 1964.

Congenital Absence of the Thumb

13. Buck-Gramcko, D.: Operativer Daumener—staz bei Aplasia und Hypoplosie. Verh. Dtsch. Orthop. Ges.,*55:*417, 1968.
14. ———: Pollicization of the index finger. Method and results in aplasia and hypoplosia of the thumb. J. Bone Joint Surg.,*53A:*1065, 1971.
15. Littler, J. W.: The neurovascular pedicle method of digital transposition for reconstruction of the thumb. Plast. Reconstr. Surg., *12:*303 1953.
16. ———: Principles of reconstructive surgery of the hand. *In* Converse, J. M. (ed.): Reconstructive Plastic Surgery, vol. 4. Philadelphia, W. B. Saunders, 1964.

Syndactyly

17. Flatt, A.: Treatment of syndactylism. Plast. Reconstr. Surg.,*29:*336, 1962.
18. Kahn, A., Jr., and Fulmer, J.: Acrocephalosyndactylism. N. Engl. J. Med.,*252:*379, 1955.

Gigantism of the Fingers

19. Barsky, A. J.: Macrodactyly. J. Bone Joint Surg., *49A:*1255, 1967.
20. Thorne, F. L., Posch, J. L., and Mladick, R. A.: Megalodactyly. Plast. Reconstr. Surg., *41:*232 1968.

Camptodactyly

21. Iselin, F., Levame, J., and Afanassief, A.: Les camptodactylies congénitales. [Soc. Med. Chir. des Hôpitaux libres de Fourier, 1966.] Arch. Hôp., *5:*1, 1966.
22. Shaff, B., and Schafer, P. W.: Camptodactyly. Arch. Surg.,*57:*633, 1948.
23. Smith, R. J., and Kaplan, E. B.: Camptodactyly

and similar atraumatic flexion deformities of the proximal interphalanageal joints of the fingers. J. Bone Joint Surg., *50A:*1187, 1249, 1968.

Trigger Thumb

24. Broadbent, T. R., and Woolf, R. M.: Flexion-adduction deformity of the thumb—congenital clasp thumb. Plast. Reconstr. Surg., *34:*612, 1964.
25. White, J. W., and Jensen, W. E.: The infant's persistent thumb-clutched hand, J. Bone Joint Surg., *34A:*680, 1952.

Congenital Absence of the Radius

26. Buck-Gramcko, D.: Pollicization of the index finger. Method and results in aplasia and hypoplasia of the thumb. J. Bone and Joint Surg., *53A:*1605, 1971.

27. Lamb, D. W.: The treatment of radial club hand. Absent radius, aplasia of the radius, hypoplasia of the radius, radial paraxial hemimelia. Hand, *4:*22, 1972.
28. ———: Radial club hand. A continuing study of 68 patients with 117 club hands. J. Bone Joint Surg., *59A:* 1977.
29. Littler, J. W.: The neurovascular pedicle method of digital transposition for reconstruction of the thumb. Plast. Reconstr. Surg., *12:*303 1953.
30. O'Rahilly, R.: Radial hemimelia and the functional anatomy of the carpus. J. Anat., *80:*179, 1946.
31. Riordan, D. C.: Congenital abscence of the radius. J. Bone and Joint Surg., *37A:*1129, 1955.
32. ———: Congenital absence of radius: a fifteen-year followup study. [Proc. Am. Orthop. Assoc.] J. Bone and Joint Surg., *45A:*1783, 1963.
33. Tachdjian, M. O.: Pediatric Orthopedics. Philadelphia, W. B. Saunders, 1972.

18 The Hip

G. Dean MacEwen, M.D., and Paul L. Ramsey, M.D.

CONGENITAL DISLOCATION OF THE HIP—EVALUATION AND TREATMENT BEFORE WALKING AGE

Early diagnosis of a congenitally dislocated hip (CDH) is essential in preventing the infant from experiencing a prolonged and involved course of treatment. The main problem in obtaining an early diagnosis is that generations of students, residents, and practitioners have been taught to examine the hips for clicks, limited abduction, asymmetrical skin creases or femoral shortening to establish the diagnosis. All of these methods for determining the presence of congenital dislocation of the hip, except asymmetrical skin folds, are, for the most part, inadequate for newborn examinations. Even the asymmetrical skin fold can be misleading because it is so often present when the hip is normal. These factors, plus the fact that the individual practitioner rarely encounters a child with a congenitally dislocated hip, account for delayed diagnosis.

EMBRYOLOGY AND ANATOMY

At 4 to 5 weeks of gestation, bulges representing the extremities develop on the anterolateral aspect of the embryo. Development of the future joint is demarcated by a line of increased density,[58] which is saucer-shaped. The cleavage of the joint cavity starts at the peripheral margins and progresses inward. Since the femoral head and acetabulum are formed from a single block of tissue, a dislocation is impossible during early developmental stages.

The blood supply to the femoral head is critical. The femoral artery gives off the profunda femoris artery, which in turn gives the lateral and medial circumflex arteries. Both are important to the circulation to the proximal femur. The lateral circumflex artery passes underneath the rectus femoris, giving off muscular branches, but most importantly a major branch supplies the anterolateral proximal femur.[37] The medial circumflex artery passes between the iliopsoas and adductor muscles, turns across the posterior aspect of the iliopsoas to reach the medial side of the femur, and passes along the femoral neck. There are two methods of extraarticular vascular compromise—with a forced positioning of the proximal femur, there is occlusion of the vessels as the acetabular rim is pressed into the intertrochanteric groove, and occlusion as the vessel passes between the muscle bellies. The anatomic path[5] of the major vessels is significant because arterial occlusions can occur with either the frog-leg or the abduction-internal rotation positions.[38]

Ogden[36] has reported that at birth the blood is supplied to the femoral head by multiple small vessels arising from both the lateral and medial circumflex vessels. With growth, this pattern changes. The lateral circumflex system recedes as a contributor to the femoral head and supplies the anteromedial metaphysis. At the same time, the medial circumflex artery changes from multiple small vessels to two larger branches called the "posterior-inferior" and "posterior-superior" vessels, which supply the major portion of the femoral head. As the pattern is changing to become more dependent on fewer but larger vessels, the amount of tissue to be supplied increases and becomes more distant because of femoral neck growth, thus maintaining the risk of avascular necrosis if the individual vessle is placed under pressure or slightly stretched.

The anatomic changes associated with dislocation represent a spectrum of abnormalities. Stability is lost when the femoral head begins to migrate laterally. An important adjunct to stability is the vacuum normally created by the snug fit of the femoral head in the acetabulum.[51] The labrum also adds stability by increasing acetabular depth. The anatomic abnormality that allows the dislocation to occur also contributes to the difficulty of regaining stability. Initially, a lax acetabular labrum (limbus) loses the vacuum, and the femoral head can be easily provoked to dislocate over the posterior acetabular rim. In the next stage, the limbus is further deformed, and the capsule and ligamentum teres are stretched. In addition, the femoral head begins to lose its spherical shape as it lies in the dislocated position. This stage of deformity is unusual for this age group. The limbus may become inverted, and there are secondary acetabular deformities. If the dislocation is present over a long period of intrauterine development, the soft tissues become contracted, preventing relocation of the femoral head. This occurrence represents the rare teratologic dislocation.

ETIOLOGY

The factors that predispose to a dislocation are genetic, hormonal and mechanical. The genetic influence is demonstrated by studies of families in which more than one child has had a dislocated hip. A dislocation in a second child occurs in approximately 22 to 50 per 1000 live births,[9, 36] which is at least 10 times the usual risk for dislocation. Andren and Borglin[1] reported an increase in uterine estrogen and content in newborns with dislocation. They postulated that failure of the liver to inactivate estrogen contributes to hormonally induced laxity of the hip capsule. Contrary to this theory, a later investigation[59] found no significant hormonal difference between controls and 16 patients with dislocation. Recently, animal studies have indicated that estrogen may be a predisposing factor.[66]

It is our clinical impression that newborns have relative joint laxity for as long as 10 days after birth. During this time a dislocation that had been present at birth often becomes stable. This is supported by Barlow's[5] study, in which 58 per cent of newborns with unstable hips developed stability spontaneously by 3$^{1}/_{2}$ days of age.

Mechanical factors also influence the occurrence of dislocation. The incidence of dislocation is greatly increased by breech position.[47] However, passage through the birth canal in the breech position does not seem to influence the dislocation, because breech-position infants delivered by Caesarean section are also prone to dislocation. This implicates intrauterine position rather than birth position as the critical factor.[64] In 1941, Chappel[9] linked fetal positions to newborn extremity malpositions. He showed that with breech positions the knees are frequently in hyperextension. Wilkinson[65] reported that full knee extension adds to hip instability, and a delay in assuming the flexed-knee position is a critical factor. The studies in which the knees of rabbits were held in extension are experimental evidence that prolonged knee extension may contribute to dislocation.[33]

The mechanical factors associated with breech malposition seem to be twofold. First, the extended knee and its associated hamstring tightness plus hyperflexion of the hip possibly increase maldirection of the forces at the hip joint. Secondly, the hyperflexed hip allows an iliopsoas contracture to develop, so that hip extension following birth promotes instability. Why the left hip should be more frequently involved than the right is unknown. However, it may be due to the positioning of the left side of the fetus adjacent to the spinal prominence, causing adduction of the left thigh.

Forced post-delivery hip extension may add to hip instability.[48, 54] This probably accounts for the frequent occurrence of dislocations in newborns in societies where infants are bundled with the hips in extension and adduction.

FIG. 18-1. Three types of dislocated hips. *(A)* Lateral diplacement occurring at birth, reduces easily and responds well to simple treatment. There is only lateral displacement of the femur with no proximal displacement. *(B)* Dislocation due to neuromuscular origin reduces easily, but tends to redislocate due to muscular imbalance. *(C)* Teratologic dislocation occurs in utero. There is frank dislocation with lateral and proximal migration of the femur at birth. A false acetabulum has developed.

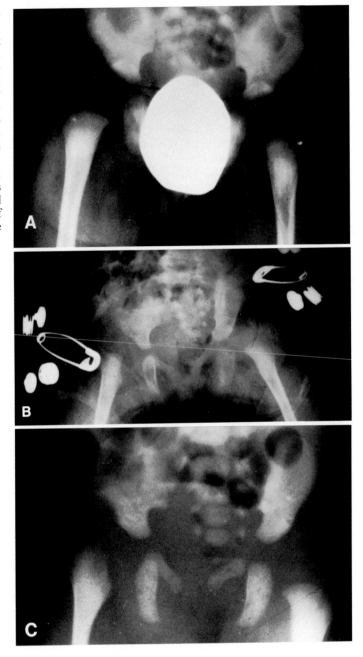

TYPES OF DISLOCATIONS

There are three types of dislocated hips (Fig. 18-1). The first type represents dislocations that occur at or near the time of birth, reduce easily and respond to simple treatment. The second type are those of neuromuscular origin. These usually reduce easily, but because of the pelvic muscular imbalance they redislocate with little provocation. Teratologic dislocations are the third type, and, contrary to the more common dislocations, these have been dislocated in utero for a prolonged period of time. Be-

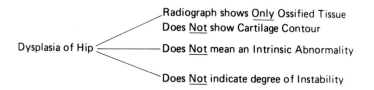

Dysplasia of Hip
- Radiograph shows <u>Only</u> Ossified Tissue
  Does <u>Not</u> show Cartilage Contour
- Does <u>Not</u> mean an Intrinsic Abnormality
- Does <u>Not</u> indicate degree of Instability

FIG. 18-2. See text.

cause of prolonged intrauterine dislocation, secondary adaptive changes of the soft tissue and bone are present at birth. The clinical characteristics of teratologic dislocations are the absence of the Ortolani sign and the inability to relocate the femoral head without traction. These dislocations are often best diagnosed by roentgenograms.

TERMINOLOGY

The terms used to describe a dislocation can lead to a misinterpretation of the anatomic deformity or degree of instability present. For example, the terms *dislocation, dislocatable, subluxation, lax, unstable,* and *dysplasia* do not have the same meaning to all clinicians. Newborns with a dislocated hip have the femoral head completely displaced from the acetabulum, and active reduction is required to reduce the hip. A dislocatable hip exists when the femoral head is in the acetabulum, but, with a provocative maneuver, it can be completely displaced from the acetabulum. Once the leg is released, the femoral head usually moves spontaneously back into the acetabulum. A subluxable hip is the most difficult to detect. Subluxation occurs when the femoral head can be moved significantly, but not completely, out of the acetabulum. Such terms as "lax" or "unstable" are most confusing because they imply that the femoral head can be moved away from the depths of the acetabulum. However, the degree of displacement is left to the imagination. Indeed, "unstable" can imply anything from minimal displacement to complete dislocation, and the term should be avoided.

"Dysplasia" indicates an abnormal development of tissue. Since the hip forms from one cartilaginous block as a spherical head and an acetabulum, "dysplasia" does not mean a primary abnormality of the developing tissue, but rather a secondary response to the dislocation. "Dysplasia" is a term commonly used to describe a greater-than-normal slope of the superior bony portion of the acetabulum. However, this finding is only a roentgenographic description and does not outline the contour of the cartilaginous acetabulum (Fig. 18-2). In fact, the underlying cartilage model may or may not be distorted. "Dysplasia" can also indicate that the femoral head on the involved side is smaller than the head of the uninvolved side. Again, as with the acetabulum, one should remember that only the bony portion of the femoral head is visible and that a large cartilaginous layer surrounds it. Therefore, abnormal roentgenograms, especially in the prewalking child, really represent secondary changes of bone development, but do not provide information regarding the contour of the cartilage.

INCIDENCE

The incidence of dislocation per 1000 live births is 1.3; dislocatable hips, 1.2; and subluxation, 9.2. Thus, with every 1000 live births, a total of 11.7 newborns have some degree of hip instability. The left hip is involved in about 60 per cent, the right hip in 20 per cent, and bilateral dislocation occurs approximately 20 per cent of the time. Seventy per cent of dislocated hips are in girls, and dislocation occurs much more frequently in the white population than the black. About 20 per cent of all dislocations occur with breech presentation, whereas the incidence of breech presentation in the general population is about 4 per cent. Females born in breech presentation are categorized as a very high risk group because both their sex and their breech position predispose them to dislocations. In fact, in a study of 25,000 newborns at our institute, this com-

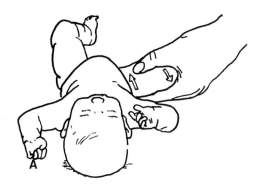

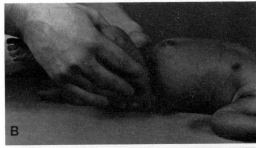

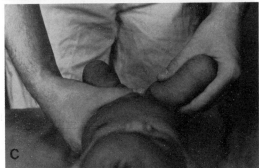

FIG. 18-3. *(A, B, and C)* The Ortolani maneuver. In this technique, the hip is gently abducted, and the thigh is raised with the fingers. This gently reduces the hip.

bination resulted in a true dislocation in one out of every 35 births. The association of torticollis with an increased risk of hip problems has been recognized. It was shown that 20 per cent of children with torticollis also have an abnormal hip.

DIAGNOSIS

The diagnosis of congenital dislocation in newborns is based on the clinical examination. For the examination, the infant needs to be lying quietly on its back with the pelvis stabilized by one hand as the examining hand flexes the thigh to 90°. The knee is flexed to an acute angle (Fig. 18-3), and the fingers are placed over the lateral aspect of the thigh, with the finger tips at the level of the greater trochanter and the thumb across the angle of the knee. The thumb should not be placed into the femoral triangle area, because pressure at this point is painful. The maneuver is performed by gently lifting the trochanter towards the acetabulum as the leg is abducted. With this motion, a proprioceptive sensation of the femoral head

sliding into the acetabulum is present. The classic jerk sign of reduction is unusual, although it is present in some newborns.

The Barlow[5] examination is a provocative test of dislocation. The extremity is grasped gently in the manner described above, but the leg is adducted slightly past the midline (Fig. 18-4), and gentle downward pressure is placed at the angle of the knee, while gentle lateral pressure is placed against the inner thigh with the thumb. A dislocatable hip then becomes completely displaced, but when the leg is allowed to abduct freely, the hip reduces. These two maneuvers alone can establish the diagnosis of a dislocation or a dislocatable hip in newborns.

A screening program in which all newborns are examined in the nursery is an efficient method to establish this diagnosis. At birth the normal infant has a hip flexion contracture and extension to within 15° or 20° of the table top. The classic clinical signs of a dislocation in an older child include limited abduction, asymmetrical thigh folds, and relative femoral shortening.[41] Contrary to popular belief, the newborn with a dislocation has a remarkably normal examination

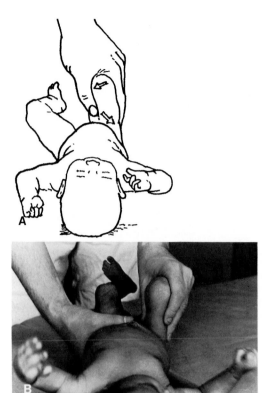

FIG. 18-4. *(A and B)* The Barlow provocative test. The thumb is placed on the inner aspect of the thigh and the hip is adducted, with longitudinal pressure exerted on the thigh, pushing it toward the table.

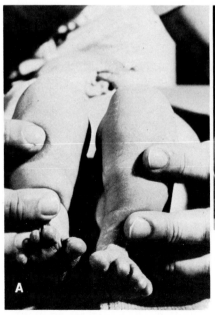

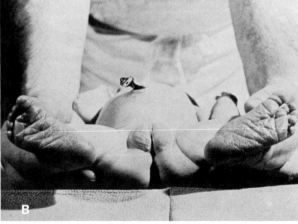

FIG. 18-5. *(A)* Newborn examination to detect limited abduction, asymmetrical thigh folds, and relative femoral shortening. *(B)* There is no limitation of abduction in this newborn, in spite of dislocation.

by these criteria (Fig. 18-5). A dislocation does not demonstrate femoral shortening, because dislocation is an event that has happened at or near birth, and the femur is slightly lateral to the acetabulum, but has not migrated proximally. Adductor tightness is also absent. Asymmetrical thigh folds are usually present if a dislocation exists; however, a large number of infants with normal hips also have asymmetry, making this method unreliable in detecting a dislocation.

ROENTGENOGRAPHIC STUDIES OF THE NEWBORN

Roentgenograms play a minor role in the diagnosis of newborns with congenital dislocation. In this group, the films often are misleading because the dislocation occurred at or near birth, and the secondary changes have not developed (Fig. 18-6). Shenton's line need not be broken and there is usually no false acetabulum. In addition, ossification of the innominate bone, which outlines the superior acetabulum, is indistinct. Therefore, the established criteria, such as the acetabular index and Hilgenreiner's line, are difficult to outline accurately.[7] Even pelvic positioning on the film makes a vast difference in the acetabular and femoral head contour and relationship. Side-to-side rotation can cause the appearance of an uncovered femoral head or abnormal acetabular index. Also, forward or posterior pelvic rotation can cause the indices to appear either increased or decreased, even when they are actually within the normal range.[56] This is particularly true with newborns because their flexion contractures cause the pelvis to rotate forward when the thighs are pressed against the roentgenography plate. A common error when taking a roentgenogram is failing to position the legs at all, allowing the hips to roll into external rotation, which disrupts the roentgenographic landmarks (Fig. 18-7). The Von Rosen[62] view taken with the legs in abduction and internal rotation is supposed to direct the femoral metaphysis above the acetabulum when a dislocation is present. However, this also is one of the positions that reduces a hip. Thus, in newborns whose hips are lax and can be placed in and

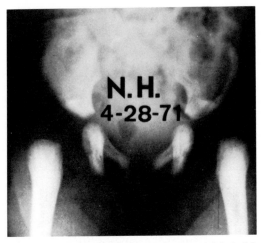

FIG. 18-6. Roentgenograms are not very helpful in detecting the newborn with congenital hip dislocation, because secondary changes have not yet occurred.

out of the acetabulum with ease, this position often reduces the hip when the hip is actually dislocated. The frog-leg position is popular to attain reduction, yet frequently a frog-leg view is obtained to determine whether a dislocation is present. This is inconsistent, because if the frog-leg position temporarily reduces the hip, the roentgenogram shows a normal hip, when in fact it may be dislocated in other positions. Another subtle but important aspect that is often forgotten is the ability of newborns to spontaneously reduce the hip by the tightening of pelvic girdle musculature, which can also give a false impression of a normal hip. (Because of the difficulties in positioning and the lack of ossification of the pelvis in newborns, one should not rely on roentgenograms for the diagnosis. A positive roentgenographic study can be helpful in the diagnosis of CDH, but a normal roentgenogram must be overruled by positive clinical findings of instability.) When the infant reaches the age of 4 to 6 weeks, roentgenograms usually are more helpful. At this time, the proximal femur has noticeable lateral and proximal displacement. Usually a false acetabulum is apparent, and Shenton's line is broken. There are numerous roentgeno-

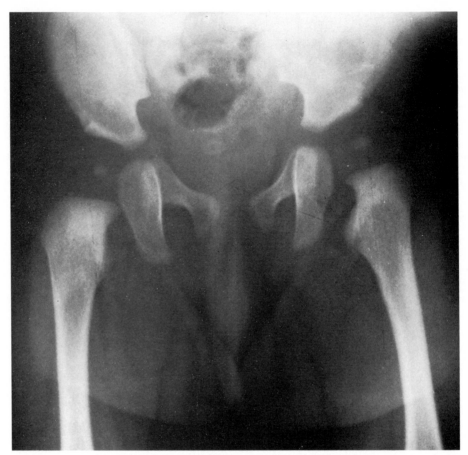

Fig. 18-7. Failure to properly position infant for roentgenograms. The roentgenographic landmarks are eliminated. Marked rotation of the thighs and rotation of the pelvis make an accurate interpretation impossible.

graphic signs,[25] as illustrated in Figure 18-8, but an important fact to remember is that they are usually absent in the newborn.

Change of Clinical Signs

Except for the ability of the examiner to reduce or displace the femoral head, the newborn examination is normal. However, between 1 and 3 months, secondary changes become readily apparent. It is at this time that the classic signs of adduction contracture and femoral shortening develop.

There is much confusion about the sign that Ortolani described in 1937.[39, 40] In his original publication he described a jerk or sudden movement as the flexed hip is ab-

ducted and the femoral head reduced. Unfortunately, the sign of the jerk or sudden movement is now commonly called a "hip click." Are hip clicks felt or heard, and is there a difference in the quality of the click? There are many high-pitched clicks or sounds about the hip and knee which are due to myofascial or ligamentous sources and are not secondary to a dislocated hip (Fig. 18-9). Although the reduction can occasionally be heard, it is far more common for it to be felt. In Ortolani's original description he stated that the jerk of reduction was not present in infants under 3 months of age. In the newborn reduction, the laterally displaced femoral head is subtly replaced into the acetabulum without a jerk. Vitally important

FIG. 18-8. Roentgenographic signs of congenital hip dislocation. (1) Horizontal Y line (Hilgenreiner's line); (2) Vertical line (Perkins' line); (3) Quadrants (formed by lines 1 & 2); (4) Acetabular index (Kleinberg & Lieberman); (5) Shenton's line; (6) Upward displacement of the femoral head; (7) Lateral displacement of the femoral head; (8) U figure of teardrop shadow (Kohler); (9) Y coordinate (Ponseti); (10) Capital epiphyseal dysplasia: (a) delayed appearance of the center of ossification of the femoral head, (b) irregular maturation of the center of ossification; (11) Bilification (furrowing of the acetabular roof in late infancy—Ponseti); (12) Hypoplasia of the pelvis (ilium); (13) Delayed fusion (ischiopublic juncture); (14) Absence of a shapely, defined, well-ossified acetabular margin, caused by delayed ossification of the cartilage of the roof of the socket; (15) Femoral shaft—Neck angle; (16) Adduction attitude of the extremity; (17) Development of the epiphyses of other joints (knees, wrists, and lumbosacral spine); (18) Radiolucent acetabular roof, limbus, joint capsule (arthrographic studies). (From Hart, V.: Congenital Dysplasia of the Hip Joint and Sequelae. Springfield, Charles C Thomas, 1952.)

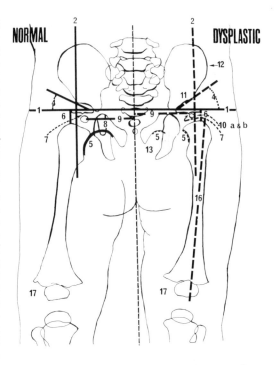

is the concept that the reduction is a proprioceptive sensation on the part of the examiner by the replacement of the femoral head. The misunderstanding of this proprioceptive concept, the extension of the jerk sign to newborns when it was originally *described* as a useful sign only for older infants, and confusion about hip clicks all contribute to undetected dislocated hips in newborns. This is not to say the jerk is never present in newborns, because occasionally it is detectable, but it is unusual. Thus, the Ortolani sign really has two characteristics; one early and one late. First, in newborns it

is a proprioceptive sensation of reduction. Secondly, in infants between 1 to 3 months, the classic Ortolani jerk sign is common (Fig. 18-10), because the soft tissues are now demonstrating more resistance to reduction than in the newborn period.

Between 3 and 6 months of age, the contractures progress until thigh shortening becomes easily detectable and tightness of the adductors is obvious (Fig. 18-11). The mother may begin to complain of difficulty with diaper changes because of an inability to spread the infant's legs, especially if the dislocation is bilateral. Bilateral dislocations

1937 Ortolani

jerk sign — sudden movement — snapping in

Not Present Under 3 Months

hip click (See, Hear, Feel)

1) Short High Frequency — Myofascial or Ligament

2) Jerk Sign — Dislocation

FIG. 18-9. See text.

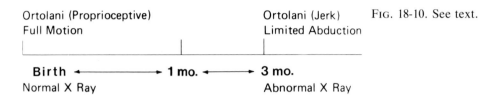

| Ortolani (Proprioceptive) | | Ortolani (Jerk) | FIG. 18-10. See text. |
| Full Motion | | Limited Abduction | |

Birth ←——————→ 1 mo. ←———→ 3 mo.
Normal X Ray   Abnormal X Ray

are often overlooked at this stage because the infant is symmetrically abnormal. At 3 to 6 months, the occurrence of the Ortolani sign decreases, because most dislocations become persistently stable in the dislocated position. As the infants become older this trend continues, so that the jerk becomes a rare occurrence by walking age.

EARLY TREATMENT

ORTHOTIC DEVICES

Treatment of the newborn is quite different from treatment of the older child, because the newborn has capsular laxity and a mildly eccentric limbus, but no abnormality of the femoral head or acetabulum. There are many devices available to facilitate reduction, but practically all are based on abduction. In newborns, full abduction is not as risky as it is in older infants, because newborns do not have adduction contractures. However, avascular necrosis can oc-

cur. A good method for treatment is the use of a Pavlik harness, which was described in 1957 by Professor Pavlik of Czechoslovakia.[41] This harness stresses the use of flexion and free abduction. Flexion begins to stabilize the hip because as the hip is flexed the femoral head is directed to the acetabulum. Often, abduction devices do not direct the femoral head toward the triradiate cartilage, but rather leave it pointing superiorly. As the hip is flexed, the head and neck axis begins to align with the acetabular axis. Although flexion is desirable, the hip should not be fully flexed. After the flexion range is adjusted, the hip is allowed to fall freely into abduction by the weight of the thighs. If the child sleeps in this device in the prone position, gradual abduction is also encouraged. In this way, the femoral head is not locked in any one position, and, actually, a controlled activity program is encouraged.

The Pavlik harness consists of an abdominal strap, two shoulder harnesses, and two leg stirrups. The stirrups have a strap that fastens to the abdominal belt, both an-

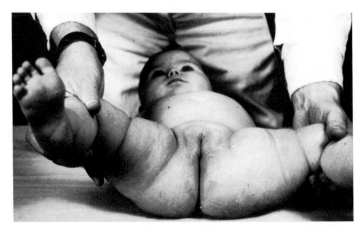

FIG. 18-11. By the age of 3 to 6 months, thigh shortening is apparent, as is tightness of the adductors, on the dislocated side.

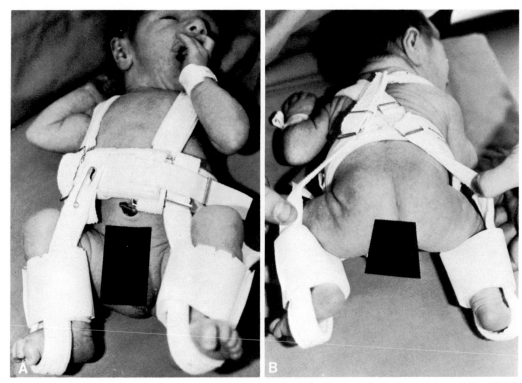

FIG. 18-12. *(A)* The Pavlik harness is applied so that baby's hips are in flexion without force. With 90° of flexion, the hips fall into abduction, *(B)* The prone position encourages gentle abduction.

teriorly and posteriorly. The posterior strap should not be pulled so tight as to force the legs into abduction (Fig. 18-12). The posterior strap should be loose enough to allow the knees to be brought within 5 cm. of the midline. Once the harness is applied, the position of the hip should be examined. Occasionally a stable reduction is not attained, and if the head remains dislocated, it usually can be felt. Secondly, a roentgenogram should be obtained with the infant in the harness. The most common error in applying the harness is to have the hips flexed less than 90° (Fig. 18-13). This may allow the femoral head to point toward the roof or the corner of the acetabulum. Once the harness is properly adjusted, the stirrups are marked at the buckles, as are the shoulder straps, so that the harness can be removed to bathe the child and to allow reapplication in the same position. The abdominal belt can be expanded as needed to allow for abdominal expansion.

There are many types of devices which basically utilize the modified frog-leg position. The Frejka pillow, the Von Rosen splint and other similar devices are successful in treating newborns with dislocation. Their success is based on the fact that newborns lack both adduction contractures and, secondary bone and cartilage changes and, therefore, there is no increased pressure on the femoral head.

Once any device is applied, one anteroposterior roentgenogram should be taken to determine that the femoral head is redirected into the acetabulum and not pushed above and against the side of the pelvis.

The anatomic deformity is more pronounced in the child over 1 to 3 months of age. At this stage, contractures are beginning to develop, roentgenograms show a slope of the bony acetabulum, and the cartilaginous portion of the acetabulum that cannot be seen on the film may also have an

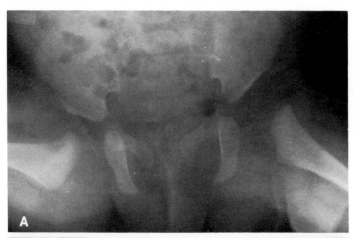

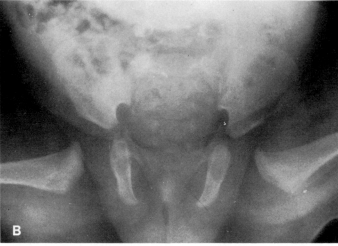

FIG. 18-13. Roentgenograms are taken with the child in the harness to insure that the hips are in flexion to at least 90°. *(A)* If this degree of flexion is not obtained, the femoral head may point to the roof or the corner of the acetabulum. *(B)* Further flexion without changing abduction corrects this problem.

abnormal slope. Therefore, the reduction in this age group is usually more unstable than in the newborn group. Whatever method is used to treat the child at this stage, these anatomic deformities must be taken into consideration, and the leg must be positioned so that the femoral head remains stable without force. At this stage it is very tempting to abduct the femur against the tight adductors to secure the reduction. However, this must be avoided at all costs because of the risk of avascular necrosis. The safe zone concept (Fig. 18-14) helps to gain reduction with minimal risk of avascular necrosis. The safe zone margins are a few degrees inside the interval between maximum abduction and the point of redislocation as the leg is brought back to the mid-

line. The Pavlik harness allows the femoral head to be stabilized, while allowing for motion within this guided range. Occasionally the femoral head points toward the triradiate cartilage with slight lateral displacement. In these cases, it is tempting to tighten the posterior strap of the Pavlik harness to bring the femoral head into a more secure, deeper position. However, this should be avoided because of the risk of producing an avascularity of the femoral head. Occasionally, an adductor tenotomy may be required. When an adduction contracture is present, it will stretch out in about 2 weeks if the femoral head is reduced (Fig. 18-15). Continued contractures are reason to suspect persistent dislocation. The Pavlik harness is left on full time and the infant is examined after a few

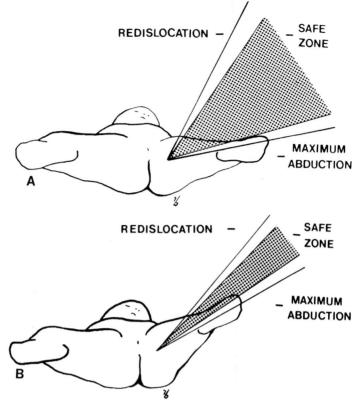

FIG. 18-14. The safe zone concept. (A) Considerable range between maximum abduction and redislocation (B) Inadequate range suggesting the need for an adductor tenotomy. (From Ramsey, P.L., Lasser, S., and MacEwen, G. D.: Congenital dislocation of the hip. J. Bone Joint Surg., 58A: 1000, 1976.)

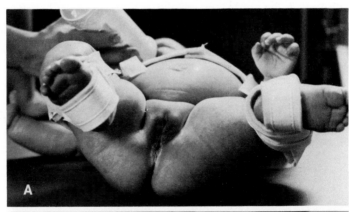

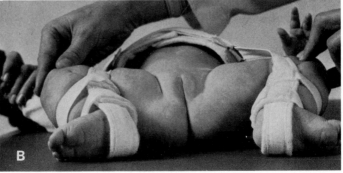

FIG. 18-15. (A) The appearrance of an infant with adduction contractures immediately after application of the harness. (B) After 3 weeks of continual wear, the adduction contractures stretch out.

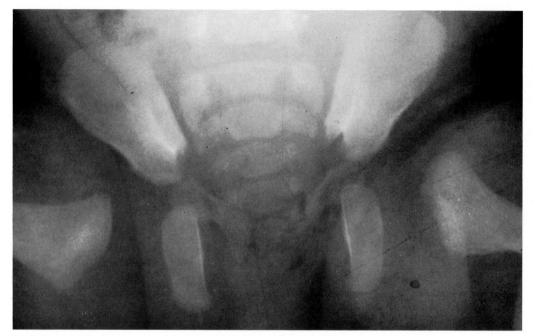

F<small>IG</small>. 18-16. Roentgenogram of an infant being treated with diapers shows that the hip is not kept in proper position. The femoral head is not directed to the acetabulum.

days to make certain that there are no complications. The clinical stability is then assessed at weekly intervals until stability is achieved. The harness is then removed for 2 hours a day. The time out of the harness is gradually increased by 2- to 4-hour increments if a neutral anteroposterior roentgenogram is consistent with reduction and if the acetabular index is stable or improving.

All children up to 6 months of age may be treated by this method without risk if the thighs are not pulled into abduction. If the femoral head does not become centered after 4 weeks, the child may be treated by traction and reduction methods.

Clinical stability in newborns is attained in 2 to 4 weeks. After the newborn period, the total length of treatment is approximately 1 to 2 times the age at which initial treatment was started.

D<small>IAPERS</small>

Diapers have no place in the treatment of a true congenital dislocation of the hip. Although multiple diapers have been used, they do not keep the hip in flexion (Fig. 18-16). In fact, the hip is in a great deal of extension most of the time. We have seen a number of children who were treated with diapers at birth with complete failure.

T<small>RACTION</small>

When the femoral head does not reduce with flexion, traction is required and skin traction is preferred. The hip and knee are flexed because of a hip flexion contracture and hamstring tightness. To apply traction, the skin is coated with an adherent material. The skin is wrapped with a Webril and the traction applied to the thighs and across the slightly bent knee. The wrapping needs to extend to and include the foot to prevent swelling. Not more than 4 to 5 lb. of skin traction are used.

Roentgenograms should be taken once a week. If there is no improvement or if there is minimal distal migration of the femoral head or metaphysis, pin traction is used. With the knee in extension, the appropriate pin placement is 1 cm. above the proximal pole of the patella. Pin stability is checked by tapping one end of the pin; the opposite

FIG. 18-17. For this infant with congenital dislocation of the hip, home treatment consists of a cast on the uninvolved side and skin traction of 1½–2 kilograms.

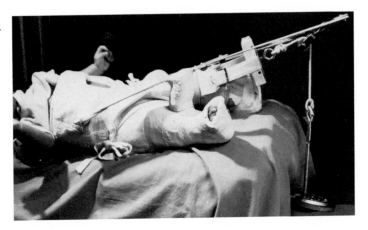

end should remain stable. If the opposite end moves while the one end is vibrating, then the pin is placed incorrectly, either in soft tissue or periosteum. Roentgenograms may be necessary to confirm the position of the pin in the femur of a young child.

To maintain sterility of the pin site, a simple gauze pad is applied, and the site is cleaned with Betadine once a day. The use of gauze or Vaseline wraps over the exit leads to retention of secretions and drainage and is not desirable.

Once there is secure skeletal fixation, it is very tempting to increase the weights. This practice is to be avoided because too much traction can cause the pin to cut into the distal femoral epiphyseal line.

In those instances where the child can be properly cared for at home, a unilateral cast with the involved leg free for skin traction over an outrigger can be used (Fig. 18-17). This program is desirable, since it keeps the child with the family and allows for gradual traction without the problems of hospitalization.

The question arises as to how long to maintain traction. Roentgenograms should be taken each week and the traction continued until the femoral head is below the level of the acetabulum.[24] An important step is to bring the femoral head well below the acetabular level to lessen the risk of avascular necrosis. Once the femoral head is down far enough, reduction can be attempted.

CASTING

Once the femoral metaphysis has been pulled well below the level of the acetabulum, the child is taken to the operating room, and, under general anesthesia, an attempt at closed reduction is made. If the hip does reduce, the most stable, yet safe, positions must be found to hold it in reduction. With the hip reduced in flexion above 90°, the leg is allowed to fall freely into abduction, and this degree of abduction is recorded. The leg is then gradually adducted back toward the midline. The point at which the hip redislocates is the instability point. The hip should be stabilized in plaster midway between its *fully* abducted position and its instability point. With this method of judging the degree of abduction, the complication of avascular necrosis can usually be avoided.

To test whether the dislocated hip is reduced, the knee is extended. When the hip is reduced, the knee cannot be fully extended unless the hip is redislocated. Another method of testing reduction is to palpate the ischium and the greater trochanter. They should be approximately on the same level; if the greater trochanter is posterior or higher, the hip is not reduced. Following reduction, a subcutaneous adductor tenotomy is performed. Most hips reduce by a closed method in this age period. The reduction of the femoral head into the acetabulum should be confirmed by roentgenogram. Arthrography is rarely helpful in this age group to determine reduction.

The application of a cast is rather complicated. Once the child is placed on the cast table, there should be one person responsible for maintaining the reduction. This may cause difficulties, since the anesthesiologist is trying to maintain the airway while an assistant is pulling at the hip to hold it in a stabilized position. Often, this results in the child sliding cephalad off the post of the table, resulting in the hips coming down into extension, which may render the previously reduced hip unstable. The knee should be in a 45° flexed position, but it must be kept in mind that the knee cannot be fully extended, or the hamstrings tighten and produce pressure on the femoral head. Once the cast is applied, it is very important that the child is comfortable during the next 6 to 12 hours. If the infant should fuss and cry uncontrollably in the cast, this is an indication of pain. If this should occur, the plaster should be removed immediately because the most frequent cause of pain in the immediate post-casting period is impending avascular necrosis of the femoral head.

Some of the most severe deformities secondary to avascular necrosis occur following cast applications without preliminary traction and without general anesthesia. This is not to say that all children need to have general anesthesia for cast application. However, usually it is difficult to apply the cast with the child awake and agitated. There is a temptation to hold the hips very snugly into place and, thus, to risk a very severe avascular necrosis. Therefore, our usual approach is to apply the cast for an unstable hip under general anesthesia.

OPEN REDUCTION

Except for the teratologic type of dislocation, very few children under walking age require open reduction, since almost all of these hips can be reduced by closed positioning or reduction methods.

If open reduction is required, the medial adductor approach of Ludloff may be used. The technique is complicated unless done by a surgeon who has had previous experience in this anatomic area. Others should use the classic anterolateral Smith-Petersen approach.

The adductor approach is appealing because the blood loss can be minimal, and it allows for an easy release of the constricted lower portion of the capsule.

If a child requires an open reduction before reaching 1 year of age, secondary procedures on the acetabulum or proximal femur are not required to maintain stability. The acetabular changes are reversible, and anteversion is not a contributing factor to instability in the under-walking-age group.

If subluxation persists after any of the previously mentioned treatment programs, a few months of abduction bracing by use of an Ilfeld or abductor brace with a pelvic band and thigh cuff usually produce stability.

CONGENITAL DISLOCATION OF THE HIP—EVALUATION AND TREATMENT AFTER WALKING AGE

After a child with an untreated congenital dislocation of the hip reaches walking age (regardless of the type of subsequent treatment), a complete recovery should not be expected. At least some stigmata will be seen in the roentgenograms of the involved hip.

The aims of treatment should be the reestablishment of the mechanics of the hip joint, thus delaying the development of osteroarthritis of the hip, and, hopefully, avoiding complications so that the patient may reach at least middle age before serious degeneration of the hip joint begins.

PATHOLOGY

In contrast to the pathology of the newborn, where there is exclusively an increased laxity of the joint capsule, the pathology in the walking child shows that all soft tissues and bony parts are distorted to a degree.

ACETABULUM

The ossification of the roof of the acetabulum is delayed and can be recognized in a roentgenogram. The acetabular labrum (limbus) may be enfolded into the posterosuperior lip of the acetabulum as a minor invagination, or in some patients it may form an almost complete diaphragm covering the acetabulum. The fat and fibrous tissue in the depths of the acetabulum may be enlarged (pulvinate), thereby obstructing reentry of the femoral head. A false acetabulum may be present and, to the less experienced surgeon, may appear to be the true acetabulum. The proximal location and the absence of an attached ligamentum teres should indicate the difference.

CAPSULE

The capsule may be constricted between the acetabulum and the femoral head to produce an hourglass deformity. This shape mainly results from the tight iliopsoas tendon indenting the capsule. The inferior surface of the capsule is stretched across the lower half of the acetabulum and, together with the intact transverse acetabular ligament, it may act as a barrier to full reduction of the femoral head below the superior acetabular roof and acetabular labrum. This is probably the most overlooked problem in relation to reduction. The capsule may also be adherent to the cartilage of the femoral head and may prevent reduction.

LIGAMENTUM TERES

The ligamentum teres may be normal, absent, or enlarged. If enlarged, it may be a relative obstruction to reduction. In the first few years of life, it is not an important source of blood supply to the hip, and, therefore, it can be sacrificed at the time of an open reduction.

FEMORAL HEAD AND PROXIMAL FEMUR

The femoral head may lose its conical form and become flattened. This change of shape is often exaggerated when the femoral head has been maintained against the side of the pelvis during an unsuccessful treatment program. The proximal femur usually demonstrates an increase in anteversion. This increase can be most accurately determined clinically by the number of degrees above the normal 45° of internal rotation that is required to produce a concentric repositioning of the femoral head.

ROENTGENOGRAPHIC EVALUATION

Roentgenographic review is most helpful in the follow-up evaluation, because most patients have few, if any, clinical symptoms in adolescence and young adult life. The evaluation of the three dimensions around the hip joint is ideal, but most emphasis is place on one dimension, the anteroposterior view, because of the difficulty in obtaining other meaningful views. Special views for anteversion have been described, but do not help much in the evaluation of an individual patient. A repeat roentgenogram with the thigh in varying degrees of internal rotation better demonstrates the subluxation that may result from anteversion of the femur (Fig. 18-18).

ACETABULAR INDEX

The acetabular index is determined by first drawing a line across the triradiate cartilages (Hilgenreiner's line).[26] This line intersects with a line from the lateral edge of the acetabulum to the triradiate cartilage. The acetabular index is the angle formed by the intersection of these two lines. In the past, the acetabular index has often been considered the absolute criterion in determining the shape of the developing acetabulum; however, it only represents the bone formation. Arthrography, however, demonstrates that the acetabulum maintains a normal cartilaginous contour much longer than was formerly believed (Fig. 18-19). Reconstructive procedures that would have been performed in past years on children at ages 3 to 4 years can be safely delayed until these children are 6 to 7 years if there is no evidence of subluxation, even though the bony outline of the acetabulum appears to be deficient.

CENTER-EDGE (CE) ANGLE

The center-edge (CE) angle is determined by finding the center of the femoral head, and marking the lateral corner of the

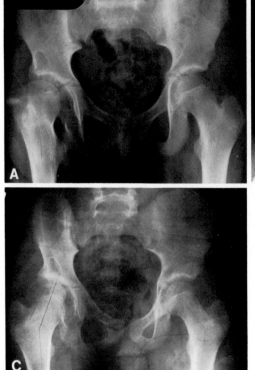

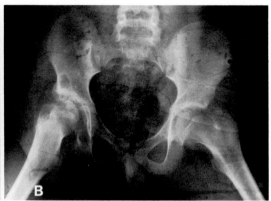

FIG. 18-18. *(A)* The neutral standing film shows deformity more of the proximal femur than of the acetabulum. *(B)* Abduction alone results in slight improvement of centering. *(C)* The internal rotation view shows more improvement. *(Continued, opposite)*

acetabulum. A horizontal line connects the two femoral head centers, and perpendicular lines are drawn from each center. A line is drawn from the acetabular edge to the center of the femoral head, and the angle formed is known as the "center-edge" angle (Fig. 18-20). The center-edge angle should be at least 20° and preferably 25° to insure normal seating of the femoral head.

After the femoral head has been reduced in the joint, an evaluation should be made regarding subluxation, as compared to a full reduction, by using the CE angle. This evaluation is relatively simple in the normal hip since the corner of the normal acetabulum can be visualized in its full aspect. An acetabular dysplasia makes the evaluation difficult because the landmarks are less distinct due to underdevelopment of the bone model, but it is still the best method to determine a slight degree of subluxation.

REDUCTION OF THE DISLOCATED HIP

A controversy still exists as to the merits of closed versus open reduction in the treatment of a child after walking age. Primary treatment of a dislocated hip in this age group is becoming rare, so that in many parts of the world surgeons are involved in the treatment of relatively few children. Of all the standard operative procedures on the hip joint, an accurate open reduction in a child of any age is probably the most difficult. It therefore should not be taken lightly. An adequate education of the surgeon is important before attempting to carry out an open reduction. In most hands, for a child up to 3 years of age, a successful closed reduction after a period of traction that has slowly pulled the femoral head to below the triradiate cartilage is usually the most successful form of treatment, resulting in the least

Fig. 18-18 *(Continued).* *(D)* Combined internal rotation and abduction results in the best centering of the hips. *(E)* A standing film after an osteotomy that combined external rotation and adduction shows the same positioning is achieved as in *(D)*.

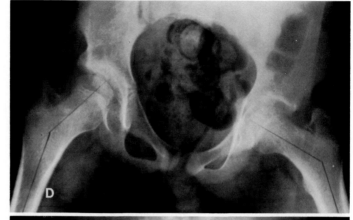

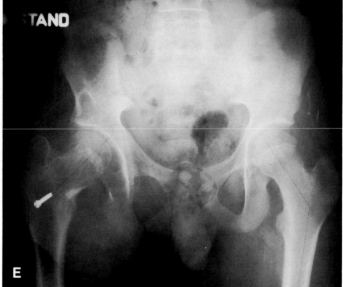

amount of stiffness and involving only a minor risk of avascular necrosis. If initially successful, redislocation is infrequent. The femoral head must be pulled down gradually with traction to below the triradiate cartilage and the position verified by roentgenograms before an attempt is made at closed reduction.

Skin traction is preferable to skeletal traction. If a pin is used, it should be placed in the distal femur instead of the tibia, just above the level of the proximal pole of the patella, with the knee in extension. After the femoral head reaches the level of the triradiate cartilage and remains there for several days, it is desirable to remove the pin and return to skin traction before reducing the hip. The reestablishment of skin traction allows the pin tract to heal and decreases the risk of infection, should an open reduction be necessary.

CLOSED REDUCTION

Gentle, closed reduction or repositioning of a dislocated hip should be performed on a child who is anesthetized to allow full muscle relaxation. The child lies in a supine posi-

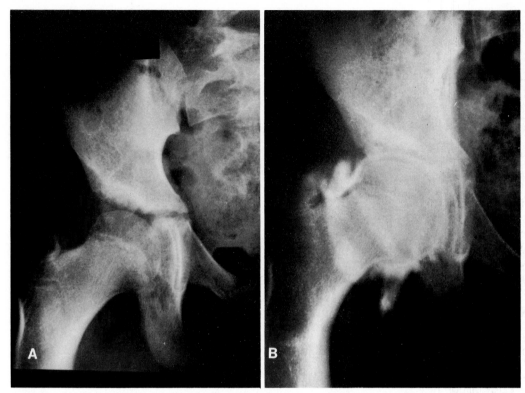

Fig. 18-19. *(A)* This roentgenogram shows a deficient bony acetabulum. *(B)* However, arthrography shows that the cartilage model is normal. Therefore, the patient has only dysplasia of the bony acetabulum.

tion with the pelvis flat on the table and the opposite extremity flexed, abducted, and stabilized by an assistant. The thigh on the affected side is flexed and adducted to relax the capsule and the adductor muscles. Manual traction is applied to the thigh while the surgeon guides the femoral head into the socket and while the thigh is abducted 50° to 60°, never approaching 80° to 90°. The thigh is gradually adducted until the femoral head again drops out of the acetabulum. This re-dislocation gives an indication of the potential stability of the joint and the chance for success of the closed reduction, as well as determining the safety zone, as outlined in the treatment program for the younger child, to decrease the risk of avascular necrosis.

All the maneuvers must be most gentle and must be carried out as a "positioning" of the leg and not a reduction in the sense of forcing the position. The total procedure should be thought of as similar to the Orto-

lani maneuver for the infant. If any tightness is demonstrated in the adductors, a sub-cutaneous adductor tenotomy should be done. This procedure is necessary in almost all children in this age group. If the arc of motion between reduction and dislocation is less than 25°, successful maintenance of re-duction is most unlikely and redislocation is to be expected. An open reduction should then be undertaken.

Roentgenograms are taken to confirm the positioning of the head in the socket, and the femoral head must point to, or slightly be-low, the triradiate cartilage. A more proxi-mal alignment of the femoral head is not compatible with a concentric reduction. Further flexion of the thigh may direct the head to the triradiate cartilage. If this is not successful, an open reduction is indicated. After closed reduction, lateral roentgeno-grams, other than to show a true redisloca-tion, have not been very useful. A plaster cast is applied with the thighs in 90° of flexion, never exceeding 60° of abduction. The modified frog-leg plaster cast is used for 6 to 9 months. An abduction brace should be used for an additional 6 months to 1 year if there are problems in maintaining centering of the femoral head. If, following this period of time, the hip still demonstrates *subluxation* with the leg in neutral position and demonstrates good centering with the leg in abduction, an evaluation should be made as to the type of extra-articular procedure which is necessary to keep the femoral head centered.

If closed reduction proves to be unsuccessful, the surgeon should be prepared to proceed with open reduction.

Slight lateral displacement of the epiphysis after closed reduction is not an indication for open reduction. The clinical signs of stability are more helpful at this stage than results of an arthrogram. After a few days or weeks the femoral head usually settles deeply into the acetabulum, as can be seen on follow-up roentgenograms. Persistent displacement at 6 weeks is an indication for open reduction.

Morel[34] of France has reintroduced and refined the technique of gradual longitudinal traction, followed by gradual positioning of the leg in abduction and internal rotation and application of a spica cast, without the need for a reduction *per se*. This technique has resulted in a concentric reduction in two-thirds of the patients, even though many are 5 or 6 years of age, and it involves a minimal risk of avascular necrosis. If after the maneuver the patient does not show full reduction at 6 weeks, open reduction is done. All of Morel's patients had innominate osteotomies a few weeks after stability had been obtained. This program has been highly successful in children up to approximately 6 years of age. It is based on the approach of gradual repositioning of the head of the femur in the acetabulum and the use of only extra-articular procedures, where possible. We agree with this concept.

OPEN REDUCTION

The indications for open reduction are: (1) if the femoral head on roentgenogram persistently lies above the triradiate cartilage; (2) if

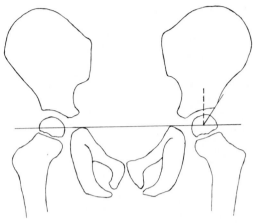

FIG. 18-20. The center-edge angle of Wiberg.

the arc of reduction and redislocation is less than 25° after an adduction tenotomy; (3) if the femoral head will not enter the acetabulum; (4) if the femoral head is still laterally placed in the acetabulum after 6 weeks of reduction; and (5) after a previously failed reduction.

In the hands of surgeons who lack extensive experience, it is probably best to consider open reduction as the only primary procedure to be carried out, reserving femoral or pelvic osteotomy for a secondary procedure. Too often redislocation has followed the combined procedures, and it is probably best to concentrate on performing a careful and complete open reduction. The secondary procedures can be carried out later, as may be required after closed reduction.

A careful open reduction should follow an organized plan, as outlined in specific textbooks, but there are several areas of prime importance.

The Smith-Petersen incision is the one usually used in this age group. The skin incision should follow along just below the iliac crest, and not over it. It should then extend in an oblique line parallel to the inguinal ligament, and it should not turn distally. This allows for the same deep exposure, but produces a much less noticeable scar. The psoas tendon should be sectioned if it is tight, but the iliacus muscle should always be left intact to preserve hip flexion.

It may be necessary to peel the capsule

from the articular cartilage of the femoral head in the older patient. This procedure should only be done with great care, and the dissection should not be carried down along the femoral neck, which risks damage to the metaphyseal vessels and increases the risk of avascular necrosis.

If the fibrofatty tissue from the acetabulum is excessive and is not thoroughly removed, it is difficult or impossible to reduce the head deeply into the socket. The use of a curette has often been suggested, however, its use can result in destruction of portions of the articular cartilage. Pituitary rongeurs have been more effective in thoroughly removing the soft-tissue material, and they do not obstruct visibility during the procedure.

The inferior half of the acetabulum is one of the most important areas of the hip and is commonly overlooked. The anterolateral exposure, which is the standard approach for open reduction in the walking child, makes the distance to the inferior capsule considerable, and, therefore, visibility of the area is limited or obscured. The inferior capsule is usually stretched upward and across the inferior acetabulum, and this capsule is best pushed downwards by blunt instruments, thus developing a potential pocket for the femoral head. The transverse acetabular ligament cannot be visualized through this approach, but with palpation and a pair of scissors, it can be felt, outlined, transected and opened, allowing the lower part of the acetabulum to widen. If a pocket is not developed inferiorly, the head will often not drop down into the lower part of the acetabulum, which is necessary for a concentric reduction. This area is the one probably most commonly overlooked in open reduction. An osteotomy is too often unwisely considered as an alternative for gaining full reduction, instead of developing the lower acetabular area. In such patients, to incorrectly use a pelvic osteotomy may only increase the intraarticular pressure and produce a redislocation or avascular necrosis. An accurate reduction must initially be obtained, and the lower acetabulum is the area of concern.

The infolding of the acetabular labrum (limbus) may also be an obstruction to a concentric reduction. This infolding can be detected at the time of open reduction by running a curved blunt instrument about the upper one-half of the acetabulum. If found, it is preferable to evert the labrum and reduce the head deeply under it. This procedure may require one or two radial cuts in the labrum before it folds outward. It is part of the normal biologic tissue and is probably required for full acetabular development. Therefore, it should not be removed unless it is impossible to unfold it outside the equator of the femoral head.

After open reduction, immobilization should not be continued for over 6 to 8 weeks, or severe stiffness may result.

The older child with bilateral hip dislocation is a most difficult problem. One should strongly consider withholding treatment in a child over 4 years of age, because the risk of stiffness in both hips is significant. This group of children has produced the greatest number of difficulties in treatment programs. Bilaterally dislocated hips, however, which are unusually mobile and in which the femoral heads pull down readily with gentle traction, may be reduced, but these are the exceptions. If roentgenograms show very high femoral heads, reductions should probably not be attempted.

The argument is put forth that, someday, better total hip joint replacement techniques may be possible if bilateral dislocated hips are reduced. To perform multiple surgical procedures in a patient that maintains bilateral dislocations throughout childhood and adolescence, in order to allow for better reconstructive replacement later, does not seem realistic. Most of these patients could get along for 25 to 40 years without treatment. Although this is not an ideal situation, it is better than having repeated, unsuccessful operations. In most instances, however, the child with unilateral dislocation is a candidate for treatment throughout childhood.

COLONNA ARTHROPLASTY

This arthroplasty is helpful for only a complete dislocation of the hip. The capsule is enclosed over the femoral head and placed in an enlarged acetabulum from which the articular cartilage has been removed. This procedure results in a significant percentage of early stiff hips. The remaining children usually develop degenerative arthritis as young adults, and the procedure is rarely, if ever, recommended. It has been essentially replaced by other procedures listed in this chapter.

COMPLICATED REDUCTIONS

If it is not possible or desirable to lower the femoral head to the level of the acetabulum with traction because of the tightness of the surrounding tissues, a technique, recently repopularized by Klisic of Yugoslavia, of shortening the femur can be used. This technique allows for the lowering of the femoral head to the acetabular level, without tension, by shortening the femur instead of elongating the muscles. If the surgeon is not very familiar with the routine methods of reduction, it is best to bring the femoral head down with traction and place the major emphasis on a careful and complete open reduction.

If shortening of the femur is employed, it is important to carry out the technique of exposure and removal of the materials preventing the reduction before transecting the femur. This allows for better control of the fragments. The femoral osteotomy is allowed to overlap the distance previously occupied by the top of the femoral head above the roof of the acetabulum (approximately 2 cm.), and some varus positioning may be desirable for stability. The anteversion may also be reduced by externally rotating the distal fragment and leaving about 10° to 15° of internal rotation. The osteotomy should be internally fixed, by pins or a plate.

PRINCIPLES OF MAINTAINING REDUCTION BY SECONDARY PROCEDURES

The ideal goal of treatment in a child first treated after walking age is to produce a reasonably perfect hip at skeletal maturity (one with no residual subluxation and only mild distortion of the acetabulum and proximal femur). Even though this goal may, at times, not be possible due to complications associated with the initial treatment, surgery may still be desirable. The types of repair and reconstructive procedures to be considered are varied. There are advantages and problems with each procedure.

As a rule, unless the hip is completely redislocated, extra-articular procedures are better directed to the proximal femur or pelvis or both, rather than using intra-articular ones, which produce a risk of stiffness in the older child.

Standing roentgenograms should always be used after a child reaches walking age. They help in evaluating a leg length discrepancy, either true or apparent. This technique can also establish the existence of subluxation, which may be present only on weightbearing, secondary to weightbearing, itself, or to a possible malalignment of the pelvis.

If a child requires a secondary procedure, it is important to consider that both the femoral and acetabular components are abnormal to some degree. Usually, one side of the joint is more distorted than the other side, so it is usually important to realign the more distorted side in an effort to produce a good result. Since both sides of the joint are not fully corrected, biologic remodeling is necessary to produce the best result. Therefore, surgery ideally should be performed when there are at least 2 to 3 years of growth potential remaining—by approximately 11 years in girls and 13 years in boys. The use of most of the procedures when the patient is skeletally mature should not be ruled out, but a less satisfactory end result should be anticipated, since little, if any, remodeling can be expected.

The abduction test, whereby the thigh is abducted to varying degrees and roentgenograms are taken, can give valuable information as to the degree of repositioning of the femoral head in the acetabulum. The test can yield information to help determine the most desirable secondary procedure (Fig. 18-21). As a rule, both the pelvis and the proximal femur lose their ability to fully remodel at approximately 7 to 8 years. After that age, in a child with a major deformity, more thought may be needed in considering a procedure to improve both aspects of the deformity.

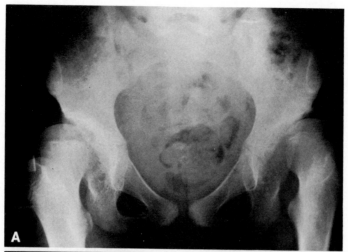

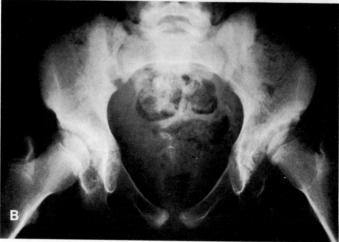

Fig. 18-21. The abduction test to determine if the femoral head will center. *(A)* The anteroposterior view shows significant subluxation of the femoral heads. *(B)* When there is abduction and internal rotation, centering results. This positioning suggests that a technique to reposition the femoral heads is appropriate.

ACETABULAR PROCEDURES

Realignment Techniques

The shelf procedure was the first extra-articular acetabular containment procedure to be developed. It allows the intact acetabular cartilage to remain in contact with the femoral head. The shelf should be thought of more as a stabilizer or buttress of the femoral head by the extension of the acetabulum rather than as an additional weightbearing surface (Fig. 18-22).

It is difficult to perform the shelf procedure at exactly the correct level. It is often placed too far proximally on the side of the pelvis. (In time, the shelf will disappear if it is not giving buttress support to the femoral head). The upper portion of the capsule must be stripped down and part of it must even be resected to give a smooth contour with the capsule over the femoral head. Only when dissection of the capsule is complete should the outer pelvic cortex be pried down and buttressed with extra bone. Wilson has reported a recent successful series in adolescents. It is a reconstructive procedure, but it is useful in the older child or young adult where little or no biologic remodeling is to be expected and where contact exists between the femoral head and the acetabulum, but the femoral head is unstable and subluxes laterally (Fig. 18-23). One-half of the femoral head must be replaceable in the acetabulum for a successful result to ensue.

FIG. 18-22. This model shows the proper level of shelf placement for the shelf procedure.

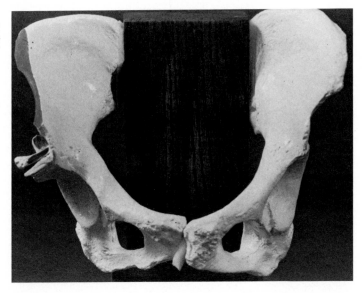

The innominate osteotomy of Salter is used to redirect the acetabulum to produce femoral head coverage laterally and anteriorly.[48] It is ideal for acetabular dysplasia and mild subluxation in children of 3 to 10 years. Anterior coverage of the femoral head is accomplished by rotation of the acetabular fragment on the symphysis. The size of the patient and the resultant distance from the midline is not important for the production of the anterior coverage (Fig. 18-24). The difficulty with this procedure arises in obtaining lateral coverage. The angulation occurs on the symphysis pubis,

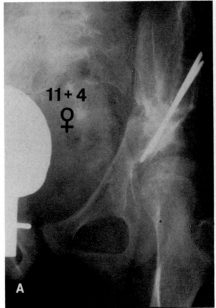

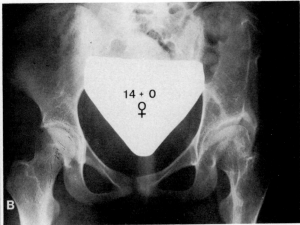

FIG. 18-23. *(A)* Immediate preoperative film of a girl 11 years and 4 months old who underwent a shelf osteotomy to salvage an inadequate Salter procedure. *(B)* Follow-up film at 14 years of age shows a contained head with the buttress effect of the shelf.

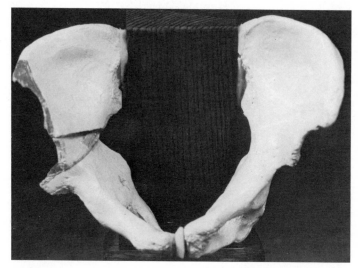

Fig. 18-24. A model of the Salter procedure, showing lateral and anterior rotation of the distal fragment and rotation at the symphysis pubis. To avoid excessive lengthening of the extremity, the graft should not separate the bony fragments posteriorly.

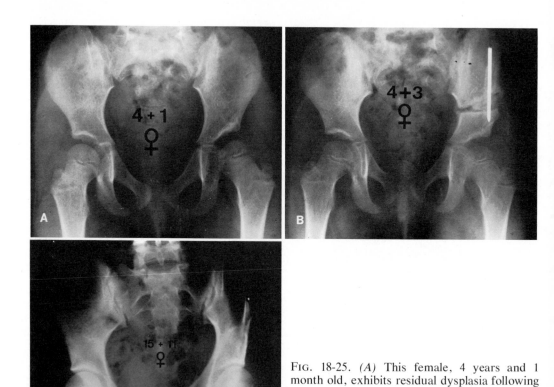

Fig. 18-25. (A) This female, 4 years and 1 month old, exhibits residual dysplasia following closed reduction. (B) A film taken immediately after Salter osteotomy shows an essentially normal acetabular roof. (C) The follow-up film taken at 15 years and 11 months shows an excellent result at skeletal maturity.

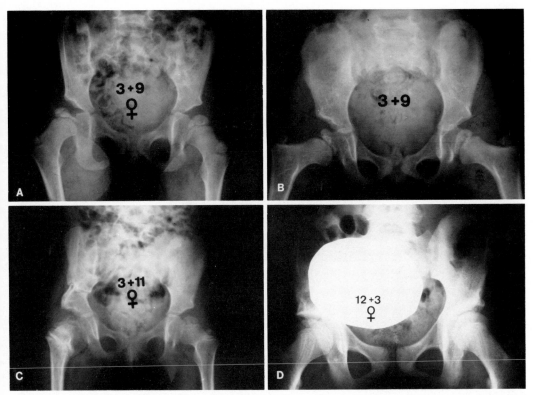

FIG. 18-26. *(A)* In this child of 3 years and 9 months, neutral-position film shows vascular changes in the femoral head and residual acetabular dysplasia. *(B)* Significant abduction is necessary to produce centering. *(C)* Film taken 2 months later, soon after the Salter procedure and intertrochanteric varus osteotomy were performed. *(D)* At 12 years of age, there is good coverage of the femoral head.

which is a significant distance from the acetabulum, limiting the possible improvement. The average change in the acetabular index that can be produced by the technique is approximately 10°. If the acetabulum must be changed significantly, this procedure is not technically feasible. An arthrogram is advisable before considering this procedure. If the cartilaginous acetabular model is normal and the hip is not subluxed, surgery can wait until the child is approximately 7 years of age, because there is a good possibility that the bony acetabulum may reconstitute and, therefore, may not require the operative procedure.

If, however, there is even a suggestion of subluxation, the procedure should be performed as soon as possible. In Salter's series, the best results were obtained in the group who had dysplasia without an associated dislocation. Ninety-four per cent of his series had an excellent result (Fig. 18-25). A disadvantage of the innominate osteotomy is that it can produce a longer extremity on the involved side, even though the osteotomy remains closed posteriorly. The osteotomy tends to lengthen the extremity by approximately 1 cm. in a patient of adult size. This change is not significant, but in a child of 6 years the problem is magnified. All follow-up roentgenograms should be taken in the standing position rather than supine to allow for a better evaluation of the hips' centering and increased leg length. If the femoral head is not fully covered after the innominate osteotomy, a heel lift on the opposite extremity may again level the pelvis. If the involved

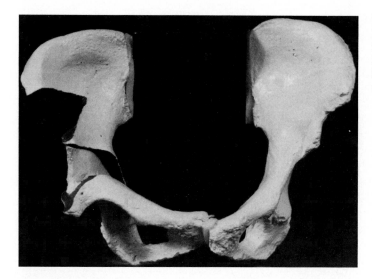

FIG. 18-27. This model of the Pemberton procedure shows the alteration in the acetabular roof achieved by angulating the hip at the triradiate cartilage.

extremity is already longer, a procedure that does not add to the length should probably be used, or a wedge of bone at the posterior section of the pelvis may be removed during the innominate osteotomy to eliminate the potential lengthening of the leg.

Some innominate osteotomies are incorrectly stabilized. The pins used are often not long enough to stabilize the distal fragment, allowing the graft to dislodge and the distal fragment to slip medially. If, after this occurs, the femoral head does not sublux, this result should be accepted. If subluxation occurs and the femoral head centers on the abduction test, a varus osteotomy is indicated rather than a second acetabular procedure (Fig. 18-26).

Pemberton Osteotomy. The acetabular roof is changed in direction and shape at the triradiate cartilage (Fig. 18-27).[42] The change in direction of the acetabular roof is, therefore, of much greater magnitude than in the innominate procedure of Salter, where the lateral rotation of the roof of the acetabulum is at the symphysis pubis. Both procedures, however, should only be done for a hip with a true, concentric reduction. This procedure is particularly indicated when there is a major, true deficiency in the angle of the cartilaginous acetabular roof. The actual deformity should be confirmed by an arthrogram, because the true cartilage model may be intact, although the bone model may appear grossly deficient. In this event, the hip would be grossly distorted by this procedure, and the procedure is contraindicated.

The Pemberton osteotomy requires extensive surgical exposure and is technically more difficult than the Salter procedure. By altering the depth of the osteotomy medially or posteriorly the distal fragment can be directed either more anteriorly or laterally, as needed for the individual patient. Since the acetabular roof is distorted, there is risk of stiffness. Therefore, as full a range of motion as possible should be obtained prior to this operation (Fig. 18-28).

Since the downward direction of the acetabular roof can be changed grossly, there is considerable risk of greatly increasing the acetabular pressure. The procedure should, therefore, be preceded by femoral traction until the femoral head is level with the final desired position, if there has been any previous upward migration.

This procedure deforms the acetabulum and produces an incongruity. However, this incongruity should correct itself in the growing child. The cut must not extend into the acetabulum and damage the articular cartilage. The Pemberton procedure may produce a stiff hip in the older child, since the acetabulum is deformed and incongruity is aggravated. Therefore, it should be ideally performed several years before skeletal

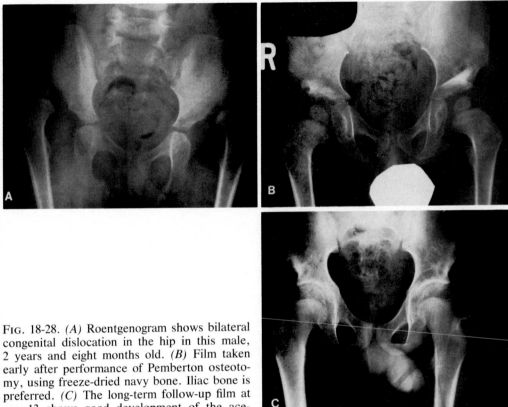

Fig. 18-28. *(A)* Roentgenogram shows bilateral congenital dislocation in the hip in this male, 2 years and eight months old. *(B)* Film taken early after performance of Pemberton osteotomy, using freeze-dried navy bone. Iliac bone is preferred. *(C)* The long-term follow-up film at age 13 shows good development of the acetabula.

maturity is reached, and postoperative immobilization should be no more than 6 weeks. Closure of the triradiate cartilage in the adolescent becomes an absolute contraindication for this procedure.

Steel Procedure. The osteotomy through the innominate bone is much like Salter's procedure, but instead of rotating on the symphysis pubis, cuts are made through both pubic rami.[56] The ischial cut is made through an incision in the buttock, and the superior ramus is sectioned from the medial aspect of the standard anterolateral Smith-Petersen approach. These extra osteotomies allow freer motion in the acetabular fragment (Fig. 18-29).

Technique. This osteotomy is much more complicated than the Salter procedure. It is indicated when the femoral head still centers on the abduction test, but where there is a major acetabular deformity (Fig. 18-30).

Contraindications. The procedure is contraindicated unless the femoral head can be reduced into the acetabulum. It is also contraindicated if the problem can be corrected by the use of simpler techniques.

Sutherland Procedure. This procedure is similar in principle and indications to the Steel osteotomy, but the osteotomy through the pubis is made from above.[58] The cut passes just medial to the obturator foramen and lateral to the symphysis pubis. A sector of bone of up to 2 cm. is removed to allow medial displacement of the distal fragment (Fig. 18-31). This osteotomy allows for somewhat less rotation than does the Steel procedure, but more than would be achieved with an innominate procedure of Salter. It can produce more medial displacement of the distal fragment than the Steel procedure because of the removal of the bone. It does, however, require pin fixation of the medial

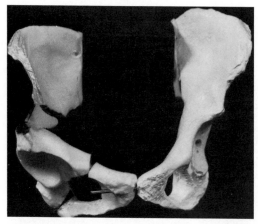

FIG. 18-29. A model of a Steel osteotomy shows cut made on the innominate bone through the three appropriate areas. The pin across symphysis is not necessary.

osteotomy, which could result in complications.

Dial Osteotomy. Principle. This procedure is a periarticular acetabular osteotomy in which a cut is made around the complete acetabulum just outside the capsule, which allows for the lateral rotation of the acetabulum (Fig. 18-32). Since the osteotomy is close to the whole acetabulum, it allows the greatest change in position of the acetabulum. There must be a concentric re-

duction in this osteotomy in order to achieve a successful result (Fig. 18-33).

Complications. It is technically difficult to cut out the whole acetabulum without either going medially through the pelvis or entering into the acetabulum. There is also a risk to the sciatic nerve and risk of producing vascular changes in the acetabular fragment, if the fragment is cut too thin. Although extensive experience by many surgeons has not been gained in the use of this operation, it would seem to be indicated in the older child and adolescent who has very severe subluxation and deformity, but where a reduction on the abduction test is still possible. This procedure, above all the procedures mentioned, should be reserved for the patients of surgeons with a large experience in hip surgery.

Reconstructive Procedure—The Chiari Method

Principle. If the femoral head does not center on abduction because of abnormality of the acetabulum, the procedure developed by Professor Chiari of Vienna, Austria may be considered.[10] It allows for good femoral coverage, but functions as an arthroplasty and a salvage procedure. It should not be considered if one of the above concentric reduction techniques is possible. If the femoral head has migrated laterally and proximally, it may no longer center on the

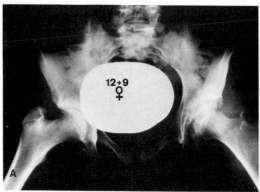
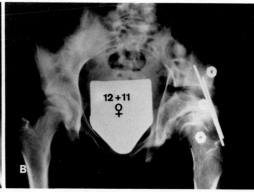

FIG. 18-30. *(A)* Preoperative film of a girl 12 years and 14 months old shows that at least 40° of abduction are required to center the femoral heads. *(B)* Film taken after Steel osteotomy shows excellent coverage.

FIG. 18-31. A model of the Sutherland osteotomy. (The arrow indicates the midline of the pelvis.)

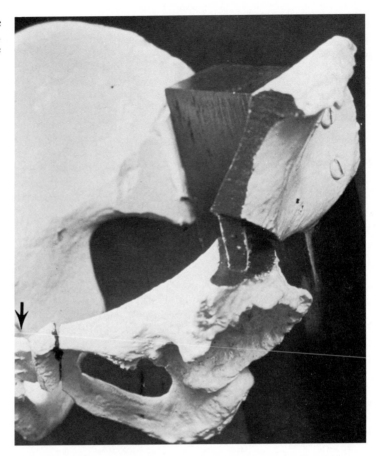

abduction test. By displacing the distal fragment medially, a roof is produced for the head underneath the lateral pelvis with the capsule interposed, thus creating an arthroplasty. By moving the femoral head toward the midline, the mechanics of the joint are improved, and therefore there is less force across the joint on weightbearing.

Technique. The osteotomy is made just above the capsule and the capsule is pushed medially, with the distal fragment, to produce an arthroplasty on top of the femoral head. In other words, it superimposes a Colonna arthroplasty lateral to the deficient contact point of the acetabulum and femoral head. It is technically exacting. Length of the extremity can rarely be regained, because the capsule is attached along the side of the pelvis. If detached, it can no longer act

as the interposing membrane. Therefore, the level of the osteotomy cannot be lowered so as to retain the capsule as an interposed tissue. The pelvic cut has to be directed medially upwards, so that the distal fragment will slide medially. This usually produces a slight shortening of the leg, and should be considered in the assessment for surgery. Ideally, the osteotomy should be domed from anterior to posterior so that the pelvic surface above the head is contoured and is as congruous as possible (Fig. 18-34). Since the pelvis is essentially cancellous bone, it will contour itself with time, to some degree. A relatively normal neck-shaft angle is an important consideration and, if not present, it should be corrected by surgery. In most surgeons' hands it is probably better to correct the femoral deformity and to proceed to the

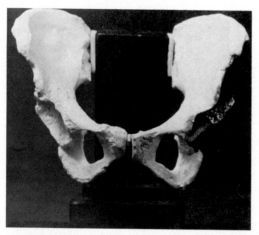

FIG. 8-32. A model of the dial osteotomy.

Chiari procedure several weeks later, after healing of the femoral osteotomy is complete (Fig. 18-35).

The displacement should be at least one-half of the width of the pelvis. Full displace-

ment, with the distal fragment displaced into the pelvis, may result in nonunion. Threaded pins placed across the osteotomy site can maintain the displacement desired and can avoid the necessity of using a spica cast postoperatively. If good pin fixation is obtained, by placing the extremity in balanced suspension, early range of motion exercises are possible within days of the procedure.

Complications. If the cut is made below the capsule, the femoral head is in direct contact with the bone of the pelvis, which is undesirable.

Evaluation. The interposed capsule, at best, will develop into fibrocartilage and will never be a true articular cartilage. This type of reconstruction should result in a 15- to 25-year period of efficient joint motion. It is a worthwhile procedure in severe subluxation where there is no possibility of centering the femoral head for patients over 8 to 10 years of age, so that they do not have to undergo a more massive procedure, such as

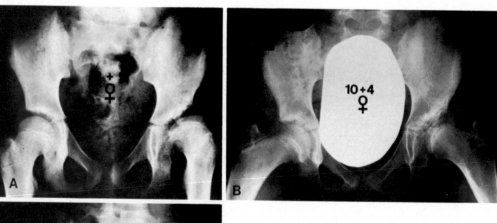

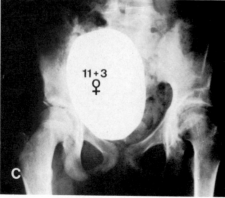

FIG 18-33. *(A)* This film shows severe hip dysplasia in this girl 8 years and 9 months old. *(B)* At 10 years and 4 months, centering is achieved on abduction. *(C)* Film taken at age 11 years and 3 months shows excellent coverage of the femoral head after dial osteotomy.

cup arthroplasty or total joint replacement.

This procedure does not preclude employing the other reconstructive procedures at a later date, and it also improves the chance of a success by improving the acetabular surface for later contact of acetabular components.

This procedure is much more mechanical than the aforementioned procedures and is less desirable because it uses the joint capsule, which is interposing substance. The articular-cartilage to articular-cartilage contact of the previous procedures is preferred.

The procedure can be done after epiphyseal closure, but there is much less remodeling potential. Also, since it is only a reconstructive procedure, it should only be carried out in the adolescent who is having pain.

Summary of Acetabular Procedures

For a surgeon to consider a pelvic procedure, he should first determine whether the major problem involves the acetabular component of the hip and whether the femoral head centers on the abduction test. If there is only mild to moderate deformity of the acetabulum and the affected extremity is not longer than the other, the innominate osteotomy of Salter is performed. If the acetabulum is increased in size or is more seriously deformed, as confirmed by arthrogram, the Pemberton procedure may be performed. The shelf procedure is occasionally indicated for the adolescent who needs only a stabilizing containment buttress. If the femoral head cannot be centered and the patient is having symptoms, the surgeon can resort to the reconstructive surgery of Chiari. If the femoral head can still be centered on the abduction test, but the deformity is severe, the Steel or Sutherland procedures should be considered, before the dial osteotomy, since this procedure is technically very difficult. If the hip problems are recognized early, these latter procedures are rarely indicated.

FEMORAL PROCEDURES

It is unrealistic to consider only one side of the pelvofemoral relationship when evaluating a child with residual deformity from a congenitally dislocated hip. There are

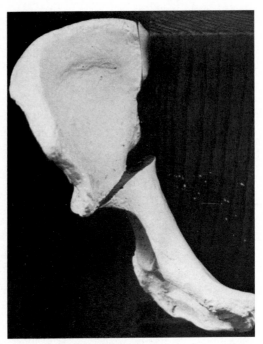

FIG. 18-34. A model of the Chiari procedure. The displacement should be at least 50 per cent of the width of the pelvis.

certain children who would benefit more from procedures performed on the femur rather than on the acetabulum.

A femoral deformity is associated with anteversion or true valgus of the femoral neck. The latter is rare unless previous surgery has disrupted the growth of the greater trochanteric epiphysis or there has been a previous avascular necrosis of the epiphysis, with damage to the lateral portion of the epiphyseal line of the femoral head and secondary growth into valgus. The effect of anteversion on hip stability is best determined by taking roentgenograms with the femur in varying degrees of internal rotation. The stabilizing effect of varus can also be similarly determined by varying the degree of abduction of the femur, as described for the evaluation of the containment potential of the acetabulum.

Femoral Surgery

Rotational Osteotomy. On rare occasions, the acetabulum may have essentially a normal contour and the proximal femur an ap-

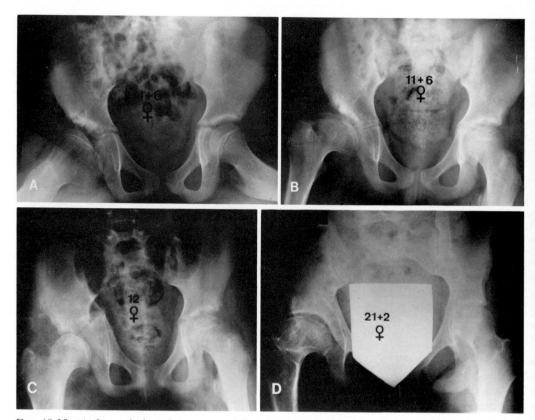

FIG. 18-35. *(A)* Lateral view shows gross deformity following avascular necrosis of the head of the femur. *(B)* Centering is not achieved on abduction. *(C)* Film taken soon after performance of the Chiari procedure shows coverage of the femoral head. *(D)* Long-term follow-up film taken at 21 years and 2 months shows good coverage of the femoral head. The patient is asymptomatic.

parent valgus, with subluxation of the femoral head. If the normal roentgengraphic alignment can be restored by simply internally rotating the lower extremity, a corrective rotational osteotomy is indicated (Fig. 18-36). This procedure can be performed at either the subtrochanteric or supracondylar area. The femur should be derotated to leave approximately 15° to 25° of residual internal rotation.

The procedure is contraindicated if the hip joint is grossly unstable, since rotation of the femur tends to redirect the distal fragment into external rotation, leaving the hip joint in the original pathologic condition.

Varus Derotational Osteotomy. If the internal rotation test of the femur is not sufficient to stabilize the hip joint, and if the thigh must be abducted to obtain the desired position of

the femoral head in the acetabulum, a varus derotational osteotomy may be indicated (Fig. 18-37). The total remodeling desired of the hip unit may not be obtained in a child under 2 years of age, because the neck-shaft angle rapidly returns to normal. If a procedure is necessary in a child under 3 years of age, an innominate osteotomy should be considered, rather than a varus osteotomy, because of its longer-lasting effect. Varus osteotomy has been a quite reliable procedure in children over 3 years. The angle should be reduced to 110° in the younger child, and, usually after age 7, to no less than 120°.

If there has been a recent avascular necrosis of the femoral head, it is better to consider the varus procedure rather than the acetabular procedure, because less pressure

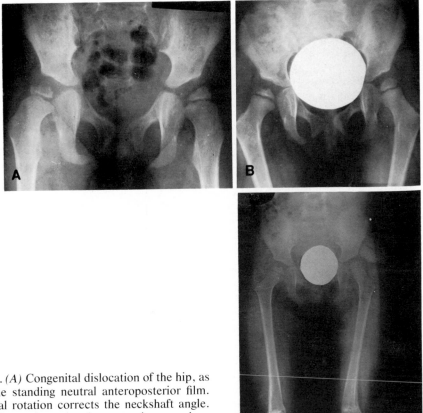

FIG. 18-36. (A) Congenital dislocation of the hip, as seen in the standing neutral anteroposterior film. (B) Internal rotation corrects the neckshaft angle. (C) Distal femoral rotational osteotomies reproduce the internal rotation position as seen in B.

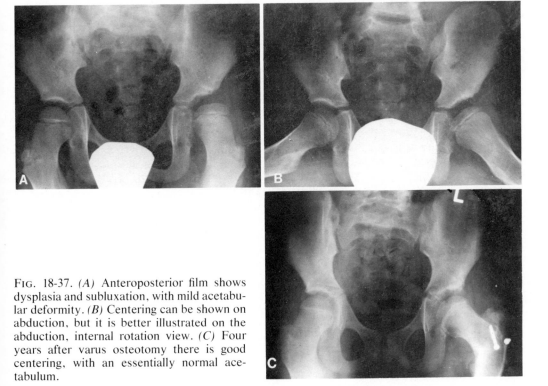

FIG. 18-37. (A) Anteroposterior film shows dysplasia and subluxation, with mild acetabular deformity. (B) Centering can be shown on abduction, but it is better illustrated on the abduction, internal rotation view. (C) Four years after varus osteotomy there is good centering, with an essentially normal acetabulum.

is produced across the hip joint with the varus procedure. However, the reduction in the angle should not be excessive because of the decreased potential of the femur to remodel into valgus position.

Summary of Femoral Procedures

Femoral deformity is much more evident than acetabular deformity in certain patients. In the younger child (under 3 years), the osteotomy correction is so rapid that the procedure is rarely indicated. If only dysplasia is present the procedure can be delayed, but if true subluxation is present, an acetabular procedure is preferred in this age group.

COMBINED PELVIC AND FEMORAL PROCEDURES

Children with marked deformities on both sides of the joint cannot be expected to obtain full correction from a realignment of only one side of the joint. The abduction test roentgenograms help to determine to what degree the hip components must be realigned to obtain centering. An arthrogram may be helpful to determine the true cartilaginous acetabular deformity. The combined procedure is more difficult, because it requires either two procedures or one difficult procedure. The question arises as to which component should be changed first. It is probably better to change the femoral component first, especially if there has been some vascular change. The femoral osteotomy decreases joint pressure, and it can be covered above with either a Salter or a Pemberton procedure, depending on the acetabular configuration. There may be other circumstances that indicate using an entirely different procedure. If the hip is not centering, a Chiari procedure is preferred. Utilization of pins and screws for rigid fixation is also preferred when carrying out procedures on both the pelvis and the femur to maintain accurate position.

COXA VARA

Coxa vara is an abnormality of the proximal end of the femur, which is characterized by a decrease in the neck-shaft angle and a presence of a primary femoral neck defect that is confined to the capital osteocar-

tilaginous plate and results in the shortening of the affected limb. Fiorani[82] in 1881 was the first to report a deformity brought about by a decrease in the angle of the neck of the femur, and Hofmeister[86] in 1894 named this condition "coxa vara." This deformity may be idiopathic or may represent a skeletal manifestation of a primary disease, such as Morquio's disease, cleidocranical dysostosis, metaphyseal dysostosis, multiple epiphyseal dysplasia or achondroplasia.[69, 85] The cause of idiopathic coxa vara is unknown. Evidence of a familial incidence lends credence to a genetic hypothesis (Fig. 18-38).[68, 78, 83, 93, 101] The genetic transmission could be autosomal dominant, while the severity would depend on the variable expressivity of the mutant gene.[83, 101]

Johanning estimated the incidence of coxa vara in the Scandinavian population to be one in 25,000 live births.[88] There is nearly an equal distribution among both sexes.[71, 79]

ETIOLOGY

Early normal growth of the proximal femur occurs from a single crescentic epiphyseal plate that differentiates into the cervical and trochanteric regions.[96] The medial cervical portion of the epiphyseal plate matures first, causing a growth spurt medially, resulting in the elongation of the femoral neck and the normal coxa valga seen in infancy. Subsequently, the lateral epiphyseal plate matures, reducing the valgus angle of the neck.[76, 96] This differential growth pattern of the capital femoral and greater trochanteric epiphyses determines the length of the proximal end of the femur and the neck-shaft angle. The delayed activity of the greater trochanteric epiphysis, concomitant with the pull of the hip abductors and the onset of walking, tends to diminish the neck-shaft angle with age.[103] The femoral neck-shaft angle is 148° at 1 year of age and gradually declines to 120° degrees in the adult. A neck-shaft angle of less than 120° indicates early coxa vara.

Currently, it is felt that coxa vara is caused by a primary endochondral ossification defect in the femoral neck, which results in unequal growth from the trochanteric apophysis and the capital epiphysis.

Compere[77] has shown experimentally with goats that any disruption between the

FIG. 18-38. Evidence of the familial incidence of coxa vara, as seen in: *(A)* mother who presented with unilateral uncorrected coxa vara with degenerative changes, and *(B)* a son who presented with bilateral uncorrected coxa vara.

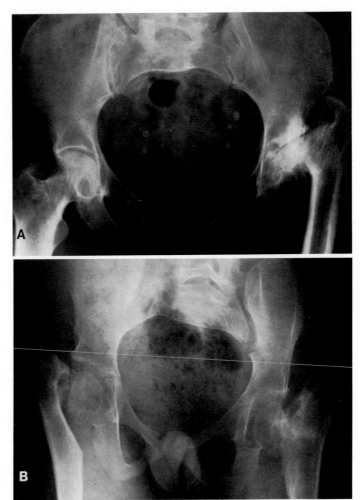

medial and lateral growth forces results in serious malformation. Arresting the growth of the capital femoral epiphysis resulted in an abbreviated femoral neck, coxa vara, an elevated trochanter, and functional limb shortening. The introduction of increased bending movement across the femoral neck with weightbearing may contribute to varus, and deformity can progress due to the structurally weakened metaphyseal bone, which bends under stress. Direct trauma had been initially blamed as the causative agent in the etiology of coxa vara.[73, 79, 88] However, the deformity is often bilateral, and it is unlikely that the neck of the femur would deform in precisely the same place (at the same time) in both hips with such frequency. Michelsson and Langenskiold have been able to induce coxa vara in rabbits atraumatically by creating a muscular imbalance of the hip through knee immobilization.[95]

Two contemporary concepts regarding the genesis of coxa vara are attempts to interpret the impedence of normal ossification. One rationale used to explain abnormal ossification suggests that the primary defect lies within the cartilaginous anlage of the femur.[91, 100] Imperfect formation of cartilage ultimately leads to delayed and often incomplete endochondral ossification. Subsequently, a structurally impoverished bone is manufactured, which is vulnerable to varus deformity.

The other popular hypothesis proposes that an embryonic vascular disturbance is responsible for faulty ossification.[70, 97]

Trueta,[102] in his studies of the circulatory supply of the femur, demonstrated that the growing head and neck of the femur depend on a highly delicate and specialized blood supply. Endochondral ossification of normal cartilage is contingent upon that blood supply; if the circulation to the femoral head and neck is arrested, the spread of ossification ceases. Local vascular interruption leads to a breakdown of ossification with secondary rarefaction along abnormal zones of strain.[88]

Both theories show agreement, however, that delayed or insufficient ossification of the medial portion of the capital femoral epiphysis results in a coxa vara. Despite their diverging avenues, both explanations show agreement that the underlying etiology of coxa vara is most likely genetic.

CLINICAL FEATURES

Appearance of this deformity coincides with the onset of walking. Patients are commonly of short stature and present with a painless limp or waddling gait.[71, 104] An excessive lumbar lordosis is often seen, particularly when the condition is bilateral. The Trendelenburg sign is positive and abduction is limited.

The greater trochanter is elevated sometimes to the degree that the tip of the trochanter impinges upon the ilium, resulting in a gluteal deficiency and, consequently, tilting of the pelvis.[72] Frequently a functional shortening of the affected limb occurs, but this generally does not exceed 2 to 5 cm.[69, 78] Mild, fixed flexion contractures of the hip and limitation of extension may be present. Pain and undue fatigue begin to become apparent in older children and adolescents.

ROENTGENOGRAPHIC FEATURES

Roentgenographs establish the existence of a femoral neck-shaft angle of less-than-normal width. They also show a triangular fragment of bone along the inferior border of the femoral neck (Fig. 18-39).[69, 70, 76, 80, 84] This triangular piece of bone is bounded medially by the nearly vertical capital epiphyseal plate and laterally by a radiolucent band, commonly called the "vertical defect" or "fissure," which traverses the neck. The epiphyseal plate and the vertical

fissure join superiorly to form an inverted "Y." The wider and more vertical the radiolucent defect and, consequently, the smaller the size of the triangular fragment, the greater the degree of varus deformity.[75, 88] This vertical defect may be misinterpreted as a fracture of the femoral neck; however, such fractures are rare in children. The femoral neck is characteristically shortened, and fragmentation is often seen near the vertical defect. The bone of the neck is osteoporotic, contributing to the varus deformity. Pylkkanen[98] has reported a decrease in the center-edge angle in children older than 10 years of age. Late roentgenographic features of coxa vara include severe varus neck-shaft angles, pseudarthrosis of the femoral neck, with fusion of the femoral head to the acetabulum, acetabular dysplasia, and arthrosis.[94, 104] All patients demonstrate a retroversion of the femur.

PROGNOSIS

Coxa vara tends to be progressive if left untreated; normal ossification rarely occurs spontaneously, and the condition may progress to an established pseudarthrosis. Some cases, however, show a tendency to recur even after operative correction. Factors that appear to influence progression and recurrence include the size of the inferomedial neck fragment, age at diagnosis and first operation and degree of correction at initial operation.

Hoyt[87] suggests that the smaller the triangular fragment, the wider the epiphyseal plate, and the more severe the ossification defect. This defect results in a greater tendency to progression. If the fragment is not incorporated into the metaphysis, recurrence of varus can be anticipated.

If a larger fragment is present, a better prognosis can be expected. Large fragments incorporate into the metaphysis more readily, suggesting that the involvement of the ossification process is to a lesser degree. Progression of the varus deformity occurs at a slower rate, and the risk of recurrence is reduced.

TREATMENT

Selecting a plan of treatment depends on the degree of deformity, the relative amount

FIG. 18-39. A large triangular bone fragment is present at the inferomedial portion of the femoral neck, with an open epiphyseal line. With osteotomy a good prognosis can be expected.

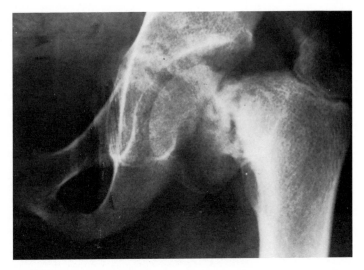

of remaining growth, the functional impairment, and the evidence as to whether the deformity is progressive. The aims of proper treatment include: (1) promotion of ossification of the cartilaginous femoral neck, (2) correction of the varus deformity, (3) reestablishment of the proper leverage-tension of the hip abductors, and (4) conversion of the nearly vertical epiphyseal plate into a more horizontal position.

Conservative treatment may be employed in mild conditions where the varus deformity has not progressed and the neck-shaft angle approaches normal. However, in the majority of instances, to accomplish all of the treatment objectives, surgical interven-

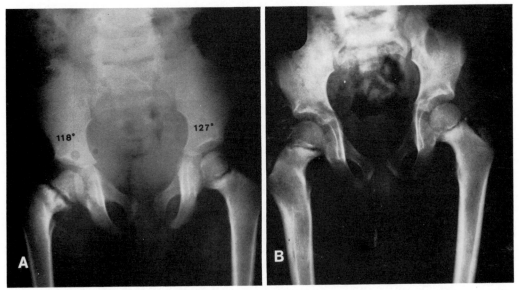

FIG. 18-40. *(A)* Congenital coxa vara seen on a standing anteroposterior film. *(B)* The neck-shaft angle is restored to normal after valgus osteotomy. The minimal defect on the right did not require surgery.

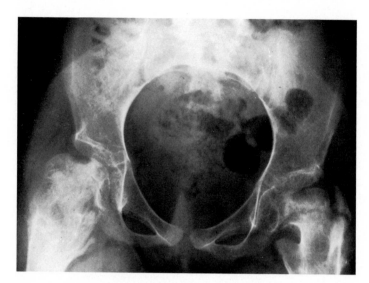

FIG. 18-41. Overcorrection led to avascular necrosis, in this case.

tion is necessary. Early surgery provides the best opportunity to achieve a painless and fully mobile hip without further shortening of the limb.[76, 98] Indications for surgery are the presence of a vertical defect, a neck-shaft angle of less than 100° to 110°, and progression of coxa vara in a young child. The latter is an extremely useful diagnostic device demonstrating the need for early surgery. Waiting until puberty or until the deformity becomes severe may hinder satisfactory improvement of the varus deformity. In addition, it may contribute to the development of acetabular dysplasia.

The intertrochanteric or subtrochanteric valgus osteotomy accompanied by internal fixation is the preferred form of treatment (Fig. 18-40).[75, 93, 98] Operative goals should include restoration of the neck-shaft angle to 140°, realignment of the capital epiphyseal plate to a more normal position, avoidance of "overpull" on the abductors by placing the hip in abduction, prevention of overcorrection, reestablishment of the normal tension leverage of the soft tissue across the hip, and avoidance of damage to the capital epiphysis or trochanteric apophyses.

MacEwen and Shands[93] introduced an oblique coronal trochanteric osteotomy that corrects the coxa vara and the femoral retroversion, simultaneously. In all surgical techniques, the surgeon must guard against the occurrence of extreme valgus and inter-

nal rotation of the distal fragment, as this may interfere with the blood supply of the femoral head, inducing avascular necrosis (Fig. 18-41).[87, 96]

CONGENITAL SHORT FEMUR WITH COXA VARA

A congenitally short femur can exist singularly or in association with other abnormalities of the femur and other segments of the lower extremity. A congenitally short femur not associated with other defects appears to be normal, except that the femur has decreased dimensions, only creating problems of limb equalization. However, a congenitally short femur with proximal femoral deformity produces marked leg length discrepancy and, in addition, mechanical hip abnormalities.

ETIOLOGY

The lower limbs appear initially as tiny buds of tissue in the lateral body wall of the fetus at 4 weeks.[109] The skeletal elements of the limbs are found as condensations of mesenchyme within the limb buds, with chondrification in a definite proximodistal sequence. By 7 weeks of gestation, all skeletal elements of limbs are present as cartilaginous models.

The etiology of the congenitally short

femur is unknown. However, it may be the result of physical or chemical trauma to the lower bud during this early development stage. Ring has suggested that this congenital anomaly is the result of endochondral ossification of defective cartilage, but the deformity may occur even earlier in the development.

CLINICAL FEATURES

The clinical findings of a congenitally short femur, with or without a defect, include, to some degree at least, a short bulky thigh, external rotation contracture of the hip and, often, limited range of motion.[110, 111, 112] In severe cases the affected leg is flexed, abducted, and externally rotated. Other parts of the body, such as the upper limb, the patella, or fibula, may be hypoplastic or absent. The affected limb may present with genu valgus[114] and the foot may be in equinus.[110] The congenitally short femur is usually diagnosed at birth. However, if the leg length inequality is slight, the deformity may not be recognized until the child reaches walking age.

ROENTGENOGRAPHIC FEATURES

Roentgenograms are of a primary importance in the diagnosis of a congenitally short femur. The deformity without associated defects appears to be abbreviated, but is virtually normal on roentgenographic examination (Fig. 18-42). The proximal femur may be in varus to a mild or severe degree. If a significant coxa vara is present in association with the congenitally short femur, the bony upper shaft, neck and capital epiphysis are usually formed imperfectly in cartilage, and may appear to be absent (Fig. 18-43). Delayed ossification of the femoral head and sclerosis in the outer femoral cortex occur.[115] The femur may also exhibit marked varus deformity in the subtrochanteric area. Stresses due to growth and an increase in weight may cause the femoral shaft to migrate posteriorly and proximally, causing a loss of continuity of the cartilage model. There is also severe shortening of the femur. Approximately 30 per cent of the affected limbs have associated fibular and tibial anomalies.

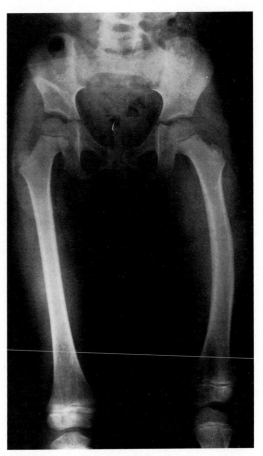

FIG. 18-42. This standing roentgenogram shows a congenitally short femur with no associated deformity. The femur is normal, but abbreviated in size, and leg length inequality can be seen.

The percentage of femoral shortening, calculated by the difference in femoral lengths divided by the length of the normal-sized femur, is found to be constant, which gives an estimation of the inhibition in growth of the femoral segment.

TREATMENT

The treatment program for a congenitally short femur without any other femoral defects is dependent on whether there exist abnormalities of the lower leg and foot. If these associated abnormalities do not exist and the total discrepancy of the length is not great, the leg length discrepancy can be

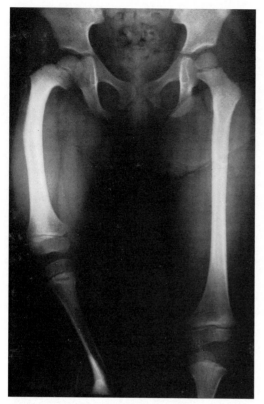

FIG. 18-43. This roentgenogram shows a congenitally short femur with coxa vara. A significant leg length inequality is apparent.

managed by standard methods of leg equalization. Epiphysiodesis or femoral shortening can be performed on the unaffected lower extremity, while shoe lifts or the leg lengthening procedure of Wagner can be used on the affected limb. Amputation followed by prosthesis fitting is usually necessary in patients with associated foot or lower leg anomalies.

In young patients with a congenitally short femur with coxa vara and a large cartilage model not yet ossified, the leg should be maintained in abduction, in order to protect the femoral head and to allow the cartilaginous acetabulum to develop, by use of a Frejka pillow or an abduction brace, usually of the Ilfeld type. A valgus osteotomy to correct the coxa vara adds length to the involved extremity. However, overcorrection must be avoided (Fig. 18-44). (See the sec-

tion on coxa vara.) Once the valgus deformity has been corrected, standard leg equalization techniques may be implemented to correct the leg length inequality and deal with abnormalities of the distal portion of the extremity.

In severe defects, the unstable hip is usually left alone and the knee fused to give a stable proximal femur and increase the lever arm. This procedure is followed by a Syme amputation of the foot and fitting with an above-knee prosthesis.

SLIPPED CAPITAL FEMORAL EPIPHYSIS

Slipped capital femoral epiphysis was first described by Paré,[144] who recognized the possibility of confusing the separation of the epiphysis of the femoral head with luxation in a dislocated hip. By the end of the 1800s many case reports of traumatic separation of the femoral epiphysis had been published. However, Royal Whitman is credited with the first description of the pathology of a spontaneous slipped epiphysis. The term "slipped capital femoral epiphysis" is somewhat misleading, because it suggests that the femoral head is displaced posteriorly and inferiorly, when, in fact, the femoral neck rotates externally and slides upward. Therefore, the goals of treatment are to keep this anatomic displacement to a minimum, maintaining motion as close to normal as possible, and to delay or prevent the onset of degenerative arthritis.

ETIOLOGY

The etiology of the slippage of the upper femoral epiphysis is still unknown. Various theories have been proposed, which include mechanical, traumatic, inflammatory, endocrine and metabolic causes.[126, 131, 135, 147]

In 1941, Howorth[130] emphasized that synovitis exists before slipping occurs, but whether this is primary or secondary is unknown. Some interesting mechanical factors are evident with the increase in the adolescent weight curve, which put extra strain on the epiphyseal line at the time when the child is most vulnerable to developing a slipped epiphysis. The epiphyseal plate normally

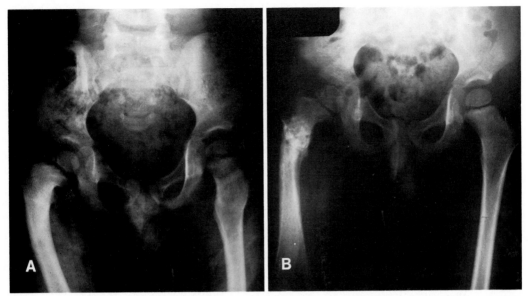

FIG. 18-44. *(A)* This preoperative roentgenogram shows a congenitally short femur with an associated coxa vara. *(B)* A successful valgus osteotomy to correct the deformity of the proximal femur was performed. Now the leg length inequality can be treated.

changes from a horizontal to an oblique position during the preadolescent and adolescent periods. The main stabilizer of the epiphysis is the periosteum of the femoral neck, which is thick in children, but atrophies during the adolescent period, thus producing a weak point at the epiphyseal line.

An endocrine basis for slipped epiphysis is suggested by the fact that the lesion is frequently accompanied by abnormalities of growth. A frequent finding associated with slipped epiphysis is the adiposogenital syndrome, a condition characterized by obesity and deficient gonadal development. Seen less often is a child with the history of very rapid growth, resulting in a tall, thin body type. In the obese children, a low level of sex hormones should be suspected, while in tall, thin children, an overabundance of growth hormone is to be found.

It is known that both growth hormones and sex hormones alter the rate of proliferation of the cartilage cells at the epiphyseal plates, with consequent changes in the thickness of the plates and the rate of skeletal growth. Sex hormones induce epiphyseal closure associated with sexual maturity. Anterior pituitary hormone stimulates the proliferation of cells of the epiphyseal plate directly, with an increase in thickness of the plates and the rate of skeletal growth.

Harris noted that between the time of activation of the gonads and the time that growth ceases, the structure of the epiphyseal plates could be dependent on the relative levels of growth hormone and sex hormone in the circulation.[126] Since it is during this interval that slipping of the femoral epiphysis occurs, it is not unreasonable to assume that an imbalance between these two hormones is the cause of structural weakness in the epiphyseal plates.

The structures of the normal epiphyseal plate responsible for its strength are: (1) the resting cartilage cells on the epiphyseal side of the plate; (2) the layer of proliferating cartilage cells in which the lacuna becomes so large that the intercellular substance remaining between them forms a thin delicate wall upon which the third layer is dependent for strength; (3) the layer of hypertrophy; and (4) the zone of provisional calcification, which strengthens the diaphyseal side of the fourth layer, thus uniting the plate firmly to the shaft and materially increasing its strength.

It may be expected that the weakest part is the third layer, where strength is entirely dependent on the thin, delicate walls of uncalcified intercellular substance. This idea was first demonstrated by Haas[125] in 1917, who found that when the periosteum about the periphery of an epiphyseal plate was removed, the epiphysis could be detached by gentle pressure. The line of separation was constant, always passing through the layer of uncalcified cartilage cells.

Recently, however, Bright and co-workers,[120] using rats, showed that the line of separation was at the bone-cartilage junction and was a weaving, irregular type of fracture. This irregularity of the fracture is also supported by work on the shear strength of the epiphyseal plate in humans.[121]

PATHOLOGY

Ponseti and McClintock[144] reported results of pathologic and metabolic studies on three patients with slipped epiphysis. Material obtained at the time of surgery showed that the growth plate was wide and greatly disturbed. The rows of cartilage cells were disorganized, the cells were grouped in clusters and the cartilage matrix seemed to have lost its cohesion. It was fibrillated, with large clefts occurring in the areas of the plate, and necrotic debris was seen in some of the clefts. The loss of cohesion of the cartilage matrix was presumably due to an alteration in the chemical composition of ground substance, and they assumed that this growth plate lesion resulted in loss of strength of the plate and was mainly responsibile for epiphyseal slipping.

Various authors have interpreted the pathologic findings in different ways, but probably the best summary of the pathology is by Howorth.[132] His study was based on gross and microscopic examinations of synovial membrane, periosteum and femoral head observed at operation in over 160 cases. During the preslipping stage, the synovial membrane is edematous and hyperemic and there is villus formation, with minimal changes in the periosteum and capsule. No changes were seen in the femoral head or the acetabulum. Microscopically, the synovial membrane shows edema and hypervascularity, with a perivascular lymphocytic infiltration. Decalcification and hypervascularity is present at the junction of the neck and growth plate. During the slipping stage, the epiphysis remains attached by periosteum and fibrous tissue, which grows over the exposed portion of the neck as the slipping occurs. The cartilaginous plate remains attached to the head, but is gradually absorbed and transformed into bone. Callus rapidly forms at the angle between the head and neck, inferiorly and posteriorly. The articular cartilage of the head and acetabulum remain normal in appearance. During the healing stage, the medial margin of the neck, which is exposed anteriorly and superiorly, gradually becomes rounded. In addition, the callus inferiorly becomes incorporated with the neck, thus changing the contour of the calcar. The epiphyseal line is gradually absorbed, and bony union occurs between the epiphysis and the neck. The synovia and periosteum become less vascular and edematous, more scarred and inelastic. The inflammatory process subsides after several months of spontaneous union of the epiphysis. The total process may require 2 to 3 years.

EPIDEMIOLOGY

Slipped capital femoral epiphysis occurs about 2 years earlier in females than males, and is closely related to puberty. In males the age range is 10 to 17 years, with an average age of 11 to 12 years. The incidence of slipped capital femoral epiphysis varies from 0.71 to 3.41 per 100,000. The black population is more frequently affected with slipped capital femoral epiphysis than the white population. Kelsey has reported an incidence of 7.79 per 100,000 in black males, as opposed to 4.74 in white males and 6.68 per 100,000 for black females, as opposed to 1.64 for white females.[138] The skeletal age in children with slipped epiphysis is usually below the chronologic age.

Males are more frequently affected than females. The range is from 1.7 to 2.6 males to one female. Rennie[145] reported a 7 per cent risk of a second family member having a slipped epiphysis. Kelsey found 49 per cent

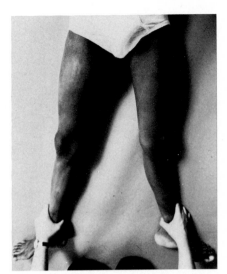

FIG. 18-45. With knees in extension, restricted abduction becomes more pronounced. This illustration shows increased external rotation of the left hip and thigh atrophy.

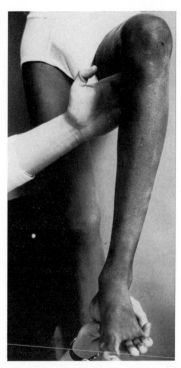

FIG. 18-46. As the thigh is flexed, it tends to roll into external rotation and abduction.

of patients with slipped epiphysis had body weights at or above the 95th percentile.[137] There is also some tendency for patients with slipped epiphysis to be tall for their age.

Slipped epiphysis occurs bilaterally in approximately one-third of the affected population, however most cases can be recognized as being bilateral at the time of the initial evaluation. Less than 15 per cent subsequently develop a slip of the second side that could not be recognized at the time of the initial examination. It can be interpreted that the risk of a second slip after discharge from the treatment of the first side is relatively slight.

CLINICAL FEATURES

The symptoms fall into three categories:

1. One form is the acute slip that occurs with significant trauma, with usually minimal or no previous complaints of pain. In this group, the pain is usually severe enough to prevent weightbearing.

2. Another form is the acute slip on an already present chronic slip. In this group the patient has already experienced some aching in the hip, thigh or knee area for weeks or even months, and may actually have been

noted to limp. With trauma the epiphysis may slip further suddenly and may give the acute symptoms, as noted in the above group.

3. The commonest form is one with chronic complaints that are usually referable to the hip or distal medial thigh in the area of the knee. Limp, pain and loss of motion are usually the presenting symptoms. In approximately 20 per cent of patients, knee pain is present in the area of the vastus medialis and often accounts for the overlooked slip. During clinical examination, loss of internal rotation is particularly notable. With the hips examined in extension, restriction of abduction becomes more pronounced as the slip increases (Fig. 18-45). As the thigh is flexed, it tends to roll into external rotation and abduction, and this represents the most clearly diagnostic feature of the examination. (Fig. 18-46). Often the diagnosis has been delayed long enough to produce significant thigh atrophy. Shortening of the leg is frequent, and it occurs before the diagnosis is made. In

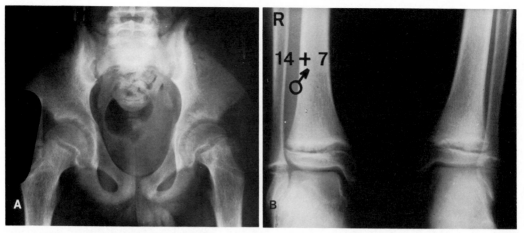

Fig. 18-47. *(A)* If slip is bilateral, as seen here, other joints should be examined roentgenographically to assist in differential diagnosis. *(B)* Note involvement of the distal fibular and tibial epiphyseal lines. This indicates the presence of a systemic condition and in this patient, an impending renal failure.

cases where there is evidence that the slip is bilateral and symmetrical, another cause for the apparent widening growth plate should be considered (Fig. 18-47), especially hypothyroidism.

ROENTGENOGRAPHIC FEATURES

The roentgenographic changes in slipped epiphysis are classic. In the earliest stages there is a widening of the epiphyseal line. The normal configuration of the femoral epiphysis on the anteroposterior film is a slight bulging of the head above and lateral to the superior border of the femoral neck. If a straight line drawn up the top of the femoral neck does not touch the femoral head, a slip must be suspected. However, when a slipped epiphysis is suspected, a frog-leg view should always be taken, because initial slipping is usually posterior, and the slipped epiphysis is often missed on an anteroposterior film (Fig. 18-48). Another helpful sign is the exclusion of the articular portion of the medial metaphysis from the acetabulum. Finally, Shenton's line is broken in the more severe slip.

The use of a three-grade evaluation is helpful, with Grade I including a displacement of the femoral level up to one-third of the width of the femoral neck, Grade II rep-resenting a femoral level with a slip greater than one-third but less than one-half the width of the neck, and Grade III including all slips of the capital femoral epiphysis of greater than 50 per cent (Fig. 18-49). It should be noted that the roentgenogram showing the maximum degree of slip, be it the anteroposterior or the frog-leg view, determines the grade.

In the acute slip, no manifestations of the healing process have occurred. However, in the chronic problem, the neck of the femur begins to develop a slight hook, which is more frequently seen on the frog-leg view, which may show layers of ossification. As the severity of the slip increases, the femoral neck comes exposed superiorly and anteriorly, and the hook or bump becomes more evident on the roentgenogram.

Recently, minor roentgenographic signs have been found, which are similar to those found in adult patients with idiopathic osteoarthritis. Often the opposite uninvolved hip develops the same configuration, indicating that it might be subject to later degeneration.

Frequently the rounded metaphysis develops a small fleck of calcification that gradually increases in size and fuses with the metaphysis (Fig. 18-50). After fusion, the previously rounded metaphysis has a classic

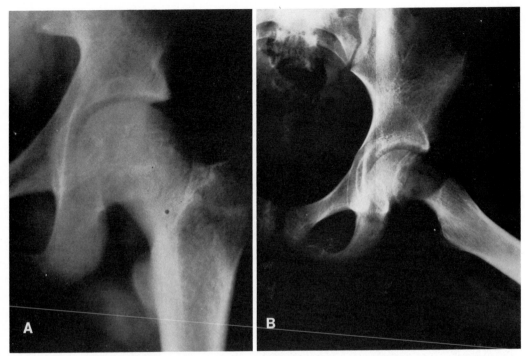

FIG. 18-48. *(A)* Slipped epiphysis can be missed on the anteroposterior projection, because it is usually posteriorly located. *(B)* Therefore, a frog-leg view should also be taken. This frog-leg view shows a Grade I slip.

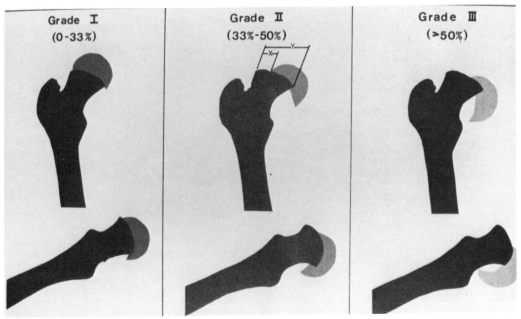

FIG. 18-49. Classification of the three grades of slip.

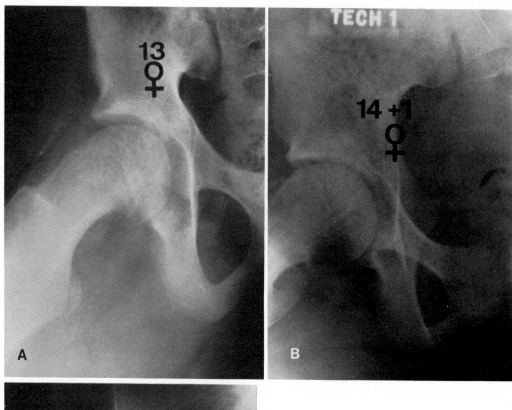

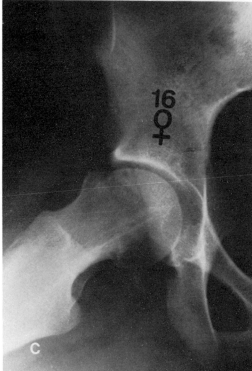

Fig. 18-50. (A, B, and C) These roentgenograms show the progression of calcification to ossification at the epiphyseal line, giving the impression of a moderate slip although only a minimal slip is present. These signs are similar to those seen in adult patients with idiopathic osteoarthritis.

FIG. 18-51. *(A)* A large pin separates the epiphyseal line from the metaphysis. *(B)* the resulting avascular necrosis.

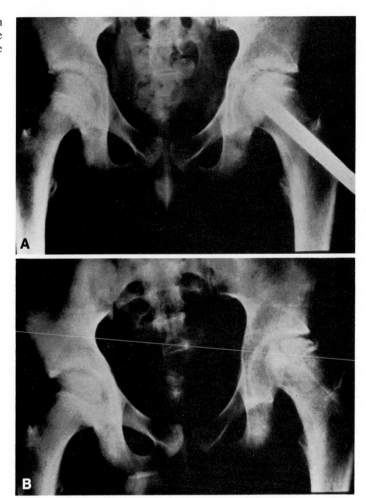

bump that is incorrectly thought to represent the original metaphysis.

TREATMENT

There have been many methods of treating slipped capital femoral epiphysis, including bedrest, osteotomy of the femoral neck, bone block of the femoral neck and growth plate, Smith-Petersen nailing, pin fixation and spica casting.

ACUTE SLIP

If the slip is acute, gentle positioning can be performed to reduce the deformity. If an acute slip has occurred on a preexisting chronic slip, it is important that the repositioning only reduce the acute aspect of the slip. If full reduction is attempted, avascular necrosis may result. If the acute slip has been present for more than 2 weeks, there is granulation tissue present, and the risk of avascular necrosis from manipulation increases rather rapidly. The question arises as to whether the reduction should be accomplished gradually by traction, or rapidly on a fracture table. Statistics favor the gradual reduction method. If the reduction is attempted on the fracture table, the repositioning should be most gentle, with minimal use of traction. Hand traction is preferred to tying the patient to the table and applying ratchet traction, because of the risk of overpull and further destruction of blood supply to the femoral head. The goal, many times, should be to produce less than a full correction, especially if an element of chronic slip has been present. The greatest threat to the hip is avascular necrosis and not incomplete reduction.

Some authors have suggested an open reduction with pegging of the femoral head through the metaphysis for an acute slip. We have had no experience with this method, but, in general, we prefer not to open the hip joint unless it is absolutely necessary. Pinning *in situ* is the most common and safest approach. The use of a heavy nail is never recommended (Fig. 18-51) because of the increased frequency of the occurrence of complications.

CHRONIC SLIP

Our treatment goal in the majority of patients with a chronic slip is to stabilize the femoral head and maintain motion. In addition to the anatomic limitation of motion, there is an associated hip irritation from synovitis, which further restricts motion. We feel that it is important to allow the synovitis to decrease by prescribing bedrest and traction before proceeding to definite treatment. This may reduce the risk of cartilage necrosis.

To pin a slipped epiphysis, usually a lateral approach is made to the proximal femur. If the head is slipped 50 per cent on both the anteroposterior and frog-leg lateral projections, the overlap of the head and the metaphysis is only 25 per cent, thus making a very small aperture for the pin to cross from the neck to the femoral head. It is then extremely difficult to place the pins without exit and reentry through the femoral neck, which is not desirable. In these situations, the pins can be placed through the anterior aspect of the base of the neck and directed posteriorly, with a better angle to engage the head. Incorrect placement of the pins is the most common error in operative management. The pins may pass posteriorly and miss the femoral head altogether, and it is not at all uncommon to have pins penetrate the articular cartilage.

The pins should preferably be placed to avoid the weightbearing area of the femoral head because of the small but definite risk of producing a segmented avascular necrosis. (Fig. 18-52) After the growth plate has closed, the pins are removed because of possible need for future hip reconstruction and the presence of local irritation. Frequently, there is great difficulty in removing the pins, and, therefore, we now use diamond-shaped, pointed, threaded Sheinmann pins cut off approximately 1.5 cm. beyond the femur.

An alternative method was developed by Howorth, where the hip joint is opened, a window placed in the neck and a small iliac bone graft placed across the epiphyseal line. This method has the advantage of earlier epiphyseal line closure, and it eliminates the need for a second procedure for pin removal. It does, however, require opening the hip joint, which always has some risk of infection.

A patient with second or third degree slip frequently has marked loss secondary to the anatomic deformity. Southwick has devised a trochanteric osteotomy, which is calculated to restore motion.[148] Although the osteotomy is ingenious and accomplishes its goal, it is complicated and has not gained wide use. It also increases the risk of chondrolysis. Another method to gain abduction and internal rotation is to resect the protruding anterior and superior aspect of the neck, as developed by Heyman and Herndon. This is indicated for the patient who, after epiphyseal line closure, may still have a mechanical block demonstrated on the lateral roentgenographic view. In our hands, this procedure has been rarely indicated.

Our preference is to pin all degrees of slip and then, later, after epiphyseal closure, to do an intertrochanteric osteotomy to realign the few hips that require it. Craig carries out the epiphyseal pinning and an intertrochanteric corrective osteotomy at the same operation. There is essentially no indication for an osteotomy of the neck, because of the 33 to 50 per cent risk of avascular necrosis.

CHONDROLYSIS

Chondrolysis, which was first described in 1930, appears to be more common in the black population, although it does occur in

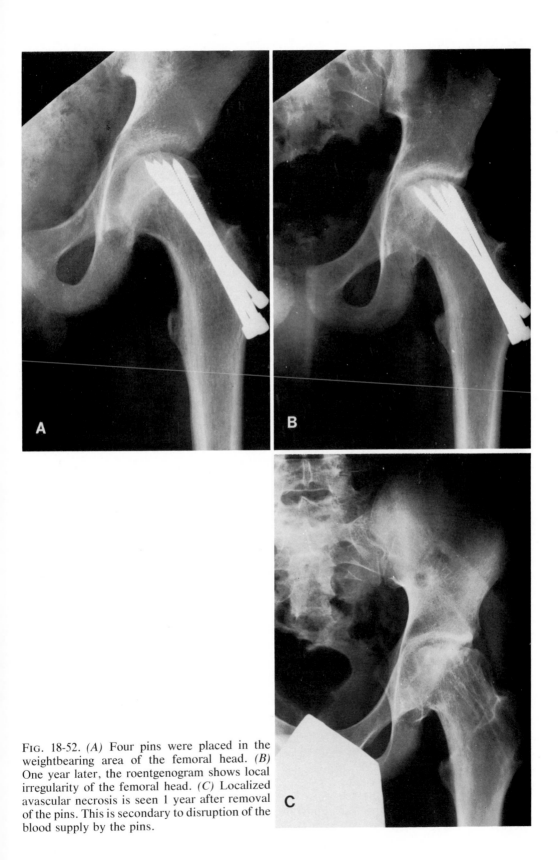

FIG. 18-52. (A) Four pins were placed in the weightbearing area of the femoral head. (B) One year later, the roentgenogram shows local irregularity of the femoral head. (C) Localized avascular necrosis is seen 1 year after removal of the pins. This is secondary to disruption of the blood supply by the pins.

whites. This troublesome occurrence progresses relentlessly until the joint space is essentially obliterated. As the chondrolysis develops, irregularity of the subchondral bone and rarefaction of both the acetabulum and femoral head progress (Fig. 18-53). The patients usually have acute pain associated with movement of the hip. With a slip of Grade II or III, the risk of chondrolysis is increased.

After initial loss of articular cartilage, there may be a gradual improvement in the joint space. However, this fibrocartilage disappears earlier than is normally expected after an uncomplicated slipped epiphysis, leading to secondary osteoarthritis.

The treatment of chondrolysis is directed toward prescribing traction and motion and salicylates, all attempting to cut down the joint reaction and to increase motion. This should be followed by a prolonged period of motion and crutch walking. If the diagnosis is made before a definite treatment program for the slip has been undertaken, this treatment should be delayed until motion can be restored and the reaction in the joint decreased. If the risk of chondrolysis is discerned in a particular person, the treatment for the slip should be as simple as possible (using pins), and attempts at regaining motion should be reinstituted within days.

TREATMENT OF THE UNINVOLVED SIDE

Since most bilateral involvement can be diagnosed at the time of the first evaluation, we do not recommend routine preoperative pinning of the second hip, because of the relatively low risk of deformity in the second hip. If, for some reason, the patient cannot be followed closely or is unreliable, it may be best to do the opposite hip.

PROGNOSIS

Long-term results using the Harris hip scale indicate that most patients in all three grades do well into middle life, if there has been no avascular necrosis or chondrolysis. This is not to imply that the hips function completely normally, because most, including those with significant Grade I slips, develop some degenerative changes. It does suggest that the simple methods of treatment, those that decrease or eliminate the risk of avascular necrosis and chondrolysis, should be those most commonly used.

LEGG-CALVÉ-PERTHES SYNDROME (COXA PLANA)

In 1909, Arthur Legg[191] from the United States presented a paper evaluating five children who developed a limp after an injury. He believed that the injury resulted in flattening of the femoral head due to the increased pressure between the femoral head and the acetabulum. This initial description was the first attempt to differentiate this condition from tuberculosis. A French orthopaedist, Jacques Calvé,[162] published an article in 1910 about a condition he believed to be noninflamatory and self-limiting, and which healed with flattening on the weightbearing surface of the femoral head. During the same year, George Perthes[196, 197] from Germany described a similar condition. The similarities of these descriptions have resulted in the naming of this condition the Legg-Calvé-Perthes syndrome. Walderström[212] first wrote about the condition in 1909, and at that time felt that it was a form of tuberculosis, but later suggested the nomenclature "coxa plana," which has also been widely accepted. It was Phemister[200] in 1921 who described the pathology as necrotic bone.

INCIDENCE AND EPIDEMIOLOGY

The condition is seen in children ages 2 to 12 years, but most of the cases are in children between 4 to 8 years of age. Males are affected four times more frequently than females, and the condition is bilateral in approximately 12 per cent of the affected children. Goff[176, 177] found that the condition occurred more frequently in the Japanese, Mongoloid, Eskimo and Central European people. He also noted that the races with the least number of reported cases were native Australians, American Indians, Polynesians

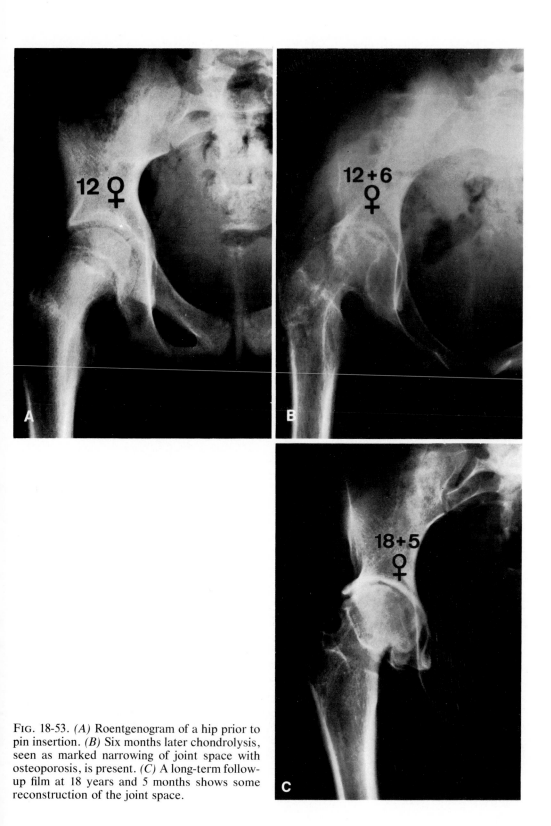

FIG. 18-53. (A) Roentgenogram of a hip prior to pin insertion. (B) Six months later chondrolysis, seen as marked narrowing of joint space with osteoporosis, is present. (C) A long-term follow-up film at 18 years and 5 months shows some reconstruction of the joint space.

and Blacks. He also found a higher incidence of the condition in the first-born child.

Fisher[17] conducted a study of 188 patients in which he found a 7 per cent incidence of more than one involved family member. Only two of his patients were black, and both demonstrated atypical changes.

Molloy[193, 194] studied single-born white affected children. Her results showed that their birth weights were usually much lower than those of unaffected children. Males with the birth weight under $5^1/_2$ lb. were five times more liable to exhibit the condition than males weighing over $8^1/_2$ lb. Molloy also found that the bone age was delayed in 89 per cent of the involved children.

Cameron and Izzat[163] compared affected children with other school-age children and found that the affected males were 1 inch shorter and the affected females 3 inches shorter in height than their respective peers. Harrison,[181] in a study of children with Perthes syndrome, found that the bone ages of these children lagged behind their respective chronologic ages. An extension of this study in siblings of children with Perthes syndrome revealed that these brothers and sisters also exhibited delayed bone ages. Therefore, it would appear that there are many unexplained constitutional factors associated with this condition, as well as the localized vascular changes.

The age of onset of Legg-Calvé-Perthes syndrome appears to be a major factor in its prognosis. Children under 5 years usually do very well if they are not affected by the unusual problem of full femoral head involvement. If onset occurs in a child after the age of 8 years, the prognosis is less favorable, and a greater area of the femoral head is usually involved.

CLINICAL FEATURES

The most frequently observed symptom of this condition is a limp, which is first noted after full activity and which gradually becomes more constant. This limp is usually painless for several weeks, which often results in a delay in visiting a physician. The pain associated with the limp is usually in the groin and inner thigh, or at times, only in the knee region. In our series, 15 per cent of the patients had knee pain, exclusively. This localization of pain often directed the clinical evaluation to the incorrect joint and further delayed the diagnosis. Muscle spasm usually occurs early in the course of the syndrome and limits abduction and internal rotation of the hip, producing a limp with each step.

ETIOLOGY

The etiology of Legg-Calvé-Perthes syndrome remains unknown, but it is in some way related to an interruption of the blood supply, in whole or in part, to the growing femoral head. The changes in the distribution of the vessels, as shown by Trueta,[57, 212, 213, 214] can be, at most, only contributing factors. A direct involvement of the vessels themselves could cause the problem. Freeman and co-worker[174] most nearly reproduced the changes of Legg-Calvé-Perthes syndrome in the femoral heads of experimental animals by repeating vascular interruption after timed intervals. A recent work showed a thrombus to be present in the inferior circumflex vessel in the femoral head of a child with Legg-Calvé-Perthes syndrome at postmortem examination. This thrombus was too recent in time of origin to produce the bone changes of Legg-Calvé-Perthes syndrome that were already present, again suggesting that more than one vascular interruption is necessary.

Legg considered that trauma to the femoral head was the cause of this condition, but it is probably a secondary factor. The trauma theory continues to have appeal, however, as shown in observations by Petrie and others. They noted that in children under treatment by the abduction method, the unaffected femoral head held deeply within the acetabulum has never developed Perthes changes, whereas it is usually expected that up to 12 per cent of affected children become bilaterally involved.

Synovitis with increased fluid pressure inside the joint is an attractive theory of the etiology of this syndrome, but only rarely (1–3%) is there a history suggesting toxic synovitis in patients that later develop Legg-Calvé-Perthes syndrome.

PATHOLOGY

Since resection of the total femoral head as a treatment method was abandoned long ago, studies of affected femoral heads are extremely rare and are based solely on accidental deaths among children with an active Legg-Calvé-Perthes condition.

The pathologic process basically involves the death of part or all of the femoral head and the gradual revascularization of the area.

Jonsater,[182] using a biopsy technique, has most completely outlined the series of events during the active process of the Legg-Calvé-Perthes syndrome, and has linked these changes with the roentgenographic stages. These findings have been confirmed by a number of other authors who have taken biopsies, most of them by drilling through the femoral neck of affected hips. Jonsater, in a study of 34 patients, found that during the initial stage the epiphysis showed pronounced necrosis of bone and grossly distorted marrow trabeculae. There were no signs of an inflammatory process. At this early stage, the roentgenograms showed only an increase in density of the femoral head, but already the bone fragments were of a soft consistency. In the next stage of fragmentation, the bone biopsy showed new-bone formation. This new bone was laid down between and on the surface of the dead trabeculae. Mattner described this bone formation as "creeping apposition," even in the early stage. This observation has also been made by Larsen and Reimann.

Biopsies taken during the fragmentation stage showed that one-half of the bony specimens were hard and the other one-half were soft. Contrary to the usual belief, the bony fragments were firmer than during the initial stage, and more normal bone marrow was also present. This finding suggests that by this stage, the femoral head is already returning to normal strength. Biopsies done later in the process show a gradual increase in the amount of living bone.

Investigations have consistently shown

that the articular cartilage is normal or, at most, is showing faint signs of degeneration in the basilar layers.

BLOOD SUPPLY TO THE FEMORAL HEAD

The deep branch of the medial femoral circumflex artery runs behind the femoral neck, between the quadratus femoris and the external obturator muscles, ending laterally on the neck. It then perforates the capsular attachment and runs up along the neck as retinacular vessels. These vessels penetrate the cartilage surface and, after branching, enter the epiphysis.

On the anterior aspect of the femoral neck, similar branches, derived from the lateral femoral circumflex artery, course along the neck in a subsynovial level to the anterior aspect of the metaphysis and epiphysis. A small branch enters the epiphysis from the ligamentum teres. Gradually, as the epiphyseal center grows, these afferent vessels assume a more peripheral position through the epiphyseal cartilage. According to Trueta,[212, 213, 214] the blood supply to the femoral head during the years 4 to 9 is limited. Distribution is greater to the posterior half of the femoral head, making the anterior part of the head more susceptible to developing necrosis. It is this part of the head that is almost always involved in the disease process. Trueta also found that the blood supply to the femoral head was more constant from the artery of ligamentum teres in black children than in white children. At the age of 4 to 6 years, first the anterior and then the distal retinacular arteries stop supplying the epiphysis. The epiphysis is then dependent on the normal function of the deep branch of the medial circumflex femoral artery and its capillaries for its blood supply. This source of blood remains until the epiphyseal line starts closing, and, thus, it no longer forms a barrier to anastomosis between the metaphyseal and the epiphyseal vascular network. Trueta concluded that this alteration in the blood distribution may be the cause for the vulnerability of the femoral head to developing Legg-Calvé-Perthes syndrome at the ages of 4 to 8 years. This study, however,

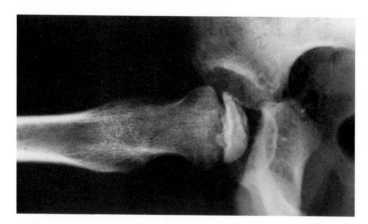

FIG. 18-54. Early segmental fracture (crescent sign), as described by Caffey.

needs to be repeated, using a much larger sample of cases, before it can be fully accepted.

ROENTGENOGRAPHIC EVALUATION

CHANGES OF THE FEMORAL HEAD

The roentgenographic appearance of the femoral head changes during the process of necrosis and revascularization. Anteroposterior and frog-leg roentgenographic views are necessary to follow the course of the process.

The earliest change of the femoral head affected with Legg-Calvé-Perthes syndrome often appears as a slightly smaller ossific nucleus on roentgenographic study. Work by Salter on 52 experimentally devascularized femoral heads in animals supported these roentgenographic findings.[206] This change is followed by an increase in the density of a part or the whole femoral epiphysis. This appearance may be caused by: (1) demineralization of the adjacent femoral neck due to disuse osteoporosis, making the femoral head appear relatively dense; (2) compaction of the necrotic femoral head bone; (3) early revascularization, with new bone being laid down over the dead trabeculae, resulting in a true increase in density. The soft-tissue changes at this time may include widening of the medial joint space and reactive thickening of the joint capsule.

The crescent sign of Caffey[161] may be the first bone change to appear. It is often not visible in the standard position. In the frog position, however, the crescent sign appears as a defined submarginal strip of decreased density on the anterolateral segment of the epiphyseal ossification center (Fig. 18-54). This radiolucent defect can replace part of the subchondral bone plate or a fragment of the superior part of the epiphysis. Caffey believes that this fragment represents a fracture.

The femoral head later breaks up into areas that are relatively dense, interspersed with areas of radiolucency. This change represents the resorption of the dead bone, with added areas of osteoid and new bone. At this stage, the whole femoral head may be displaced laterally in the acetabulum. Attention should also be given to the lateral half of the femoral head, which may extrude from its normal location. This extrusion is accompanied by the roentgenographic appearance of flattening of the bone portion of the epiphysis caused by absorption of bone, but the cartilage model is usually only slightly altered. True deformity is present in the later stages of Legg-Calvé-Perthes syndrome. Gradually, over 3 to 4 years, the femoral head regains a homogeneous density. The last area to fill in is the anterior portion of the femoral head, as shown on the frog-leg view.

ARTHROGRAPHY

Roentgenographic evaluation of anteversion shows that almost all hips with the Legg-Calvé-Perthes syndrome have anteversion within normal limits at the start of the process. Therefore, anteversion cannot be implicated in the etiology of the condition. Also, in follow-up, patients with increased anteversion had the same results as patients without increased anteversion. Therefore, increased anterversion *per se* does not seem to adversely affect the end result.

ARTHROGRAPHY

Schiller and Axer[208] found the femoral head to be enlarged early in the disease process, which is shown by arthrography. This enlargement could account for the inability of the acetabulum to contain the femoral head in some patients. Arthrography can also demonstrate the change in the spherical shape of the femoral cartilaginous surface, which can occur early in the "fragmentation" phase or in the latter portion of the increased density phase, if sufficient underlying bone is involved.

Arthrography in the regenerative phase can show the true joint deformity, which is helpful in outlining a treatment program. In the residual stage, after full regeneration has occurred, arthrography is of little help, since the joint contour follows that of the regenerated subchondral base of the femoral head.

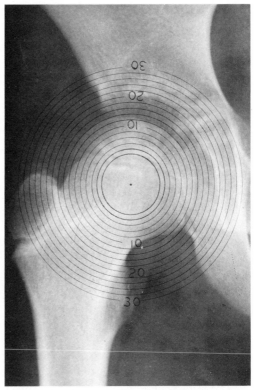

FIG. 18-55. The Mose template superimposed on a roentgenogram to evaluate the degree of sphericity of femoral head. It should be used on the anteroposterior and the frog-leg projections.

PROGNOSIS

The great variability in the end result intrigues students of this syndrome. Ingenious methods have been devised to assess the end result of the hip affected with Legg-Calvé-Perthes syndrome. It is generally agreed that the more spherical the femoral head at the end of treatment, the better the end result, and there is less risk that arthritis will ensue. The different quotients obtained by measuring various parameters of the femoral head are good methods of evaluation, but these are time-consuming and impractical for use with the individual patient. The most practical technique seems to be the method of Goff,[176] further developed by Mose,[195] which consists of drawing concentric circles 2 mm. apart on a transparent template (Fig. 18-55). The template is superimposed on the anteroposterior and lateral roentgenograms and gives a satisfactory evaluation of the degree of sphericity. If the outline of the head is a perfect circle on both projections, the result is rated "good." If the outline of the head varies from a perfect circle by one 2 mm., the result is rated "fair." If the outline of the femoral head varies from the circle by more than 2 mm. in either the anteroposterior or lateral projection, the result is rated "poor." This method of measurement is rigid and quite reproducible. The center-edge (CE) angle of Wiberg can also be recorded to assess the acetabular coverage. However, from a practical viewpoint, the hip will be rated "poor" by the method of Mose before the CE angle will be altered.

CATTERALL CLASSIFICATION

Catterall,[164, 165] in an attempt to classify patients according to the amount of femoral epiphysis involvement, studied the natural

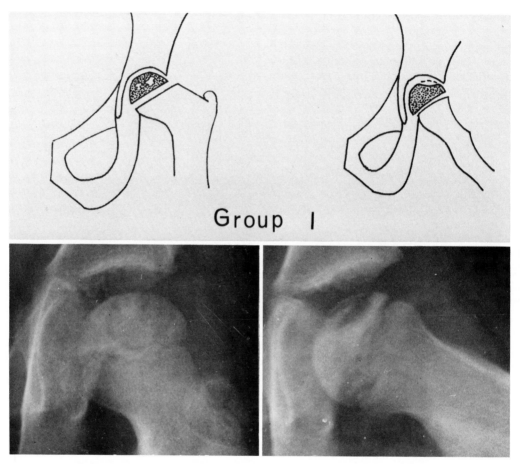

FIG. 18-56. Catterall classification, Group I. There is no significant change in density of the femoral head on the anteroposterior projection.

history of the process within a series of patients. By studying the evolution of the disease in a group of untreated patients, Catterall presented the following classification:

Group I

The anterior part of the head is involved. There is no collapse in the involved segment. Metaphyseal changes do not occur, and the epiphyseal plate is not involved. Healing occurs without significant sequelae (Fig. 18-56).

Group II

The involved segment undergoes increased density, and this fragment can be recognized best on the anteroposterior roentgenogram. However, the uninvolved pillars of normal bone can be seen medially and laterally, and they prevent significant collapse (Fig. 18-57). The presence of an intact lateral column in the femoral head seen on the lateral roentgenogram is of great prognostic significance. Metaphyseal changes may be seen, but the epiphyseal plate is usually protected by an uninvolved tongue of epiphyseal bone that reaches anteriorly. In Group II, regeneration occurs without much loss of epiphyseal height. With an intact epiphyseal plate, the remodeling potential is not affected, and the end result is usually good, especially if several years of growth remain after the process has finished (Fig. 18-58).

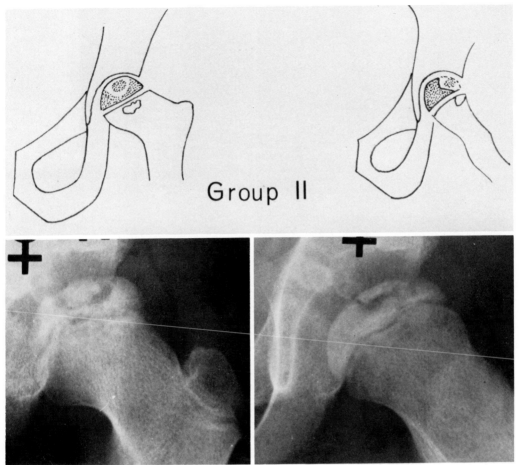

FIG. 18-57. Catterall classification, Group II. There is an intact lateral pillar on the anteroposterior projection, with minimal involvement of the epiphyseal line and metaphysis.

Group III

Up to three quarters of the femoral epiphysis is affected in this group. There is no intact support laterally, and the metaphysis is usually involved. The epiphyseal plate is unprotected and is often actively involved in the process (Fig. 18-59). Collapse is more severe, and the collapsed fragment itself is larger. The process takes longer and the results are usually poorer (Fig. 18-60).

Group IV

The entire epiphysis is affected. Collapse occurs early and is often severe (Fig. 18-61). Restoration of the femoral head is slower and usually is less complete. The epiphyseal line is usually involved directly in the process, and if it is severely damaged and can no longer grow normally, it may greatly limit the ability of the femoral head to remodel. This may contribute to a poor result, in spite of the treatment method employed. Treatment, however, in most of these patients, prevents a severe deformity with a grossly deformed femoral head from occurring (Fig. 18-62).

This classification focuses on the degree of involvement of the femoral head. However, patients are encountered that fall between these groups. Our evaluation shows that the degree of involvement has a definite prognostic significance. For example, pa-

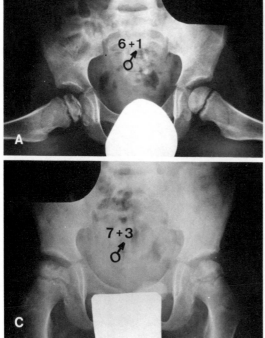

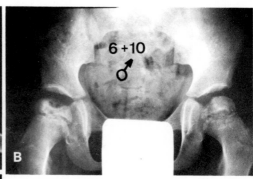

FIG. 18-58. *(A)* Catterall Group II. This child was first seen with Legg-Calvé-Perthes disease at 6 years and 1 month. *(B)* The anteroposterior view 9 months later, showing intact lateral pillar. *(C)* Treatment was discontinued early. Follow-up films taken at 7 years and 3 months showed a good result.

tients with Group III or Group IV involvement are more prone to poor results, and a Group I or Group II type of involvement may need very little treament. This method of evaluation is limited, however, because the physiciam must wait for months to determine the true extent of the involvement, and the classification may appear to change during this interval (Fig. 18-63). There are, however, other factors that contribute to a less-than-ideal result.

IMPORTANT FACTORS INFLUENCING PROGNOSIS

The loss of motion in the early stage of the disease process is due to soft-tissue reaction or actual contracture. Later it may result from established bony deformity, in which case it may not be reversible. If loss of motion is allowed to persist or if it recurs after successful early treatment and is not corrected, a good result is not to be expected.

Lateral subluxation, seen as increased distance between the medial joint line and the femoral head, with an associated decrease in coverage of the femoral head, is a well-recognized feature of Legg-Calvé-Perthes syndrome. If allowed to persist, it results in abnormal stresses on a vulnerable femoral head, and a good result cannot be obtained, no matter how small the area of femoral head involvement. In addition, in some patients, especially those showing Group III and Group IV involvement, some of the epiphysis is actually extruded laterally. If extrusion occurs, the amount of proximal femur which is uncovered is larger than that expected by the effect of an increased medial joint space, alone. The changes secondary to extrusion of the lateral portion of the femoral head are usually much more significant and are much more common than in true subluxation of the total femoral head. This extruded portion is first seen roentgenographically as faint flecks of calcification. This is the major factor in the development of an enlarged femoral head during regeneration (Fig. 18-64). The lateral calcifications are within the cartilage model and are indications that part of the femoral head will regenerate outside the

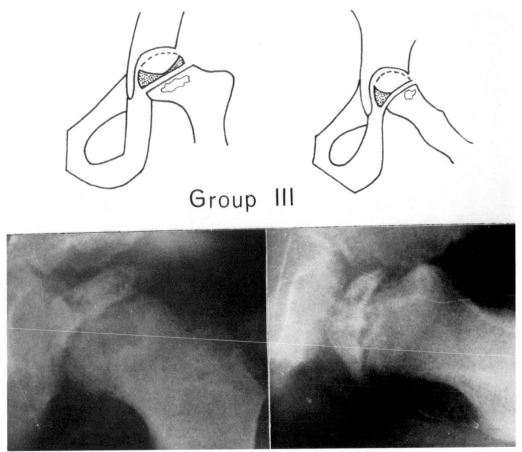

FIG. 18-59. Catterall classification, Group III. There is loss of lateral support on the anteroposterior projection and involvement across the epiphyseal line in the frog-leg projection.

acetabulum. The total head will be larger and will be distorted unless this extruded portion can be kept reduced within the acetabulum during the soft stage of change. In an extreme case, the head can appear to be actually split by the acetabular margin. Early lysis of the lateral portion of the epiphysis usually indicates loss of support laterally and vulnerability to abnormal stresses, meaning that the involved hip will fall into a Catterall Group III or Group IV classification.

A metaphyseal cyst may appear early in the fragmentation stage and may disappear during regeneration. Biopsy of a cystic lesion shows some immature connective tissue, blood vessels, and formation of a few giant cells (only reactive-type tissue). A biopsy is rarely, if ever, indicated. In more severe involvement, the epiphyseal line may appear to be more horizontal.

These roentenographic changes have been described by Catterall as producing a "head at risk" for serious deformity. However, persistent loss of motion is probably the most important early sign of impending serious problems.

DIFFERENTIAL DIAGNOSIS

In the early stage, before bone roentgenographic changes occur, toxic synovitis and pyogenic arthritis or osteomyelitis of the femoral neck must be considered as differential diagnoses. In Legg-Calvé-Perthes syndrome, there is little

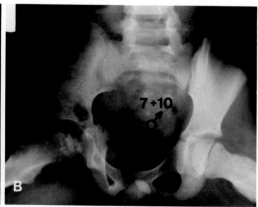

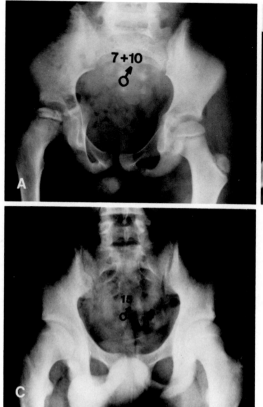

FIG. 18-60. *(A and B)* Catterall Group III. Initially this child was seen at age 7 years and 10 months, and was treated in concentric reduction. *(C)* Follow-up film taken at age 15 show fair results by Mose the Mose method.

change in white blood cell count and little, if any, increase in the sedimentation rate. If true doubt exists as to the diagnosis of the syndrome, the hip should be aspirated, as for any joint suspected of harboring infection. If no fluid is recovered, injection of a small amount of contrast fluid, followed by taking of a roentgenogram, verifies that the joint had been entered. If there is an unusual, fuzzy appearance of the femoral heads or if the child has generalized retardation, a thyroid study may be helpful, but it is rarely indicated.

A major problem is differentiating Legg-Calvé-Perthes syndrome from multiple epiphyseal dysplasia. The latter should be suspected in bilateral involvement, especially when involvement is symmetrical and when the femoral heads do not have a characteristic appearance of Legg-Calvé-Perthes syndrome. All hip joints that do not follow the classic picture of increased density, and presence of the crescent sign followed by fragmentation should be considered suspect. A family history may often be obtained. Roentgenograms of other joints, especially a tunnel view of the knee and an anteroposterior view of the ankles showing lateral tilt of the ankle motion, helps to determine the diagnosis.

TREATMENT

PRINCIPLE

Treatment in Legg-Calvé-Perthes syndrome should be to achieve a favorable environment in which the process can run its self-limited course. All affected femoral heads heal, and the only principle of treatment is to try and minimize the distortion during the active stages of the process.

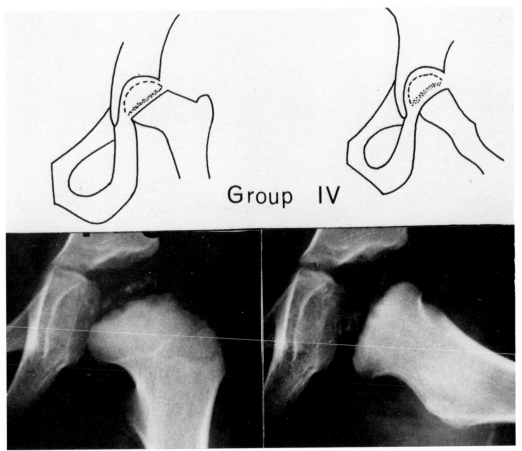

FIG. 18-61. Catterall classification, Group IV. There is total involvement of the femoral head, with exposure of the epiphyseal line.

The most important initial treatment principle is to rapidly regain and maintain a range of motion. This is too often overlooked in the enthusiasm to proceed with a treatment program. Traction and bedrest are most helpful in regaining motion. Full abduction should be restored and internal rotation should be regained, although the last 10° of internal rotation may not be essential. Two to 3 weeks of treatment may be necessary, and only after this period of time should an adductor release be considered. The traction program may be carried out at home if the family situation allows. In approximately 20 per cent of the patients, an inflammatory-like reaction persists and oral salicylates may reduce the reaction. Only after the motion has been established should a bracing program be instituted.

Formerly the major treatment efforts were directed towards non-weightbearing. In recent years it has been recognized that if the femoral head can be maintained deeply within the acetabulum during the soft vulnerable phase of the disease process, a more normal femoral head will result. It is to be remembered that the acetabulum is not involved in the early phase of the disease and, therefore, it can serve as an excellent mold. However, it must be recognized that even with a full treatment program, either containment orthosis or surgery, a less-than-

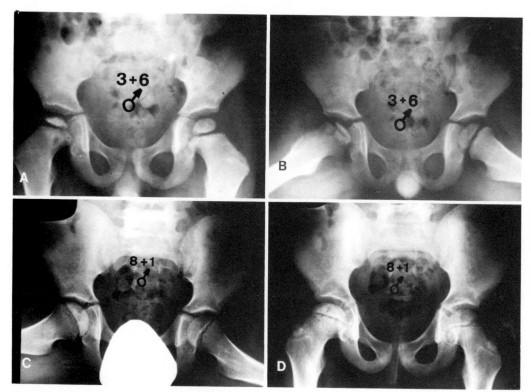

Fig. 18-62. *(A and B)* Catterall Group IV. There is total femoral head involvement in this young child, with no resultant restriction of motion. *(C and D)* After treatment, minimal residual deformity is present, as seen at age 8 years and 1 month.

excellent result should be expected in patients that are older and have major femoral head involvement (Fig. 18-65).

THE NON-WEIGHTBEARING METHOD

Non-weightbearing treatment includes bedrest with or without traction, an ischial weightbearing brace, and a Snyder sling. Bedrest, for longer than is necessary to regain motion in the hip, is no longer practical. Ischial weightbearing braces truly are not weight-relieving. On occasion they may actively increase the pressure across the hip joint, and, therefore, they are contraindicated. Successful use of the Snyder sling and Forte harness depends solely on the cooperation of the patient. These devices are of little help other than for the occasional problem where the diagnosis has not been confirmed and the treatment program is planned to continue for only a few weeks.

CONTAINMENT METHODS

The concept of treatment is to keep the femoral head deeply seated within the acetabulum throughout its vulnerable weakened period and to maintain a full range of hip motion. If the femoral head is placed deeply into the acetabulum, weightbearing *per se* does not seem to be an important consideration, except possibly in the older child with major femoral head involvement. In abduction, the hip abductors are at a gross mechanical disadvantage, and they cannot apply strong force across the joint. Also, the soft femoral head is stabilized on all sides by the intact acetabulum.

Abduction should be of such a degree that the lateral aspect of the epiphyseal line reaches the lateral margin of the acetabulum. This lateral coverage should be confirmed by a standing roentgenogram in the holding device used for treatment (Fig.

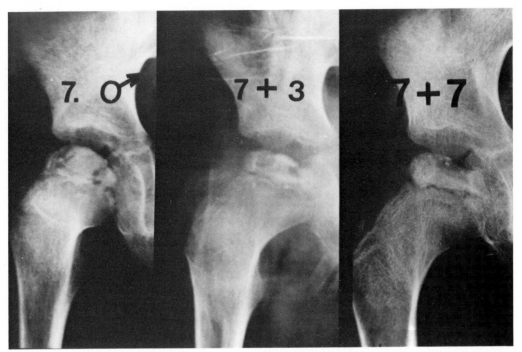

FIG. 18-63. The roentgenogram of a 7-year-old child suggests that there is major femoral head involvement. Three months later, the degree of involvement is questionable. By the time the child is 7 years and 7 months old, he is diagnosed as having Catterall Group II involvement, and can bear weight without a brace.

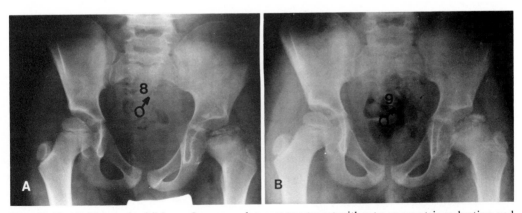

FIG. 18-64. *(A)* This male child, age 8 years underwent treatment without a concentric reduction and presented with extrusion of the lateral portion of the epiphysis with lateral flecks of calcification and ossification. *(B)* At age 9 years, well-established reossification of the lateral flecks results in a union with and enlargement of the femoral head.

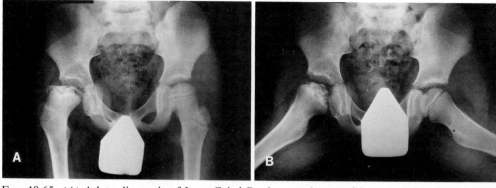

Fig. 18-65. *(A)* A late diagnosis of Legg-Calvé-Perthes syndrome with gross deformity was made and confirmed by roentgenograms. *(B)* However, since the hip can abduct to 15°, surgery to remove the extruded portion of the femoral head is not necessary.

18-66). Thirty-five to 55° of leg abduction may be necessary to achieve this coverage, depending on the neck-shaft angle of the femur and the tilt of the epiphyseal line in the particular patient. Inadequate degrees of abduction can result in formation of a pressure point laterally and may do more harm than good. Maintaining an internal rotation position beyond a few degrees of rotation is probably not important, since anteversion is not normally increased in the early stages of Legg-Calvé-Perthes syndrome. The subluxation, collapse and extrusion that may occur in the early stages of the process can be decreased or eliminated with adequate early containment. Various methods of holding the thigh in abduction and internal rotation include: non-weightbearing abduction braces, abduction casts of Petrie and Harrison, and, the ones most recently introduced, abduction weightbearing braces of Craig, Newington, Toronto and Atlanta (Fig. 18-67).

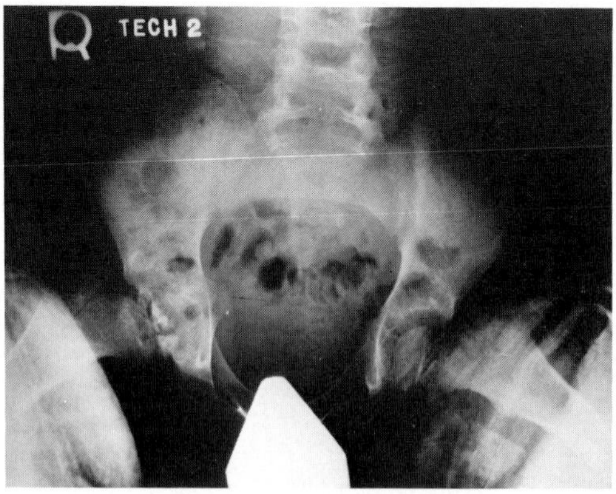

Plaster Method

It is important to always remember that an essentially full range of motion must exist in the hip prior to placing the child in an abduction device. As soon as a child is active in any type of containment device, a *standing* anteroposterior roentgenogram of the pelvis is necessary to confirm that the femoral head is fully covered, as planned.

The use of Petrie[199] abduction casts has been very helpful as a short-range form of treatment. The casts can be applied as soon as a full range of motion is achieved, with no delay being necessary for fabrication of a brace. The casts also give the physician an opportunity to evaluate the total problem over a period of a few months, without a serious financial commitment for a brace, and, particularly, it allows for time to determine the severity of the femoral head involvement. A child should not remain in the cast for more than 2 to 3 months at a time, and it is usually removed after 2 months. If casting

Fig. 18-66. Lateral coverage is confirmed by a standing roentgenogram in a holding device. The superior portion of the epiphyseal line is abducted to within the border of the acetabulum to prevent extrusion.

is to be continued, the child should remain out of the cast for several days, in order to regain full knee motion. It is recommended that, except on rare occasions, no more than two or three sets of casts be used before other containment methods are attempted or the treatment program is abandoned because of the mild involvement of the femoral head. If the casts are not changed frequently, there may be risk of damage to the articular cartilage of the knees. The casts must also fit snugly about the thighs to minimize stress on the medial collateral ligament. In our patients, no late problems from this method have resulted.

Orthosis Method

There are many types of braces and orthoses available, all of which are basically designed for the same containment purpose. There is little difference in efficiency amoung the methods. However, the local bracemaker or orthotist must be familiar with the method used, and the need for repairs must be kept to a reasonable level. When required, these repairs should be made promptly to minimize the time out of the brace. Each time that the child is reevaluated the device should be removed and the hip examined to see if a full range of motion is still present. If motion has decreased, the child should be returned to a temporary traction program. If the hip remains slightly painful, the child may use in addition a nights-only home traction setup.

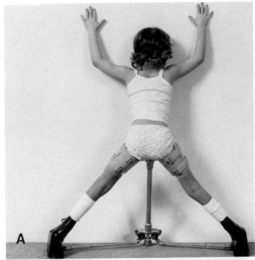
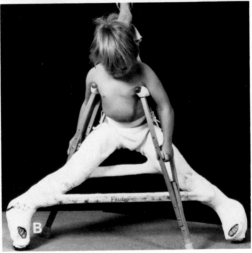

FIG. 18-67. *(A)* The Toronto brace—an abduction containment orthosis. *(B)* The Petrie cast achieves abduction with mild internal rotation.

TIMING THE END OF TREATMENT

In the past, most treatment programs were continued until the femoral head had filled in, as was indicated by both anteroposterior and lateral roentgenograms, or at least until the subchondral bone plate had been reestablished in both views. This process requires at least 18 months and sometimes up to 4 years, making the program undesirable, because its duration is both very indefinite and lengthy.

Our clinical and roentgenographic evaluations of the patients that discontinued their treatment program early, of their own desire, have allowed us to observe that little, if

any, distortion of the femoral head occurs if weightbearing is resumed after the increased density in the femoral head disappears (Fig. 18-68). This reconfirms a similar observation by Ferguson.[172] The increased density disappears essentially at the completion of the fragmentation stage, which is after approximately 1 year of the process. The studies of Jonsater also demonstrated that there was increased strength in the biopsy fragments by the time the fragmentation stage was reached. The term *fragmentation* suggests

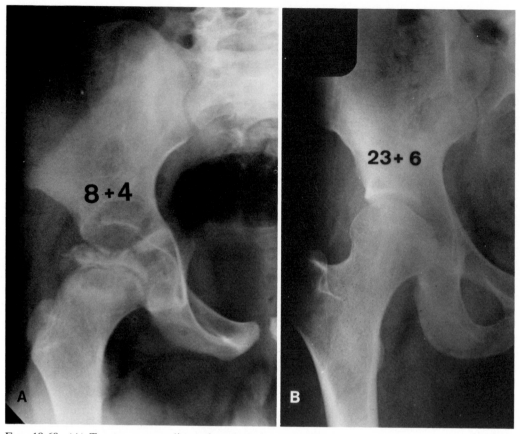

FIG. 18-68. *(A)* Treatment was discontinued at the end of the sclerotic phase for this child of 8 years and 4 months. *(B)* Long-term follow-up film taken at 23 years and 6 months shows excellent remodelling with no further collapse.

to the clinician a fragile and defective phase and is inappropriate, since new bone is already returning to the epiphysis.

In most patients it requires 6 months of observation to determine the full extent of involvement of the femoral head by the Catterall classification. Up until that time, especially in the older child, there is the risk of a Group II involvement changing to Group III involvement. Studies with radioactive isotopes may allow earlier diagnosis of the full extent of the involvement, but they are not generally available at the present time. If it can be determined that the involvement is only Group II and the patient has a full range of motion, the treatment can be stopped even before the dense segment is eliminated. Thus, many patients can be allowed to walk unassisted by the end of the first 6 months.

If the involvement is Group III or Group IV, usually the increased density areas have vanished by 12 to 15 months, and weight-bearing can again be allowed.

To graduate the child from a brace program, we suggest allowing him to remove the brace for a few hours and to ambulate only in the house. The child should be evaluated within a week to determine if loss of motion has occurred. If full motion remains, the time out of the brace can be increased and the motion frequently rechecked. Loss of motion is an indication that a longer period of full-time wear is necessary. It appears that at any stage in the process of Legg-Calvé-Perthes syndrome the retention of a full range of motion is probably the most important sign that the program is under control.

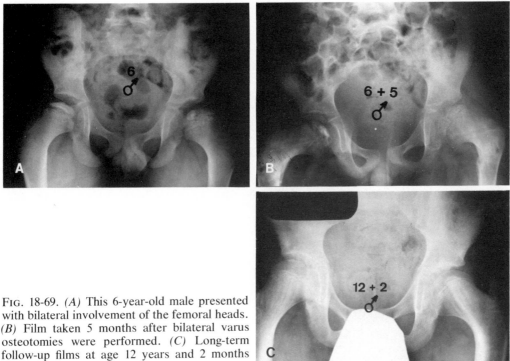

FIG. 18-69. *(A)* This 6-year-old male presented with bilateral involvement of the femoral heads. *(B)* Film taken 5 months after bilateral varus osteotomies were performed. *(C)* Long-term follow-up films at age 12 years and 2 months show good results.

SURGICAL PROCEDURES

In principle, a surgical procedure may be considered for only two separate indications. It is either done early in the process, to prevent the deformity and replace a nonoperative containment method, or later in the process in an effort to improve an established but, at least to some degree, reversible deformity.

Replacement for Nonoperative Methods

The principle of containment by operative means involves placing the femoral head deeply within the acetabulum by some form of surgery. This containment can be produced by either altering the acetabulum to provide further coverage (usually the innominate osteotomy of Salter) or decreasing the angle of the proximal femur (varus osteotomy). Both surgical and nonoperative containment methods should produce the same end results, if they are carried out correctly. Surgery is more often indicated when the prognosis indicates that the healing phase may be prolonged (the older child with a more severely involved femoral head). Since no real deformity is expected with Group I and Group II involvement, except for the rare hip with subluxation, the surgery need only be considered for Group III and IV involvement.

Geographic and social factors influence greatly the indications for surgery. In some areas, proper abduction braces or orthoses may not be available. Some children and families do not have the proper attitudes to follow a full bracing program. A surgical program should probably not be introduced unless the child can be properly followed and reevaluated for possible complications.

It must be emphasized that the child must have an essentially full range of motion. This motion must be present for some weeks or months before considering surgery. A cast or a brace will ideally be required for a few months to produce the desired motion. It also allows a time period during which the

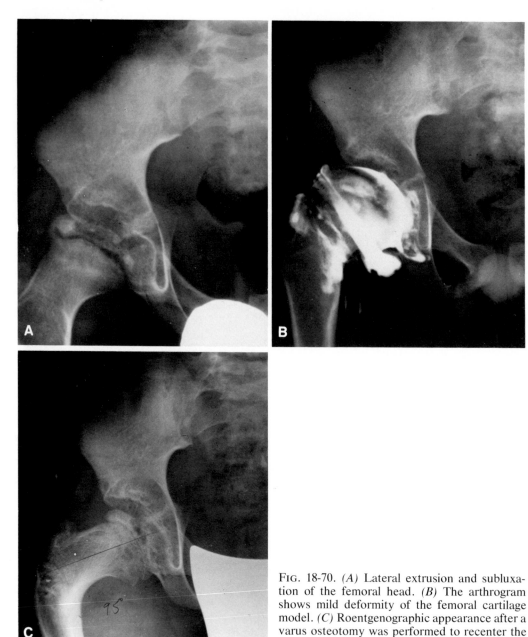

FIG. 18-70. *(A)* Lateral extrusion and subluxation of the femoral head. *(B)* The arthrogram shows mild deformity of the femoral cartilage model. *(C)* Roentgenographic appearance after a varus osteotomy was performed to recenter the head.

extent of involvement of the femoral head can be determined, especially if the process is in the earliest stages.

The varus osteotomy is usually preferred to allow full centering of the head (Fig. 18-69). The angle should be reduced to no more than 110°, because if the epiphyseal line is in-

volved, a more normal angle may not reestablish later (Fig. 18-70). Derotation may be carried out, but this should usually be only a few degrees unless the child has an abnormal increase in anteversion.

The Salter osteotomy has value in the primary treatment of Legg-Calvé-Perthes syn-

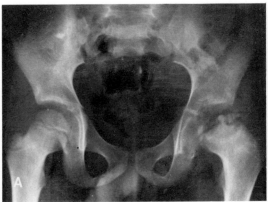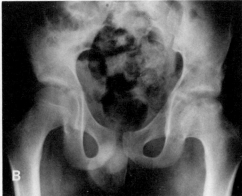

FIG. 18-71. *(A)* Preoperative roentgenogram shows total femoral head involvement. The spherical outline of the femoral head was verified by arthrogram. *(B)* Four years after Salter osteotomy was performed, a satisfactory result can be seen.

drome, but difficulty may occur in regaining motion after this procedure, especially in the older child with total head involvement (Fig. 18-71). It is also difficult to get enough lateral coverage if the head centers fully only after 20° of motion on the abduction test. The procedure should be preceded by an arthrogram, and moderate distortion of the cartilage model is a contraindication. The patient with an uncontrolled subluxation of a Group II type or the younger child with free motion can be treated by the procedure.

Reconstruction

An operation performed late in Legg-Calvé-Perthes syndrome to correct an already present deformity may cover the femoral head, reshape it, or translate motion into a more useful range. The improved mechanical environment hopefully allows further remodeling, if potential for growth still remains. If no growth potential remains, most patients with the syndrome are best left alone, unless they are having significant pain symptoms, which are usually rare until middle life (Fig. 18-72).

If the goal of the reconstructive surgery is to reestablish containment by an indirect approach on the proximal femur or the acetabulum, it is mandatory that the final position be demonstrated before the surgical procedure be performed. An abduction test roentgenogram should be used to verify the position, and if it is not satisfactory, a traction program to attempt to produce reduction is indicated. If this is not accomplished, the surgical procedure will fail, and the malalignment may be worsened.

If Legg-Calvé-Perthes syndrome is recognized and treated early, the need for late reconstructive procedures is lessened.

Varus Osteotomy. If the femoral head can be replaced within the acetabulum, a varus osteotomy may be done, as in the primary treatment group. If, however, there has already been considerable loss in height of the epiphysis, the varus will exaggerate this total loss. The child may later require an epiphysiodesis of the distal femur on the opposite leg to achieve final leg length equality. The neck-shaft angle should only be reduced to 120°, because children requiring this procedure are usually older and often experience involvement of the epiphyseal line, and, therefore, they do not regain the normal angle.

Salter Innominate Osteotomy. This is seldom indicated as a reconstructive procedure, since there is usually already significant deformity in the femoral head. If it is to be considered, it should be preceded by an arthrogram to check the sphericity of the head. If sphericity has been lost, the procedure should not be done.

The Chiari Procedure is only rarely indicated for children with Legg-Calvé-Perthes syndrome. There is probably no indication

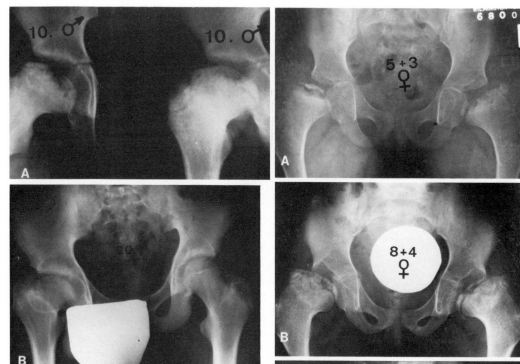

Fig. 18-72. (A) This 10-year-old male shows total head involvement, with major involvement through the epiphyseal line to the metaphysis. (B) At age 20 years, there is premature closure of the epiphyseal line, with ineffective modeling and overgrowth of greater trochanter.

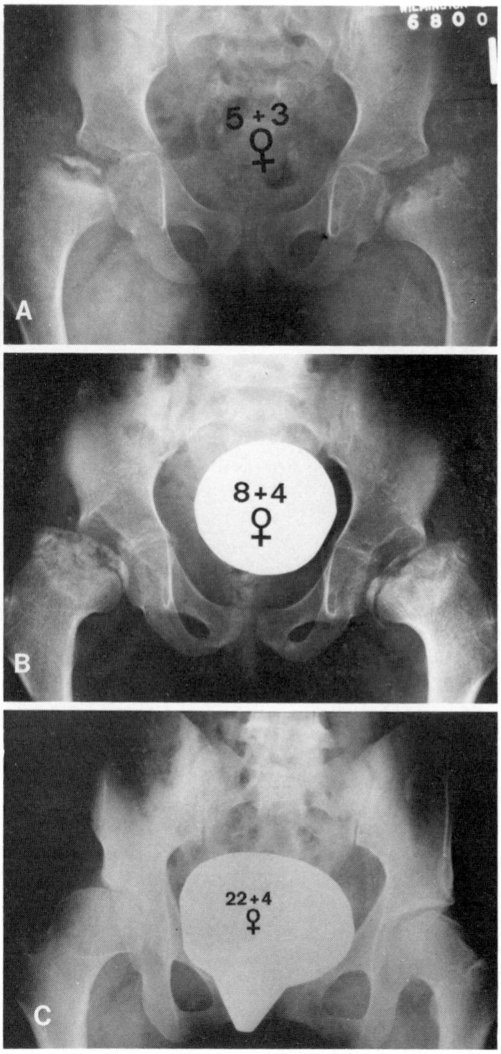

Fig. 18-73. (A) Roentgenogram of the hip of a child 5 years and 3 months old, showing gross extrusion. Containment methods are not possible. Resection should not be performed at this stage. (B) The epiphysis should be partially reconstituted, as was seen on roentgenogram when the child was 8 years and 4 months old, before considering resection. (C) Long-term follow-up film showing an improved contour.

for this procedure in an older child or adolescent who does not have pain. It may be considered for the rare case of an older child with coxa magna who is having considerable pain from a mechanical obstruction to motion.

Garceau Procedure. Garceau described a removal of the part of the femoral head that extrudes out beyond the acetabulum to such a degree that it locks the thigh in adduction or neutral position. This procedure can be considered for the hip where no abduction is possible from a mechanical block. The procedure should not be considered until there has been adequate buildup of new bone in the weightbearing area (Fig. 18-73 A, B, C). If done too early, the soft weightbearing area of the femoral head may extrude again and result in further deformity and, there-

fore, surgery must wait well into the reconstructive phase (Fig. 18-74). The procedure is rarely indicated and is never needed if containment methods are used in the earlier phases of the process.

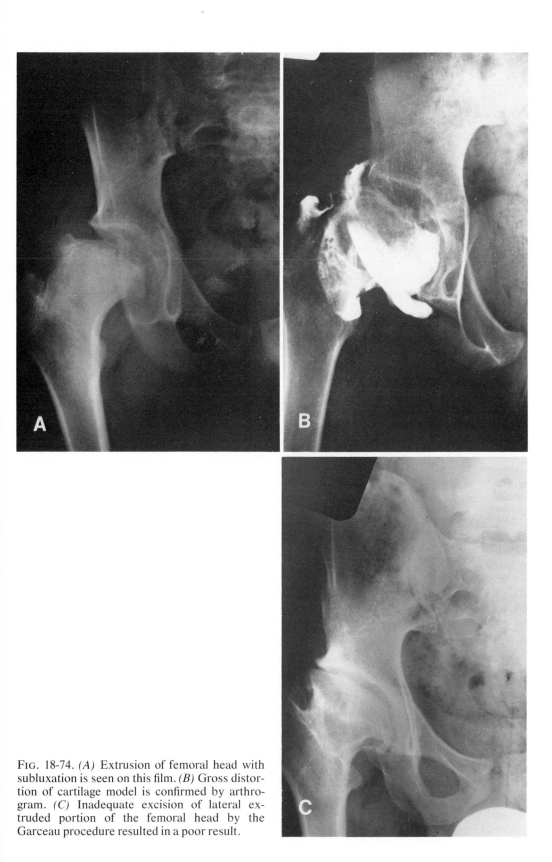

FIG. 18-74. (A) Extrusion of femoral head with subluxation is seen on this film. (B) Gross distortion of cartilage model is confirmed by arthrogram. (C) Inadequate excision of lateral extruded portion of the femoral head by the Garceau procedure resulted in a poor result.

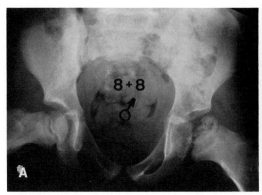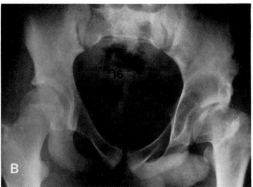

Fɪɢ. 18-75. *(A)* Total femoral head involvement seen with secondary acetabular dysplasia. However, the femoral head centers on abduction. *(B)* Salter and varus osteotomies were performed, and long-term follow-up shows improved positioning.

Combined Procedures

The rare patient who has had an extrusion or subluxation of the femoral head for many months may also have a true secondary dysplasia of the acetabulum. If the femoral head still centers on the abduction test, the dysplasia may be improved by a combined innominate osteotomy and varus osteotomy of the proximal femur (Fig. 18-75). If this combination is to be considered, it should be preceded by an arthrogram to show the extent of the cartilage change of the acetabulum. If the cartilage model is intact, only femoral surgery is indicated.

PLANS OF MANAGEMENT

The following plan of management is suggested. For Group I involvement, regardless of the age of the patient, no specific treatment appears to be indicated, as long as a full range of motion is maintained. Changes in range of motion may herald a more severe form of the condition, so the patient must be watched initially for 2 to 4 weeks and the program changed if necessary. In Group II involvement, there are rarely poor results for patients under 7 years of age, regardless of the type of treatment. Therefore, for the young child, containment efforts are probably not necessary unless there is true subluxation. In the child 7 years of age, early containment should be achieved by an orthosis, and care should be taken to maintain range of motion because of the risk of the hip's changing to more serious involvement or slight subluxation. If the condition remains as a Group II type, treatment can be discontinued gradually by approximately 6 months.

For Groups III and IV, regardless of the patient's age, emphasis should be placed on maintaining containment and full range of motion. In very young children, those of 3 to 4 years, if there are no signs of irritation in the joint, and if there is no suggestion of subluxation, a course of observation can be carried out. However, frequent observations are indicated. In Group III and Group IV involvement in the child of 7 years, the surgeon, may consider the surgical program because of the family. The recent work of Klisic and McKibbon suggests that in older children with total involvement the results are usually poor, so an active motion program and no surgery is probably the best treatment program. Weight-relief abduction treatment may be of help in the latter group, but to date there is no real proof that this is so.

CONCLUSIONS

It can be stated that Catterall's classification is prognostically significant. Different types of deformities have different natural histories. Early energetic treatment is very important in preventing deformity, and it should be in the form of containment of the femoral head and maintenance of the range of motion. Finally, treatment can be discontinued long before reestablishment of the subchondral plate is observed. Once the dense bone has disappeared, walking can again be allowed if motion is not impaired. Therefore, the typical child with Legg-Calvé-Perthes disease can go through a treatment program of usually less than 14 months in duration and usually does not require a surgical procedure for defects seen as part of the disease process.

TRANSIENT SYNOVITIS

Transient synovitis is a very common hip ailment in children. Despite its frequency, however, it is not well understood. The multitude of names for transient synovitis indicates the varying attitudes towards this condition (i.e., transitory arthritis, observation hip, toxic synovitis, transitory coxitis, coxitis serosa seu simplex, acute transitory epiphysis and intermittent hydrarthritis). However, "transient synovitis" is the name most commonly used, primarily because of its noncommittal nature.

The painful hip and joint stiffness is caused by non-specific, non-pus-forming inflammation of the synovial membrane of the joint capsule, Jacobs explored three hips with transient synovitis and found normal articular cartilage with marked synovial hypertrophy and congestion both on gross and microscopic examination.[228]

ETIOLOGY

The etiology of transient synovitis remains unknown. Trauma, infection, and allergic hypersensitivity are several of the proposed causes for the inflammation. There has been evidence supporting and contradicting each of these causes.

There are many ligaments and muscular insertions about the hip joint and the joint capsule itself which lend themselves to strain from the extraordinary movement, allowed by the ball-and-socket hip joint.[223] The articular cartilage itself is also vulnerable, and damage to it may explain the frequent finding of acute pain at one point in the range of motion. If there is joint bleeding as the result of trauma, there is synovial inflammation due to vascular engorgement, with undesirable effects upon the articular surface. Blockley and Porter[221] noted that the painful hip is often first noticed in the morning when a child is waking. They suggested that minor trauma may have occurred while the child was sleeping when the hip joint was fully relaxed. If minor subluxation occurs, it may give rise to a muscular spasm similar to the "pulled elbow" of a younger age group, with normal roentgenograms and symptoms that clear within a few days. Symptomatic pain is not always limited to the hip joint. Donaldson[224] stated that 55 per cent of his patients who complained of pain situated it in the anterior hip region, 20 per cent also had pain in the knee of the affected extremity, and the rest had diffuse pain usually localized in the affected thigh. Trauma was always a predisposing factor in his series.

Spock[231] proposed that a concurrent infection was responsible for the synovial inflammation. Seventy per cent of his cases with transient synovitis had upper respiratory infections within a 2-week period prior to the onset of symptoms. Six of his patients had sera titered against viral antigens, and three showed elevated titers. One of the three patients had a fourfold increase in Coxsackie B antigen titer. Paired sera was determined for 10 patients, and 4 showed elevated antibody levels. Also, 30 per cent of the patients who had throat cultures taken showed evidence of harboring beta-hemolytic streptococci, as compared to 10 per cent of the control asymptomatic group. Spock concluded that Coxsackie B virus and beta-hemolytic streptococci were concomitant infections of transient synovitis. The large number of patients with transient synovitis who have a history of predisposing upper respiratory infections gives support to this argument. Forty-eight per cent of Spock's cases had nasopharyngitis. Gledhill[227] found that 22 out of 111 cases had upper respiratory infections. Twenty per cent of Donaldson's patients had this infection or infected tonsils. However, Spock treated 78 per cent of his patients with antibiotics, with no results. Blockley and Porter found that only two out of 17 patients had evidence of rising antibody titers. They also completed a virologic investigation and concluded that a virus was not responsible for transient synovitis.

The third possible cause of transient synovitis is allergic hypersensitivity of the synovium. Edwards[226] believes that the synovium is sensitized due to an allergic condition and may be affected by a focus of infection elsewhere in the body, as opposed to a metastatic process. Four of his 13 patients exhibited some form of allergy. Also, 5 of his patients had histories of frequent colds, sore throats, nasal discharge, and, in one case, otitis media, all of which he thought could have been caused by undetermined allergies. It is necessary to find the possible focus of the interacting infection. Hypertrophied and infected tonsils were found in eight of Edwards' 13 cases. In one case, the only focus for infection was a partially healed furuncle in the thigh. Further, two patients with a history of allergy were given steroids, and both exhibited dramatic recoveries within 1 day and remained well. On the other hand, Spock found only a normal occurrence of allergy in his 47 cases and found no evidence that transient synovitis was due to allergic antigen contact. Donaldson states that he cannot substantiate toxic or allergic hypersensitivity to an infection in relation to the onset of transient synovitis.

In summation, no single causative factor has been isolated for transient synovitis. Since transient synovitis merely describes a temporary inflammation of the synovium, trauma, infection and allergic hypersensitivity may play a part singly or in combination, resulting in the characteristic synovial condition.

SEQUELAE

Although transient synovitis is relatively mild, it can have lasting effects on the involved joint. DeValderrama[223] conducted a follow-up study of 23 patients who had been diagnosed to have transient synovitis 15 to 20 years earlier. Four of his patients had coxa magna, three had osteoarthritis without coxa magna, three had minor coxa magna without osteoarthritic change, and two showed broadening of the femoral neck

without evidence of change in the femoral head. He concluded that degenerative arthritis may be a sequel and that the vascular engorgement associated with the inflammation of the synovium increases the blood supply to epiphyseal cartilage. The increase not only produces a varying degree of decalcification, but also stimulates the growth and subsequent enlargement of the corresponding epiphysis.

On the other hand, Nachemson[230] could find no correlation between age, sex, and preliminary severity of the transient synovitis and the later hip abnormalities. These abnormalities consisted of mild motion limitation, coxa magna, and cysts and roentgenographic dark spots of the femoral neck. These effects were found to be mild and rare. Therefore, although there is some correlation between transient synovitis and later complications, the exact relationship cannot be pinpointed.

CLINICAL FEATURES

Although its etiology is still unknown, transient synovitis is a definite clinical entity with recognizable symptoms, signs, and evolution. Transient synovitis occurs in children between the ages of 2 and 12 years, with an average age of onset being 6 years.[228] However, most of the patients seem to be under 7 years of age. Males are affected slightly more often than females.[224, 231] Either hip may be involved, but both are never involved simultaneously, nor is there involvement of other joints. The primary symptoms and signs are pain, limp, and the restriction of passive motion in the hip joint. About 65 per cent of the patients complain of pain either in the hip or radiating downward to the knee or thigh, but seldom does it radiate to the lower leg.[226, 227] Tenderness can often be localized anteriorly, although seldom is it over the greater trochanter. There is no soft-tissue "thickening" over the anterior hip or trochanter.[224] A noticeable limp may accompany the complaint of pain, but Gledhill noted that a third of his patients had a painless limp. Thus, pain or a limp is almost always present with transient synovitis.

Limitation of passive hip motion is always

present and is due to protective muscle spasms. There is restriction in all directions, particularly in abduction, internal rotation, external rotation and extension.[224, 225, 228] Muscular spasms about the hip accompany the motion limitation, and most of the spasms occur in the flexors and adductors; however, there is no muscular weakness, atrophy or inguinal adenopathy. Aspiration of the joint results in sterile joint fluid, which is either clear, slightly cloudy, yellow, or bloodstained.[226, 228] A low-grade temperature of 99 to 100° is often present, which rarely goes as high as 103°. A biopsy of the synovium of the hip joint reveals a nonspecific synovitis.

One of the most notable characteristics of transient synovitis is the speed with which the symptoms appear and disappear. Edwards claims that the symptoms may be insidious as well as acute. Gledhill usually diagnosed synovitis within 1 week of the onset of symptoms, and the subsequent duration was 1 to 4 days. Spock's average duration of illness was 13 days, with a range of 4 to 65 days. One characteristic of transient synovitis is its self-limiting nature and speed of recovery. However, this may not be used for differential diagnosis of transient synovitis, for it is similar to the first stages of other more serious hip disease, such as Legg-Calvé-Perthes disease. The more serious diseases, however, seem to have a more repetitious, chronic nature, and if the painful stiff hip returns, a primary diagnosis of transient synovitis must be held with deep suspicion.

ROENTGENOGRAPHIC FEATURES

Roentgenographic analysis is important in the diagnosis of transient synovitis, for the lack of bony abnormalities can rule out advanced stages of other diseases of the hip joint. Both frontal and lateral roentgenograms should be taken. Most roentgenographic examinations yield normal films, but these negative findings are usually due to examination of bony material.

There may be widening of the medial joint space, with lateral displacement of the femoral head. There may be evidence of capsular distension.[222] However, there is difficulty in identifying soft-tissue signs due to the variation in quality of the films and in the positioning of the child. The important point is that there is a basically normal roentgenogram of the hip in children with transient synovitis, and this can differentiate it from the more advanced stages of other more serious hip diseases.

DIAGNOSIS

The basic criteria for diagnosis of transient synovitis are: (1) pain at the hip joint, thigh or knee; (2) passive restriction in the range of hip motion; (3) lack of bony abnormalities in the roentgenographic examination; and (4) complete recovery after a maximum period of 2 months of therapy. The importance of transient synovitis is not in the disease itself, but rather in its role as a precursor to most other diseases of the hip. In this respect, transient synovitis is diagnosed through the systematic elimination of the other more serious hip disorders. Only when this is done may physicians conclude that they are dealing with transient synovitis.

Laboratory tests generally produce negative results, however, there does seem to be a slight elevation of the erythrocyte sedimentation rate and leukocyte count.[229]

Serious hip diseases which must be differentiated from transient synovitis are: Legg-Calvé-Perthes syndrome, osteomyelitis, septic arthritis, osteoid osteoma, syphilis, tuberculosis, slipped capital femoral epiphysis, and rheumatoid arthritis.

Legg-Calvé-Perthes syndrome involves necrosis of the capital femoral epiphysis, with the result being a residual epiphyseal deformity seen on a roentgenogram as a flattening of the femoral head. The seriousness of this disease and the radically different treatment program makes Legg-Calvé-Perthes identification critical during the process of diagnosis of possible transient synovitis. This is difficult due to the clinical similarities between the first stages of Legg-Calvé-Perthes disease and transient synovitis. Both of these diseases affect the same age group, with identical distribution and frequency in males and females, and both result in the same symptoms. The child with transient synovitis usually has a normal bone age, whereas the child with Legg-Calvé-Perthes syndrome almost always has a significant retardation of bone age.

Osteomyelitis is accompanied by acute swelling of the joint. An increased leukocyte count and a positive blood culture should reveal the septic involvement. The more advanced stages show a definite roentgeno-graphic change in bone characteristics.

Septic arthritis involves an infectious process and has an acute, febrile clinical picture. There is usually more restriction of hip motion. Joint aspiration is diagnostic.

Osteoid osteoma may be recognized by roentgenographic examination. Tubercular synovitis is a more chronic disease than transient synovitis. A history of contact with tuberculosis may help in diagnosis, and there is an eventual change in the joint structure. Joint aspiration, with smear and culture, should confirm the diagnosis. A slipped capital femoral epiphysis occurs more commonly in older children, and can be recognized by roentgenographic examination.

Rheumatoid arthritis and rheumatic fever are more chronic diseases than transient synovitis, and they often affect more than one joint, as opposed to the monoarticular affectation of transient synovitis. Furthermore, rheumatic fever has characteristic cardiac signs.

TREATMENT

There is some slight variation in the treatment of transient synovitis, but the central goal of treatment is the prevention of weightbearing until the patient is asymptomatic. A characteristic of transient synovitis is its remarkable resolution with rest. However, the child should be followed for at least 18 months after he becomes asymptomatic. Traction may be helpful to reduce spasm, but should be applied in line with the position in which the child holds the leg. This decreases the risk of increasing the joint pressure and causing possibly secondary vascular compromise to the femoral head. Aspiration of the joint should be carried out in the patient with acute and significant symptoms where a true infection is suspected.

REFERENCES

Congenital Dislocation of the Hip

1. Andren, L., and Borglin, M. E.: A disorder of estrogen metabolism as a causal factor of congenital dislocation of the hip. Acta Orthop. Scand., *30:*169, 1960.
2. Averett, J. E., and MacEwen, G. D.: Innominate osteotomy as a reconstructive procedure. South. Med. J., *61:*1212, 1968.
3. Badgley, C. E.: Correlation of clinical anatomical facts leading to a conception of the etiology of congenital hip dysplasias. J. Bone Joint Surg., *25:*503, 1943.
4. ———: Etiology of congenital dislocation of the hip. J. Bone Joint Surg., *31A:*341, 1949.
5. Barlow, T. G.: Early diagnosis and treatment of congenital dislocation of the hip. J. Bone Joint Surg., *44B:*292, 1962.
6. Botting, T. D. J., and Scrase, W. H.: Premature epiphyseal fusion at the knee complicating prolonged immobilization for congenital dislocation of the hip. J. Bone Joint Surg., *47B:*280, 1965.
7. Caffey, J., Ames, R., Silverman, W. A., Ryder, C. T., and Hough, G.: Contraindication of the congenital dysplasia predislocation hypotheses of congenital dislocation of the hip through a study of the normal variation in acetabular angles at successive periods in infancy. Pediatrics, *17:*632, 1956.
8. Carter, C., and Wilkinson, J.: Persistent joint laxity and congenital dislocation of the hip. J. Bone Joint Surg., *46B:*40, 1964.
9. Chapple, C., and Davidson, D.: A study of the relationship between fetal positions and certain congenital deformities. J. Pediatr., *18:*483, 1941.
10. Chiari, K.: Ergebnisse mit der Beckenosteotomie als Pfannendach plastik. Z. Orthop., *87:*14, 1955.
11. Chuinard, E. G.: The relationship and treatment of congenital dysplasia of the hip and degenerative arthritis. J. West. Pacific Orthop. Assc. *1 x 2,* 9(2):48, 1972.
12. Chuinard, E. G., and Logan, M. D.: Varus-producing and derotational subtrochanteric osteotomy in the treatment of congenital dislocation of the hip. J. Bone Joint Surg., *45A:*1397, 1963.
13. Coleman, S. S.: Treatment of congenital dislocation of the hip in the infant. J. Bone Joint Surg., *45A:*1322, 1963.
14. ———: Treatment of congenital dislocation of the hip in the older child. Curr. Prac. Orthop. Surg., *6:*99, 1975.
15. Coleman, S. S., and MacEwen, G. D.: Congenital dislocation of the hip in infancy, AAOS Instruc. Course Lect., *21:*155, 1972.
16. Colonna, P. C.: Capsular arthroplasty for congenital dislocation of the hip; indications and technique. J. Bone Joint Surg., *47A:*437, 1965.
17. Compere, E. L., and Schnute, W. J.: Treatment of congenital dislocation of the hip. J. Bone Joint Surg., *28:*555, 1946.
18. Crenshaw, A. H.: Cambell's Operative Orthopaedics, ed. 5. St. Louis, C. V. Mosby, 1971.

19. Dickson, F. D.: The shelf operation in the treatment of congenital dislocation of the hip. J. Bone Joint Surg., *46B:*198, 1964.

20. Dunn, P.: Congenital dislocation of the hip (CDH): Necropsy studies at birth. Proc. R. Soc. Med., *62:*1035, 1969.

21. Ferguson, A. B.: Primary open reduction of congenital dislocation of the hip using a median adductor approach. J. Bone Joint Surg., *48B:*682, 1966.

22. Gage, J. R., and Winter, R. B.: Avascular necrosis of the capital femoral epiphysis as a complication of closed reduction of congenital dislocation of the hip: A critical review of twenty years' experience at Gillette Children's Hospital. J. Bone Joint Surg., *54A:*373, 1972.

23. Gill, A. B.: Plastic construction of an acetabulum in congenital dislocation of the hip—the shelf operation. J. Bone Joint Surg., *17:*48, 1935.

24. ———: Congenital dislocation of the hip. AAOS Instruc. Course Lect., *1:*146, 1943.

25. Hart, V. L.: Congenital Dysplasia of the Hip Joint and Sequelae. Springfield, Charles C Tomas, 1952.

26. Hilgenreiner, J.: Zur Frühdiagnose und Frühbehandlung der angeborenen Hüftverrenkung. Med. Klin., *21:*1385, 1425, 1925.

27. Kawamura, B.: Personal communication, 1976.

28. Langenskiold, F.: Technical aspects of the operative reduction of congenital dislocation of the hip. Acta Orthop. Scand., *20:*8, 1950.

29. MacEwen, G. D., and Shands A. R., Jr.: Oblique trochanteric osteotomy. J. Bone Joint Surg., *49A:*345, 1967.

30. McKibbin, B.: Anatomical factors in the stability of hip joint in the newborn. J. Bone Joint Surg., *52B:*148, 1970.

31. Michelsson, J. E., and Langenskiold, A.: Dislocation or subluxation of the hip. J. Bone Joint Surg., *54A, 6:*1177, 1972.

32. Mitchell, G. P.: Arthrography in congenital displacement of the hip. J. Bone Joint Surg., *45B:*88, 1963.

33. ———: Problems in the early diagnosis and management of congenital dislocation of the hip. J. Bone Joint Surg., *54B:*4, 1972.

34. Morel, G.: The treatment of congenital dislocation and subluxation of the hip in the older child. Acta Orthop. Scand., *46,*364, 1975.

35. Muller, G. M., and Seddon, J. J.: Late results of treatment of congenital dislocation of the hip. J. Bone Joint Surg., *35B:*342, 1953.

36. Ogden, J. A.: Changing patterns of proximal femoral vascularity. J. Bone Joint Surg., *56A:* 941, 1974.

37. ———: Treatment positions for congenital dysplasia of the hip. J. Pediatr., *86:*732, 1975.

38. O'Malley, A. G.: Congenital dislocation of the hip. J. Bone Joint Surg., *47B:*188, 1965.

39. Ortolani, M.: Un segno poco noto e sua importanza per la diagnosi precoce di prelussazione congenita dell 'anca. Pediatria, *45:*129, 1937.

40. ———: Le diagnostic clinque fait par la recherche du signe du ressaut est la seul moyen permettant le traitement vraiment précoce et total de la luxation congénitale de la hanche. Bull. Acad. Nat. Med., *141:*188, 1957.

41. Pavlik. A.: De funktionelle Behandlungsmethode mittels Riemenbugel als Prinzip der konservativen therapie bei angeborenen (Hüftgelenksuerren kungen) der Säuglinge. Z. Orthop. *89:*341, 1957.

42. Pemberton, P. A.: Capsular arthroplasty for congenital dislocation of the hip: indications and techniques. Some long-term results. J. Bone Joint Surg., *47A:*437, 1965.

43. Petrie, J. G.: Congenital dislocation of the hip in infancy. J. Bone Joint Surg., *47A:*607, 1965.

44. Plattou, E.: Rotation osteotomy in the treatment of congenital dislocation of the hip. J. Bone Joint Surg., *35A:*48, 1953.

45. Ponsetti, I. V.: Congenital dislocation of the hip in the infant. AAOS Instruc. Course Lect., *10:*151, 1953.

46. ———: Non-surgical treatment of congenital dislocation of the hip. J. Bone Joint Surg., *48A:*1392, 1966.

47. Ramsey, P. L.: Congenital hip dislocation before and after walking age. Postgrad.Med., *6(4):*114, 1976.

48. Salter, R. B.: Role of innominate osteotomy in the treatment of congenital dislocation and subluxation of the hip in the older child. J. Bone Joint Surg., *48A:*1413, 1966.

49. Salter, R. B., and Dubos, J.: The first fifteen years' personal experience with innominate osteotomy in the treatment of congenital dislocation and subluxation of the hip. Clin. Orthop., *98:*72, 1974.

51. Shands, A. R.: Handbook of Orthopaedic Surgery, ed. 7. St. Louis, C. V. Mosby, 1948.

52. Somerville, E. W.: Development of congenital dislocation of the hip. J. Bone Joint Surg., *35B:*568, 1953.

53. ———: Open reduction in congenital dislocation of the hip. J. Bone Joint Surg., *35B:*363, 1953.

54.———: Some mechanical factors in causation of congenital dislocation of the hip. Dev. Med. Child Neurol. *4:*147, 1962.

55. Stanislavljevic, S.: Diagnosis and Treatment of Congenital Hip Pathology in the Newborn. Baltimore, Williams & Wilkins, 1964.

56. Steel, H. H.: Triple osteotomy of the innominate bone. J. Bone Joint Surg., *55A:*343, 1973.

57. Strayer, L. M.: Embryology of the human hip joint. Yale J. Biol. Med., *16:*13, 1943.

58. Sutherland, D. H.: Personal communication, 1975.

59. Thieme, W. T., Wynne-Davies, R., Blair, H. A. F., and Loraine, J. A.: Clinical examination and urinary estrogen assays in newborn children with congenital dislocation of the hip. J. Bone Joint Surg., *50B:*546, 1968.

60. Tronzo, R. G.: Surgery of the Hip Joint. Philadelphia, Lea & Febiger, 1973.

61. Utterback, T. D., and MacEwen, G. D.: Comparison of pelvic osteotomies for the surgical correction of the congenital hip. Am. Orthop., *98:*104, 1974.

62. Von Rosen, S.: Early diagnosis and treatment of

congenital dislocation of the hip joint. Acta Orthop. Scand., *26:*136, 1957.

63. Wagner, H.: Erfahrungen mit der pfannenosteotomie bei der Korrektur der dysplastischen Hüftgelenkpfanne. Der Orthopäde, *2(4):*253, 1973.

64. Watanabe, R. S.: Embryology of the human hip. Clin Orthop., *98:*8, 1974.

65. Wilkinson, J. A.: Prime factors in the etiology of congenital dislocation of the hip. J. Bone Joint Surg., *45B:*268, 1963.

66. ————: Post-natal survey for congenital displacement of the hip. J. Bone Joint Surg., *54B:*40, 1972.

67. Yamamuro, T., Hama, J., Shilcato, J., Sanada, H., and Takeda, T.: Connective tissue of the joint capsule and sex hormones. Conn. Tissue. (Tokyo), *6:*151, 1974.

Coxa Vara

68. Almond, J. G.: Familial infantile coxa vara. J. Bone Joint Surg., *38B:*539, 1956.

69. Amstutz, H. C., and Freiberger, R. H.: Coxa vara in children. Clin. Orthop., *22:*73, 1962.

70. Babb, F. S., Ghormley, R. K., and Chatterton, C. C.: Congenital coxa vara. J. Bone Joint Surg., *31A (1):*115, 1949.

71. Barr, J. S.: Congenital coxa vara. Arch. Surg., *18:*1909, 1929.

72. Becton, J. L., and Diamond, L. S.: Persistent limp in congenital coxa vara. South. Med. J., *60:*921, 1967.

73. Blockey, N. J.: Observation on infantile coxa vara. J. Bone Joint Surg., *51B:*106, 1969.

74. Blocksom, J. P.: Personal communication. 1977.

75. Blount, W. P.: Blade-plate internal fixation for high femoral osteotomies. J. Bone Joint Surg., *25:*319, 1943.

76. Calhoun, J. D., and Pierret, F.: Infantile coxa vara. Am. J. Roentgenol. Radium Ther. Nucl. Med., *115:*561, 1972.

77. Compere, E. L., Garrison, M., and Fahey, J. S.: Deformities of femur resulting from arrestment of growth of capital or greater trochanteric epiphysis. J. Bone Joint Surg., *22:*909, 1940.

78. Duncan, G. A.: Congenital coxa vara occurring in identical twins. Am. J. Surg., *37:*112, 1937.

79. Elmslie, R.: Injury and deformity of the epiphysis of the head of the femur: Coxa vara. Lancet, *1:*410, 1907.

80. Fairbank, J. A. T.: Infantile or cervical coxa vara. *In* Robert Jones Birthday Volume. A Collection of Surgical Essays. London, Milford, 1928.

81. Ferguson, A. B.: Developmental coxa vara. *In* Ferguson, A. B. (ed.): Orthopaedic Surgery In Infancy and Childhood, ed. 4. Baltimore, Williams and Wilkins, 1975.

82. Fiorani, F.: Concerning a rare form of limping. Gazz. d. osp., *2:*717, 1881.

83. Fisher, R. L., and Waskowitz, W. J.: Familial developmental coxa vara. Clin. Orthop., *86:*2, 1972.

84. Hark, F. W.: Congenital coxa vara. Am. J. Surg., *80:*305, 1950.

85. Hasue, M., Kimura, F., Funayama, M., and Ito, R.: An unusual case of coxa vara, characterized

by varying degrees of metaphyseal changes and multiple clipped epiphyses. J. Bone Joint Surg., *50A:*373, 1968.

86. Hofmeister, F.: Coxa vara: A typical form of curvature of the femoral neck. Beitr. Klin. Chir., *12:*245, 1894.

87. Hoyt, W.: Personal communication, 1974.

88. Johanning, K.: Coxa vara infantum. I. Clinical appearance and aetiological problems. Acta Orthop. Scand., *21:*273, 1951.

89. ————: Coxa vara infantum. II. Treatment and results of treatment. Acta Orthop. Scand., *22:*100 1952.

90. Knowles, K. G.: Congenital coxa vara; presentation of a case. R.I. Med. J., *46:*594, 1963.

91. LeMesurier, A. B.: Developmental coxa vara. J. Bone Joint Surg., *30B:*595, 1948.

92. Letts, R. M., and Shokeir, M. H. K.: Mirror-image coxa vara in identical twins. J. Bone Joint Surg., *57A:*117, 1975.

93. MacEwen, G. D., and Shands, A. R., Jr.: Oblique trochanteric osteotomy. J. Bone Joint Surg., *49A:*345, 1967.

94. Magnusson, R.: Coxa vara infantum. Acta Orthop. Scand., *23:*248, 1954.

95. Michelsson, J. E., and Langenskiold, A.: Coxa vara following immobilization of the knee in extension in young rabbits. Acta Orthop. Scand., *45:*399, 1974.

96. Morgan, J. D., and Somerville, E. W.: Normal and abnormal growth at the upper end of the femur. J. Bone Joint Surg., *42B:*264, 1960.

97. Noble, T. P., and Hauser, E. D.: Coxa vara. Arch. Surg., *12:*501, 1926.

98. Pylkkanen, P. V.: Coxa vara infantum. Acta Orthop. Scand. [Suppl.], *48:*1, 1960.

99. Ring, P. A.: Congenital Short Femur. J. Bone Joint Surg., *41B:*73, 1959.

100. ————: Congenital abnormalities of the femur. Arch. Dis. Child., *36:*410, 1961.

101. Say, B., Taysi, K., Pirmar, T., Tokgozoglu, N., and Inan, E.: Dominant congenital coxa vara. J. Bone Joint Surg., *56B (1):*78, 1974.

102. Trueta, J.: The normal vascular anatomy of the human femoral head during growth. J. Bone Joint Surg., *39B:*358, 1957.

103. Von Lanz, T., and Mayet, A.: Die Gelenkkörper des menschlichen Hüftgelenkes in der progredienten Phase ihrer umwegigen Ausformung. Z. Anat., *117:*317, 1953.

104. Zadek, I.: Congenital coxa vara. Arch. Surg., *30:*62, 1935.

Congenital Short Femur With Coxa Vara

105. Aitkin, G. T.: Amputation as a treatment for certain lower-extremity congenital abnormalities. J. Bone Joint Surg., *41A (7):* 1267, 1959.

106. Amstutz, J. C., and Wilson, P. O., Jr.: Dysgenesis of the proximal femur (coxa vara) and its surgical management. J. Bone Joint Surg., *44A (1):* 1, 1962.

107. Bevan-Thomas, W. H., and Millar, E. A.: A review of proximal focal femoral deficiencies. J. Bone Joint Surg., *49A (7):*1376, 1967.

108. Fixsen, J. A., and Lloyd-Roberts, G. C.: The natural history of early treatment of proximal

femoral dysplasia. J. Bone Joint Surg., *56B:*86, 1974.

109. Fock, G., and Sulamaa, M.: Congenital short femur. Acta Orthop. Scand.,*36:*294, 1965.
110. Frantz, C. H., and O'Rahilly, R.: Congenital skeletal limb deficiencies. J. Bone Joint Surg.,*43A (8):*1202, 1961.
111. Freund, E.: Congenital defects of femur, fibula and tibia. Arch. Surg.,*33 (3):*349, 1939.
112. Kim, K., and Cowell, H.: Personal communication, 1977.
113. McKenzie, D. S.: The prosthetic management of congenital deformities of the extremities. J. Bone Joint Surg.,*39B (2):*233, 1957.
114. Ollerenshaw, R.: Congenital defects of the long bones of the lower limb. J. Bone Joint Surg., *7:*528, 1925.
115. Ring, P. A.: Congenital short femur. J. Bone Joint Surg.,*41B (1):*73, 1959.
116.———: Congenital abnormalities of the femur. Arch. Dis. Child.,*36:*410, 1961.

Slipped Capital Femoral Epiphysis

117. Badgley, C. E., Isaacson, A. S., Wolgamat, J. C., and Miller, J. W.: Operative therapy for slipped upper femoral epiphysis. An end result study. J. Bone Joint Surg.,*30A:*19, 1948.
118. Bousseau, M.: Disjonction épiphysaire traumatique de la tête du fémur et des épines iliaques antérieures, mort; autopsie. Bull. Soc. Anat. Fr., *42:*283, 1867.
119. Burrows, J. J.: Slipped upper femoral epiphysis. J. Bone Joint Surg.,*39B:*641, 1957.
120. Bright, R. W., Burstein, A. H., and Elmore, S. M.: Epiphysealplate cartilage. A biomechanical and histological analysis of failure modes. J. Bone Joint Surg.,*56A:*688, 1974.
121. Chung, S. M. K., Batterman, S. C., and Brighton, C. T.: Shear strength of the human femoral capital epiphyseal plate. J. Bone Joint Surg., *58A:*94, 1976.
122. Cordell, L. D.: Slipped capital femoral epiphysis. Postgrad. Med.,*60 (4):*135, 1976.
123. Cowell, H. R.: The significance of early diagnosis and treatment of slipping of the capital femoral epiphysis. Clin. Orthop.,*48:*89, 1966.
124. Ferguson, A. B., and Howorth, M. B.: Slipping of the upper femoral epiphysis. J.A.M.A., *67 (25):*1867, 1931.
125. Haas, S. L.: The localization of the growing point in the epiphyseal cartilage plate of bones. Am. J. Orthop. Surg.,*15:*563, 1917.
126. Harris, W. R.: The endocrine basis for slipping of the upper femoral epiphysis. An experimental study. J. Bone Joint Surg.,*32B:*5, 1950.
127. Herndon, C. H.: Treatment of minimally slipped upper femoral epiphysis. AAOS Instruc. Course Lect.,*21:*188, 1972.
128. Herndon, C. H., Heyman, C. H., and Bell, D. M.: Treatment of slipped capital femoral epiphysis by epiphyseodesis and osteoplasty of the femoral neck: A report of further experiences. J. Bone Joint Surg.,*45A:*999, 1963.
129. Heyman, C. H.: Treatment of slipping of the

upper femoral epiphysis. Surg. Gynecol. Obstet., *89:*559, 1949.
130. Howorth, M. B.: Slipping of the upper femoral epiphysis, Surg. Gynecol. Obstet.,*73:*723, 1941.
131. ———: Slipping of the upper femoral epiphysis. J. Bone Joint Surg.,*31A:*734, 1949.
132. ———: Pathology: Slipping of the capital femoral epiphysis. Clin. Orthop., *48:*33, 1966.
133. Jacobs, B., and Wilson, P. D.: The treatment of slipping of the upper femoral epiphysis. A follow-up study of 300 cases. Arch. Orthop. Unfall-Chir., *56:*349, 1964.
134. Jerre, T.: Early complications after osteosynthesis with a three flanged nail in situ for slipped epiphysis. Acta Orthop. Scand.,*27:*126, 1958.
135. Joplin, R. J.: Slipped capital femoral epiphysis. The still unsolved adolescant hip lesion. J.A.M.A.,*188:*379, 1964.
136. Kelsey, J. L.: Epidemiology of slipped capital femoral epiphysis: A review of the literature. Pediatrics, *51 (6):*1042, 1973.
137. Kelsey, J. L., Acheson, R. M., and Keggi, K. J.: The body builds of patients with slipped capital femoral epiphysis. Am. J. Dis. Child., *124:*276, 1972.
138. Kelsey, J. L. Keggi, K. J., and Southwick, W. O.: The incidence and distribution of slipped capital femoral epiphysis in Connecticut and Southwestern United States. J. Bone Joint Surg., *52A:*1203, 1970.
139. Klein, A., Joplin, R. J., and Reidy, J. A.: Treatment of slipped capital femoral epiphysis. J.A.M.A.,*136:*445, 1948.
140. Kleinberg, S., and Buchman, J.: The operative vs. the manipulative treatment of slipped femoral epiphysis. J.A.M.A.,*107:*1545, 1936.
141. Lindstrom, M.: Surgical treatment of epiphyseolysis capitis femoris. Acta Orthop. Scand.,*28:*131, 1958.
142. Moore, R. D.: Conservative management of adolescent slipping of the capital femoral epiphysis. Surg. Gynecol. Obstet., *80:*324, 1945.
143. Paré, A.: Fracture of the neck of the femur. *In* Cinq Livres de Chirurgie Paris, 1572.
144. Ponseti, I. V., and McClintock, R.: The pathology of slipping of the upper femoral epiphysis. J. Bone Joint Surg.,*38A:*71, 1956.
145. Rennie, A. M.: Familial slipped upper femoral epiphysis. J. Bone Joint Surg.,*49B:*535, 1967.
146. Scham, S. M.: Capital femoral epiphysiolysis treated by plugging with cortical beef bone. Acta Orthop. Scand.,*39:*171, 1968.
147. Sorenson, K. H.: Slipped upper femoral epiphysis. Acta Orthop. Scand.,*39:*499, 1968.
148. Southwick, W. O.: Osteotomy through the lesser trochanter for slipped capital femoral epiphysis. J. Bone Joint Surg.,*49A:*807, 1967.
149. Stulberg, S. D., Cordell, L. D., Harris, W. H., Ramsey, P. L., and MacEwen, G. D.: Unrecognized childhood hip disease: a major cause of idiopathic osteoarthritis of the hip. *In* The Hip Society, The Hip. St. Louis, C. V. Mosby, 1975.
150. Tillema, D. A., and Golding, J. S.: Chondrolysis following slipped capital femoral epiphysis in Jamaica. J. Bone Joint Surg.,*53A (8):*1528, 1971.
151. Wagner, L. C., and Donavan, M. M.: Wedge os-

teotomy of neck of femur in advanced cases of displaced upper femoral epiphysis. A ten year study. Am. J. Surg., *78:*281, 1949.

152. Waldenstrom, H.: On necrosis of the joint cartilage by epiphyseolysis capitis femoris. Acta Chir. Scand., *67:*936, 1930.

153. Wiberg, G.: Epiphyseolysis capitis femoris. Acta Orthop. Scand., *12:*179, 1941.

154. ———: Pinning for slipping of the epiphysis of the femoral head. Acta Orthop. Scand., *18:*4, 1948.

155. ———: Considerations on the surgical treatment of slipped epiphysis with special reference to nail fixation. J. Bone Joint Surg., *41A:*253, 1959.

156. Wilson, P. D., Jacobs, B., and Sheeter, L.: Slipped capital femoral epiphysis. J. Bone Joint Surg., *47A:*1128, 1965.

Legg-Calvé-Perthes Syndrome

157. Axer, A., and Schiller, M. G.: The pathogenesis of the early deformity of the capital femoral epiphysis in Legg-Calve-Perthes Syndrome (L.C.P.S.). Clin. Orthop., *84:*106, 1972.

158. Axer, A., Schiller, M. G., Segal, D., Rzetelmy, V., and Gershuni-Gordon, D. H.: Subtrochanteric osteotomy in the treatment of Legg-Calve-Perthes Syndrome (L.C.P.S.). Acta Orthop. Scand., *44:*31, 1973.

159. Bobechko, W. P., and Harris, W. R.: The radiographic density of avascular bone. J. Bone Joint Surg., *42B:*626, 1960.

160. Broder, H.: The late results in Legg-Perthes Disease and factors influencing them. A study of one hundred and two cases. Bull. Hosp. Joint Dis., *14:*194, 1953.

161. Caffey, John: The early roentgenographic changes in essential coxa plana; their significance in pathogenesis. Am. J. Roentgenol. Radium Ther. Nucl. Med., *103:*620, 634, 1968.

162. Calvé, J.: Sur une forme particulière de coxalgie greffée sur des déformations caractéristiques de l'extremité supérieure du fémur. Rev. Chir., *42:*54, 1910.

163. Cameron, J. M., and Izatt, N. N.: Legg-Calve-Perthes disease. Scott. Med. J., *5:*148, 1960.

164. Catterall, A.: The natural history of Perthes disease. J. Bone Joint Surg., *53B:*37, 1971.

165. ———: Coxa plana. Mod. Trends. Orthop., *6:*122, 1972.

166. Danielsson, L. G., *et al.:* Late results of Perthes disease. Acta Orthop. Scand., *36:*70, 1965.

167. DeCamargo, F. P.: Revascularization of the neck of the femur in Legg-Calve-Perthes Syndrome. Clin. Orthop., *10:*79, 1957.

168. Dolman, C. L., *et al.:* The pathology of Legg-Calve-Perthes disease; a case report. J. Bone Joint Surg., *55A*, 184, 1973.

169. Eaton, G. O.: Long-term results of treatment in coxa plana. J. Bone Joint Surg., *48A:* 1031, 1967.

170. Edgren, W.: Coxa plana. Acta Orthop. Scand. [Suppl.]: *84,* 1965.

171. Evans, D. L., Lloyd-Roberts, G. C.: Treatment in Legg-Calve-Perthes disease. J. Bone Joint Surg., *40B:*182, 1958.

172. Ferguson, A. B., *et al.:* Coxa plana and related conditions at the hip. J. Bone Joint Surg., *16:*781, 1934.

173. Fisher, R. L.: An epidemiological study of Legg Perthes disease. J. Bone Joint Surg., *54A:*769, 1972.

174. Freeman, M. A. R., and England, J. P. S.: Experimental infarction of the immature canine femoral head. Proc. R. Soc. Med., *62:*431, 1969.

175. Friberg, S.: The roentgenological end results after caliper treatment of coxa plana with varying degrees of epiphyseal involvement. Acta Orthop. Scand., *46:*234, 1975.

176. Goff, C. W.: Recumbency versus nonrecumbency treatment of Legg-Perthes disease. Clin. Orthop., *14:*50, 1959.

177. ———: Legg-Calve-Perthes syndrome (L.C.P.S.). Clin. Orthop., *22:*93, 1962.

178. Gower, W. E., *et al.:* Legg-Perthes disease. J. Bone Joint Surg., *53A:*759, 1971.

179. Graham, J., *et al.:* Perthes disease involving the hip joint. J. Bone Joint Surg., *53B:*650, 1971.

180. Harrison, M. H. M., Turner, M. B., and Nicholson, F. J.: Coxa plana. J. Bone Joint Surg., *51A:*1057, 1969.

181. Harrison, M. H. M., Turner, M. H., and Jacobs, P.: Skeletal immaturity in Perthes disease. J. Bone Joint Surg., *58B:*37, 1976.

182. Jonsater, S.: Coxa plana; a histo-pathologic and arthrographic study. Acta Orthop. Scand. [Suppl.]: *12,* 1953.

183. Kamhi, E., MacEwen, G. D.: Treatment of Legg-Calve-Perthes disease: Prognostic value of Catterall's classification. J. Bone Joint Surg., *57A:*651, 1975.

184. Karadimas, J. E.: Conservative treatment of coxa plana. J. Bone Joint Surg., *53A:*315, 1971.

185. Katz, J. F.: Conservative treatment of Legg-Calve-Perthes disease. J. Bone Joint Surg., *49A:*1043, 1967.

186. ———: Legg-Calve-Perthes disease. Clin. Orthop., *71:*193, 1970.

187. ———: Osteochondroma of the neck of the femur in Legg-Calve-Perthes Disease. Clin. Orthop., *68:*50, 1970.

188. ———: Recurrent Legg-Perthes disease. J. Bone Joint Surg., *55A:*833, 1973.

189. Langenskiold, A., and Salenius, P.: Epiphysiodesis of the greater trochanter. Acta Orthop. Scand., *38:*199, 1967.

190. Lauritzen, J.: Legg-Calve-Perthes disease: A comparative study. Acta Orthop. Scand. [Suppl.]: *159,* 1975.

191. Legg, A. T.: An obscure affection of the hip joint. Boston Med. Surg. J., *162:*202, 1910.

192. Marklund, T., *et al.:* Coxa plana: a radiological comparison of the rate of healing with conservative measures and after osteotomy. J. Bone Joint Surg., *58B:*25, 1976.

193. Malloy, M. K., and MacMahon, B.: Birth weight and Legg Perthes disease. J. Bone Joint Surg., *49A:*498, 1967.

194. Molloy, M. K., and MacMahon, B.: Incidence of Legg-Calve-Perthes disease (osteochondritis deforans). N. Engl. J. Med., *275:*998, 1966.

195. Mose, K.: Legg-Calve-Perthes disease. Acta Orthop. Scand. [Suppl.]:*86*, 1966.

196. Mussbichler, J.: Angiography of the hip refion. Acta Radiol. [Diagn.] (Stockh), *11*:593, 1971.

197. Perthes, G.: Uber arthritis deformans juvenilis. Dtsch. Z. Chir., *10*:111, 1910.

198. ———: Uber osteochondritis deformans juvenilis. Arch. Klin. Chir., *101*:779, 1913.

199. Petrie, J. G., and Bitenc, I.: The abduction weight bearing treatment in Legg-Perthes disease J. Bone Joint Surg., *53B*:54, 1971.

200. Phemister, D. B.: Perthes disease. Surg. Gynecol. Obstet., *33*:87, 1921.

201. Ponsetti, I. V.: Legg-Perthes disease. J. Bone Joint Surg., *38A*:739, 1956.

202. Ponsetti, I. V., and Cotton, R. L.: Legg-Calve-Perthes disease; pathogenesis and evolution. J. Bone Joint Surg., *43A*:261, 1961.

203. Ratliff, A. H. C.: Pseudocoxalgia. J. Bone Joint Surg., *38B*:598, 1956.

204. ———: Perthes disease. J. Bone Joint Surg. *49B*:102, 1967.

205. Salter, R. B.: The pathogenesis of deformity in Legg-Perthes disease. J. Bone Joint Surg., *48B*:389, 1966.

206. ———: The pathogenesis of deformity in Legg-Perthes disease; an experimental investigation. J. Bone Joint Surg., *50B*:436, 1968.

207. Sanders, J. A., and MacEwen, G. D.: A long-term follow-up on coxa plana at the Alfred I. duPont Institute. South. Med. J., *62*:1042, 1969.

208. Schiller, M. G., and Axer, A.: Hypertrophy of the femoral head in Legg-Calve-Perthes syndrome (LCPS). Acta. Orthop. Scand., *43*:45, 1972.

209. ———: Legg-Calve-Perthes syndrome (LCPS). Clin. Orthop., *86*:34, 1972.

210. Siffert, R. S.: The growth plate and its affections. J. Bone Joint Surg., *48A*:546, 1966.

211. Somerville, E. W.: Perthes disease of the hip. J. Bone Joint Surg., *53B*:639, 1971.

211a. Trueta, J.: The normal vascular anatomy of the human femoral head during growth. J. Bone Joint Surg., *39B*:358, 1957.

212. Trueta, J., and Amato, V. P.: The vascular contribution to osteogenesis. III. Changes in the growth cartilage caused by experimentally induced ischaemia. J. Bone Joint Surg., *42B*:571, 1960.

213. Trueta, J., and Little, K.: The vascular contribution to osteogenesis. II. Studies with the electron microscope. J. Bone Joint Surg., *42B*:367, 1960.

214. Trueta, J., and Morgan, J. D.: The vascular contribution to osteogenesis. I. Studies by the injection method. J. Bone Joint Surg., *42B*:97, 1960.

215. Walderstrom, J.: Der obere tuberkulöse cullumherd. Z. Orthop. Chir., *24*:487, 1909.

216. Wansbrough, R. M., *et al.*: Coxa plana, its genetic aspects and results of treatment with the Ling Taylor walking caliper. J. Bone Joint Surg., *4*:169, 1929.

217. Wilkins, K. E.: Current concepts in Legg Perthes disease. U. of Texas Health Science Center, San Antonio, Texas.

218. Wolcott, W. E.: The evolution of the circulation in the developing femoral head and neck; an anatomic study. Surg. Gynecol. Obstet., *77*:61, 1943.

219. Zahir, A., England, J. P. A., and Freeman. M. A. R.: Studies of articular cartilage following infarction of the capital femoral epiphysis in the puppy. Proc. R. Soc. Med., *63*:583, 1970.

220. Zemansky, A. P.: The pathology and pathogenesis of Legg-Calve-Perthes disease (osteochondritis juvenilis deformans coxae). Am. J. Surg., *4*:169, 1929.

Transient Synovitis

221. Blockley, N. J., and Porter, B. B.: Transient synovitis of hip; a virological investigation. Br. Med. J., *4*:557, 1968.

222. Brown, I.: A study of the "capsular" shadow in disorders of the hip in children. J. Bone Joint Surg., *57B*:1975.

223. deValderrama, J.: The "observation hip" syndrome and its late sequelae., J. Bone Joint Surg., *45B*:462, 1963.

224. Donaldson, W.: Transient synovitis of the hip joint. Ped. Clin. North Am., 1073, Nov., 1955.

225. Drey, L.: A roentgenographic study of transitory synovitis of the hip joint. Radiology, *60*:588, 1953.

226. Edwards, E.: Transient synovitis of the hip joint in children; a report on 13 cases. J.A.M.A., *148*:30, 1952.

227. Gledhill, R.: Transient synovitis and Legg-Calve-Perthes disease; a comparative study. Can. Med. Assoc. J., *100*:311, 1969.

228. Jacobs, B.: Synovitis of the hip in children and its significance. Pediatrics, *47*:558, 1974.

229. Lucas, L.: Painful hips in children. AAOS Instruc. Course Lect., *5*:144, 1948.

230. Nachamson, A.: A clinical and radiological follow-up study of transient synovitis of the hip. Acta Orthop. Scand., *40*:479, 1969.

231. Spock, A.: Transient synovitis of the hip joint in children. Pediatrics, *24*:1042, 1959.

19 Lower Limb Length Discrepancy

Sherman S. Coleman, M.D.

In this chapter on the management of inequalities in length of the lower limb, the term "limb length discrepancy" will be used, rather than the term "leg length inequality" because of its greater accuracy and specificity. Since the leg is, by definition, only that part of the lower limb extending from the knee to the ankle, and since lower limb inequality may be manifest in any segment from the pelvis to and including the foot, it seems more appropriate to refer to the "lower limb" rather than to the "leg."

Proper management of the problem of limb length inequality is mainly contingent upon three factors. First, all the available data surrounding and having bearing on the case must be examined and cross-evaluated in order to arrive at a competent decision of whether or not the inequality warrants some form of surgical correction. Second, the various methods of surgical equalization must be understood, and it must be decided which method or combination of methods would be most desirable for the case in question. Finally, a comprehensive understanding of all the technical aspects of surgical equalization must be mastered.

The problem of limb length discrepancy is common, and its importance will likely not diminish, despite the fact that the etiological factors have changed considerably during the past 15 years. Prior to the advent of the poliomyelitis vaccine, lower limb length discrepancies due to muscle paralysis of poliomyelitis were the most common. However, in the United States and in those countries where the poliomyelitis vaccine has been effectively employed, the problem of limb length inequality due to poliomyelitis has almost vanished, and other causes of discrepancy have assumed greater importance (see below).

Minor discrepancies in limb length are often seen, and many can be either ignored or treated with a small shoe lift. Yet when the discrepancy approaches 2 cm., some form of surgical equalization should be considered.

NORMAL GROWTH AND BEHAVIOR OF A LONG BONE

It is essential that one understand the normal process of longitudinal growth of the long bones of the lower limb in order to appreciate not only the mechanisms by which limb length inequality can be produced but also the current methods of treatment. The appendicular skeleton is preformed in cartilage and longitudinal growth of a bone takes place by interstitial cartilage proliferation, both at the physeal plate and at the articular cartilage, followed by gradual and orderly replacement of the cartilage by bone. This has been called "endochondral ossification." In the femur and tibia, each has a primary center of ossification (diaphysis) and two secondary ossification centers, one at each end (epiphyses). The physeal plate makes a much greater contribution to the length of any long bone than does its companion articular cartilage. Yet, chondrogenesis and chondral ossification of the proliferating articular cartilage are essential for

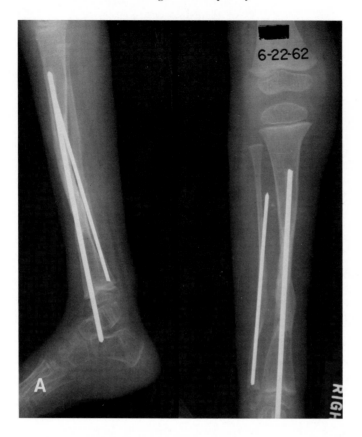

6-22-62

A

FIG. 19-1. A patient with congenital pseudarthrosis of the tibia who was treated with intramedullary rodding and autogenous bone grafting. *(A)* Early postoperative film, taken 1 year following surgery. The smooth rod is passing through the epiphyseal plate, as well as the articular surfaces of the talocalcaneal and talotibial joints. *(Legend continued on facing page.)*

normal epiphyseal growth, both longitudinal and peripheral. Studies have shown that the femur contributes 54 per cent of the total length of the lower limb and the tibia contributes 46 per cent. Furthermore, the distal femoral and proximal tibial physeal plates provide a greater length increment to their respective bones than do the proximal femoral or distal tibial growth centers. In the femur the distal end provides approximately 70 per cent of the ultimate total length of that bone, and the proximal end of the tibia contributes about 60 per cent of the total longitudinal growth of that bone. Therefore, injuries and diseases affecting the growth centers about the knee result in much greater alteration in growth than do similar insults occurring elsewhere in the lower limb.

The portion of these physeal growth cartilages that is most sensitive to insult is the germinal layer, since irreparable damage to this layer of cartilage cells, either from trauma or infection, can lead to complete growth arrest. Different kinds and degrees of injury are tolerated differently. For example, a smooth metal device of considerable size can be passed through the center of a physeal plate and remain there indefinitely without significant or irreparable influence upon growth (Fig. 19-1). However, a similar sized threaded device may interrupt growth permanently, if it is left for several weeks or months. Furthermore, damage to the peripheral (perichondral and periosteal) areas of the growth plate are poorly tolerated, whereas small areas of the central portion may be traumatized without significant alteration in growth. The exception is a crushing injury to the physeal plate, which may totally destroy its growth potential, leading to early epiphyseal-metaphyseal closure. Significantly displaced epiphyseal fractures which affect the germinal and proliferating layers of the cartilage can also cause growth arrest, unless appropriately treated. This is because the physeal

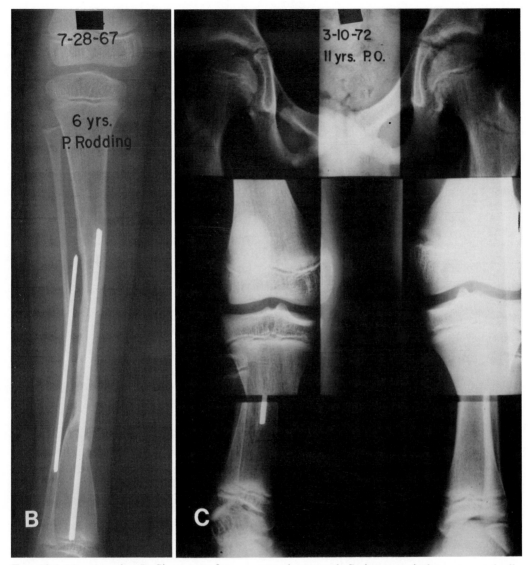

FIG. 19-1 *(Continued)*. *(B)* Six years after surgery, the smooth Steinmann pin has now gradually migrated into the tibia by virtue of continued growth of the distal and proximal physeal plates. *(C)* Eleven years postoperatively, the tibia remains solidly united and limb lengths are equal, indicating that there has been no interference with epiphyseal growth, despite the fact that a smooth rod passed through the physeal plate for several years.

plate becomes effectively bridged by the bone of either the metaphysis or the epiphysis. Limb length discrepancies can also be produced by any chronic process that stimulates excessive chondrogenesis in these growth centers. Any condition that produces hyperemia of the entire limb or of even a single bone can cause overgrowth to such a degree that a treatable limb length discrepancy results. The amount of additional skeletal growth expected at the time of injury or affliction also has great influence on the amount of discrepancy to be expected. It is, therefore, apparent that the cartilaginous growth centers play a vital role in the problem of limb length inequality, and the degree of discrepancy and the nature of the discrepancy (shortening or angulation) are a reflection not only of the type of injury or noxious influence, but also of the skeletal age at which such insult occurs.

FACTORS GOVERNING THE DECISION FOR EQUALIZATION

There are many factors that govern the need for equalization of a limb length discrepancy, especially when surgical equalization is being considered. As each case must be approached on an individual basis, it is essential that all the circumstances be evaluated, both singly and in conjunction with the other factors involved, when any method or combination of methods for correction of any inequality is being considered.

The factors include the following:

1. Cause of the discrepancy (etiology)
2. Degree of discrepancy
3. Skeletal age
4. Progression of the discrepancy
5. Anticipated adult height
6. Strength and balance of the musculature
7. Status of the foot and ankle
8. Localization or predominant site of the inequality (thigh or leg)
9. Sex of the patient
10. General or extenuating health factors
11. Needs and desires of the patient and the parents

CAUSE OF THE DISCREPANCY

There are five broad etiological categories which embrace the majority of instances of limb length discrepancy. These can be listed as follows:

Etiologies of Limb Length Discrepancy

Congenital and Developmental
  Terminal limb deficiencies
    Paraxial hemimelias
    Proximal femoral focal deficiencies
  Congenitally short femur
  Hemiatrophy or hemihypertrophy
  Posterior bow of tibia
  Ollier's disease
  Congenital dislocation of the hip
Paralytic
  Poliomyelitis

  Encepalopathy (cerebral palsy)
  Myelopathy
  Miscellaneous other causes of flaccid paralysis
Infections of Bone and Joint
  Causing growth retardation or arrest
    Osteomyelitis; acute
    Pyarthrosis
  Causing growth acceleration
    Osteomyelitis, chronic
Trauma of Bones and Joints
  Causing growth retardation or arrest
    Injuries to physeal plate
  Causing growth acceleration
    Fractures of metaphysis and diaphysis
  Resulting in shortening
    Malunion (excessive overriding) of fractures
Miscellaneous
  Tumors & tumorous conditions producing "overgrowth"
    Fibrous dysplasia
    Osteoid osteoma
    Hemangiomatosis
    Neurofibromatosis
  Tumor or tumorous conditions producing growth retardation
    Solitary enchondroma
    Solitary bone cyst
    Neurofibromatosis

The cause of the limb length discrepancy is extremely important when contemplating surgical corrections of that discrepancy. Each etiological type can accomplish shortening or lengthening in a different manner and to a different degree. There also exists a broad spectrum with respect to the type and significance of other limb abnormalities associated with each cause. These factors carry much of the weight in evaluating the indications for or against surgical equalization. Subsequently, and as will be discussed in more depth later in this chapter, the type of corrective measure utilized will be greatly contingent upon the cause of the shortening.

CONGENITAL AND DEVELOPMENTAL CAUSES

As noted above, *congenital and developmental* causes of limb length discrepancy include a wide variety of conditions. Nearly all terminal limb deficiencies, whether unilateral or bilateral, result in some discrepancy of limb length. Paraxial hemimelia of the fibula, either partial or complete, is the most com-

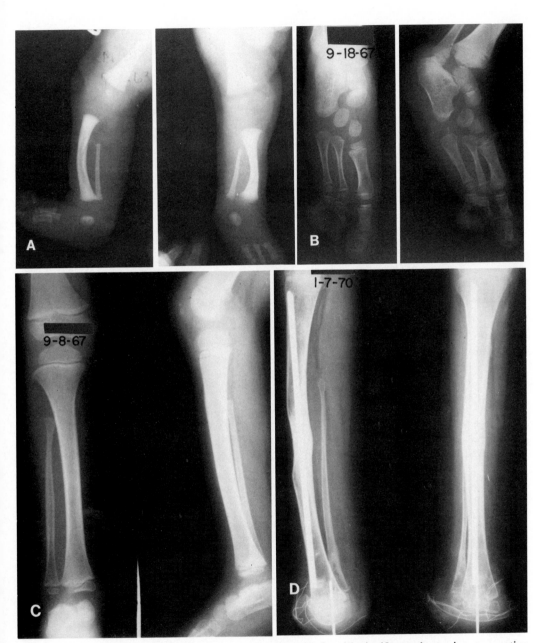

Fig. 19-2. (A) A patient with a partial hemimelia of the fibula with significant shortening, presenting shortly after birth. (B) Gross abnormality of the foot, with only three rays and tarsal coalition. (C) Preoperatively the tibia is foreshortened, with some 6 cm. of discrepancy in limb lengths. The foot, however, is still not plantigrade. (D) The success of tibial lengthening following bone grafting is evident; however, a disarticulation of the ankle was accomplished. Thus, in this case even though equalization was achieved, the foot was so deformed that the results of the surgery were negated. It would have been far better to disarticulate this foot in the beginning, rather than to subject her to the multiple lengthening procedures. The importance of the need for a plantigrade foot prior to lengthening is evident in this patient.

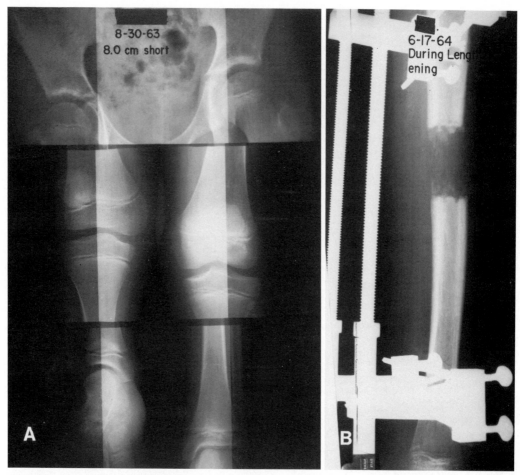

FIG. 19-3. A 10-year-old female with complete paraxial hemimelia of the fibula on the right side, having 8 cm. of discrepancy. She had a plantigrade foot, despite the shortening. *(A)* An orthoroentgenogram showing the site of her shortening. *(B)* The result of a 4.5-cm lengthening in the tibia. Satisfactory union ensued, but it eventually required osteotomy for valgus deformity. She also underwent a distal femoral epiphyseal arrest on the long side, but it was done too late to achieve complete equalization. *(Legend continued on facing page.)*

mon cause of excessive congenital shortening. Often the shortening is severe and the foot and ankle are deformed. Therefore, most often, ablation of the foot is required, and equalization of the length discrepancy is achieved by means of an orthosis or a prosthesis (Fig. 19-2). However, some select patients, wherein the shortening is not severe and the foot and ankle are in good condition, can be treated by equalization procedures that preserve the foot (Fig. 19-3).

Proximal femoral focal deficiency is less common, but far more dramatic in its manifestations. It is a very challenging and unique condition which, in unilateral cases, virtually always requires ablation of the foot. Limb length equalization is then achieved by use of a prosthesis (Fig. 19-4). Monographs have been written about this subject, emphasizing the many complicated problems which this abnormality poses and underscoring the need for individualized treatment.

Instances of the congenitally short femur are often accompanied by an anterolateral bow of the femur, which is usually located

FIG. 19-3 *(Continued). (C)* An orthoroentgenogram showing the discrepancy at skeletal maturity, with correction, by means of tibial lengthening and epiphyseal arrest, of approximately 9 cm. This illustrates that the simple presence of paraxial hemimelia of the fibula does not necessarily contraindicate tibial lengthening or other equalization procedures. The essential requirement is that there be a very good plantigrade foot.

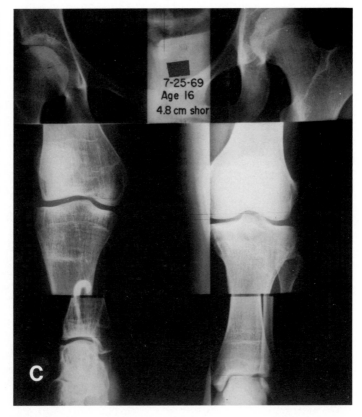

7-25-69
Age 16
4.8 cm short

at the subtrochanteric level or in the region of the proximal third of the femur. Such instances are also frequently accompanied by shortening of the tibia and fibula. Usually there is a normal foot and ankle, and the degree of shortening is quite variable. The solution must, therefore, be approached individually.

Discrepancies due to hemiatrophy or hemihypertrophy (Fig. 19-5) are uncommon, but they are significant in that they may be due to some other underlying cause. For example, in the case of hemiatrophy, associated factors may exist, such as neurofibromatosis, an obscure neurological disorder, or even a Wilms' tumor. In hemihypertrophy, localized neurofibromatosis or excessive proliferation of subcutaneous fat are frequently encountered.

Ollier's disease (enchondromatosis of bone) is very rare, but it almost always results in some degree of limb length discrepancy because of its variable, but predomin-

antly unilateral, manifestation (Fig. 19-6). Likewise, hemangiomata, lymphangiomatosis, and hemangiomatosis can produce limb length discrepancies by hyperemia and resultant overgrowth or, rarely, by progressive bone dissolution which produces shortening (Fig. 19-7).

Congenital dislocation of the hip causes an unusual type of shortening. It is unique in that its treatment largely is directed toward reducing the dislocation. Only when reduction is contraindicated or impossible, or when complications of treatment such as epiphyseal necrosis or physeal arrest become evident, do methods of correction other than reduction of the dislocation become serious considerations.

PARALYTIC CAUSES

These causes of limb length discrepancy include poliomyelitis, unilateral flaccid paralysis due to other causes, and hemiplegia

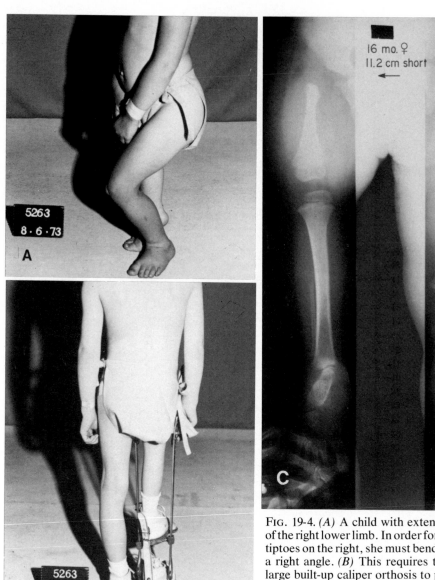

FIG. 19-4. *(A)* A child with extensive shortening of the right lower limb. In order for her to stand on tiptoes on the right, she must bend the left knee to a right angle. *(B)* This requires that she wear a large built-up caliper orthosis to permit more effective ambulation. *(C)* The discrepancy, as seen on scanogram. In such a case, ablation of the foot and use of a prosthesis are indicated.

FIG. 19-5. This orthoroentgenogram shows approximately 4-cm. difference in limb length due to simple hemihypertrophy or hemiatrophy. The musculature and the bones and joints are all normal, but they simply differ in size from one side to the other.

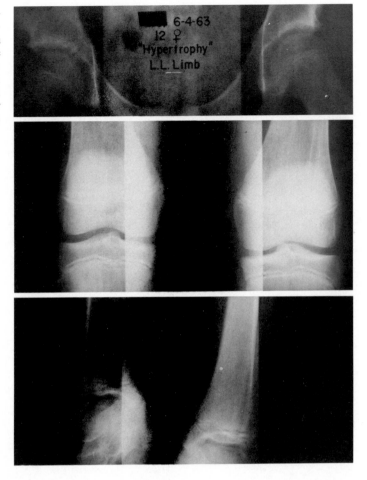

due to spastic paralysis. As noted earlier, poliomyelitis, though rare in the United States, will continue to offer occasionally the problem of shortening (Fig. 19-8). The cause of the shortening is two-fold: the first and most significant factor is the muscle atrophy, the accepted belief being that this results in reduced stimulation of normal skeletal growth. On the other hand, there are studies, such as those by Haas, which suggest that growth is not necessarily dependent upon muscle function. The second factor is a peculiar coldness of the limb, which in some instances seems to produce even further atrophy or lack of growth. The latter is a highly variable manifestation, due to some poorly understood disturbance in vasomotor control. This peculiar vascular manifestation seems to be the best explanation for the unpredictable degree of shortening seen in various patients with poliomyelitis who have similar degrees of muscle weakness or paralysis (see p. 844). Encephalopathy (cerebral palsy) or myelopathy with spastic paralysis, on the other hand, rarely produces a degree of discrepancy which requires an equalization procedure. In the past 17 years at the Intermountain Unit of the Shriners Hospital, only two surgical equalization procedures (both were epiphyseal arrests) have been performed upon children having a limb length discrepancy due to cerebral palsy. This indicates that a degree of discrepancy requiring surgical equalization is seldom encountered in cerebral palsy. The explanation for this is

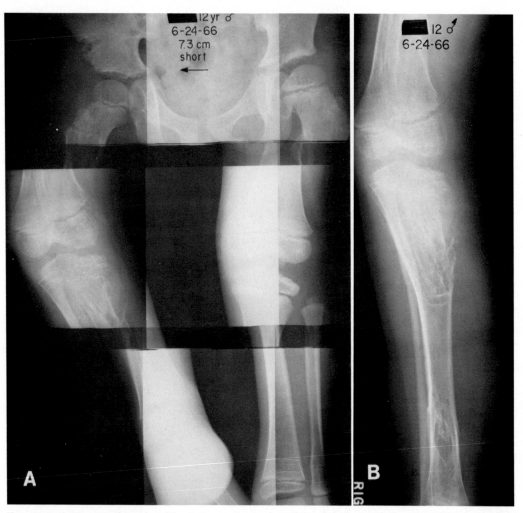

FIG. 19-6. A 12-year-old male with a 7.3-cm. shortening of the right lower limb, secondary to multiple enchondromatosis. *(A)* The orthoroentgenogram. *(B)* A more detailed view of the tibia, with its multiple cartilaginous lesions.

that, first, the paralysis is often rather symmetrical, and, second, there is usually an intact reflex motor arc with preserved functioning anterior horn cells innervating muscles that continue to function, even though at a spastic, somewhat reflex level. Thus, a degree of muscle atrophy comparable to that seen in poliomyelitis is much less likely to occur.

INFECTIOUS CAUSES

Pyogenic disease of the skeleton will very likely continue to occur, despite the fact that prudently prescribed and effective antibiotic therapy is available. Depending upon the location, degree and duration of a bone or joint infection, a limb can become either shortened or lengthened. Epiphyseal arrest due to bone infection may occur as the result of pyogenic disruption of the physeal plate (Fig. 19-9). Similarly, destruction of part or all of the epiphysis due to pyarthrosis is not rare, especially in the hips of infants and young children (Fig. 19-10). Destruction or premature closure of normal growth centers in this age group can produce impressive and challenging limb length discrepancies. On the other hand, stimulation of longitudinal limb growth can be produced by chronic osteomyelitis, wherein the long-standing hyperemia of chronic infection serves to stimulate epiphyseal growth (Fig. 19-11). Discrepancies resulting from overgrowth due to chronic infection, however, rarely are of significant magnitude to justify or require surgical equalization.

TRAUMATIC CAUSES

Trauma can produce three different types of discrepancies. First, overgrowth may occur due to stimulation of bone growth following fracture of the femur or tibia. This seems to be the result of the hyperemia invoked by the trauma and the resultant healing process. Overgrowth is commonly seen in children under the ages of 10 or 12 having fractures, even though a slight amount of overriding usually follows most fractures of the lower limb. Longitudinal overgrowth of bone following trauma, especially in fractures of the femur, has always been of interest and importance to orthopaedic surgeons. David[37] and Gatewood and Mullen[41] were

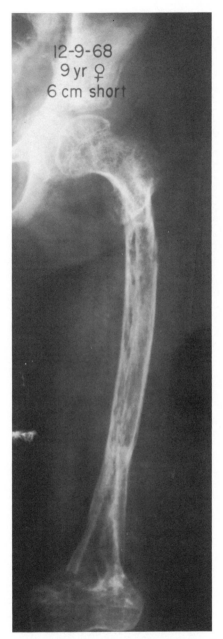

FIG. 19-7. Extensive hemangiomatosis of the femur may produce significant shortening.

among early observers. Cole,[31] Phemister,[74] and Barford and Christensen[9] maintained that overgrowth resulting from fracture was a natural compensatory phenomenon. Those holding that overgrowth was secondary to hyperemia were Aitken, Cia-

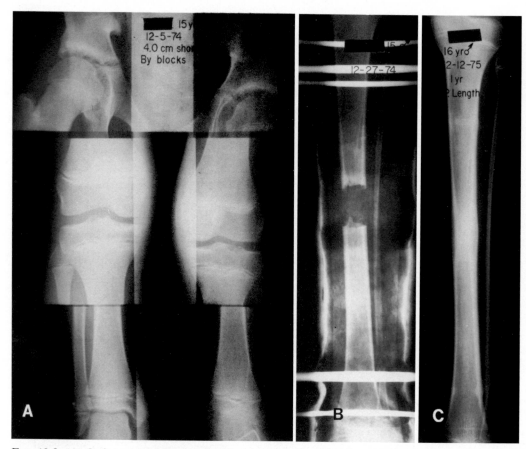

FIG. 19-8. *(A)* Orthoroentgenogram of a 15-year-old male with 4 cm. of shortening as the result of poliomyelitis acquired when he was a young child. A pantalar arthrodesis had been done because of the completely flail foot and ankle. *(B)* The results of a tibial lengthening. *(C)* One year following the tibial lengthening, the tibia is solidly united, and the patient has been bearing full weight for 6 months.

cotti and Blackett,[3] and Speed.[84] Compere and Adams[36] agreed, and also felt that the increased length was possibly the result of medullary blood supply interruption. Furthermore, on the basis of experimental studies on rabbits, they found that the period of overgrowth lasts only as long as the healing period. Bisgard's[14] animal experiments supported those of Compere and Adams. Trueta[93] was among those to note that the greater the extent of overriding of the fracture fragments, the greater the subsequent overgrowth. Recently, Staheli[85] showed in his clinical observations that greater stimulation of overgrowth occurs in fractures of the proximal one-third of the femur, with the

least amount of stimulation being found in the distal one-third.

Shortening, on the other hand, may be produced as the result of significant angulation or excessive overriding following fracture. Also, excessive growth retardation can occur as the result of irreversible damage to the physeal plate, producing premature epiphyseal-diaphyseal fusion.

It is very important to distinguish between different types of limb length discrepancy following infection or trauma, because treatment may vary significantly from one type to the other. For example, in cases of shortening due to fracture with overriding or malunion of the fragments, the degree of shortening will very likely remain static due to the fact that the epiphyses on the short side can be expected to grow at the normal and equal rate of the opposite member. Discrepancy in these situations can be corrected by epiphyseal arrest on the long side, accomplished during the time of skeletal development when continued growth of the short side corrects the discrepancy. Conversely, and correspondingly, when shortening is the result of epiphyseal arrest, due to trauma or bone infection, the shortening will not be static but, rather, will be progressive as long as the patient grows. Surgical arrest of the opposite companion physeal plate under these circumstances will *not* effect any correction, but rather only stops the inevitable progression of the discrepancy. Any correction must, therefore, be accompanied by arrest of additional growth centers or by some other means of equalization. The above circumstances underscore and emphasize the most important basic principle involved in correcting limb length discrepancy by growth arrest, namely, that any correction of the discrepancy is predicated upon continued normal longitudinal limb growth on the shortened side.

Shortening due to traumatic growth arrest is the result of irreversible damage to a growing physeal plate in the lower limb following fracture. The type of epiphyseal injury has a direct relationship to the possibility of epiphyseal-metaphyseal fusion (growth arrest). Salter and Harris [80] have developed an anatomical classification of these injuries, which enables the surgeon not only to define the nature of the injury, but also, more importantly, to have some idea of the prognosis following injury (Fig. 19-12). Five different anatomical types have been outlined, but, from a practical clinical standpoint, only two major clinical types are useful. Functionally and clinically, Types 1 through 3 can be grouped together, because if appropriate treatment is administered, growth arrest is very unlikely to occur. Conversely, Types 4 and 5 can be similarly grouped because growth arrest is very likely to develop, either symmetrically or asymmetrically (shortening or angulation), regardless of the treatment instituted.

In the majority of patients the anatomical

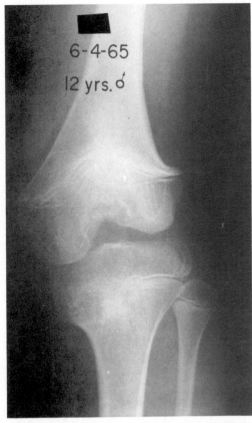

FIG. 19-9. Partial distal femoral and proximal tibial growth arrests have been produced by acute osteomyelitis in this 12-year-old male. He has had osteotomies of the distal femur and the proximal tibia to maintain alignment.

nature of the injuries can be readily ascertained by means of roentgenographic examination. In some situations, however, more than one anatomical type may occur in the same injury (Fig. 19-13). These episodes of multiple epiphyseal injuries require that several months be allowed to pass before a prognosis is made, in order to observe the functional behavior of the physeal plate. Unfortunately, Type 5 cannot often be detected by roentgenographic examination in the early posttraumatic period, and Type 4 may not respond favorably to conscientious efforts at closed or open reduction. It is also suggested by Speed[84] and others that traumatic epiphyseal displacement may

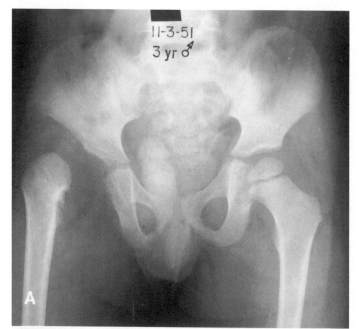

FIG. 19-10. (A) Results of pyogenic arthritis of the right hip with complete loss of the femoral head and complete hip dislocation. (B) The limb is 5 cm. short, and a hip fusion has been accomplished. (C) A distal femoral epiphyseal arrest was performed. At skeletal maturity, limb lengths were within 1 cm.

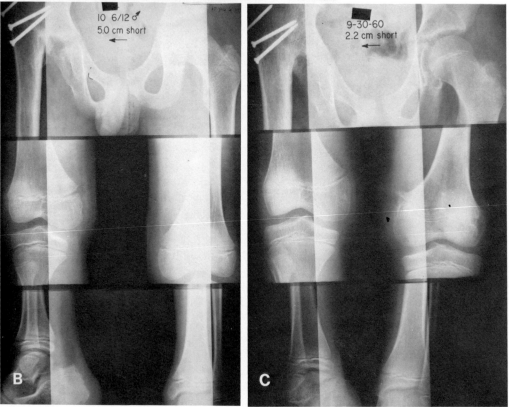

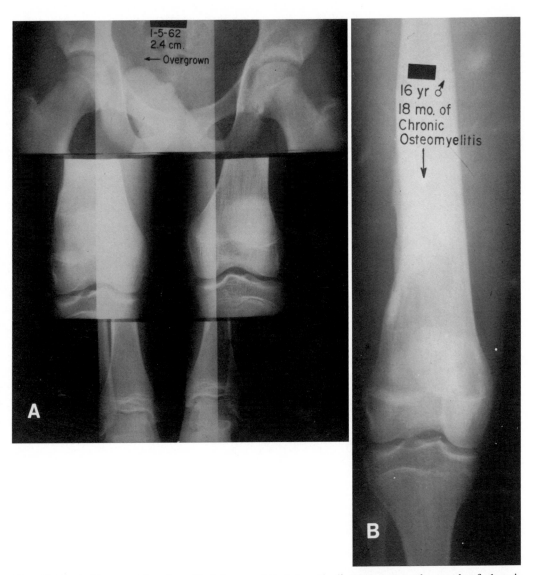

Fig. 19-11. A 13-year-old male with 2.4 cm. of limb length discrepancy as the result of chronic osteomyelitis of the right distal femur. *(A)* An orthoroentgenogram, showing that the discrepancy is located exclusively in the femur. *(B)* A better view of the chronic inflammatory process can be seen. Unfortunately, this young man was seen too late to achieve equalization by simple epiphyseal arrest.

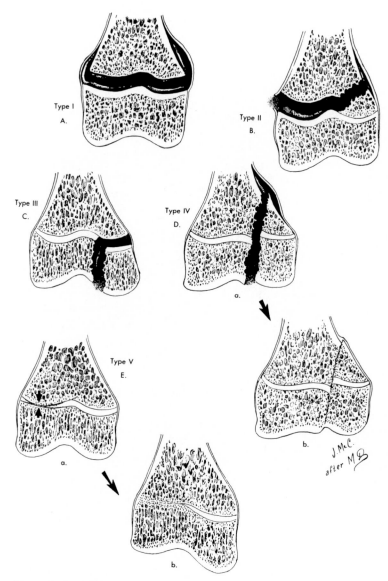

FIG. 19-12. Salter-Harris classification of epiphyseal injuries. (Redrawn after Salter, R. B., and Harris, W. R.: Injuries involving the epiphyseal plate. J. Bone Joint Surg., *45A:*587, 1963.)

incur overgrowth in some cases, just as it occurs in shaft fractures.

MISCELLANEOUS CAUSES

Miscellaneous causes of limb length discrepancy include a variety of unusual conditions which may stimulate or retard bone growth. Any tumor or tumorous condition which invokes a chronic increase in vascularity of the limb or a major bone can produce a limb length discrepancy requiring consideration of correction.

Examples of conditions which may stimulate bone growth include fibrous dysplasia (Fig. 19-14), osteoid osteoma (Fig. 19-15) and soft-tissue hemangiomatosis and neurofibromatosis. Conversely, conditions result-

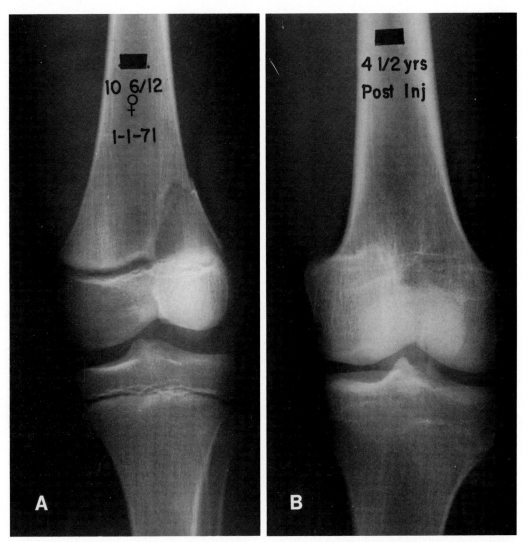

FIG. 19-13. A 15-year-old female who, 4¹/₂ years previously, sustained a complex epiphyseal fracture in the left distal femur. *(A)* The combination of a Type 2 and a Type 4 epiphyseal injury. Complete arrest of the epiphyseal plate occurred, resulting in a 4.2-cm. shortening at skeletal maturity. *(B)* The x-ray film of the distal femur at maturity. This case demonstrates how a combination of epiphyseal injuries can occur, and in such situations predictions with respect to future behavior of a growth plate must be guarded. It would have been better had the arrest been recognized early so that the opposite companion epiphysis could be arrested. At skeletal maturity a femoral shortening by resection had to be accomplished.

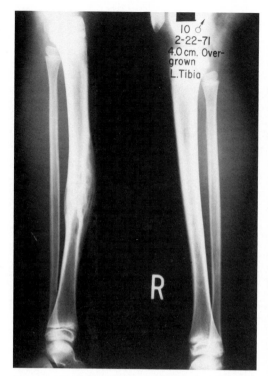

FIG. 19-14. A case of fibrous dysplasia of the tibia known to be present for 8 years. The resulting 4 cm. of overgrowth of the tibia is evident.

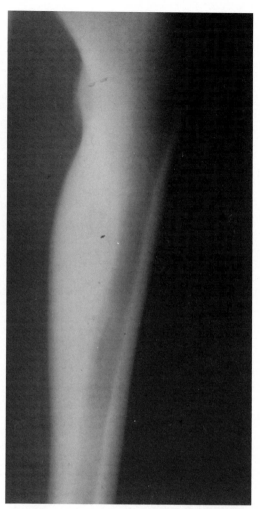

FIG. 19-15. Osteoid osteoma of the proximal femur, with symptoms of at least 2 years' duration. The chronic hyperemia produced a 2.5 cm. increased length of this involved left femur.

ing in retardation or shortening of the limb include solitary bone cyst, enchondroma, hemangiomatosis of bone (Fig. 19-7) and neurofibromatosis (Fig. 19-16). Most often, discrepancies produced by such lesions are not great, and because of their rarity they are not particularly important.

Thus, the importance of the etiology of any limb length discrepancy is evident, and it must be a major consideration when contemplating surgical correction. Whether the inequality is due to growth retardation, growth acceleration, growth arrest, fracture with overriding and malunion, or congenital dislocation of the hip, has a significant influence upon what form of equalization program might be required. As a specific example, highly divergent therapeutic considerations would be exercised when dealing with a limb length discrepancy due to poliomyelitis and an inequality resulting from a traumatic epiphyseal arrest.

THE DEGREE OF DISCREPANCY

This is a most significant factor in deciding the appropriate management of limb length discrepancy. Differences of less than 2.0 cm. (under 0.75 inches) are customarily accepted and can be treated by nonsurgical methods, such as a shoelift or no treatment at all. At the other end of the scale, any projected inequality exceeding 15 cms. (over 6.0 inches) is usually in excess of the amount that any combination of procedures can be effectively or predictably employed to

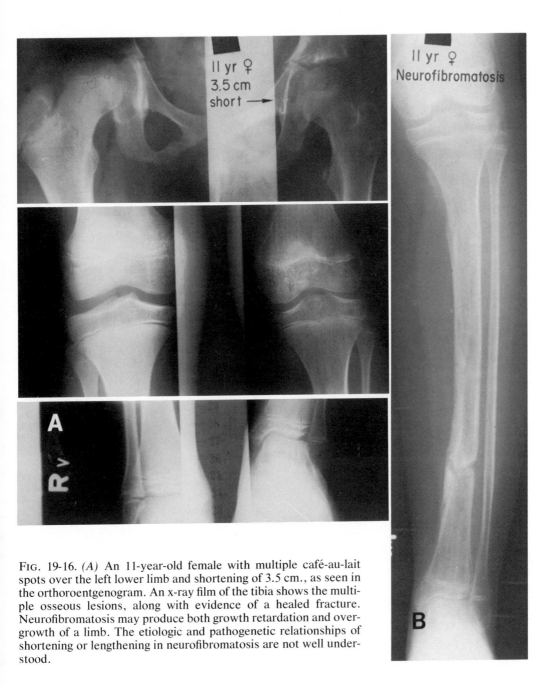

FIG. 19-16. (A) An 11-year-old female with multiple café-au-lait spots over the left lower limb and shortening of 3.5 cm., as seen in the orthoroentgenogram. An x-ray film of the tibia shows the multiple osseous lesions, along with evidence of a healed fracture. Neurofibromatosis may produce both growth retardation and overgrowth of a limb. The etiologic and pathogenetic relationships of shortening or lengthening in neurofibromatosis are not well understood.

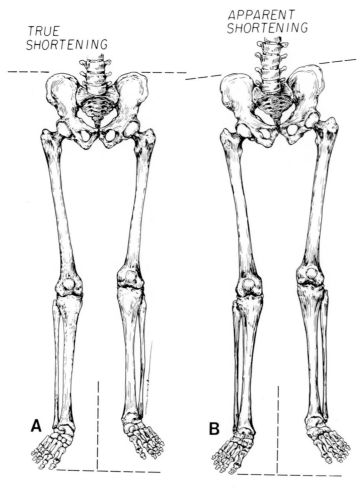

TRUE
SHORTENING

APPARENT
SHORTENING

A

B

Fig. 19-17. The difference between true shortening, *(A)*, and apparent shortening, *(B)*. In the case of true shortening, the limb from the hip joint to the ankle is truly short by actual measurement. In *(B)*, as a result of pelvic obliquity, adduction contracture of the apparent short side, or abduction contracture of the apparent long side, the side on which the pelvis is elevated appears shorter than its opposite member. The limb lengths, however, are actually the same.

equalize the discrepancy. The only exception is when surgical conversion (amputation or disarticulation) and application of a prosthesis are employed. For the most part therefore, only a limb length inequality between 2.0 and 15 cms. warrants serious consideration toward surgical correction. These are not rigid figures, and they represent only practical guidelines which may be modified by the many other factors involved in the deliberation.

It is critically important to distinguish between a relative (apparent) and an absolute (true) limb length discrepancy. An absolute limb length discrepancy is defined between the iliac crest and the foot. Relative (apparent) shortening or lengthening can be produced by an abduction contracture of the apparently long limb or an adduction contracture of the apparently short limb (Fig. 19-17). This situation is commonly seen in neurologic disorders, such as poliomyelitis and cerebral palsy. The apparent shortening or lengthening is basically the result of pelvic obliquity, which can sometimes cause a significant functional lower limb length discrepancy. In such instances, all efforts at treatment should be directed towards correcting the pelvic obliquity, and its cause, by whatever means is necessary. Correspondingly, implementation of limb shortening or lengthening procedures in relative disorders of limb length is nearly always contraindicated, because the real problem—the pelvic obliquity—will remain uncorrected.

After identifying the nature of the discre-

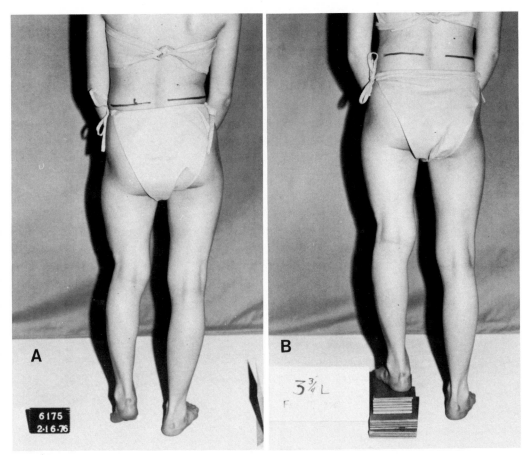

FIG. 19-18. *(A)* A child with nearly 4 inches of shortening, due to traumatic distal femoral and proximal tibial epiphyseal arrests. *(B)* The amount of lift needed under the heel to achieve a level pelvis. The exact height of the blocks necessary to achieve equalization is included in the photograph.

pancy, the next step is to document accurately the amount of discrepancy by means of photographs and roentgenograms. To ascertain the amount of discrepancy, three techniques should be employed, namely: (1) leveling the pelvis with an appropriate elevation under the shoe; (2) measuring the limbs by tape measure and (3) measuring the limbs by roentgenographic examination (scanogram or orthoroentgenogram).

The first and most practical procedure is that of placing elevations of variable thickness under the short limb in order to level the pelvis when the patient is standing in bare feet. The amount of elevation required to level the pelvis is easily determined. This is the most reliable method, because

it accomplishes the ultimate goal of equalization—a level pelvis. It readily accounts for any variation in bony landmarks and differences in pelvic size and shape, as well as foot size and shape. A photograph should be made of the patient, showing that the pelvis is level and recording the precise amount of lift required to achieve this (Fig. 19-18). The best roentgenographic technique for determining limb length discrepancy is the orthoroentgenogram. This procedure utilizes three separate roentgen exposures, with the beam sequentially centered directly over the hip, the knee and the ankle joints (Fig. 19-19). The distances between the major joint surfaces are calibrated by means of a centimeter rule placed at the

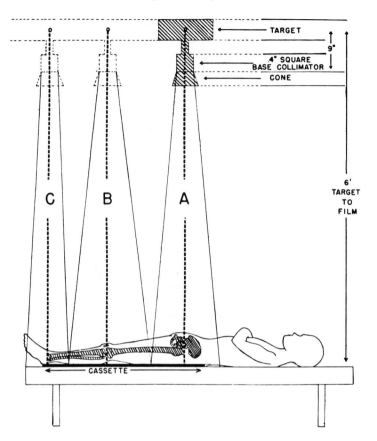

Fig. 19-19. Method of making an orthoroentgenogram. (From Tachdjian, M. O.: Pediatric Orthopedics. Philadelphia, W. B. Saunders, 1972.)

same level as that upon which the patient lies. The resultant film can be used to establish with reasonable accuracy not only the total amount of discrepancy between the hip and ankle joints, but also the location of the discrepancy, that is, whether it is in the femur, the tibia, or both. There are two deficiencies of orthoroentgenography which offer potential errors in measurement. First, the technique ordinarily does not take into account any variation in size of the pelvis or the foot, and these must be calculated into the final determination of discrepancy. Second, if the patient's position is altered between any of the roentgen exposures, the examination is invalidated. Thus, the need to double check the orthoroentgenogram by other methods of measurement is evident.

The tape measure should be employed to provide corroborative measurements of various bony prominences, measured from the pelvis to the lower limb. Conventionally, the anterosuperior iliac spine is utilized on the pelvis, and the medial malleolus is the standard prominence used in the lower limb. Measurements from the umbilicus to the malleolus and to the heel are frequently used, because this latter measurement takes into account any variation in size of the foot and pelvis and any abnormalities or variations in the bony prominences. This technique also assists in determining whether the discrepancy is true or apparent. Care must be exercised to ascertain that the pelvis is level. Even though it is the determination most subject to error, and is the one which lends itself least well to documentation, one of the most important values of the tape measurement is that of confirming and double checking the values derived from the other examinations. Ideally, all three should validate and complement each other. In this way any errors can be detected and accurate determination of the discrepancy is virtually assured. It is essential to remember that any flexion contracture of the hip or knee, and any equinus contracture of the ankle may seriously influence any of these determinations. It is essential that a careful and comprehensive effort be made to measure and record the exact amount of discrepancy. Without this measurement, a responsible approach to the problem of limb length inequality is impossible.

SKELETAL AGE

Once the degree of discrepancy has been established accurately, it is necessary to determine the skeletal age of the patient, especially if correction by growth arrest is being contemplated.

The skeletal age of the patient is important for several reasons. First, if skeletal maturity has been reached (or nearly so), correction by growth arrest is impossible. Furthermore, if skeletal age is grossly different from chronological age, or if the patient is skeletally very immature, correction of limb length discrepancy by growth arrest may be unpredictable or impractical. In patients having limb length inequality who are approaching skeletal maturity, in order to achieve equalization safely and effectively, one must resort to either shortening of the long limb by bone resection or employing some selective lengthening process. In the instance where unpredictability of correction by epiphyseal arrest exists, or when the patient is very young, equalization can be accomplished by mechanical lengthening, application of a shoe lift, amputation and prosthesis or, in rare cases, temporary growth arrest (stapling), depending upon the degree of discrepancy and the cause of the discrepancy. In some cases a combination of lengthening and shortening may be employed. It is obvious that there are a challenging number of variables that must be dealt with in assessing the factor of skeletal age.

There are several ways in which skeletal age can be assessed, none of which is critically accurate. In all of the methods, there is a relatively wide standard of deviation (12 months). The most popular method of determining skeletal age is the use of a single

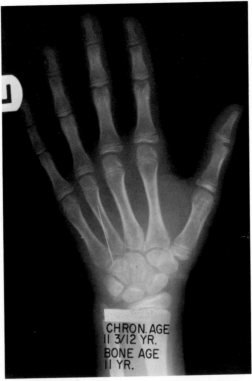

FIG. 19-20. An x-ray film of the wrist and hand in a young female whose chronological age is 11³/₁₂ years and whose skeletal age is 11 years. This determination is essential when contemplating any form of equalization by growth arrest.

anteroposterior roentgenogram of the wrist and hand (Fig. 19-20). By comparing the patient's wrist and hand film with a known standard, a reasonably accurate determination of skeletal age can be achieved. The Greulich and Pyle Atlas[46] is the most highly accepted documentation of skeletal age. Standards of skeletal age for both males and females are based upon the stage of development of various primary and secondary ossification centers in the wrist and hand. There are other methods of determining skeletal age, an example being interpretation of the state of epiphyseal development of the long bones of the lower limbs. None of these methods, however, has been as well accepted or universally utilized as evaluating the roentgenogram of the wrist and hand.

By appropriately utilizing this data, a

sufficiently accurate assessment of skeletal age, can be made and from a clinical standpoint, a soundly based therapeutic program can be devised. When wide and erratic variations are encountered between chronologic and skeletal age, greater care must be exercised in formulating a therapeutic program, especially when permanent epiphyseal arrest is being contemplated as a method of equalization. This is because epiphyseal arrest relies upon critical calculations of skeletal age and relatively predictable growth patterns in order to obtain appropriate correction and to avoid over- or undercorrection.

Studies such as those by Green and Anderson[43] and Bayley[11] agree that skeletal age is a far more accurate measurement than chronological age in evaluating and predicting the status of a discrepancy. In addition, they cite a very close correlation between skeletal age and sexual maturity.

PROGRESSION OF THE DISCREPANCY

Once the discrepancy has been documented and the patient's skeletal age has been identified as well as it can be, this knowledge can be effectively applied in reaching some understanding as to the progressional qualities of the discrepancy.

Progression of the discrepancy is important for several reasons. On one hand, if a difference in limb length is static or relatively so, the best form of equalization treatment can be planned more accurately and more specifically. On the other hand, if the discrepancy is progressive, it is extremely important that it be accurately documented and its progression plotted. By this means it can be ascertained whether the shortening is along a linear, rather predictable course or whether it is following a more erratic and unpredictable course. It should be recognized that on rare occasions, minor limb length discrepancies may stabilize or largely correct themselves spontaneously, and in such rare situations it is probable that no treatment will be needed.

Throughout the literature, many methods of plotting the factors surrounding a limb length discrepancy have been described. They represent efforts to correlate the rela-

tive rates of growth of the long and short limb, the sex variables, the degree of skeletal maturity, the chronological age, and the degree of limb length discrepancy. From this data one attempts to determine what types of equalization procedures would best suit the individual case and when the procedures should be performed. At present one of the most widely used growth prediction methods is that which was published (as revised from an earlier study) by Green and Anderson.[45] The "growth remaining" method, as it is called, employs a chart depicting the amount of additional growth to be expected from a normal proximal tibia and distal femur in different sexes and at different skeletal ages (Fig. 19-21).

In addition, the percentage of growth inhibition of the shorter limb is determined over a given time interval (suggested as at least 3 months) by subtracting the amount of growth in the short limb from the amount of growth in the normal limb, dividing the remainder by the amount of growth in the normal limb, and then multiplying by 100:

$$\frac{\text{growth normal} - \text{growth involved} \times 100}{\text{growth normal}}$$

This ratio, used in conjunction with the growth remaining chart, is evaluated and the patient's growth curves are manipulated in an effort to decide upon a course of action and the optimal time to pursue that course.

The second method of evaluating a limb length inequality has been very recently developed by Moseley.[69] It is referred to as the "straight line" graph for limb length discrepancies. Although the author has not yet had the opportunity to employ it, the method appears to have significant advantages over other methods. The parameters for its use are essentially the same as those for the "growth remaining" method. Skeletal age is determined by the Gruelich and Pyle method,[46] as the corresponding limb lengths (of both short and long limbs) are recorded. It is recommended that several determinations be made, as in the Anderson-Green method. The advantages of the "straight line" method are the following: no mathematical calculations are necessary; the growth rates of the short and long sides can be easily compared at a glance; the pa-

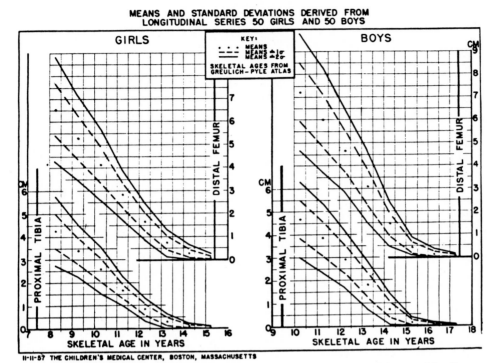

FIG. 19-21. The Green-Anderson growth-remaining chart. (From Anderson, M., Green, W. T., and Messner, M. B.: Growth and predictions of growth in the lower extremities. J. Bone Joint Surg., *45A:*10, 1963.)

tient's height, relative to his or her skeletal age group, is quickly determined, as are lengths of the limbs at maturity. One can also see graphically exactly when and where the best equalization procedure should be accomplished. In addition to the simplicity of the method, it appears that it is significantly more accurate than the alternative methods. The reader is urged to consult the Moseley article for details.[69]

ANTICIPATED ADULT HEIGHT

Anticipated adult height is one of the most elusive factors to determine accurately. This also requires a periodic skeletal age determination, provided that the patient's growth is plotted against normal height and growth patterns, and this information is compared to genetic data. Even when parental stature is known, ultimate stature is difficult to predict with a high degree of confidence. All determinations must be considered estimates,

as evidenced by earlier studies. For example, a study of Bayley[11] in 1946 noted that skeletal age is much more highly correlated with relative size than is chronological age. She presented a series of tables for use in approximating expected adult heights from skeletal age and relative heights. Some general relationships with respect to relative maturity and adult height were outlined. These are: (1) early maturing girls are usually large when young, their growth slows down to about an average rate at 13 years, and they complete growth rapidly, becoming smaller adults; (2) late-maturing girls are more often small when young, catching up to the average at about age 13, and becoming tall adults; (3) early maturing boys do not exhibit the abrupt curtailment of growth as in girls (this is attributed to the action of sex hormones), but the rate of growth slows down more gradually. They seem to have an equal likelihood of becoming tall, medium, or short; however, they tend to be of a larger, broader, or heavier build at all ages than do late-maturing boys; and (4) late-maturing boys continue to grow, some even into their early twenties, and more often than not they become tall adults. They are usually slender and long-legged, their greater adult height being due primarily to continued growth of the lower limbs.

In any event, the importance of this factor is related not only to its consideration in accurate plotting of the progression of an inequality, but also to the assumption that a patient of anticipated significantly short stature will more likely desire some form of lengthening rather than shortening procedure. Conversely, a patient with predictable ultimate stature of normal or taller-than-average proportions will be more amenable to, and probably more appropriately treated by, some form of shortening procedure, if the discrepancy does not exceed 4 or 5 cms.

STRENGTH AND BALANCE OF THE MUSCULATURE

The strength and balance of the musculature in the shortened limb is important for two reasons. First, it is a questionable practice to lengthen a short limb where an above-knee brace is already required for independent ambulation. Second, to elongate a very weak, shortened limb may possibly create a situation where an above-knee brace may be required for independent ambulation, whereas prior to lengthening a brace was not necessary. This unfortunate circumstance may result from one of two mechanisms: (1) weakening existing musculature by elongation, or (2) producing a longer lever arm with a resultant mechanical disadvantage. Alternatively, there is some valid concern that lengthening of a limb having completely normal musculature may result in some degree of paresis of muscles, due to neuropraxia (temporary), muscle stretch (probably temporary), or to ischemic necrosis (permanent). Finally, by virtue of a combination of the above circumstances, any previously existing imbalance of muscle strength may be accentuated by lengthening. Thus, an accurate knowledge of the strength and balance of the musculature of the limb must be ascertained prior to considering any form of equalization procedure

which requires elongation of the shorter limb.

STATUS OF THE FOOT AND ANKLE

The status of the foot and ankle becomes of major importance when discrepancies exist which may require tibial lengthening for equalization. Foot and ankle deformities existing prior to lengthening almost invariably are accentuated by the elongation process, and any uncorrected preexisting ankle equinus almost always is made worse by lengthening. Therefore, in contemplating a lengthening procedure in the tibia, the patient should have a plantigrade foot and a stable ankle, and there must be no fixed or uncorrectable ankle equinus.

Conversely, when the shorter side has a foot that is neither plantigrade nor capable of being made plantigrade, or when there is an unstable ankle, tibial lengthening is contraindicated. Therefore, when discrepancies exist which are correctable only by a combination of epiphyseal arrest and some form of lengthening, it is essential that the status of the foot and ankle be carefully appraised.

LOCALIZATION OF PREDOMINANT SITE OF THE INEQUALITY (THIGH OR LEG)

The principal site of the shortening (or lengthening) is important for the simple reason that it is desirable to keep the segments of the lower limb as equal as possible. Thus, any discrepancy in the thigh or leg portion would be most appropriately corrected by equalizing the corresponding segment of the opposite member. This is not always possible, nor necessarily desirable, but it is a factor that must be taken into account.

SEX OF THE PATIENT

The sex of the patient is significantly less important than skeletal age when considering equalization. However, in some instances it can be a very significant factor. Generally speaking, a girl will accept a shorter ultimate anticipated stature than a boy. Correspondingly, a boy would likely prefer lengthening to shortening, when confronted with the alternative of being significantly shorter than his peers. This factor is subtle, but one which can not be ignored and must be weighed carefully in all instances of inequality.

GENERAL OR EXTENUATING HEALTH FACTORS

Evaluation of general or extenuating health factors of each patient, with respect to the indications and the techniques for correcting limb length inequality, is frequently not given appropriate attention. However, if this issue is given proper consideration from the first evaluation, a significant number of physical and psychological complications can be prevented, or at least anticipated. The ultimate goal in the treatment of unequal limb lengths is to give the patient as great a degree of normality of function as is possible. When the welfare of the patient as a whole is not taken into account, complications worse than the limb length discrepancy may be encountered.

PHYSIOLOGIC FACTORS

The organic problems of the patient being considered for limb length equalization are usually easier to evaluate than are those stemming from psychological problems, which may be covert. In an effort to uncover and define such problems, it is, of course, essential that a complete history be taken and a comprehensive physical examination be given. It should be ascertained that the patient is in the best possible physical and psychological condition prior to any attempt at major methods of equalization. This is especially true in situations which involve extensive surgery or prolonged hospitalization. Certain physical and medical factors may even be considered as possible contraindications to the use of a particular procedure. Some of the more obvious examples are hypertension, heart disease, any previous osteomyelitis of the limb, angular or flexion deformities, muscle weakness in borderline cases, extensive scarring of soft tissues, and neurologic or vascular abnormalities. These and other disturbances must be evaluated whenever considering any major equalization procedure. Furthermore, if it is elected to undertake correction, all of these factors must be monitored carefully throughout the treatment program.

PSYCHOLOGICAL FACTORS

Whenever contemplating a major equalization procedure, the psychological condition of the patient is a subject of considerable importance. Even to a patient who is psychologically healthy, the ordeal of long-term treatment and a convalescence which may involve prolonged immobilization can be an emotionally draining experience. When either the patient or the parents suffer from psychological problems, as may often be the case in children having a deformity, major surgery and prolonged convalescence may be less well tolerated. Little satisfaction can be gained by improving the patient's physical condition while his emotional condition deteriorates. A patient who is very frightened or poorly prepared, or one who is undergoing great psychological stress, very often experiences more pain during treatment, and may often exhibit many psychosomatic manifestations, such as depression, irritability, anorexia and weight loss. On the other hand, patients filled with abnormally strong feelings of inadequacy and insecurity that they attribute to the deformity often view surgery as the whole answer to their problems, and they may be overzealous, almost desperate, for treatment. Any complications encountered during treatment of this type of patient could be disastrous. Also, they are more likely to find fault with the operative procedure or result. This type of problem might be manifest in a patient with a minor discrepancy, but one who is highly conscious of the discrepancy, and who is convinced that it is conspicuous to others. Therefore, the patient may insist that treatment be effected for its correction. Naturally, medical care should not be withheld from these patients, but the many factors involved must be given serious consideration. In an instance where the patient is not strong enough emotionally to endure an extended ordeal, perhaps the lengthening procedure should not be employed, even at the expense of losing some height by means of the alternate method of limb shortening.

Furthermore, it may be desirable that in some cases the patient, as well as the parents, undergo professional counseling, initially and throughout the convalescent period.

In any problem as complex as the treatment of limb length inequality, early and careful attention to all of the general and extenuating health factors of the patient can very possibly lessen or prevent many potential problems, not only for the patient but also for the surgeon.

NEEDS AND DESIRES OF THE PATIENT AND PARENTS

The final and very important factor that must be evaluated in arriving at a satisfactory approach to treatment of limb length discrepancy is the issue of the *personal needs and desires* of the patient and parents. Most often the patient is not mature or knowledgeable enough to weigh all facets of the problem to the extent that an informed opinion can be expressed. However, this does not mean that a full explanation of all the ramifications of the problem and its treatment should not be given. The parents must be informed as to all of the advantages, disadvantages and potential complications of all appropriate and feasible techniques of equalization. Once the many facts and subtleties of each procedure have been thoroughly discussed, often the decision becomes apparent. It is not uncommon to have several evaluation and discussion periods before a satisfactory conclusion is reached by the three parties concerned (patient, parents, and physician). Therefore, in formulating a therapeutic program, the needs and desires of the patient and parents must be given strong consideration, provided that they have been fully informed and understand the advantages and disadvantages of the treatment modalities.

The treatment of limb length inequality has traditionally involved a multiplicity of approaches which are enormously dissimilar and, in many instances, are controversial in principle, technique and result. It is essential that the surgeon be as well informed and as objective as possible, in order that all methods for equalization may be evaluated according to their relative merit. Only in this way can the surgeon choose the method most appropriate for the patient, while also considering the other factors surrounding the discrepancy and the decision to correct it.

METHODS OF EQUALIZATION OF LIMB LENGTHS

Equalization of limb lengths can be achieved by several techniques, both nonsurgical or surgical. Nonsurgical methods include shoe lifts and a variety of braces and prosthetic devices. Surgical modalities can be grouped into four broad categories, namely, those which (1) convert a limb with a terminal deficiency, by ablation of a portion of the limb, to a limb that will facilitate use of an artificial limb; (2) shorten the long side; (3) lengthen the short side; (4) utilize a combination of lengthening and shortening. As mentioned earlier, any solution to a problem of limb length inequality requires a sound knowledge of all of these technical procedures, in order to arrive at the best possible therapeutic program.

NONSURGICAL METHODS

A shoe lift is a simple method of equalizing limb lengths, but children often refuse to wear it or are unhappy if forced to do so. Furthermore, the indications for a shoe lift prescription are difficult to define accurately. Large discrepancies, those in excess of 5 or 10 cms., require cumbersome and unattractive shoe alterations in order to equalize a limb length discrepancy, but such lifts are often accepted because, by their use, ambulation is made easier. On the other hand, smaller lifts of 2.0 cm. or less usually are refused. A shoe elevation of 2 cm. or less exerts its effect only during the act of walking or standing with the knees extended. Once the knee on the long side is flexed, the effect of the lift is lost. Correspondingly, when the patient sits or lies down, a shoe lift obviously exerts no effect. The ultimate need for the lift must then be based either upon the effect of the shortening upon gait or upon any symptoms which might possibly result from a discrepancy. These may include low back discomfort and lumbosacral and lower lumbar scoliosis. Lowback pain during childhood is rarely caused only by a limb length discrepancy. Whether limb discrepancies, by themselves, cause significant structural scoliosis is controversial. The duration and amount of limb length discrepancy necessary to produce a structural scoliotic curve of significance is not accurately known, but it is reasonable to assume that the greater the discrepancy and the earlier it occurs during the period of a child's growth, the more likely it is that a structural curve may result. Still, it is not known whether such a curve is clinically significant. Therefore, whether to equalize limb lengths by shoe lifts in order to forestall the onset of the development of scoliosis is a moot issue, and specific guidelines are impossible to contrive. It largely becomes a matter of philosophy. I am not convinced that the presence of a limb length discrepancy necessarily means that a shoe lift should be prescribed. Furthermore, it is extremely difficult to establish how much of a lift to prescribe, although some elaborate and detailed tables have been devised as guidelines for shoe lifts.[38] In some cases complete equalization is undesirable, such as in cases of muscle weakness about the hips, knees or ankles, because equalization may make the limb so long that foot clearance is made difficult. Thus, it becomes difficult to outline any specific solution to such a highly individualized problem. On the other hand, if ambulation is prevented or compromised because of shortening, an elevation of some sort is undoubtedly required and indicated. Also, if the patient has significant symptoms of limb length inequality, he needs or wants the lift, and his symptoms are relieved by the lift, then this also represents a positive indication. These are obviously situations which may vary greatly from one patient to the next.

SURGICAL METHODS

Surgical Conversions to an Artificial Limb

Very large shoe lifts, orthoses, and caliper extensions may provide a practical aid to ambulation in cases of extreme limb length discrepancy, deformity, or terminal deficiency. However, a child or parent rarely desires permanent use of an orthosis such as that shown in Figure 19-4. Almost always, a more definitive equalization procedure is desired. Cosmetically, as well as functionally, the most satisfactory solution is frequently ablation of the foot or a portion of the limb in order to facilitate the use of an artificial limb. From a practical point of view the earlier this decision can be confidently reached, the sooner one can enable the patient to accept the conversion to a prosthesis. As emphasized by Aitken[3] conversion to a prosthesis is indicated and most appropriately accomplished when the natural history of the deformity is sufficiently well known that the surgeon is confident of the need for ablation and is convinced that other methods of equalization of limb lengths are either impossible or impractical.

Shortening of the Long Side

Shortening of a limb can be accomplished in one of three ways: (1) the physeal growth centers of the distal femur or the proximal tibia and fibula can be arrested prematurely by epiphyseodesis; (2) the same centers can be arrested temporarily or premanently by epiphyseal stapling; or (3) either the femur or the tibia (or both) can be shortened by resection of bone. As with all surgical procedures, each has its advantages and disadvantages, and each has its prerequisites, indications and contraindications.

Epiphysiodesis

The primary goal of epiphysiodesis is to achieve surgical epiphyseal growth arrest in the distal femur or the proximal tibia and fibula, or both. If physeal closure is successfully accomplished, and if the short limb continues to grow, gradual correction of the inequality takes place according to the amount of growth remaining in the short limb.

History. Early studies, such as those by Gatewood and Mullen[41] showed that the cartilaginous epiphyseal lines were responsible for nearly all the longitudinal growth in bones of the lower limbs, and that their fusion, even if premature, is sufficient to stop any subsequent growth, except for that small portion contributed by the articular cartilages. Prompted by such studies,

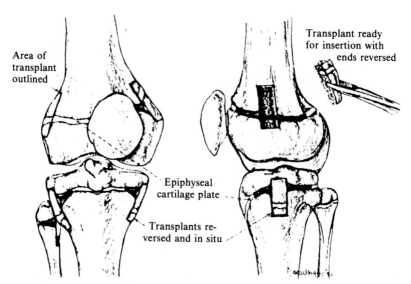

Area of transplant outlined

Transplant ready for insertion with ends reversed

Epiphyseal cartilage plate

Transplants reversed and in situ

Fig. 19-22. Epiphyseal arrest by epiphysiodesis, according to Phemister. (Courtesy C. Howard Hatcher, M.D. From Phemister, D. B.: Operative arrestment of longitudinal growth in bones in the treatment of deformities. J. Bone Joint Surg., *15:*1, 1933.)

Phemister[73] developed a simple technique for epiphyseal-diaphyseal fusion. In his procedure, fusion is accomplished by excising a block of the cortex on both sides of the physeal plate and reinserting it with the ends reversed (Fig. 19-22). Except for minor modifications, such as those suggested by Green and Anderson[43] and Eyre-Brook, who recommend removal of a block of bone containing much more than just the cortex (which thus accomplishes a wider, longer and thicker fusion), the Phemister technique has survived with very little alteration. Other variations from the Phemister technique include the White modification (Fig. 19-23)[99] and the modifications of the White and Stubbins technique (Fig. 19-24),[100] as cited by Blount,[17] both of which strive to achieve a greater degree of operative simplicity.

Other early literature dealt mainly with various aspects of epiphyseodesis. Green and Anderson[43] stress the importance of accurate assessment of skeletal maturity and expected growth, with respect to the time at which the procedure is accomplished. Straub, Thompson and Wilson,[88] who careful documented their cases, signified that "a

good result" could be claimed if final length differed by less than 3/4 inch, if there was 75 per cent or better correction of the total discrepancy. They found that 10 per cent of their cases developed angular deformities, ultimately requiring surgical correction. This closely paralleled other early results, such as those by Regan and Chatterton,[78] who found that 11 per cent of their cases developed significant deformities. Since that time more exact operative technique and improved, more knowledgeable planning of the cases have greatly decreased the incidence of deformities resulting from this procedure. Thus, Phemister's simple yet ingenious method of equalizing limb lengths by permanently arresting growth of the appropriate physeal center on the long side in growing patients persists as one of the most effective means of equalizing modest discrepancies in limb lengths.

Indications. Generally speaking, equalization of lower limb length inequality by permanent epiphysiodesis is the most commonly accepted method of equalizing moderate limb length inequalities in North America. This procedure is indicated when the limb length discrepancy is not great, and

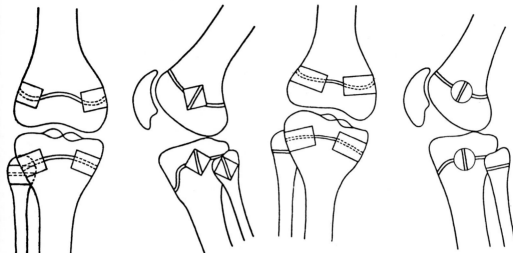

FIG. 19-23. The White modification of the Phemister epiphysiodesis. (From White, J. W., and Stubbins, S. G., Jr.: Growth arrest for equalizing leg lengths. J.A.M.A., *126:*1146. Copyright 1944, American Medical Association.)

FIG. 19-24. A modification of White's technique of epiphysiodesis. (From Blount, W. P.: Trauma and growing bones. Septième Congrès de la Société Internationale de Chirurgie Orthopédique et de Traumatologie. Barcelona, 1957.)

when there is sufficient anticipated growth of the opposite long limb, so that correction of the inequality can be reasonably expected. If expected growth on the long side is insufficient to produce adequate correction, this procedure is obviously not indicated.

Prerequisites. To qualify for this operation, the patient should have a discrepancy not exceeding 5 cms. However, in patients whose anticipated ultimate stature may be greater than normal, limb length inequalities in excess of 5 cms. may still be appropriately treated by epiphysiodesis. On the other hand, when the expected adult height is less than normal, or when there is significant discrepancy between chronological age and skeletal age, correction by epiphysiodesis may be inappropriate or unacceptable. Thus, even though certain broad and general guidelines can be recognized, latitude of interpretation must be exercised when considering equalization by epiphyseal arrest. It must be remembered also that epiphysiodesis is permanent and irreversible, and its purpose is to produce a calculated, premature physeal plate closure. It is necessary that the growth potential of the short

side (see p. 829), the skeletal age of the patient (see p. 827), and the anticipated adult height (see p. 829) be predicted with a high degree of certainty to achieve a good result.

Technique. As noted earlier, arresting growth of a major physis requires that a symmetrical bony bridge be created between the epiphysis and the metaphysis. It must be strong enough to produce a permanent and ultimately complete bony fusion. This is not difficult to accomplish, provided certain basic orthopaedic surgical principles are followed. The medial and lateral aspects of the distal femur or proximal tibia and fibula (or all three, if indicated) are exposed through a 2-inch vertical, transverse or oblique incision placed over the center of the epiphyseal plate. The physis is identified by passing a Keith needle through the overlying periosteum and perichondrium into the plate. A flap of periosteum and perichondrium is elevated, exposing at least 1 square inch of the femur, including equal portions of the metaphysis and epiphysis on either side of the epiphyseal plate. A generous-sized square plug of bone (approximately ³/₄ inch square and ¹/₄ inch thick) is removed, which contains the physis and adjacent portions of the epiphysis and metaphysis. The plate is then thoroughly curetted and drilled, leaving only the peripheral portions intact. The defect is packed with bone taken from the adjacent metaphysis, and the bone plug is replaced after rotating it 90°, thus bridging the plate with solid bone. The periosteum and perichondrium are then closed snugly to help hold the plug in place. The same procedure is accomplished on the opposite side of the bone.

The fibular epiphysiodesis is done by simply a radical curettage. The bone is so small that removing a plug of bone is more difficult and is usually not necessary, provided the curettage is thorough.

Appropriately and thoroughly accomplished, epiphyseal-diaphyseal fusion ordinarily occurs within 3 months. There is some evidence to show that a brief period of growth stimulation occurs immediately after this procedure, but from a practical standpoint, it has not been of significance in the ultimate clinical result.

Advantages and Disadvantages. The advantages of this procedure include the following: (1) it is technically relatively simple and has a low morbidity; (2) the correction of the inequality is accomplished by normal growth of the short side; (3) the rate of acceptable corrections is attractively high (more than 90 per cent); and (4) significant complications are rare.

The disadvantages are as follows: (1) the patient's ultimate stature is shortened; (2) often the unaffected (longer) limb is operated upon; and (3) the operation is virtually irreversible.

Complications. Aside from the usual complications of any major surgery on bone, there are specific potential complications inherent in this procedure. These include: (1) failure to calculate bone age accurately, resulting in over- or undercorrection; (2) asymmetrical growth arrest, producing valgus or varus deformity; and (3) failure to effect an epiphysiodesis at all. Most of these complications are fortunately rare or their effect is insignificant with respect to the end result.

Epiphyseal Plate Stapling

Haas[49] showed that by encircling the epiphyseal plate of the femurs of growing dogs with wire loops, retardation of lon-

gitudinal growth of the involved limb was effected. When the loops were untied, growth resumed. Staples were then used in a similar study[50] in 1948. Stimulated by this work, Blount and Clark[20] published a paper outlining the use of stainless steel staples to correct limb length inequalities and angular deformities such as knock knees (Fig. 19-25). Green and Anderson[45] observed that inhibition of growth with staples is less rapidly facilitated than when epiphysiodesis is employed. They also noted the potential complications related to stapling, especially the danger of premature epiphyseal fusion. They suggested that stapling be regarded as simply another method of complete growth arrest. Most of the remaining pertinent literature, such as works by Poirier,[75] May and Clemens,[65] and Brockway, Craig and Cockrell,[24] deals with the numerous complications which can arise from the stapling procedures. In his review of the number of complications reported in the literature, Tachdjian[89] recommended that stapling be discarded in favor of epiphysiodesis for growth arrest.

Thus, Blount's procedure of correcting limb length inequality by stapling the physeal plate has achieved dubious acceptance. It was developed with the concept that correction could be accomplished in a younger patient with limb length inequalities without expecting a permanent growth arrest. The staples placed across the physeal plate are of sufficient strength that they are able to interrupt growth of this growth center. If equalization takes place prior to skeletal maturity, the staples are removed, and normal growth is then expected to resume. Conceptually, therefore, the stapling procedure is a method of temporarily interrupting growth, which can be applied to younger children who have a significant limb length discrepancy on whom a shortening procedure is considered acceptable.

Indications. According to Blount and others, the best indication for the use of staples to correct a limb length inequality is a situation in which the discrepancy, preferably one that is not progressive, occurs in a child who is skeletally immature, so that sufficient additional growth will take place in the short limb to correct the discrepancy after stapling is accomplished.

It might be noted that the ideal indication

for the use of staples in the growing skeleton is for the correction of developmental angular deformities about the knee (Fig. 19-25). However, the author prefers to delay use of the staples until the patient is almost skeletally mature, so that the staples will not have to be removed prior to cessation of growth. This avoids the possibility of overcorrection, in the event that permanent growth arrest occurs.

Because there is some potential latitude in the age at which stapling can be done, and because stapling may be safe to accomplish in children who have not yet reached the skeletal age for permanent epiphysiodesis, the operation *may* be indicated in other circumstances, such as: (1) children with limb length discrepancies in whom there is a difference between skeletal and chronological age of more than 18 months and (2) children with *proven* static limb length discrepancies who are too young for permanent epiphysiodesis. In light of these indications, the need for physeal stapling is obviously rare, but in these occasional instances, the procedure may offer a valuable method of temporarily interrupting longitudinal growth.

Advantages of Stapling. When properly executed, according to the strict procedural techniques outlined and emphasized by Blount, this operation is relatively simple, though technically demanding. Since the subperiosteal and interior portions of the bone are not openly violated, the morbidity is less than in epiphysiodesis. Convalescence is much more rapid because there is less surgical trauma, and the bone is not temporarily weakened, as with epiphysiodesis. The patient may resume full activities as soon as the wound is healed and full range of motion of the knee has returned.

Theoretically the principal advantage that the operation offers over permanent epiphysiodesis is the latitude it permits for errors in calculations of skeletal age or limb length discrepancy. If it appears that overcorrection might occur, the staples may be removed in the anticipation that normal growth will resume on the operative side. Blount has shown that this can occur, but whether resumption of growth consistently occurs following staple removal has not been proven in a statistically useful series of patients, and, in fact, much evidence points

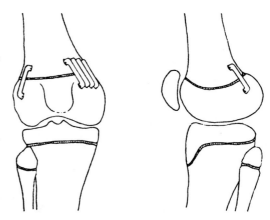

FIG. 19-25. The stapling procedure for angular deformity at the knee. (From Blount, W. P., and Zeier, F.: Control of bone length. J.A.M.A., *148:*451. Copyright 1952, American Medical Association.)

to the contrary. Thus, although this procedure possesses a distinct potential advantage over epiphysiodesis because of its proposed safety factor, the reliability of this procedure is not really proven.

Disadvantages of Stapling. As implied above, there are some uncertainties about this procedure, which represent potentially serious disadvantages. Whether or not resumption of growth occurs following staple removal can pose a serious problem. However, this applies only if stapling has been done in a younger child, wherein resumption of growth is critical to maintenance of limb length equality. If the physeal plate closes prior to normal skeletal maturity, an obvious overcorrection may occur, resulting in excessive shortening. Conversely, if compensatory acceleration of growth takes place upon removal of the staples, the procedure will not have achieved its purpose. The occurrence of these adverse situations is unpredictable, and the possibility of their occuring may reflect much more the technique by which the procedure is done, rather than the procedure itself. If the staples do not have to be removed prior to skeletal maturity this disadvantage is largely vitiated.

Another disadvantage has to do with the operative procedure required to remove the staples. Even though it appears minor, this operation is essentially of the same extent as the procedure employed to insert the staples. Most often the devices must be removed, even after skeletal maturity is achieved, because they frequently are the source of discomfort due to the formation of overlying bursae or simply the palpable presence of metallic structures under the subcutaneous tissues. Sometimes the removal can be difficult, especially if the cross member of the staple is initially sunk into the bone, resulting in its subsequent burial. However, if they have been properly inserted outside the periosteum this is usually not a problem.

This operation is demanding on the technical skills of the surgeon, because the staples must be precisely inserted under roentgenographic control. It requires much more meticulous attention to detail than epiphysiodesis, because any significant injury to the physeal plate must be assiduously avoided in the stapling procedure in order to avoid permanent growth arrest. There is also the possible consequence, as stated by Tachdjian, of damaging the periosteum and the epiphyseal vessels during stapling. Therefore, because of the greater technical demands placed upon the surgeon in the stapling procedure, a relative disadvantage exists, when compared to the operation for permanent physeal arrest, as described earlier.

Complications. Since this procedure carries with it some uncertainties, the number of possible complications is somewhat greater than those encountered in epiphysiodesis. The most significant are those which are clearly related to the technical aspects of the procedure, listed as follows: (1) premature growth arrest resulting in excessive shortening; (2) asymmetrical growth arrest, either temporary or permanent, producing valgus or varus deformity; and (3) failure of the devices, or the techniques by which they are inserted, resulting in no growth retardation or correction.

Bone Shortening (Resection)

This method of equalization is reserved for those patients who have a significant limb length inequality, but who are not candidates for lengthening or are skeletally too old to qualify for equalization by growth arrest. This is a much more formidable method of equalization, as compared to simple growth arrest, since it requires resection of a generous portion of the shaft of either the femur or the tibia and fibula, coupled with appropriate rigid internal fixation and local autogenous bone grafting. Nevertheless, it represents a valuable and practical method of equalization in skeletally mature patients whose needs justify its execution.

History. As cited by Goff,[42] the first recorded case of bone shortening was accomplished by Rizzoli in 1846, when he allowed the fractured fragments of a femur to override. The patient was a woman whose unfractured limb was over 10 cm. shorter than the other. The results of Rizzoli's procedure were such that they seemed to justify the use of this method in achieving correction of limb length inequality, in some cases. Throughout the history of bone shortening procedures, a multitude of different approaches are cited (mainly with respect to femoral shortening), which differ more in technical details than in philosophy. Calvé and Galland[27] described an oblique osteotomy with overriding. White[99] proposed a femoral shortening by simple overlap of a transverse osteotomy and internal fixation with screws. The use of tibial onlay graft following resection of a stepout osteotomy of the femur was favored by J. R. Moore [67] and by Phalen and Chatterton.[72] Harmon and Krigsten[53] also suggested that the excised bone portion be used in creating an onlay bone graft, when performing tibial and femoral resection. Howorth[55] utilized an end-to-end or step-cut resection, with the internal fixation being accomplished by use of a metal plate. Blount[16] recommended that the shortening be done in the subtrochanteric region, whereas R. D. Moore[68] suggested a method of supracondylar shortening of the femur. Thompson, Straub and Campbell[90] and Stirling[87] summarized their preference for an oblique osteotomy with multiple screw fixation. Cameron[28] dealt with resection by parallel V-shaped osteotomies, followed by screw fixation. Although not original with them, Merle D'Aubigne and Dubousset[66] preferred using a step-cut osteotomy, with resection of both ends and internal fixation with an intramedullary rod and screws.

Indications. As noted above, only those individuals who are nearing skeletal maturity or those who are skeletally mature should be subjected to this procedure. Prior to skeletal maturity, the previously described growth arrest procedures performed alone, or in combination with some form of lengthening (when excessive discrepancy exists), are usually more appropriate than bone resection.

As a general rule such a major procedure as this is not justified unless the discrepancy exceeds 2.5 or 3 cms. On the other hand, no rigid minimal figure should cause a patient to be denied the operation if the discrepancy is less than that, provided the patient strongly desires it and fully understands all of the potential complications of the operation. I personally have never performed resection of bone for lower limb length equalization unless the discrepancy exceeded 2.5 cm.

Clearly, shortening by resection alone is indicated only when the procedure can effect equal or nearly equal limb lengths through resection of less than 5 or 6 cms., which is about the maximum amount of shortening tolerated in the femur. Therefore, any discrepancy greater than 5 or 6 cms. probably should not be corrected by resection alone, but rather in combination with a lengthening procedure. In the case of the tibia, the maximum amount of shortening safely tolerated is about 3.0 cm. In my opinion, the ideal indication for equalization by resection of bone is a skeletaly mature patient who is of acceptable height, and whose discrepancy can be fully corrected by femoral rather than tibial resection.

Femoral Versus Tibial Resection. Other things being equal, it is far easier and safer to shorten the femur rather than the tibia and fibula. Femoral resection, recommended to be performed at the subtrochanteric level, enjoys the following advantages over tibial resection: (1) there is relative ease of accomplishment; (2) it lends itself well to internal fixation; (3) it requires no external fixation; (4) union is usually rapid; and (5) there is little weakening of the thigh or hip musculature, and any resultant weakness rapidly disappears. Finally, (6) correction up to 6.0 cms. is technically possible and is safe.

In the tibia, on the other hand, one has to deal with two bones. There are complicated fascial planes and muscle compartments, which render the neurovascular bundle more susceptible to injury during sudden shortening of any significant degree. The level of shortening must be accomplished in the middle or upper shaft, which is below the major areas of origin of the leg musculature. This makes at least temporary weakness of the musculature almost inevitable, and recovery of strength takes much longer, if it ever recovers completely. A cast is usually necessary, which temporarily compromises ankle and knee motion. Furthermore, the limb is usually restricted to a maximum of about 3 cms. of correction.

It is evident from my experience that femoral resection is much preferable to tibial-fibular shortening, and I have done this almost exclusively, regardless of the portion of the lower limb having the maximum discrepancy (Fig. 19-26). Nevertheless, an occasional instance may arise where the discrepancy is exclusively in the leg segment (below the knee) and where equalization of knee levels is highly desirable. Ordinarily this is in an adolescent girl or young woman whose circumstances may justify the increased risks attendant upon tibial shortening. When it is done I strongly recommend that a radical fasciotomy be performed in the anterior compartment, and even possibly the posterior compartment, in anticipation of potential neurovascular complications.

Technique. For equalization of limb length discrepancy by femoral resection, the author prefers the technique illustrated in Figure 19-27. The shortening is done at the intertrochanteric or the subtrochanteric level, and a compression nail plate or screw plate combination is employed for internal fixation. It embraces all the advantages of the various methods of femoral shortening and capitalizes on the advantages outlined on page 842.

With the patient on a fracture table, an appropriate lateral incision is made over the proximal thigh, with the upper limb of the incision extending to the level of the greater trochanter. The fascia lata is split longitudinally and the vastus lateralis and underlying periosteum is elevated from the base of the greater trochanter, distally, for about 5

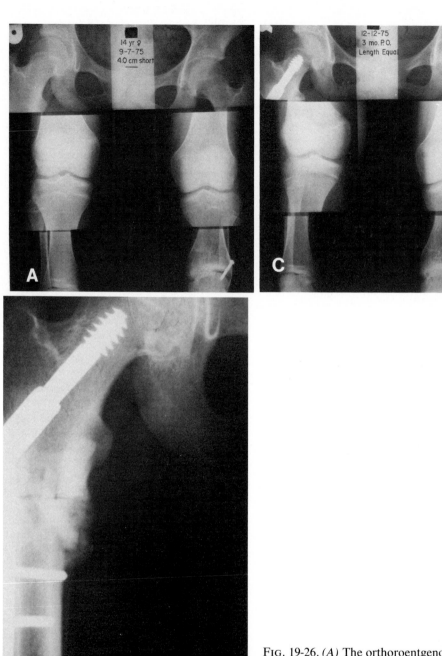

Fig. 19-26. *(A)* The orthoroentgenogram of a 14-year-old female whose limb length difference is 4 cm. as a result of a traumatic distal tibial epiphyseal arrest. Correction of the angular deformity in the ankle has been achieved. *(B)* Three months following femoral shortening to achieve equalization, the osteotomy has healed. *(C)* The orthoroentgenogram shows the limb lengths to be exactly equal.

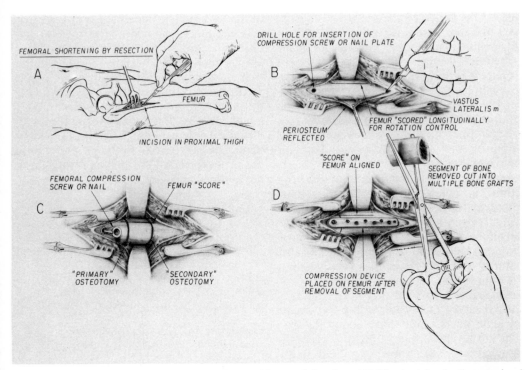

FIG. 19-27. Femoral shortening by resection and internal fixation. *(A)* The incision in the proximal thigh must be adequate in length to receive the internal fixation device. *(B)* The periosteum has been reflected, and a linear score has been made on the femur throughout the area of resection. The score assists in orientation of rotation. *(C)* The femoral compression device has been placed into the head and neck of the femur, and the amount of femoral shaft to be resected is identified. The two osteotomies are then accomplished. The osteotomies must be made precisely parallel to each other to permit good apposition of the fragments when they are approximated. *(D)* The side plate has been affixed, with appropriate shortening having been accomplished. The score on the femur is aligned, and the resected bone is cut into bone grafts.

inches. A drill hole is made for passage of a guide pin into the femoral head and neck, just as in the nailing of a femoral neck or an intertrochanteric fracture. The placement of this guide pin is checked roentgenographically for position. A small trough or "score" about $2^{1}/_{2}$ inches long is made parallel to the long axis of the femur, which is used as reference for control of rotation after the femur is sectioned. The "score" must extend at least one-half inch proximal to the site of initial osteotomy and well below the lowest point of resection. The periosteum is elevated completely around that portion of the femur to be excised. The compression screw is placed into the head and neck, and its length and position are verified by roentgenogram. The primary osteotomy is

accomplished, and the appropriate length of femur is resected. The distal end of the femur is brought proximally and clamped to the barrel and sideplate of the compression device. Accuracy of rotation is verified by aligning it with the "score" previously made on the femur, and the sideplate is screwed to the distal fragment. A compression mechanism may be used prior to placement of the screws, thus assuring impaction of the fragments.

After verifying the position of the compression screw plate device by roentgenographic examination, the segment of bone removed is cut into small grafts, which are placed about the osteotomy site. The wound is then closed in layers. At this point the thigh appears more bulky than it did previously. This is due to the increased muscle mass over the area of resection. This bulkiness gradually recedes as the muscles adapt to their new length.

No cast is necessary, and the patient can be ambulatory with crutches and non-weighbearing on the operated side as soon as comfort permits. Graduated weightbearing is begun in about 3 months, or when early union of the osteotomy is evident on roentgenograms.

Advantages. Despite the fact that this procedure is much more formidable than growth arrest operations, there are certain distinct advantages to equalization by bone resection, even in this comparison. First of all, it can be done at any time after skeletal maturity and, therefore, there are no time constraints for accomplishing the procedure. Secondly, a highly accurate equalization can be accomplished, without having to calculate or be concerned about the patient's exact skeletal age. Finally, if properly done in the skeletally mature patient, overcorrection cannot occur.

Disadvantages. The fact that a major resection of bone is required along with a large metal implant or internal fixation device, as well as the attendant potential complications, represent the major disadvantages to the operation. Therefore, the preoperative evaluation must be very thorough in order to insure that the indications and the needs of the patient justify undertaking this major procedure.

CORRECTION OF LOWER LIMB LENGTH INEQUALITY BY LENGTHENING

Conceptually, lengthening of the short side in treatment of limb length inequality is, in most instances, the most attractive approach to this problem. Unfortunately, because of the many problems and uncertainties inherent in lengthening, this method of equalization has justifiably become relegated to a position where it is only occasionally indicated. At the present time, lengthening by any technique is indicated *only* when the simpler methods of shortening are, by themselves, either unacceptable or inappropriate. However, because there always is the occasional patient who requires both lengthening of the short side and shortening

of the long side, or lengthening of the short side alone, this method of equalization will always occupy a small but important sector of our therapeutic armamentarium in the treatment of limb length inequality.

There are two conceptually different methods of lengthening a limb; these are (1) lengthening by stimulation of growth and (2) mechanical lengthening. They are widely divergent approaches to the problem, both as to concept as well as technique, and these are outlined as follows:

Lengthening by Stimulation of Growth
  Stimulation by creation of arteriovenous fistula
  Stimulation by subepiphyseal implantation of dissimilar foreign materials
  Periosteal stripping
  Stimulation by multiple surgical insult
  Stimulation by ganglionectomy (sympathectomy)
Lengthening by Mechanical Means
  Lengthening by osteotomy and gradual distraction
  Femoral lengthening and tibial lengthening
  Lengthening by osteotomy, sudden distraction and implantation of bone or foreign materials, such as a "spacer"
  Iliac osteotomy (modified Salter osteotomy)
  Femoral osteotomy

Lengthening by Stimulation of Growth

Arteriovenous Fistula. It has long been known that children with congenital or acquired arteriovenous fistulae or hemangiomata of a limb often develop increased growth in the involved limb. (see p. 820). In some situations the vascular lesions have produced lower limb length discrepancies requiring surgical correction. It is, of course, also well established that disease conditions which produce increased vascularity by means of hyperemia also may produce overgrowth of the limb (see p. 815). On the strength of these observations it was felt that a surgically created arteriovenous fistula in the superficial femoral vessels could result in stimulation of growth in the shorter limb, with resultant gradual "physiological" correction of the discrepancy. In concept this seems logical, but, from a practical standpoint, the long-term results have not stood up to critical analysis.

In general, the disadvantages and complications have outweighed the value of any correction achieved.

History. Janes and Musgrove[57, 58] began experimental work on dogs in 1949. Their experiments indicated that bone growth might be accelerated by the creation of an arteriovenous fistula to increase the blood supply. Janes and Jennings,[56] as well as associates Vanderhooft, Kelly, Janes and Peterson,[94] later continued this research by applying the operative procedure to children. They should be credited with the most comprehensive studies in the field, although other contributions have been made by Vesely and Mears,[95] who present a particularly objective evaluation of the problem.

The major advantage of this procedure is basically conceptual, being that correction of the lower limb length inequality can be achieved by a process of increasing blood supply to the shorter limb. This could be a very great advantage if the results were not vitiated by several significant disadvantages and complications. Other advantages include the lack of need for any skeletal transfixion or external appliances, and the relative simplicity of the procedure.

The disadvantages and complications are serious, unfortunately. It is because of these that the procedure has been almost completely abandoned. The most serious problem created by this operation is the cardiovascular abnormality resulting from increased cardiac output. Instances of definitely increased heart size have not been unusual; and even though it is considered a reversible situation upon closure of the fistula, it is a worrisome and objectionable feature. Other documented complications include murmurs, hypertension, mild edema, varicosities, ulceration, cramps and failure to establish a fistula. Another disadvantage includes the need for a second operation to take down the fistula. Granted, this is not a serious procedure, but it does involve surgery upon two major lower limb vessels. A distressing disadvantage also involves the unpredictability of the results. Janes and Jennings[56] reported that in a well-documented group treated by an arteriovenous fistula, 32.5 per cent achieved equalization and 32.5 per cent achieved some degree of correction, and in the remaining 35 per cent an actual increase in the discrepancy was observed. The approximate, expected *maximum* decrease in discrepancy was only around 3.5 cm. and the accomplishment of this took up to 6 years. Similar results were cited by Vesely and Mears.[95] Furthermore, because failure to achieve correction may not be convincingly evident for several years, it is possible that in some instances the ideal time will have passed when some other simpler, more predictable method of equalization, such as growth arrest, may be undertaken.

Currently, therefore, I feel that it is not appropriate to continue use of the AV fistula in the treatment of lower limb length inequality. If the discrepancy is great (more than 5.0 cm.), the operation will not achieve correction and if the difference in length is small (2.0 cm.), simpler, more reliable and less complicated methods are more acceptable.

Metaphyseal Stimulation by Subepiphyseal Implantation of Foreign Material. Based upon the observation that hyperemia and other irritative metaphyseal lesions can produce increased physeal growth, Pease[71] believed that a shortened lower limb could be stimulated to grow faster than the opposite limb by means of implanting dissimilar metals (the battery effect) and other foreign materials in the metaphyseal region of the distal femur or the proximal tibia. In a followup review of the patients operated upon, the following observations are significant: He found that ivory was the most suitable material for implantation. However, his results were extremely variable. In one case, he achieved 3 cm. of correction, but for most of his patients insignificant or nonexistent correction was obtained. Pease concluded that no valid predictions could be drawn from his endeavors. In addition, Haas,[51] Bohlman,[21] Carpenter and Dalton[29] and Tupman[93] all experienced disappointments in use of this technique because of its lack of reliability. In many cases there was actually a loss of growth in the treated limb. The possibility of infection also posed a threat, and in some cases foreign body reactions produced such ill effects as flexion contractures of the knee.

It is clear that the complications and unpredictability of results obtained render the Pease procedure obsolete, and it is only being mentioned here for historical interest and to emphasize that it should not be done.

Periosteal Stripping. Ollier[70] in 1867 showed that periosteal stripping of the tibia stimulated growth. Since that time there has been periodic interest in the procedure as a possible mode of treating limb length inequality. Wu and Miltner in 1937 reported a substantial increase in growth of the tibia in rabbits after stripping the whole periosteum. Trueta in 1953 felt that periosteal stripping was a factor influencing overgrowth in unreduced fractures. Yabsley and Harris,[103] in experiments on the tibial shaft of young rabbits, noted some stimulation of growth following closed fractures that were accompanied by periosteal damage. Khoury[61] and associates did extensive experimentation on dogs and monkeys and produced some lengthening through periosteal stripping. A second stripping, however, proved unreliable. It appears that the merit of the procedure is negligible, since the effect of stripping lasts only a few weeks following the operation. Also, subsequent surgery to extend its effectiveness is rarely helpful and, at best, the most length that can be gained is but a few millimeters.

Multiple Surgical Insults. It is well known that "overgrowth" of the limb often follows fracture repair in the long bones of young children (see p. 815). This can be observed clinically, especially in patients with femoral fractures who are under 12 years old. If the fractured ends are anatomically reduced, a limb length discrepancy may result due to overgrowth, presumably as the result of hyperemia of the reparative process. Such overgrowth is not uniformly predictable, even though a rather consistent pattern is identified following certain fractures of the femur. Although overgrowth following a variety of limb fractures has been reported (p. 816), it would appear that the greatest incidence of overgrowth follows fractures of the proximal diaphysis. Most records show an average of about 1 cm. overgrowth occurring in the first year following the fracture. However, more extensive lengthening has been reported in cases where the fracture initially resulted in shortening of 1 cm. or greater. Most investigators feel that accelerated growth lasts only as long as does the healing process, usually about one year.

A more radical approach to treatment of the shortened limb has been recommended by Sofield,[83] who utilized repeated osteotomies of the tibia or femur, accompanied by intramedullary fixation. Results were negligible. Such repeated osteotomies were also recommended by Blount.[16] Early experiments utilizing drilling and curetting and attempts at stimulation of growth, such as those by Compere and Adams[36] in 1937 (in long bone fractures in rabbits) resulted in minimal overgrowth of the bone. A strong advocate of the procedure was Goff[42] who reported the use of a "splinter" osteotomy (a series of oblique perforating cuts across the long bone shaft), to gain from 0.5 to 1.5 cm. in length. Agerholm[2] in 1959 also reported good results with his step-cut osteotomy for stimulating growth.

However, because of its unpredictability and the equivocal success in producing growth stimulation, the procedure has not gained favor and the results have clearly not justified the magnitude of the surgical exercises.

Currently, therefore, there is little statistically valid evidence to support continuing a program involving surgical procedures that are designed to stimulate bone growth by surgical trauma alone. The greater reliability and predictability of mechanical lengthening makes it a much more acceptable method of gaining increased length, as compared with stimulation procedures.

Ganglionectomy or Sympathectomy. Due to the frequent "coldness" associated with the polio limb, wherein there frequently is shortening, and in view of the contrary observation that lesions associated with increased vascularity sometimes produce overgrowth of an involved limb, it has been proposed that sympathectomy might enhance growth or shortened limbs. The literature on treatment of the limb inequalities associated with poliomyelitis by means of sympathetic ganglionectomy is dotted with controversy. Harris and MacDonald[54] failed to effect growth stimulation by this means in animals, but they observed favorable results in children, under highly controlled conditions. Barr[10] also reported some degree of success, but advocated that the procedure be used only in conjunction with other equalization procedures. Opponents to the use of sympathetic ganglionectomy for limb growth stimulation include Bisgard,[13] Fahey,[40] and Green.[44] It is my opinion that the procedure is unreliable in producing limb growth stimulation and should be used only when it is otherwise desirable to stimulate circulation to the limb.

Mechanical Lengthening

It is my opinion that this method of lower limb elongation is the most proven and reliable, despite the many controversies surrounding the indications and potential complications of the procedure. Historically, lower limb lengthening by osteotomy and distraction has been highlighted by alternating periods of enthusiasm and almost total rejection. In order to understand and appreciate the qualified acceptance of mechanical limb lengthening, it is essential to review the historical features surrounding its evolution, with respect to both tibial lengthening and femoral lengthening.

History. Codivilla[30] introduced the concept of femoral lengthening in 1905. His technique included an oblique osteotomy, with skeletal traction applied to the calcaneus. Others who employed Codivilla's method modified the traction device, such as Magnusson[64] who facilitated traction in femoral lengthening by use of a Hawley table. Putti[76, 77] accomplished limb lengthening by initially placing the patient in traction on a Braun frame, passing Kirschner wires through the proximal and distal ends of the bones to be lengthened, and applying traction to opposite ends of an oblique osteotomy. He then used his special "osteotone," which consisted of two pins connected with a telescoping tube and a spring extension device. Abbott and Crego,[1] finding that Putti's device was unstable and offered no control of bone fragments, devised an apparatus consisting of four stainless steel drill pins (two above and two below), a pin guide and a device that combined traction with a supporting splint. They also suggested a method of tibial and fibular lengthening using a similar device, while emphasizing the need for release of soft tissue prior to lengthening. Both Putti and Ab-

bott stressed the importance of directly applying both traction and countertraction to the bone to be lengthened. Despite further improvements made on the lengthening device, Compere[35] in 1936, dissatisfied not only with the length of convalescence following lengthenings but also with the high incidence of delayed or nonunion, recommended bone grafting at the time of femoral lengthening. This consisted of an onlay graft of cortical tibial bone applied on the proximal fragments of the femur. He also outlined the complications of limb lengthening. Harmon and Krigsten[53] and Phalen and Chatterton[72] felt that bone shortening should be used in place of lengthening, because of the many poor results following lengthening. Bost,[22] like Abbott, stressed the need for release of soft tissues prior to femoral lengthening. Later, in 1956,[23] he and Larsen proposed a technique of femoral lengthening using an intramedullary rod. Brockway and Fowler's[25] review in 1944 of 105 limb lengthening operations, showed that they were in favor of tibial lengthening (Abbott method) and that femoral lengthenings were far too dangerous. McCarroll[63] wrote that the Phemister technique of epiphyseal arrest had essentially made limb lengthenings, especially femoral lengthening, obsolete. He recommended that when indicated, femoral lengthening should be done using a slotted blade and a subtrochanteric Z-type osteotomy. Crego in 1957, as cited by Goff,[42] felt that tibial lengthening, because of the frequent necessity of secondary heel cord lengthenings, and because of muscle weakness resulting from the lengthening, should be completely discarded in deference to bone shortening or femoral lengthening. Sofield[82] also cited numerous cases of subsequent muscle weakness and felt that limb lengthening was too hazardous to continue. Goff[42] also had given up the procedure almost entirely in favor of other simpler modes of equalization. Allan[7] discussed simultaneous lengthening of the tibia and femur, but emphasized that knee stiffness often ensues. He also dealt extensively with the complications of lengthening.[5, 6]

Despite the fear and unacceptance shown by many surgeons with respect to mechanical limb lengthening, much has been accomplished in the last 25 years to greatly improve the techniques, results and acceptance of the procedure. In 1952, Anderson[8] published a paper which rekindled much of the lost enthusiasm for tibial lengthening. His procedure consisted of distal fibular osteotomy, a distal tibiofibular synostosis, division of the tibia by percutaneous drilling and osteoclasis, and slow lengthening by means of transfixion pins held in a distraction device. This will be discussed in more detail later in the chapter along with my own modifications. Westin[98] described a method of femoral lengthening using a periosteal sleeve to bridge the gap in the bone fragments. His findings indicated that the sleeve was at least partly responsible for increased rapidity of bridging the distraction gap with new bone during and and immediately following lengthening. Gross[47] and Kawamura[59] both recommended bone grafting as early as 8 weeks, in the event of delayed union or nonunion. Kawamura[59, 60] further broadened our understanding of the complications in his studies of 1968 and 1969. It is reasonable to assume that the improvements in our knowledge and technical expertise make this procedure increasingly more useful and practical, as long as the indications and prerequisites are clearly defined and strictly followed.

Osteotomy and Gradual Distraction. Throughout the evolution of lengthening procedures, the method which has remained most consistently acceptable is osteotomy followed by gradual distraction. A variety of techniques has been employed, but the fundamental principles have remained more or less constant in all. These technical principles include: (1) a semi-open or open transverse, oblique or step-cut osteotomy in the femur or tibia, (2) application of a mechanical distraction device, and (3) gradual (usually daily) distraction of approximately 1–2 mm. per day. Variations in these basic issues results largely from minor differences in concepts regarding the physiology of bone repair, and differences in approaches to the biomechanics of the hardware employed. It is reasonable to predict that as our technical knowledge and skills become further refined current methods may soon become outmoded. However, the basic mechanical approach to the solution of this problem will

likely be unchanged for some time to come. Since nearly all of the principles apply equally to operations done on the femur and the tibia, the discussion of those principles can, therefore, encompass procedures done on either bone.

The Osteotomy. For many years the technique of osteotomy involved subperiosteal exposure of the shaft of the tibia or femur, followed by either a step-cut or an oblique osteotomy. This technique is still preferred in some modern lengthening procedures. By serendipity, Anderson developed a method of percutaneous osteoclasis when one of his patients scheduled for a tibial lengthening sustained a closed, transverse fracture of the tibia of the short limb. He applied the distraction device and proceeded to lengthen the tibia without open surgery. Rapid union ensued, and since that time the technique of percutaneous drilling and "semi-closed" osteoclasis has become a well-established method of osteotomy. The potential advantages of this technique over the open method are theoretical, and they can be listed as follows: (1) the magnitude of the surgery is lessened, (2) wide exposure of bone is avoided, and (3) the environment of a closed fracture is simulated. The obvious disadvantage is that the ends of the bone become much more widely spaced during the distraction process than in the step-cut or the open, oblique osteotomy. Despite the arguments which may support one method over the other, it has not been unequivocally proven that union is more rapid or more certain with any one of these techniques of osteotomy. There is evidence to support any of the techniques. Therefore, as far as can presently be determined, the surgeon may confidently choose that osteotomy which lends itself best to the specific technical aspects of a particular lengthening technique or device.

The Distraction Device. A multiplicity of distraction devices has been developed over the years in an effort to provide a reliable, simple and uncomplicated means of separating the bones. All of the devices currently being used have several features in common: (1) two skeletal transfixion pins above and below the osteotomy; (2) some mechanism for controlling angulation, rotation and displacement during distraction;

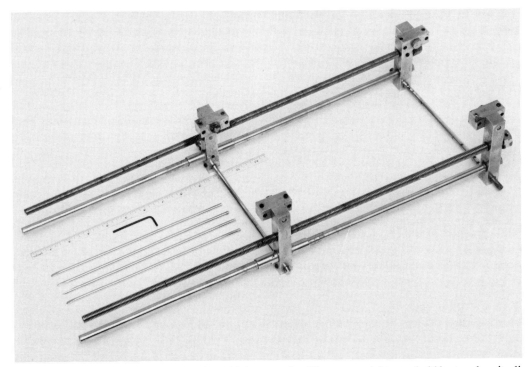

FIG. 19-28. The tibial lengthening device which we prefer. The two uprights are held by two longitudinal steel rods, one smooth and one threaded. The uprights are then connected by two transverse steel rods, which maintain the uprights perpendicular to each other. Also illustrated are the ⁵/₃₂-inch smooth Steinmann pins, and the Allen wrench.

and (3) parallel longitudinal threaded rods for systematic and controlled separation of the transfixed bony fragments (Fig. 19-28).

The Program of Distraction. There are two well-accepted axioms regarding the distraction process. One has to do with the rate of lengthening and the other has to do with the ultimate limits of distraction (or lengthening). The guidelines regarding rapidity of lengthening are less well established, and there is a fairly wide degree of latitude governing this parameter. On the other hand, some reasonably sound clinical and experimental data is available, which may be of assistance in governing the total amount of lengthening that may be safely achieved.

Limits of Distraction. In 1968, Kawamura[60] and his associates published their findings from extensive research in the field of limb lengthening. Their experiments, which involved blood chemical, histological, and electromyographic studies, put forth suggestions governing technique, rate, and limits, of lengthening. The recommended technique was tibial lengthening, utilizing a small incision, a tube-like elevation of the periosteum, and an oblique "subcutaneous" osteotomy. Electromyography of the lengthened muscles indicated that a 10 per cent lengthening of the bone's initial total length was a safe limit, with 15 per cent being the absolute maximum. Beyond this any increased length resulted in a significantly increased number of complications.

Until Kawamura's study, which established some defensible guidelines, the amount of ultimate length to be gained by lengthening had been arbitrarily set at 5.0 cm., or 2 inches, in either the femur or the tibia. Unfortunately, this figure was utilized regardless of the age of the patient or the initial length of the bone. Consequently, many complications were encountered that might otherwise not have occurred (see p. 850). My personal experience holds that the maximum amount of total distraction should not exceed 15 per cent of the original length of the bone. This applies equally well to the femur and the tibia. Even with this maximum limit, great care must be exercised so as to avoid untoward complications, which may compromise not only the end result but also the viability of the limb itself.

Rate of Lengthening. Kawamura's findings (using biochemical studies of enzymes of the elongated muscles) concluded that slow lengthening should be done in several stages, with the first lengthening being limited to 3 per cent of the total bone length. This should be done during the first 2 weeks or more. He felt this was the best compromise between the need for rapid lengthening, which theoretically insures against nonunion, and the need for slower lengthening, which protects soft tissues.

Some children tolerate a more rapid rate of lengthening than do others. Also, some types of discrepancies, such as that due to poliomyelitis, lend themselves to more rapid lengthening than do discrepancies from congenital causes. These are individual circumstances which must be treated accordingly. As a general rule, however, in consideration of all of the factors outlined below the standard accepted rate of lengthening is $^1/_{16}$ inch or about 1.6 mm. per day. As noted earlier, this may be exceeded in some situations, or in other instances this rate of distraction may not be tolerated (especially in the femur). Each patient must be managed individually, utilizing certain subjective and objective observations.

Some clinical guidelines are available, which are especially helpful in governing the rate of distraction; these are: (1) the development of muscle paresis, (2) the degree of pain, (3) the development of a sensory or motor neurologic deficit, (4) any alterations in local circulation, and (5) any significant elevation of diastolic blood pressure (above 95 mms.). These facts must be monitored at regular intervals throughout each day of lengthening, and, if adverse signs appear, the distraction must cease or be reversed, if necessary. The reasons for most of the local

alterations appear rather obvious; however, an exact explanation of any alterations in the muscles to lengthening has until just recently been somewhat vague.

In a very sophistocated study utilizing electromicroscopy, Calandriello[26] has shown that in order for muscles to be elongated, the fibrils actually have to rupture and then become restored by regeneration. This phenomenon occurs readily under circumstances of slow lengthening, but if rapid lengthening is accomplished, there may be failure of the muscle fibrils to repair themselves, and hemorrhage will occur, followed by cicatrix formation. Therefore, care must be exercised in the rapidity with which lengthening is accomplished. Conceptually, because of the greater length and excursion of thigh musculature, it would appear that more rapid lengthening could be tolerated in the femur than in the tibia, wherein the muscles are shorter and have less excursion.

Femoral Lengthening by Osteotomy and Gradual Distraction

This surgical procedure is more formidable than tibial lengthening, has more potential complications and usually has a higher morbidity rate. Consequently, I believe that femoral lengthening, as herein described, should be reserved for only those patients whose limb length inequality cannot be corrected by any other currently acceptable means. Utilizing this rather rigid criterion, the indications for the femoral lengthening operation will be extremely uncommon. Nevertheless, there will undoubtedly always be a few instances where the procedure is justified and desirable. Before this procedure is seriously considered, however, all prerequisites must be satisfied and all of the technical aspects must be thoroughly understood. In addition, the indications and contraindications, the advantages and disadvantages, as well as all of the potential complications must be throughly known by the surgeon and the patient.

Indications. As noted above, correction of limb length inequality by lengthening of the femur is indicated when no other method or combination of methods of equalization are acceptable or appropriate. If one reviews the many considerations which are operative in a case of limb length inequality, it appears impossible to provide a concise list of indications with any practical value. Nevertheless, some broad guidelines can be set down which may be of assistance in determining whether femoral lengthening is feasible. These should not be viewed as restrictive considerations, because each patient will present different problems, both physical and psychological all of which must be put into proper perspective.

It is convenient to group the guidelines under four broad categories having to do with: (1) degree of the discrepancy, (2) etiology of the discrepancy, (3) location of the discrepancy; and (4) established or anticipated height of patient.

Degree of Discrepancy. When inequalities of length exceed 10.0 cm., it becomes very difficult to achieve equalization by epiphyseal arrest alone, or even in combination with tibial lengthening. In such instances, femoral lengthening may be indicated. If a discrepancy approximates 15.0 cm., the only way in which surgical equalization can possibly be achieved is with a combination of epiphyseal arrest, tibial lengthening, *and* femoral lengthening. Thus, if one employs the degree of discrepancy as a major parameter, femoral lengthening *may* be indicated in individuals having 10.0 cm. or more of limb length discrepancy, femoral lengthening is *necessary* in those patients with 15.0 cm. of length discrepancy, if surgical equalization is to be accomplished without ablation.

Etiology of Discrepancy. As mentioned earlier, there are some instances of limb length inequality which lend themselves well to femoral lengthening on the basis of their underlying cause. Adolescents and young adults whose shortening is the result of poliomyelitis, fracture with overriding of the fragments (malunion) and premature epiphyseal arrest due to trauma or infection.[76, 96] The reasons why these patients tolerate femoral lengthening so well may be due to the fact that the soft tissues and neurovascular elements were at one time longer (in overriding fragments) or were destined to be longer (in retarded or arrested growth). On the other hand, femoral shortening of congenital or developmental origin responds less well to lengthening. In these instances there may be a more difficult lengthening process, and a greater likelihood of the need for bone grafting and subsequent operative procedures.

Location of Discrepancy. Clearly it is desirable to have equal thigh and leg segments. Thus, if the discrepancy is largely in the femur, it can be argued that the equalization procedure should take place in the femur. Conceptually this is fundamental, but practically the problems of femoral lengthening must be weighed against the desirability of equal knee heights. When all of the factors support the need or desirability of equalizing the femoral lengths, lengthening of the femur may be indicated.

Established or Anticipated Adult Height. In patients who have completed growth, this factor can be accurately established. In growing patients, some latitude with respect to the final determination must be exercised. The principal issue has to do with whether it is more appropriate to lengthen or shorten the limb by surgery on the femur. Faced with comparable degrees of discrepancy, it is clear that in any male patient having 5.0 cm. of femoral shortening, and in one who is or can plan to be 72 inches tall, shortening of the femur by 4 to 5 cm. is preferable to a lengthening procedure. Correspondingly, if the patient is a female and less than 62 inches tall, or a male and shorter than 68 inches, femoral lengthening may be the more desirable therapeutic program.

Prerequisites. If it is determined that femoral lengthening is indicated, it is necessary that all prerequisites be met before the procedure is undertaken, in order to avoid catastrophic and disabling complications. First of all, it is essential that there be a stable, preferably normal hip joint. If this does not exist, the possibility of dislocating the femoral head during distraction is a serious concern. Second, the knee joint must have a normal range of motion, or nearly so. Mechanical lengthening of the femur exerts a tremendous force across the knee joint by means of the stretch on the quadriceps and hamstring muscles. Therefore, any prior compromise of motion or function of the knee will undoubtedly be accentuated by femoral lengthening. Third, the musculature and soft tissues of the thigh must be pliable and distensible in order to permit lengthening. Severe scar or cicatrix formation in the skin, subcutaneous tissues or muscles renders effective lengthening difficult or impossible. Finally, the patient must be normotensive and must have no vascular compromise in the limb to be lengthened. As noted earlier, hypertension may be a serious complication during femoral lengthening. If the patient has an elevated blood pressure prior to lengthening, the possibility that further elevation might occur must weigh heavily against lengthening.

Contraindications. It is clear that in any patient whose clinical situation does not meet the indications and the prerequisites for lengthening, as outlined above, lengthening is contraindicated. Also, any aspect of the patient's general health, either psychological or physiological, which might seriously compromise the femoral lengthening procedure must be considered a contraindication to the technique.

Advantages. There are two circumstances where femoral lengthening has an advantage over other methods of surgical equalization. These include those situations where (1) the major or entire amount of shortening is in the femur and where (2) the discrepancy is so great that any other method or combination or other methods cannot effectively or acceptably accomplish equalization. In the former case, its advantage applies to those instances where it is important to achieve equalization in that particular portion of the limb which is short, and in the latter case the procedure has an advantage because it can possibly provide additional length unobtainable by any other means. To equalize discrepancies residing primarily in the femur by femoral lengthening has more than just a philosophical advantage. The alternative is shortening; and shortening the femur in a child who is already short has serious cosmetic and psychological drawbacks. Shortening of the long femur in an effort to equalize a discrepancy in the thigh in a short person may impart a simian appearance to the patient. This is because the upper limbs and the leg segment of the lower limb may thereafter appear disproportionately long when compared with the entire lower limb.

The disadvantages of gaining lower limb length equalization by femoral lengthening are the complications of the procedure. It is the threat of complications and the seriousness of them when they occur that argue against doing the procedure. These complications are multiple and are probably reflective of the fact that such an operation, generally speaking, is unphysiologic. Because of the importance of these complications, it is essential that they be discussed completely.

One of the major disadvantages of femoral lengthening is inherent in the fact that the technical aspects of the operation are still undergoing refinement. Until the procedure can be made technically simpler, and until greater agreement can be reached regarding the best surgical approach, this disadvantage will continue to remain a serious drawback.

One of the major complications includes the effect femoral lengthening has upon the knee joint. Prolonged and occasionally permanent restriction of knee motion is a major concern following this procedure. Knee motion is always seriously restricted during the lengthening process, and in some cases it has required as long as 12 months or more for motion to return to preoperative levels. To what extent articular cartilage necrosis is produced by the pressure exerted across the knee joint and whether it is reversible are unknown factors. Treatment of such a complication requires prolonged efforts at regaining knee motion by physiologic motion of the knee joint.

A second complication is delayed union or nonunion of the lengthened area. Although such an occurrence may be considered an expected development in the lengthening procedure, it usually requires a second operation, consisting of bone grafting and internal fixation. If this becomes necessary, it represents a technical challenge, due to the fact that it is preferable to do the grafting operation with the distraction device in place. This requires great care, not only in preparation of the operative field, but also in clinical judgement to avoid another dreaded complication, namely, a deep wound infection.

Hypertension not infrequently develops during the lengthening process, especially after femoral lengthening, and it represents one of the most worrisome problems of all. The cause of the elevated blood pressure is not well established, but it has been the subject of several studies. The elevation is seen in both the diastolic and the systolic levels.

Badgley[101] was among the first to report an increase in blood pressure during bone lengthening, especially in the femur. He noted increases from normal to 185 mm. Hg systolic pressure and to 140 mm. Hg diastolic pressure. In 1967 Yosipovitch and Palti[104] studied the phenomenon by experiments with dogs, and they examined records of patients undergoing limb lengthening. Their results suggested that the more immediate rise in blood pressure was probably the result of a reflex response to the rapid tension developed in the sciatic nerve in the upper portion of the thigh during lengthening. The condition was aggravated by the common sitting posture in bed assumed by patients during lengthening. A later manifestation of hypertension has also been suggested as being due to ischemia of the kidney caused by an increased afferent activity in the sciatic nerve, a condition long known to cause reflex spasms in renal blood vessels. Recently Harandi[52] and his coworkers reported development of hypertension in two patients following correction of severe hip and knee flexion contractures due to polio. They concluded that the elevation of blood pressure was mediated by the sympathetic nerves accompanying the femoral and popliteal arteries. Therefore, it is still uncertain as to whether the cause of the hypertension is mediated through the large nerve trunks or the sympathetic nerves that accompany the major vessels. In any event, upon the development of hypertension specific treatment is indicated. Treatment consists primarily of one thing—cessation of the lengthening process. Occasionally antihypertensives may be indicated. Most often the pressure elevation is transient, and usually when lengthening is interrupted the pressure returns to normal levels within a 24- or 48-hour period, at which time lengthening may safely be resumed. Although no permanent, irreversible, catastrophic changes have been reported as a result of lengthening-induced hypertension, it nevertheless represents a serious and treacherous complication.

Pin tract infections of significance are rare, but serous drainage about the pins is common. Unless a deep infection occurs, the only unattractive aspect of the transfixion pins is the subsequent scarring, which is almost always unavoidable. Because of the large muscle mass through which the pins pass in the thigh, pin tract problems and resultant scarring can be somewhat troublesome. Once a deep pin tract infection occurs, removal of the pin or pins may be required. Obviously, if union has not occurred at the time the pin tract problem is recognized and treatment is aggressively instituted, a major problem exists with respect to maintaining increased length of the femur. Furthermore, such an infection temporarily contraindicates any bone grafting procedure which is designed to gain union. Treatment of deep pin tract infections, which force premature removal of the pins, requires massive antibiotic therapy and skeletal traction to maintain length while awaiting a surgical environment receptive to a delayed surgical approach to grafting and internal fixation. This potential problem has encouraged me to do early bone grafting (at 8–10 weeks) and plating of the distracted fragments, in order to avoid loss of length in the event that a pin or pins has to be removed prematurely. My technique of bone grafting and plating, utilizing the Wagner method of femoral lengthening, is discussed on p. 857.

There is a miscellaneous group of complications that can be very troublesome, but because of their singular nature they must be handled on an individual basis. These include: (1) fracture of the lengthened area; (2) angulation with malunion; (3) temporary neurovascular disturbances during the lengthening process; and (4) the occurrence of some degree of knee instability. All of these adverse situations must be thoroughly defined in order to provide appropriate treatment.

Methods. Many techniques of femoral lengthening have been utilized over the past 70 years, ever since Codivilla of Italy performed a femoral lengthening in 1905. Most of these earlier methods have been abandoned because of serious technical problems and serious complications. In recent years the technical aspects of the procedure have become more refined, but the operation still offers a serious challenge to anyone desirous of mechanical elongation of a short

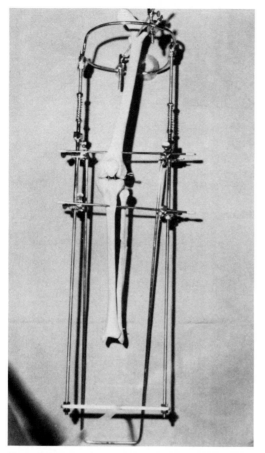

FIG. 19-29. The Bost device for femoral lengthening.

femur. The fact that newer and more innovative techniques are being developed simply re-emphasizes the persistent need for a safer, more effective and more proven technique for femoral lengthening. Currently, the most well-accepted and proven methods of femoral lengthening are the techniques of Bost and his associates[23] and Wagner.[96] Although the Bost technique deserves mention because of its widespread acceptance, the author's current preference is the Wagner procedure.

The Bost-Larsen procedure[23] was introduced in 1955, and it has been one of the most popular techniques utilized over the past 25 years. A vertical through-and-through pin is placed in the proximal femur near the femoral neck, and a transverse pin

is placed through the supracondylar region. These skeletal fixation devices are attached to a spring-loaded distraction mechanism designed for gradual lengthening (Fig. 19-29). An open, transverse osteotomy is made at the subtrochanteric level of the femur, and alignment, angulation and displacement are controlled by means of an intramedullary rod placed downward from the greater trochanter. A periosteal "sleeve" is created at the level of the osteotomy, through which the distal fragment is distracted (Fig. 19-30). Conceptually, this preserves an intact periosteum in the area of distraction, therefore promoting more rapid bone desposition. A pin is also placed in the proximal tibia in order to maintain a fixed position of the femur and tibia across the knee joint. This is done with the intent of reducing the pressure on the articular surfaces of the distal femur and proximal tibia during lengthening. An illustration of a patient who has undergone femoral lengthening conducted by this method is seen in Figure 19-31.

Despite the time-proven value of this technique, there are two specific disadvantages to the operation: (1) the problems encountered in nursing care of a patient with a vertical proximal pin and the large circular device to which the pin is attached; and (2) the difficulty in placing internal fixation across the osteotomy site if delayed or nonunion ensues or if the pins have to be removed prematurely because of loosening or infection.

Wagner. The limb to be lengthened is approached from the lateral side (Fig. 19-32). A sandbag placed under the buttock is helpful during the procedure. The greater trochanter is identified, and a small stab wound is made through the skin at about the level of the lesser trochanter, or slightly above. A template is placed over the stab wound, and a drill guide is inserted through the proximal hole of the template. The guide is placed against the outer cortex of the femur as close as possible to the center of the anterioposterior diameter of the femur. A long $\frac{1}{8}$-inch drill is then placed through the guide, and the femur is drilled transversely through both cortices. It is extremely important that the direction of the drill hole be perpendicular to the long axis of the femur. A Shanz screw of appropriate length is then

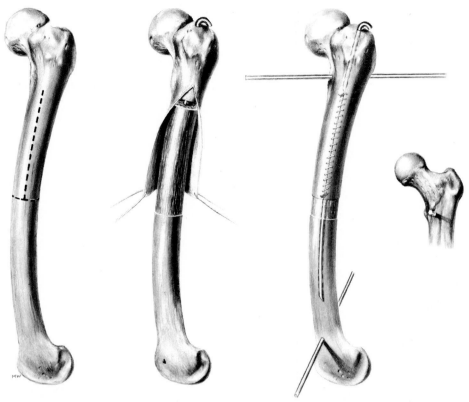

FIG. 19-30. The Bost technique for femoral lengthening, as modified by Westin. (From Westin, G. W.: Femoral lengthening using a periosteal sleeve. Report of 26 cases. J. Bone Joint Surg., *49A:* 83, 1967.)

inserted into the drill hole until it firmly engages both cortices of the femur. Verification of its depth and location should be made by roentgenograms. Utilizing the template, a second stab wound is made at a proper distance from the first so as to receive the proximal portion of the distraction device. A Schanz screw is placed into the femur, exactly parallel to and in the same manner as the first screw. Its depth can be verified by comparing it to the first screw.

A template is then used in the same manner over the distal femur, or alternatively the distraction device may be used, if desired. I find it easier to insert the drill guide through the template. Exercising care to avoid the distal femoral epiphysis, if open, two Schanz screws are inserted into the distal femur parallel to the previous two screws. Depth can usually be verified by palpation over the medial aspect of the distal femur.

After all four screws are appropriately inserted, the distraction device is applied, and if the femur is still intact, all lock nuts are secured. This is necessary so that after the femur is osteotomized, proper orientation of the fragments will be achieved upon replacement of the distraction device. The device is then removed in order to facilitate the osteotomy.

A lateral incision of appropriate length is made parallel to the long axis of the femur, centering over the midpoint between two sets of screws. The fascia lata is exposed, and a portion at least 2 inches wide is excised, both anteriorly over the quadriceps and posteriorly as far as the hamstring muscles. The lateral intermuscular septum is also excised down to the periosteum of the femur. The vastus lateralis is then elevated *extraperiosteally,* so as to preserve the periosteum as a "sleeve." The periosteum is

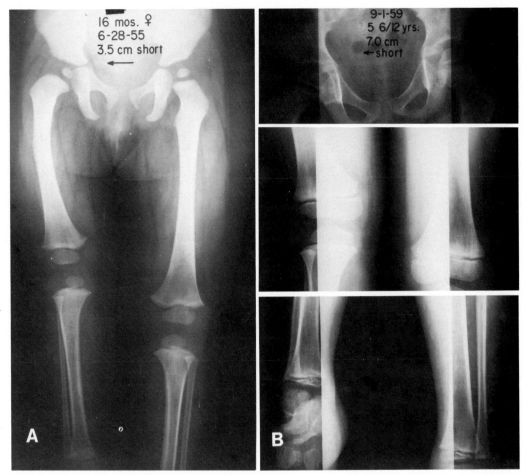

FIG. 19-31. *(A)* This 16-month-old female was initially measured to have 3.5 cm. of shortening, due to a congenital short femur on the right, as seen in the scanogram. *(B)* At age 5½ years, the orthoroentgenogram shows 7 cm. of shortening. *(Legend continued on facing page.)*

next incised and elevated over a distance of at least 2 inches, and a transverse osteotomy is made midway between the two sets of screws and at the *proximal level* of the periosteal "sleeve." There are two reasons why the osteotomy is best made transversely at this location. First, the possible need for subsequent bone grafting and plating is greatly assisted by having comparable lengths of the full thickness of the femur on both sides of the distraction defect. Clearly, a step-cut osteotomy would grossly complicate the subsequent use of a plate, if needed. Secondly, the distal fragment must lie in the periosteal "sleeve," therefore, the os-

teotomy must be proximal with respect to the "sleeve." I have had greater difficulty doing the sleeve in the midshaft area than in the subtrochanteric area, possibly because the periosteum is thinner in this area of the bone.

Before closing the wound, the distraction device is reapplied exactly as it was stabilized before the osteotomy. Once locked into place, the osteotomy site can be inspected to verify the position of the fragments. At this point, I turn the distraction knob eight full turns, which distracts the fragments about ½ inch (1.25 cm.), with the knee flexed 45°. The peripheral pulses are

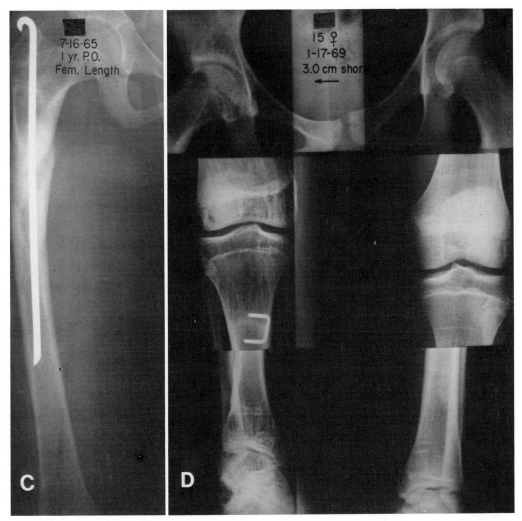

FIG. 19-31 *(Continued)*. *(C)* Due to increasing discrepancy, a femoral lengthening was accomplished by the Bost technique at age 12. *(D)* The final orthoroentgenogram, taken at skeletal maturity. In the interim, a right tibial lengthening had been accomplished, in addition to a left distal femoral arrest.

palpated and the blood pressure is checked. If these are normal, then the osteotomy site is again exposed to make sure the alignment is satisfactory. The wound is closed, but the fascia lata cannot and *should not* be closed. Wagner recommends flexing the knee fully at the close of the operative procedure in order to loosen any fibers of the quadriceps which might be pierced by the distal screws.

Postoperatively, no lengthening is performed until the second postoperative day. Thereafter the distraction knob is turned one full turn daily (¹/₁₆ in. or 1.6 mm.). The peripheral pulses, motor and sensory functions and blood pressure must be monitored at least four times daily. Any compromise of the neurovascular status or any elevation of the diastolic pressure over 105 mm. Hg requires immediate temporary cessation of the lengthening and may even require reversing the mechanism by one or two turns. A graph of the daily and the total lengthening accomplished, and the neurovascular and blood pressure status, should be at the pa-

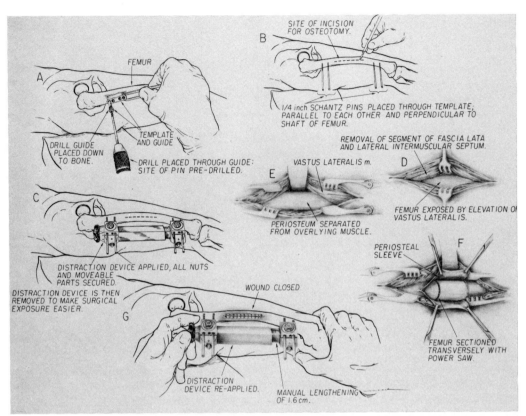

FIG. 19-32. Technique of femoral lengthening by the Wagner method. *(A)* The template and guide are placed over the proximal femoral shaft. Through a stab wound the femur is drilled transversely, just about at the level of the lesser trochanter. *(B)* The four Shanz pins are in place, two above and two below the intended site of the osteotomy. The incision for femoral osteotomy is indicated. *(C)* The distraction device is then applied to the Shanz screws, and measurements are taken. This assures that upon reapplication of the device after osteotomy that the femoral fragments will be in the same position as before. *(D)* The exposure of periosteum after resection of the fascia lata and intermuscular septum. *(E and F)* The development of a periosteal envelope; the site of the osteotomy can be seen. *(G)* Following osteotomy, the periosteum is closed, as is the remainder of the wound, and the distraction device is applied. Manual lengthening of approximately 1.6 cm. is then accomplished. Sterile dressings are applied. *(Legend continued on facing page.)*

tient's bedside at all times. Also, it is a good rule that only one person accomplish the lengthening in order to avoid failure to lengthen or overlengthening.

Active and active assistive knee motion and quadriceps setting should be carried out daily, as soon as symptoms permit. Most often the knee motion is sharply reduced to about 30° immediately postoperatively and during the period of distraction. Even this amount of motion is essential in order to avoid pressure necrosis of cartilage and to provide nourishment to the articular cartilage.

Throughout the elongation process, a weekly roentgenogram should be taken to verify the position of the fragments and to confirm the amount of distraction achieved. As long as the screws are in place, daily attention is essential. I prefer a daily alcohol wash, followed by application of Neosporin ointment.

I feel that hospitalization for the duration of the distraction process is essential. Once

FIG. 19-32 *(Continued). (H)*
The lengthening device.

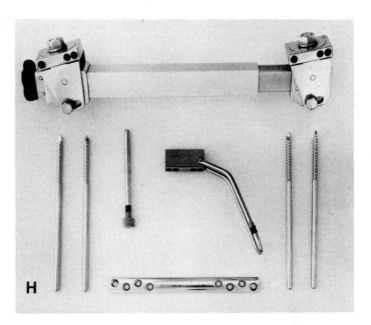

the desired length has been achieved, however, and the neurovascular blood pressure status is stabilized and normal, the patient may be discharged to a responsible home. Ambulation with crutches is optional, but I discourage any activities other than ambulation within the home. Active knee motion is encouraged and should be done as often as possible. At least 45° to 60° of knee motion must be maintained during and immediately after lengthening.

An x-ray film is taken 8 weeks after cessation of the lengthening, and a determination must be made regarding the need for bone grafting and plating. If there is failure of bony bridging, or if there is inadequate bony bridging, I favor immediate bone grafting and plating. This permits removal of the distraction device and enhances bony union, and gives greater assurance of solid, strong union. It also makes increased knee motion possible, because the pins are removed from their location in the distal portion of the vastus lateralis muscle.

Bone Grafting and Plating of Wagner. If it is elected to graft and plate the distraction defect, I prefer to accomplish it with the distraction device in place. This can only be done safely, however, if the pin tracts are clean and there is no sign of a pin tract in-

fection. This is another reason why an early decision is helpful when contemplating grafting. The longer the pins remain in, the greater the likelihood of pin tract problems.

The iliac crest and the entire length of the anterior aspect of the thigh are surgically prepared (Fig. 19-33). The distraction device is carefully sealed out of the field by sterile adhesive drapes *prior* to the surgical preparation. This renders the field clean over the anterolateral aspect of the femur. Prior to making the thigh incision, a generous quantity of iliac bone is obtained through an incision over the iliac crest. This wound is then closed, and the second incision is made on the thigh. The remaining and regrown fascia lata is incised, and the interval between the vastus lateralis and the vastus intermedius is developed. The proximal and distal fragments are exposed subperiosteally for a distance long enough to receive the specially designed eight-hole plate, with four holes for each fragment. The defect between the bone is cleaned of any soft tissue, and the ends of the bone are appropriately denuded, so as to receive the bone graft. The plate is applied, using specially designed screws, and the defect is filled with the iliac bone. The wound is closed routinely and the distraction device is removed. Usually no cast is necessary (Fig.

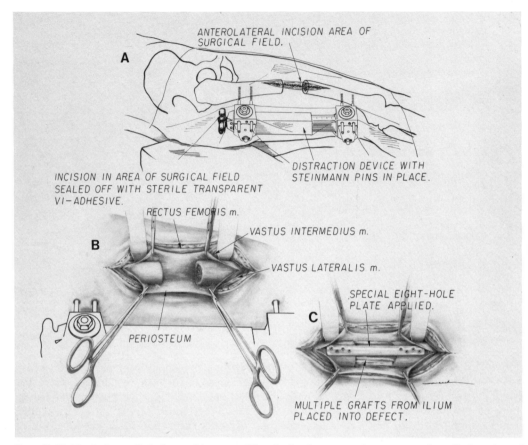

FIG. 19-33. Technique of plating and bone grafting for inadequate union or nonunion of a lengthened area. The iliac crest and anterolateral aspect of the thigh are surgically prepared. The distraction pins are carefully draped out of the operative field and out of the field of surgical preparation. The distraction device is purposely left intact, as long as the pins are clean and if they can be adequately excluded from the operative field. *(A)* The incision and its relationship to the distraction device. *(B)* The bone is shown, with a periosteal tube elevated for reception of the bone graft. *(C)* The special eight-hole plate is applied on the anterolateral aspect of the femur, and the defect is filled with iliac grafts. Periosteum is then closed as well as is possible, and the wound is closed in layers. Fixation by the special plate is usually sufficiently strong so that the distraction device may be removed safely. This encourages greater knee motion, since the pins are removed from the quadriceps muscle.

19-34). An alternate surgical approach is done with the patient prone. A postero-lateral incision is made, and grafts are obtained from the posterior ilium.

Postoperatively, active knee motion is begun. Complete knee motion may not be achieved for several months. In the meantime, solid strong union of the lengthened femur should have occurred. Weightbearing is permitted, according to the judgement of the surgeon. Because of the rigidity and strength of the plate, its removal is advise-able at a time when its need has been exceeded.

Osteotomy and Sudden Distraction. Codivilla's[30] initial effort to increase the limb length by femoral elongation involved a principle of sudden or rapid distraction. This was accompanied by a significant number and variety of complications. Since then several techniques have been practiced, which conceptually have been designed to

FIG. 19-34. A 13-year-old male with a congenital shortening of the right lower limb who had previously undergone tibial lengthening for a shortening of 8 cm. *(A)* The orthoroentgenogram shows that the lower limb is still 4 cm. short. *(B)* Ten weeks after Wagner femoral lengthening, the amount of bone bridging the distracted fragments is obviously inadequate and, therefore, an autogenous bone grafting and plating of the femur were accomplished. *(C)* The results of the plating and grafting procedure.

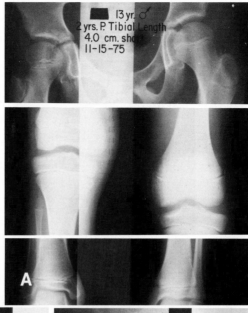

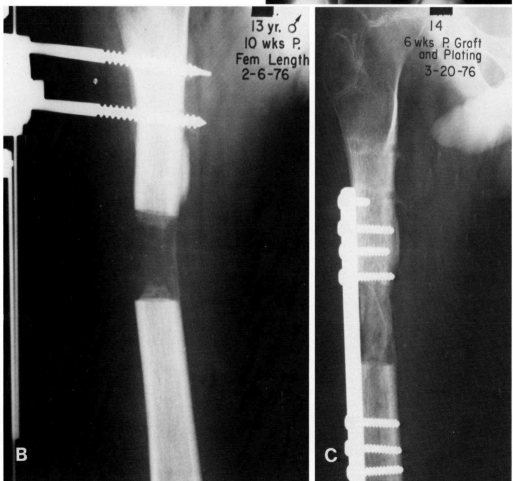

achieve lengthening without the prolonged morbidity and technical challenge of gradual distraction. As far as popularity and acceptance is concerned, however, none has achieved or maintained the level of acceptance of the techniques outlined above. It is appropriate, however, that each be mentioned with reference to the original source.

Sudden, immediate lengthening of the femur on the short side, along with simultaneous shortening of the contralateral femur has been recently suggested by Merle d'Aubigne and Duboussett[66] The technique involves removal of an approximately 1-inch long full segment of femur on the long side, with insertion of this autograft into an 1-inch distraction defect on the short side. The osteotomized fragments are internally fixed by an intramedullary rod. It was felt that this procedure could accomplish 2 inches of correction in a single operative exercise. The two negative features which have vitiated the value of this operation include the facts that both limbs had to undergo simultaneous major surgery, and that the bone graft placed in the lengthened side frequently underwent some degree of resorption. The increased morbidity occasioned by the bilateral surgical procedure and the lack of predictable equalization is self-evident, and this operation has, therefore, largely been abandoned.

In 1912, Magnusson[64] attempted a femoral lengthening on a Hawley table by distracting the bone fragments all at once. He experienced disastrous results, and one patient actually died of shock. Since that time, no convincingly favorable results have been reported with the sudden distraction technique. Furthermore, as shown by Calandriello,[26] sudden stretch on muscles may produce extensive scarring and ultimate compromise of muscle function. The methods utilizing sudden elongation of the femur, therefore, have not been well accepted, not only because of the uncertainty with respect to the degree of lengthening that can be expected, but also because of the serious potential complications inherent in the techniques. I have had no personal experience with any of the foregoing technical procedures involving sudden lengthening, and I recommend that they not be employed.

Pelvic Osteotomy. Although uncommonly practiced, the indication for its use occurring infrequently, pelvic osteotomy can be utilized to gain up to 1 inch of length by sudden separation of the distal fragment of a complete innominate osteotomy. With downward and outward displacement of an appropriately executed osteotomy, little resistance to the lengthening is encountered. The tendinous portion of the iliopsoas muscle must be released, and the abductors must be recessed downward from the iliac crest. All else then moves distally with the inferior fragment. A trapezoid- rather than a triangular-shaped graft is removed from the iliac crest and it is placed in the osteotomy defect in the same manner as described by Salter.[79] Two large threaded pins must be used to hold the fragments in the corrected position while union occurs. A one and one-half hip spica cast must be employed for at least 8 weeks, followed by nonweightbearing and crutch walking, until firm union and maturation of the bridged defect has occurred (Fig. 19-35). The same technical pitfalls exist as for Salter's innominate osteotomy.

When the acetabulum is normal, this procedure should probably be used only in instances of severe shortening, as an adjunct to other equalization procedures. The uncertainty inherent in altering the relationships of a normal acetabulum does not warrant its routine use; however, for obvious reasons, the procedure may be indicated in the rare case exhibiting a dysplastic acetabulum. As an extension of this concept, the innominate osteotomy may be required before femoral lengthening whenever a dysplastic acetabulum exists. This is done in order that a stable hip can be achieved. It is clear that the need for such a procedure is rare indeed, if the above indications are followed.

Tibial Lengthening by Osteotomy and Gradual Distraction

Historically, this is the most time-proven and consistently reliable method of elongating the lower limb. As noted earlier, Abbott[1] is given credit for developing the basic concepts of tibial lengthening and proving that it is a feasible procedure, in certain instances. It has survived the many controversies surrounding lengthening procedures in general,

FIG. 19-35. An anteroposterior view of the pelvis, showing a 1-inch gain in elongation of the left lower limb by means of a modified Salter osteotomy. A large trapezoid-shaped graft was used, with no specific effort made towards rotation of the distal fragment. The gain in length from the iliac crest to the floor was 1 inch.

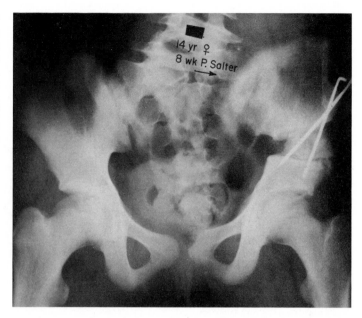

and currently it remains a very valuable procedure when properly done under the right circumstances. More recently, Anderson[8] introduced a novel variation in the technique whereby the osteotomy is accomplished through a percutaneous drilling operation (see p. 846). This has simplified the procedure and has minimized some of the complications which were so feared when the open osteotomy was done. The transverse, percutaneous "semi-open" osteotomy is currently the procedure most commonly used, and it is the one preferred by the author.

Indications. This procedure may be indicated in one of the situations listed below. It is essential, however, that all of the factors mentioned earlier be reviewed prior to reaching a decision to perform this operation. The possible indications are as follows: (1) in a patient with shortening in excess of 4.0 cm., preferably with the majority of the discrepancy being located in the tibia; (2) in a patient whose discrepancy justifies surgical equalization, but who is skeletally too old for epiphyseal arrest; (3) in a patient who has a major discrepancy exceeding that which can be acceptably corrected by epiphyseal arrest or shortening alone; and (4) in patients in whom amputa-

tion (and prosthetic prescription) is a likely alternative. In evaluating the indications, it is essential that the prerequisites for tibial lengthening be identified.

Prerequisites. Several criteria must be met before tibial lengthening can be seriously considered. The prerequisites can be listed as follows: (1) a plantigrade foot or one that can be made so; (2) a stable ankle; (3) good muscle balance in the foot and ankle; (4) normal vasculature of the limb; (5) a stable knee with a normal range of motion; and (6) a patient who is normotensive, with no serious and evident extenuating physical or emotional problems.

Contraindications. Clearly, this procedure is contraindicated in anyone not meeting the indications or the prerequisites for tibial lengthening. In addition, severe soft-tissue scarring, poor skin condition, sclerotic bone, and instances where there is a prior history of bone infection or nonunion or pseudarthrosis may represent contraindications. However, even these must be viewed with circumspection, since Stelling[86] has safely and effectively performed tibial lengthening in a case of shortening due to congenital pseudarthrosis, once union had been achieved. However, this is not recommended except for the surgeon who is con-

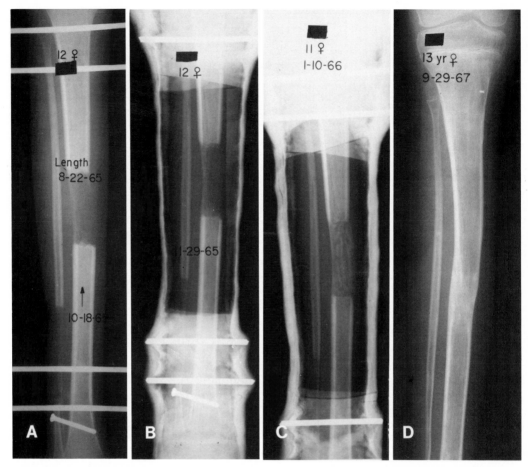

FIG. 19-36. *(A)* Tibial lengthening, approximately 10 weeks following the initial lengthening procedure. Note that there is little bone evident in the lengthened area. *(B)* Six weeks later, there is little increase in bridging of the lengthened area. *(C)* The iliac bone grafts placed between the bone ends in the defect are seen. *(D)* Solid union is seen not only in the tibia but also in the fibula 9 months after the grafting procedure.

versant with all of the problems inherent in tibial lengthening, as well as with those accompanying the treatment of congenital pseudarthrosis. The need for concern regarding the other soft tissues and bones is self-evident.

Advantages. Because of the subcutaneous location of the tibia, and because of the usual presence of the fibula, certain advantages are obtained by tibial lengthening, as compared to femoral lengthening. First of all the procedure is technically less complicated; secondly, the hardware employed is much more uniformly designed; and thirdly, the procedure has fewer major complications,

and treatment of them is rendered simpler by the unique anatomy of the leg.

Disadvantages and Complications. Lengthening is an unphysiologic operation, and it results in a variety of complications, which must be anticipated whenever this procedure is done. These complications represent the disadvantage of this procedure, as opposed to simpler forms of equalization, such as shortening by resection or growth arrest. The complications and their treatment represent a very important feature of this section, because it is with these issues that the surgeon and the patient must contend when considering tibial lengthening.

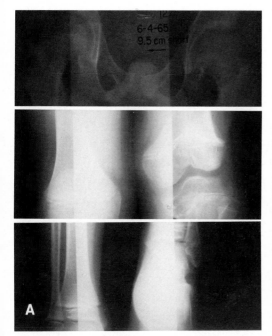

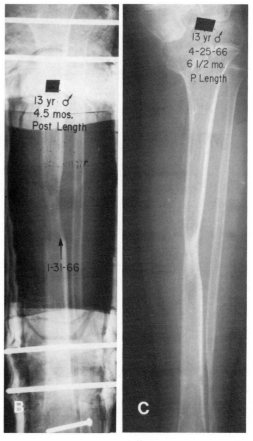

FIG. 19-37. *(A)* The orthoroentgenogram of a 12-year-old male with excessive shortening as the result of pyogenic osteomyelitis and arrest of the proximal tibial and distal femoral epiphyses on the left. *(B)* A tibial lengthening was accomplished, and in 4¹/₂ months following lengthening, the fragments had united, but were not quite solid enough for weightbearing. *(C)* Six and one-half months after lengthening, with no intervention by bone grafting, solid union ensued, with sufficient strength to permit protected weightbearing. If progressively increasing strength of the bone bridging the defects is evident, bone grafting probably is not necessary.

In the skeletally mature patient, the complication rate from tibial lengthening is greater than in the skeletally less mature patient. Also, as noted earlier, patients whose shortening is the result of congenital problems have a higher incidence of complications than those whose discrepancy is due to paralysis or the complications of skeletal infection or trauma. It is convenient to group the complications of lengthening as follows: (1) systemic; (2) local, at the tibial osteotomy site or in the pin tracts; (3) local, at the fibular osteotomy site; (4) regional, in the adjacent bones or joints; (5) neuromuscular; (6) vascular (compartment syndromes).

Systemic complications include emotional lability, mental depression, hypertension, anorexia and weight loss. These are all temporary conditions, and respond dramatically to cessation of lengthening. In rare instances weight loss and anorexia persist for several months, but once normal activity is resumed, these symptoms gradually subside. Hypertension does not seem to be as much of a problem in tibial lengthening as in femoral elongation.

Local complications most frequently consist of inadequate union, delayed union and nonunion of the tibial osteotomy site. Judgement is required to determine the indications for bone grafting. In cases of "inadequate union," the distracted area requires grafting when the bridging bone fails to hypertrophy over a period of 8 to 12 weeks (Fig. 19-36). In cases of delayed union, usually the bridged area strengthens with judicious use of weightbearing casts

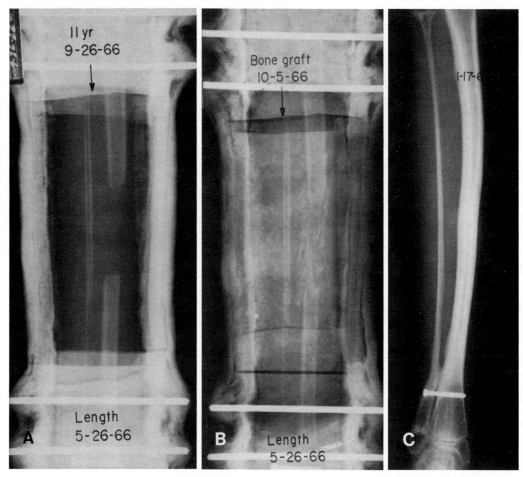

Fig. 19-38. *(A)* Four months after lengthening, there is no evidence of bone formed between the two distracted fragments. *(B)* The immediate postoperative film through the cast shows the bone grafts in place. *(C)* The final result demonstrates solid bony union and the reformed medullary cavity.

(Fig. 19-37). When nonunion exists, there is no evidence of bridging bone 6 to 8 weeks following cessation of lengthening, and grafting is mandatory (Fig. 19-38). Other complications include seepage about the pin tracts, which is very common, but a true pin tract infection is rare if appropriate care is given to the pins during and immediately following lengthening. Infection of the tibial osteotomy site occurred only once in our series. When it occurs, treatment must be given according to the usual principles of bone infection. Local complications may also occur in the area of the fibular osteotomy or resection. If the osteotomy fails to unite, and there is remaining skeletal

growth, then the transfixion screw between the tibia and fibula must not be removed unless union of the fibula is achieved by bone grafting, or unless the distal fibula is fused to the distal tibia. Since the fibula does not grow normally unless solidly united, failure of fibular union in this area results in progressive valgus deformity of the ankle, as a result of continued tibial growth and reduced growth of the distal fibula. Correction of this complication requires distal tibial osteotomy and creation of a tibio-fibular synostosis (Fig. 19-39).

Regional problems include knee flexion contractures, equinus of the ankle, accentuated valgus of the subtalar joint, and valgus deformity of the tibia. Most of these are reversible and respond well to an exercise program. On occasion, triple arthrodesis is necessary to correct the subtalar valgus of the foot.

Neuromuscular complications of any significance have been rare in our experience. Occasionally temporary interruption of lengthening has been necessitated because of the development of transient sensory changes in foot and leg. None has persisted. Significant motor loss occurred in one of our patients who sustained an anterior compartment syndrome and lost function of all of her dorsiflexors. This is discussed below under vascular complications.

Vascular complications of significance are rare. One patient in our series developed an anterior compartment syndrome and lost her entire anterior compartment as a result of muscle ischemic necrosis. The diagnosis was delayed and clouded by the relative absence of pain and the presence of a palpable dorsalis pedis pulse. We have had several instances of cavus foot developing following lengthening, and this seemingly is the result of unrecognized ischemia occurring in the intrinsic musculature of the foot. Because of this experience, as noted earlier, I now routinely perform an anterior compartment fasciotomy at the time of the initial lengthening procedure. It may be that fasciotomy of the posterior compartment is indicated, as well.

Technical Aspects. The surgical technique involved in tibial lengthening has been recorded in depth below, but the author feels that some innovations and qualifications in the technical details deserve special mention, as illustrated in Figure 19-40. In recent years I have modified the procedure of tibial lengthening in two ways. First, I no longer resect the fibula, as described earlier, rather, a long, oblique osteotomy is performed just above the tibial fibular transfixion. This is done in order to reduce the amount of separation of the fibula required following lengthening; it is believed that this discourages delayed and nonunion of the fibula (Fig. 19-39). Secondly, I routinely perform anterior compartment fasciotomy. Since doing this I have had no early or late sequelae traceable to neurovascular compromise of this compartment. As mentioned

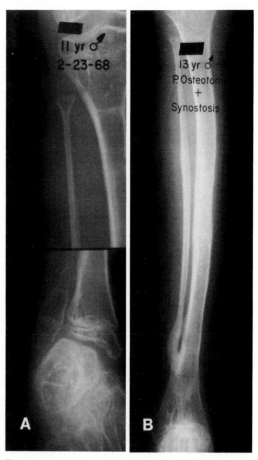

FIG. 19-39. *(A)* A valgus deformity of the ankle and deformation of the distal tibial epiphysis secondary to failure of union of the fibula. *(B)* Osteotomy of the distal tibia and synostosis of the fibula to the tibia resulted in correction of the deformity.

previously, possibly even a posterior compartment fasciotomy may be indicated in some cases, but I have not yet performed it.

It is also very important to monitor the blood pressure during tibial lengthening, just as in femoral lengthening. Occasionally it will be necessary to cease lengthening due to transient hypertension, but in over 100 lengthening procedures performed by me, permanent cessation of the elongation procedure due to this circumstance has not been required.

Technique. A 1½-inch incision is made over the lateral aspect of the distal fibula,

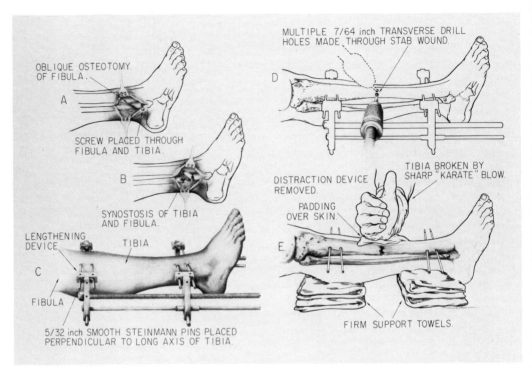

FIG. 19-40. Technique of tibial lengthening. *(A)* My preferred technique for stabilizing the ankle mortise. A screw is placed across the fibula into the tibia to stabilize the mortise, and a long oblique osteotomy of the fibula is accomplished just proximal to the screw. No bone from the fibula is removed, and the wound is closed. *(B)* An alternate method, originally suggested by Anderson, wherein a synostosis is created between the tibia and fibula. Six weeks must be allowed between creation of the synostosis and the subsequent tibial lengthening in order for synostosis to become solid. The objection to this approach is twofold: it requires two operative procedures, and it creates a permanent synostosis between the tibia and fibula. *(C)* The Steinman pins and the distraction device are in place. *(D)* The percutaneous drilling, which weakens the tibia through its midpoint. This is done through a small stab wound. Following effective weakening, the tibia is broken by means of a sharp "karate" blow. The distraction device is then reapplied precisely in the same fashion as shown in *(C)*, and distraction of approximately four turns is accomplished. A short cast is applied, extending from the toes to just below the upper pins. Not illustrated is the important step of a fasciotomy of the anterior compartment. (See text.)

just above the level of the distal tibial epiphysis. The fibula is exposed subperiosteally and a $^{7}/_{64}$-inch screw is placed across the fibula into the tibia at least $^{1}/_{4}$ to $^{1}/_{2}$ inch above the distal tibial epiphysis. This stabilizes the mortise of the ankle joint, and protects the fibular epiphysis during lengthening. A long, oblique fibular osteotomy is then made just above the screw. This is necessary to allow fibular distraction during the tibial lengthening process. The wound is closed.

Next, a vertical incision about 2 inches in length is made over the anterior aspect of the leg, centered over the anterior tibial muscle. The fascia of the calf is exposed and split longitudinally as far proximally and distally as possible to accomplish a decompression of the anterior compartment. Then, *only the skin and subcutaneous tissues* are closed. The purpose of this is to anticipate and possibly avoid the development of an anterior compartment syndrome during lengthening. With the distraction device in place, a stab wound is made over the lateral aspect of the proximal tibia, just below the tibial tubercle. Through the proximal hole of the distraction device, a smooth $5/32$-inch Steinmann pin is placed transversely through the long axis of the tibia in such a way that it passes through the companion hole of the distraction device on the medial side. It is very important to place this pin properly, because all other pins have to align with this pin. Care must also be exercised so that the pin pierces both cortices of the tibia. The second pin is then placed in the lower hole of the distal portion of the distraction device. At this point it is wise to pull the skin towards the midpoint of the tibia to reduce the stretch on the skin about the pin tracts during lengthening. This pin should be exactly parallel to the first pin in all directions. Similarly, the other two pins are placed so that the tibia is firmly transfixed above and below. The device is then squared in all directions, and the lock nuts are secured. This assures the surgeon that when the device is replaced following osteotomy, the fragments will be in the same alignment as the intact tibia. The device is then removed, leaving the pins in place.

A stab wound is made over the anterior crest of the tibia at its midportion. Using a $7/64$-inch drill, the tibia is drilled transversely and percutaneously many times so as to weaken the bone. The leg is then suspended between two elevations of sterile surgical drapes, and the tibia is broken by means of a sharp, direct blow over the drilled portion. The pretibial skin should be well padded to protect not only the skin of the tibia, but also the surgeon's hand. If excessive difficulty is encountered in fracturing the tibia, a small osteotome can be inserted to complete the osteotomy.

After the percutaneous osteotomy has been accomplished, the lengthening device is reapplied exactly as it had been placed in the intact tibia. Palpation of the subcutaneous crest of the tibia usually verifies the absence of any offset or angulation. The device is secured to the pins, and six turns of the lengthening screws are made. This accomplishes two things: it separates the fragments, which may reduce the immediate postoperative pain, and it reduces the duration of subsequent elongation. If the heel

cord is tight, a percutaneous lengthening may be done, if it had not been done earlier in the surgery. The pins are sealed with collodion over sterile sheet wadding. A short cast is applied, which extends up to *but not including* the proximal pins. The ankle and foot should be held in a neutral position. If there is any tendency to valgus or varus angulation, a transverse pin may be placed through the calcaneus, and this is incorporated in the cast. When the cast is dry, that portion of the cast over the dorsum of the foot and ankle is removed to enable the surgeon to keep close watch over the neurovascular status of the foot and limb.

Postoperatively the lengthening is begun on the second day, and the same postoperative routine is exercised here as in femoral lengthening (see p. 855). Eight weeks after the completion of lengthening, windows are removed from the anterior and posterior aspects of the cast. A roentgenogram is taken at that time to determine the status of union. If failure of union or inadequate union exists, prompt bone grafting is indicated. If union is satisfactory, the pins and cast may be removed and a new, snug, above-knee cast is applied. If union appears good, but not quite strong enough for pin removal, an additional 6 weeks of transfixion may be indicated. This requires good judgement on the part of the surgeon. Eventually a below-knee, patella-tendon-bearing (PTB) walking cast can be utilized, and gradually a removable polypropylene brace may be employed until recanalization of the medullary canal takes place.

Bone Grafting Following Tibial Lengthening Procedures. It is well known that a certain number of tibial lengthening procedures results in failure of union or develops "inadequate union." In these cases, bone grafting is necessary. My technique for this procedure is illustrated in Figure 19-41.

A large window is taken out of the anterior aspect of the cast, and the cast is thoroughly sealed away from the operative field by adhesive drapes. Great care must be exercised in the operative preparation and draping of the field, since the surgical procedure is done through a window in the cast.

A vertical incision approximately $2^{1}/_{2}$ inches long is made directly over the site of

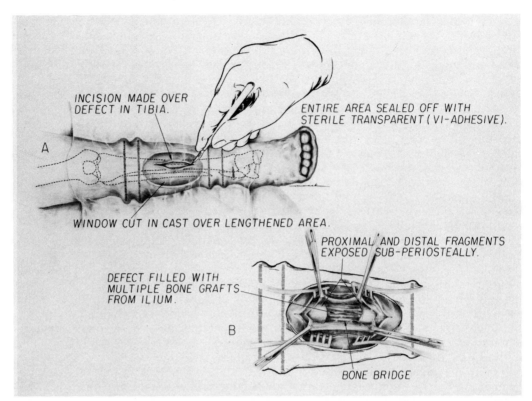

FIG. 19-41. Technique of bone grafting in the event of inadequate union or nonunion after tibial lengthening. Through a window in the cast lying over the anterior aspect of the tibia, the central one-third of the tibial crest is prepared and draped, utilizing sterile adhesive VIdrape. The cast must be assiduously draped out of the field to preserve sterility. A small 2-inch incision is made vertically over the defect in the tibia. The periosteum is reflected over the proximal and distal fragments, and the defect between the bone ends is thoroughly cleaned of all debris. *(B)* The defect is filled with bone grafts taken from the iliac crest. The periosteum is closed, along with the skin and subcutaneous tissues, and a compression dressing is applied.

the tibial defect. The exposure is very simple, because the bone is so subcutaneous in its location. The proximal and distal fragments are identified, and the intervening tissue between the two bone ends is thoroughly cleaned of soft tissue. I try to make a flap of soft tissue which will receive the bone grafts obtained from the iliac crest, just as was done in femoral grafting.

The bone grafts are then laid in the defect, and the skin and subcutaneous tissues are simply closed. This is a relatively simple operative procedure, but it must be emphasized that great care must be exercised in the operative preparation.

Usually within 8 weeks there is solid union of the tibia, and the pins may then be removed. At that time the same follow-up care is utilized as when the tibia unites without grafting.

LIMB LENGTH INEQUALITY DUE TO ANGULAR DEFORMITIES

Angular deformities can produce alterations in limb lengths in three ways, namely: (1) shortening, as a result of an asymmetrical growth arrest due to trauma or infection; (2) elongation, as a result of asymmetrical stimulation of growth following fracture or infection; or (3) angulation, following malunion of a fracture. The most significant problem in limb length discrepancy is that associated with asymmetrical growth arrest, because this may, depending upon the age at which it occurs, result in a very challenging therapeutic problem. Shortening of a lower limb due to an asymmetrical growth arrest means that a significant portion of the epiphyseal plate has been closed as a result of trauma or infection. The most common etiological factor is trauma, which may be surgical or nonsurgical (Fig. 19-42). The problem differs from symmetrical growth arrest in that there is not only a true limb length discrepancy, but also there is an angular deformity. The solution to the problem, therefore, must take into account both abnormalities.

The degree of limb length discrepancy, and to a comparable extent the degree of angulation, depends not only upon the age at which the insult occurs, but also upon the particular growth centers involved. Thus, growth centers about the knee, at comparable skeletal ages, produce greater degrees of limb length discrepancy and angular deformity than those at the hip or ankle, simply because of the differences in their contribution toward longitudinal growth of the limbs (see p. 806). In principle, however, the length and angular alterations must be approached similarly, regardless of their skeletal location.

In treating conditions involving limb shortening due to asymmetrical growth arrest, therefore, two fundamental problems surface: (1) correction of the angular deformity, and (2) correction of the limb length discrepancy. The solution to the length discrepancy embodies all of the fundamental issues which have been discussed earlier. The problem of the angular deformity, on the other hand, poses several different philosophical, biological, and technical questions. Philosophically, the issue centers around the factors of ultimate height, the need or tolerance for repeated operations such as osteotomies, and willingness to accept an operation in which the results cannot be accurately predicted. Biologically, the question involves such issues as the reversibility of an asymmetrical skeletal growth arrest, and the ability of a surgeon to alter a growth aberration in the bone after it has undergone such an arrest. Technically, of course, the issues focus on the various procedures available for correcting limb length

inequalities and angular deformities. Acquired deformities are almost always possible to correct from a technical standpoint, but deciding upon the procedure or procedures best suited to accomplish correction can tax the ingenuity of the most experienced surgeon. All of the factors mentioned in the earlier section on limb length inequality must be taken into account and, in addition, the technical problem of correcting angulation must be considered.

The special philosophical issues principally concern the willingness of the patient (and the parents) to undergo multiple operative procedures in order to correct angulation and shortening. In turn, this has a direct relationship to the problem of the ultimate length of the limb, as well as limb-trunk proportions. On the one hand, some degree of increased length can be achieved by multiple corrective angulation (opening wedge) osteotomies. By this means, the degree of discrepancy can be minimized, but probably can never be completely corrected, unless the child sustained the growth arrest towards the end of skeletal maturity. Conversely, by arresting growth completely by means of an angulation osteotomy through the physeal plate, prevention of the recurrence of deformity can be assured. However, ultimate total height will automatically be reduced on that side, and almost surely some form of major shortening or lengthening procedure will become necessary to achieve correction, especially if the initial asymmetrical arrest occurred when the possibility of significant skeletal growth remained. In summary, therefore, the complexity of the problem is even greater than in cases of pure limb length inequality, because decisions occasionally have to be made, which, by virtue of unique growth and skeletal age characteristics, may create new and different problems.

Biologically, there is some evidence to show that an asymmetrical bony bridge across the growth plate can be excised, and the deforming and shortening process can be reversed. Langenskiold[62] reported instances wherein resection of the osseous bridge, accompanied by replacement of the resected defect by fat, resulted in resumption of normal longitudinal growth. In Langenskiold's series, even some degree of cor-

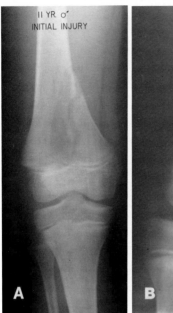

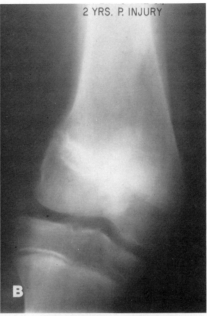

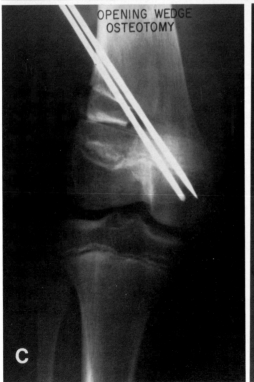

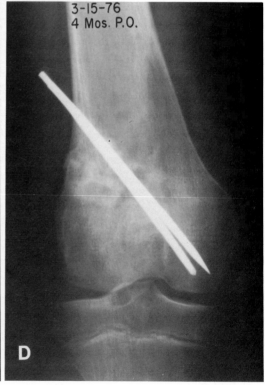

Fig. 19-42. *(A)* Roentgenogram of the distal femur and proximal tibia of a 10-year-old male who sustained a Type 2 epiphyseal injury. *(B)* Two years following injury the lateral aspect of the distal femoral epiphyseal plate is obviously fused, and there is an angular deformity of nearly 30°. There is also a 2-cm. shortening of the same limb. *(C)* The results of an opening wedge osteotomy. The angular deformity is corrected and there is a 2-cm. gain in length. *(D)* Four months postoperatively, the healed osteotomy is evident.

Fig. 19-43. *(A)* Roentgenogram of a child born with a congenital posterior bow of the left lower limb. *(B and C)* Ten months later, much of the deformity had corrected. *(D)* By the age of 7 years, almost complete correction had taken place, but there was 4.5 cm. of shortening of the left lower limb, predominantly in the tibia. This young girl was 59 inches tall at age 14, and because of the discrepancy being located predominantly in the tibia, a tibial lengthening was accomplished. *(E)* Bone grafting was required for union, but a satisfactory union with equal limb lengths is evident.

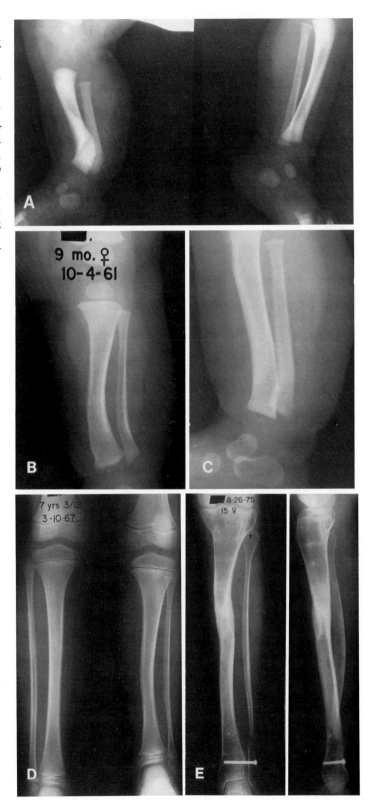

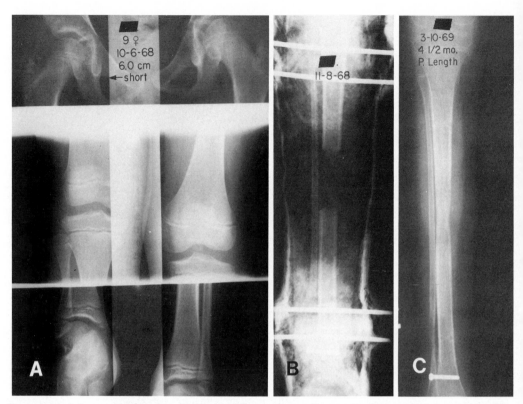

FIG. 19-44. A 9-year-old female with 6 cm. of shortening as the result of congenital shortening of the right lower limb. *(A)* Approximately equal shortening exists in both the femur and the tibia, as seen in the orthoroentgenogram. *(B)* The results of a 5.0-cm. tibial lengthening. *(C)* Four and one-half months after lengthening, the tibia is solidly united, and the patient is fully ambulatory without protection. *(Legend continued on facing page.)*

rection of the angular deformity occasionally occurred. This surgical procudure requires a very precise analysis and location of the anatomical abnormality and resection of the bony bridge requires not only great technical skill and experience with a dental bur, but also the need for a dissecting microscope. Also, because of the close proximity of some physeal plates to their adjacent articular cartilages, the operation is probably only technically practical in the physeal plates about the knee and ankle.

Although I have had no surgical experience with the operation, I feel that the results of this operative procedure are unpredictable, and at the present time the operation must be considered as exploratory and uncertain. Nevertheless, it has promise, especially in younger children, when the freightening magnitude of the potential length discrepancy and angular deformity may justify its use. I feel in older children, over the skeletal age of 12 or 13 years, however, that the more conventional and proven methods of correction are preferred.

Technically, all of the various procedures discussed under correction of limb length inequality may be utilized at one time or another in different circumstances to correct the limb length discrepancy. In addition, the use of angulation osteotomy (both opening and closing wedge) or asymmetrical epiphyseal plate stapling (temporary growth arrest) is almost always required for correction of the angular component of the prob-

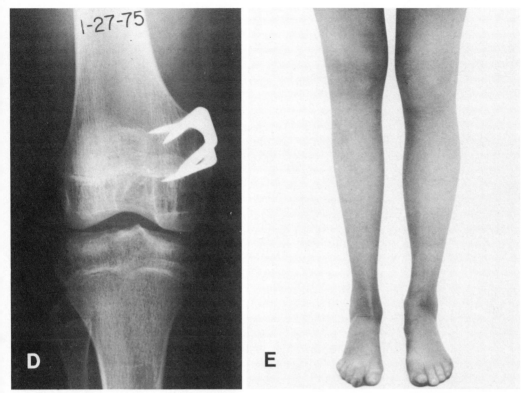

FIG. 19-44 *(Continued). (D)* Because of an angular deformity of the knee and the residual shortening, a simultaneous medial femoral stapling on the short side and an arrest of the longer distal femoral epiphysis was accomplished. *(E)* A standing photograph shows equal limb lengths. It demonstrates that a slight difference in knee levels is not cosmetically significant. This illustrates the value of utilizing bone lengthening procedures, shortening procedures (epiphyseal arrest), and epiphyseal stapling for correction of angular deformities.

lem. These procedures have been well proven, and they are predictable as well as versatile.

Treatment

In approaching the problems of limb length inequality and angular deformity, due to malunion or fracture or asymmetrical growth arrest, each patient presents with a singular set of anatomical facts, variables and circumstances. The solutions to the problem are equally variable and versatile. It is impossible to design a specific program of treatment which will satisfactorily solve all problems. One must take all factors into account, weigh the importance of each facet of the problem, and fabricate a solution which best meets the needs and desires of the patient and the parents. The analysis of the problem and the fabrication of the solution clearly requires, in each instance, knowledge and compassionate consideration of the philosophical issues, thorough understanding of the biology of the physeal plate, and well-founded technical expertise and experience in performing the various operative procedures.

IMPLEMENTATION OF EQUALIZATION PROCEDURES

It is impossible to provide explicit guidelines for any given method of equalization. This becomes particularly obvious when the

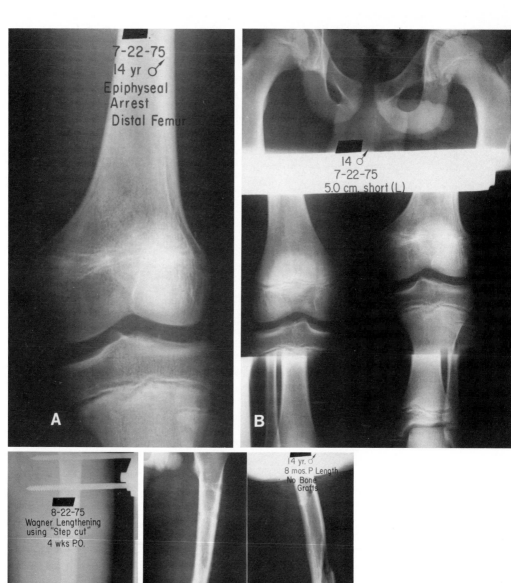

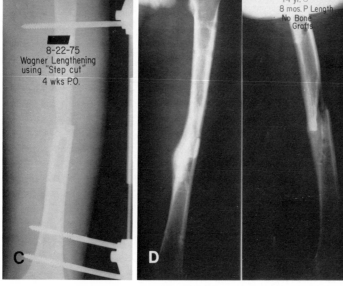

wide variety of techniques are reviewed and the many factors influencing the decision for or against equalization are considered. However, in addition to those situations described earlier in the text, a few examples of how certain specific procedures and combinations of equalization procedures may be employed are illustrated below.

Tibial Lengthening Only

Tibial lengthening for congenital shortening of the tibia was accomplished in a skeletally mature 14-year-old girl. She was born with a posterior bow of the tibia and fibula, and at skeletal maturity the bones straightened spontaneously, but there was 4.0 cm. of limb shortening, all in the tibia. Because her height was only 59 inches, and because she did not want to be further shortened, it was elected to accomplish a tibial lengthening, as described in the text. She required a bone graft for ultimate union, but bone grafting is not unusual following lengthening of any congenitally short bone.

The salient point to emphasize in this patient is that tibial lengthening alone is suitable for one of unusually short stature, especially when the shortening is predominantly in the tibia (Fig. 19-43).

Tibial Lengthening, Contralateral Distal Femoral Epiphysiodesis and Ipsilateral Medial Femoral Stapling

Tibial lengthening was felt indicated in a 9-year-old girl whose congenital lower limb shortening of 6.0 cm. was located predominantly in the tibia. The lengthening procedure was successful, and this was followed by epiphysiodesis of the distal femur on the long side. Because of an angular deformity at the knee on the congenitally short side, a stapling of that distal femoral physeal plate was accomplished, as described in the text (Fig. 19-25). At skeletal maturity her limb

lengths were equal, despite a slight discrepancy in the knee heights.

This patient demonstrates the occasional need for a combination of equalization procedures that are appropriately timed (Fig. 19-44).

Femoral Lengthening Only

A femoral lengthening alone was accomplished in a 14-year-old boy whose 5.0 cm. limb length discrepancy was confined to the femur. The shortening was due to traumatic premature physeal plate arrest in the distal femur. His anticipated adult height was 67 inches, and the patient preferred lengthening to shortening. This etiologic type of acquired shortening is most appropriately suited to a lengthening procedure, if indicated. Union rapidly occurred in this patient, whose femur was lengthened by a modified Wagner technique.

When the shortening is located predominantly in the femur and is acquired rather than congenital in etiology, femoral lengthening is preferred over tibial lengthening (Fig. 19-45).

Femoral and Ipsilateral Tibial Lengthening and Contralateral Distal Femoral Epiphysiodesis

Femoral lengthening (Bost type), tibial lengthening (Anderson type) and distal femoral physeal arrest on the long side were necessary in a 12-year-old boy to achieve satisfactory equalization. The shortening was due to partial physeal plate arrest secondary to osteomyelitis, and the projected discrepancy was in excess of 16.0 cm. He previously had distal femoral and proximal tibial osteotomies in order to correct angular deformities.

This patient illustrates how multiple equalization procedures may occasionally be justified, even when the projected discrepancy

FIG. 19-45. *(A)* A 14-year-old male presenting with a 5 cm. shortening due to arrest of the distal femoral epiphysis following trauma. *(B)* The scanogram reveals the amount of discrepancy and shows that it is entirely in the femur. This patient was only 66 inches tall, with an anticipated adult height of 68 inches. It was his desire that his femur be lengthened on the short side, rather than shortened on the long side. *(C)* Four weeks postoperatively, the distraction device can be seen in place, with lengthening of 5 cm. *(D)* Eight months postoperatively, solid union of the femur has been achieved. This step-cut lengthening is not recommended for the Wagner technique, since it compromises the technique of plating and bone-grafting, if it is necessary.

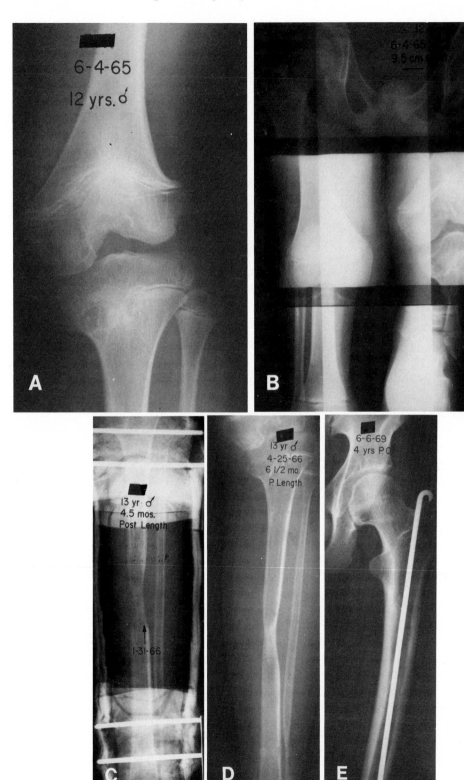

FIG. 19-46. A 12-year-old male was seen initially for lower limb shortening secondary to pyogenic osteomyelitis of the distal femur and proximal tibia, resulting in arrest of the distal femoral epiphysis and partial arrest of the proximal tibial epiphysis. Osteotomies of the distal femur and proximal tibia had been done to correct angular deformities. *(A)* The deformity of both physeal plates and the angular deformity of the knee joint. *(B)* The limb length inequality by orthoroentgenogram measures 9.5 cm. *(C)* The results of tibial lengthening. *(D)* The appearance some 6¹/₂ months postoperatively. *(E)* A Bost-type femoral lengthening was accomplished, and the results of that procedure are shown.

(F) An orthoroentgenogram shows the discrepancy at skeletal maturity. In the interim, a distal femoral epiphyseal arrest had been accomplished, and the combined procedures, therefore, resulted in equalization of some 14 cm., with 5 cm. of correction in the tibia and 5 cm. in the femur by lengthening, and a 4-cm. correction was achieved by distal femoral arrest. This illustrates how a variety of equalization procedures may be employed to achieve satisfactory correction.

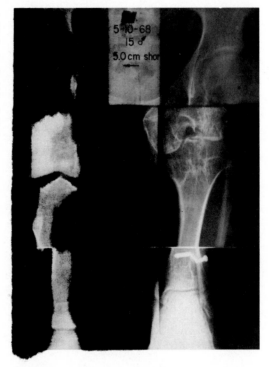

exceeds the conventional upper limits of 15.0 cm (Fig. 19-46).

These cases demonstrate how the various equalization procedures can be employed under a variety of circumstances. In each instance, all factors influencing the choice of equalization procedures were evaluated in depth. In addition to these deliberations, all indications and prerequisites of each procedure had to be met, and the patient and parents were sufficiently well informed so that they could intelligently participate in the decision to proceed with the operative program. It is sometimes extremely difficult to arrive at these decisions, and often repeated discussions are required to clarify the various aspects of the problem. It is impossible to devise a "cookbook" equalization program on the basis of x-ray films and physical examination alone. The need for individualization and selective evaluation of an equalization program cannot be overemphasized, because only by carefully weighing *all* of the facets of a problem of limb length inequality is it possible to arrive at the appropriate solution.

The author wishes to express appreciation and gratitude to his research assistant, Mrs. K. A. Morton, for her valuable assistance and helpful suggestions in preparation of the manuscript.

REFERENCES

1. Abbott, L. C., and Crego, C. H.: Operative lengthening of the femur. South. Med. J., *21:*823, 1928.
2. Agerholm, J.: The zig-zag osteotomy. Acta Orthop. Scand., *29:*63, 1959.
3. Aitken, A. P., Blackett, C. W., and Ciacotti, J. J.: Over-growth of the femoral shaft following fractures in childhood. J. Bone Joint Surg., *21:*334, 1939.
4. Aitken, G. T.: Personal communication, 1976.
5. Allan, P. G.: Bone-lengthening. J. Bone Joint Surg., *30B:*490, 1948.
6. ———: Leg lengthening. Br. Med. J., *1:*218, 1951.
7. ———: Simultaneous femoral and tibial lengthening. J. Bone Joint Surg., *45B:*206, 1963.
8. Anderson, W. V.: Leg lengthening. J. Bone Joint Surg., *34B:*150, 1952.
9. Barford, B., and Christensen, J.: Fractures of the femoral shaft in children with special reference to subsequent overgrowth. Acta Chir. Scand., *116:*235, 1958-59.
10. Barr, J. S., Stinchfield, A. G., and Reidy, J. A.: Sympathetic ganglionectomy and limb length in poliomyelitis. J. Bone Joint Surg., *32A:*793, 1950.
11. Bayley, N.: Tables for predicting adult height and skeletal age and present height. J. Pediatr., *28:*49, 1946.
12. Bianco, A. J.: Personal communication, 1975.
13. Bisgard, J. D.: Longitudinal bone growth, the influence of sympathetic deinnervation. Ann. Surg., *97:*374, 1933.
14. ———: Longitudinal overgrowth of long bones with special reference to fractures. Surg. Gynecol. Obstet., *62:*823, 1936.
15. Blount, W. P.: Blade-plate internal fixation for high femoral osteotomies. J. Bone Joint Surg., *25:*319, 1943.
16. ———: Fractures in Children. Baltimore, Williams & Wilkins, 1954.
17. ———: Trauma and Growing Bones. Septiéme Congres de la Société Internationale de Chirurgie Orthopédique et de Traumatologie. Barcelona, 1957.
18. ———: Unequal leg length in children. Surg. Clin. North Am., *38:*1107, 1958.
19. ———: Unequal Leg Length. AAOS Instruc. Course Lect., *17,* 1960.
20. Blount, W. P., and Clark, G. R.: Control of bone growth by epiphyseal stapling. Preliminary report. J. Bone Joint Surg., *31A:*464, 1949.
21. Bohlman, H. R.: Experiments with foreign materials in the region of the epiphyseal cartilage plate of growing bones to increase their longitudinal growth. J. Bone Joint Surg., *11:*365, 1929.
22. Bost, F. C.: Operative lengthening of the bones of the lower extremity. AAOS Instruc. Course Lect., *1,* 1944.
23. Bost, F. C., and Larsen, L. J.: Experiences with lengthening of the femur over an intramedullary rod. J. Bone Joint Surg., *38A:*567, 1956.
24. Brockway, A., Craig, W. A., and Cockrell, B. R., Jr.: End result of 62 stapling operations. J. Bone Joint Surg., *36A:*1063, 1954.
25. Brockway, A., and Fowler, S. B.: Experiences with 105 leg-lengthening operations. Surg. Gynecol. Obstet., *72:*252, 1942.
26. Calandriello, B.: The behavior of muscle fibres during surgical lengthening of a limb. Ital. J. Orthop. Traumatol., *1:*231, 1975.
27. Calvé, J., and Galland, M.: A new procedure for compensatory shortening of the unaffected femur in cases of considerable symmetry of the lower limbs (fractures of the femur, coxalgia, etc.). Am. J. Orthop. Surg., *16:*211, 1918.
28. Cameron, B. M.: A technique for femoral shaft shortening. A preliminary report. J. Bone Joint Surg., *39A:*1309, 1957.
29. Carpenter, E. B., and Dalton, J. B., Jr.: A critical evaluation of a method of epiphyseal stimulation. Followup notes on article previously published. J. Bone Joint Surg., *45A:*642, 1963.
30. Codivilla, A.: On the means of lengthening in the lower limbs, the muscles and tissues which are shortened through deformity. Am. J. Orthop. Surg., *2:*353, 1905.
31. Cole, W. H.: Results of treatment of fractured femurs. Arch. Surg., *5:*702, 1922.
32. Coleman, S. S.: Management of Complications of Tibial Lengthening. Proc. of the 11th Congress, Soc. Internat. de Chirurgie Orthopedique et de Traumatologie. Mexico City, 1969.
33. ———: Current concepts of tibial lengthening. Orthop. Clin. North Am., *3:*201, 1972.
34. Coleman, S. S., and Noonan, T. D.: Anderson's method of tibial lengthening by percutaneous osteotomy and gradual distraction. Experiences with 31 cases. J. Bone Joint Surg., *49A:*263, 1967.
35. Compere, E. L.: Indications for and against the leg lengthening operation. J. Bone Joint Surg., *18:*692, 1936.
36. Compere, E. L., and Adams, C. O.: Studies of the longitudinal growth of long bones; the influence of trauma to the diaphysis. J. Bone Joint Surg., *19:*922, 1937.
37. David, V. C.: Shortening and compensatory overgrowth following fractures of the femur in children. Arch. Surg., *9:*438, 1924.
38. Diveley, R. L.: Foot appliances and shoe alterations. Orthopedic Appliances Atlas, *1:*471, 1952.
39. Eyre-Brook, A. L.: Bone shortening for inequality of leg lengths. Br. Med. J., *1:*222, 1951.
40. Fahey, J. J.: The effect of lumbar sympathetic ganglionectomy on longitudinal bone growth as determined by the teleoroentgenographic method. J. Bone Joint Surg., *18:*1042, 1936.
41. Gatewood, and Mullen, B. P.: Experimental observations on the growth of long bones. Arch. Surg., *15:*215, 1927.
42. Goff, C. W.: Surgical Treatment of Unequal Extremities. Springfield, Charles C Thomas, 1960.
43. Green, W. T., and Anderson, M.: Experiences with epiphyseal arrest in correcting discrepancies in length of the lower extremities in infantile paralysis. J. Bone Joint Surg., *29:*659, 1947.
44. ———: The problem of unequal leg lengths. Pediatr. Clin. North Am. *2:*1137, 1955.
45. ———: Skeletal Age and Control of Bone Growth. AAOS Instruc. Course Lect., *17,* 199, 1960.

46. Greulich, W. W., and Pyle, S. I.: Radiographic Atlas of Skeletal Development of the Hand and Wrist, ed. 2. Stanford University Press, 1959.

47. Gross, R. H.: An evaluation of tibial lengthening procedures. J. Bone Joint Surg., *53A:*693, 1971.

48. Haas, S. L.: The relation of the blood supply to the longitudinal growth of bone. Am. J. Orthop. Surg., *15:*157, 305, 1917.

49. ———: Retardation of bone growth by a wire loop. J. Bone Joint Surg., *27:*25, 1945.

50. ———: Mechanical retardation of bone growth. J. Bone Joint Surg., *30A:*506, 1948.

51. ———: Stimulation of bone growth. Am. J. Surg., *95:*125, 1958.

52. Harandi, B. A., and Zahir, A.: Severe hypertension following correction of flexion contractures of the knee. A report of 2 cases. J. Bone Joint Surg., *56A:*1733, 1974.

53. Harmon, P. H., and Krigsten, W. M.: The surgical treatment of unequal leg length. Surg. Gynecol. Obstet., *71:*482, 1940.

54. Harris, R. I., and McDonald, J. L.: The effect of lumbar sympathectomy upon the growth of legs paralysed by anterior poliomyelitis. J. Bone Joint Surg., *18:*35, 1936.

55. Howorth, M. B.: Leg-shortening operation for equalizing leg length. Arch. Surg., *44:*543, 1942.

56. Janes, J. M., and Jennings, W. K.: Effect of induced arteriovenous fistula on leg length. Ten-year observations. Proc. Mayo Clinic, *36:*1, 1961.

57. Janes, J. M., and Musgrove, J. E.: Effect of arteriovenous fistula on growth of bone. Preliminary report. Proc. Mayo Clinic, *24:*405, 1949.

58. ———: Effect of arteriovenous fistula on growth of bone. Surg. Clin. North Am., *30:*1191, 1950.

59. Kawamura, B.: Leg Lengthening, Principles Involved and the Limiting Factors. Proc. of the 11th Cong., Soc. Internat. de Chirgurie et de Traumatologie. Mexico City, 1969.

60. Kawamura, B., Mosona, S., Takahaski, T., Yano, T., Kobayashi, Y., *et al.*: Limb lengthening by means of subcutaneous osteotomy. J. Bone Joint Surg., *50A:*851, 1968.

61. Khoury, S. C., Silberman, F. S., and Cabrine, R. L.: Stimulation of the longitudinal growth of long bones by periosteal stripping. J. Bone Joint Surg., *45A:*1679, 1963.

62. Langenskiold, A.: Personal communication, 1975.

63. McCarroll, H. R.: Trials and tribulations in attempted femoral lengthening. J. Bone Joint Surg., *32A:*132, 1950.

64. Magnuson, P. B.: Lengthening of shortened bones of the leg by operation. Surg. Gynecol. Obstet., *17:*63, 1913.

65. May, V. R., Jr., and Clemens, E. L.: Epiphyseal stapling with special reference to complications. South. Med. J., *58:*1203, 1965.

66. Merle D'Aubigne, R., and Dubousset, J.: Surgical correction of large length discrepancies in the lower extremities of children and adults, J. Bone Joint Surg., *53A:*411, 1971.

67. Moore, J. R.: Tibial lengthening and femoral shortening. Pa. Med. J., *36:*751, 1933.

68. Moore, R. D.: Supracondylar shortening of the femur for leg length inequality. Surg., Gynecol. Obstet., *84:*1087, 1947.

69. Moseley, C. F.: A straight line graph for leg length discrepancies. J. Bone Joint Surg., *59A:* 174-179, 1977.

70. Ollier, L.: Traite experimental et clinique de la regeneration des os et de la production artificielle du tissu asseux. Paris, Masson, 1867.

71. Pease, C. N.: Local stimulation of growth of long bones, a preliminary report. J. Bone Joint Surg., *34A:*1, 1952.

72. Phalen, G. S., and Chatterton, C. C.: Equalizing the lower extremities: a clinical consideration of leg lengthening versus leg shortening. Surgery, *12:*678, 1942.

73. Phemister, D. B.: Operative arrestment of longitudinal growth of bones in the treatment of deformities. J. Bone Joint Surg., *15:*1, 1933.

74. ———: Bone growth and repair. Ann. Surg., *102:*261, 1935.

75. Poirier, H.: Epiphyseal stapling and leg equalization, J. Bone Joint Surg., *50B:*61, 1968.

76. Putti. V.: The operative lengthening of the femur. J.A.M.A., *77:*934, 1921.

77. ———: Operative lengthening of the femur. Surg. Gynecol. Obstet., *58:*318, 1934.

78. Regan, J. M., and Chatterton, C. C.: Deformities following surgical epiphyseal arrest. J. Bone Joint Surg., *28:*265, 1946.

79. Salter, R. B.: Innominate osteotomy in the treatment of congenital dislocation and subluxation of the hip. J. Bone Joint Surg., *43B:*518, 1961.

80. Salter, R. B., Harris, W. R.: Injuries involving the epiphyseal plate. J. Bone Joint Surg., *45A:*587, 1963.

81. Sofield, H. A.: Leg lengthening. Surg. Clin. North Am. *19:*69, 1939.

82. ———: Personal communication, 1965.

83. Sofield, H. A., Blair, S. J., and Millar, E. A.: Leg lengthening. A personal follow-up of 40 patients some years after the operation. J. Bone Joint Surg., *40A:*311, 1958.

84. Speed, K.: Longitudinal overgrowth of long Bones. Surg. Gynecol. Obstet., *37:*787, 1923.

85. Staheli, L. T.: Late femoral and tibial length inequality following femoral shaft fractures in childhood. J. Bone Joint Surg., *43A:*1224, 1966.

86. Stelling, F. H.: Personal communication, 1975.

87. Stirling, R. I.: Equalization of limb length. J. Bone Joint Surg., *37B:*511, 1955.

88. Straub, L. R., Thompson, T. C., and Wilson, P. D.: The results of epiphysiodesis and femoral shortening in relation to equalization of leg length. J. Bone Joint Surg., *27:*254, 1945.

89. Tachdjian, M. O.: Pediatric Orthopedics, vol. 2. p. 1469. Philadelphia, Saunders, 1972.

90. Thompson, T. C., Straub, L. R., and Campbell, R. D.: An evaluation of femoral shortening with intramedullary nailing. J. Bone Joint Surg., *36A:*43, 1954.

91. Truesdell, E. D.: Inequality of the lower extremities following fractures of the shaft of the femur in children. Ann. Surg., *74:*498, 1921.

92. Trueta, J.: The influence of the blood supply in controlling bone growth. Bull. Hosp. Joint Dis., *14:*147, 1953.

93. Tupman, G. S.: Treatment of inequality of the lower limbs. The results of operations for stimulation of growth. J. Bone Joint Surg., *42B:* 489, 1960.

94. Vanderhoeft, P. J., Kelly, P. J., Janes, J. M., and Peterson, L. F. A.: Growth and structure of bone distal to an arteriovenous fistula: Quantitative analysis of the tetracycline-induced transverse growth patterns. J. Bone Joint Surg., *45B:*582, 1963.

95. Vesely, D. G., and Mears, T. M.: Surgically induced arteriovenous fistula. Its effect upon inequality of leg length. So. Med. J., *57:*129, 1964.

96. Wagner, H.: Operative Beinverlängerung. Der Chirurg, *42.(6):*260, 1971.

97. ———: Personal communication, 1977.

98. Westin, G. W.: Femoral lengthening using a periosteal sleeve. Report of 26 cases. J. Bone Joint Surg., *49A:*83, 1967.

99. White, J. W.: Overlapping procedure for shortening bone defects. A.A.O.S. Instruc. Course Lect. *2:*201, 1949.

100. White, J. W., and Stubbins, S. G., Jr.: Growth arrest for equalizing leg lengths. J.A.M.A., *126:*1146, 1944.

101. Wilk, L. H., and Badgley, C. E.: Hypertension, another complication of leg lengthening procedure. Report of a case. J. Bone Joint Surg., *45A:*1263, 1963.

102. Wu, Y. K., and Miltner, L. J.: A procedure for stimulation of longitudinal growth of bone. An experimental study. J. Bone Joint Surg., *19:*909, 1937.

103. Yabsley, R. H., and Harris, W. R.: The effect of shaft fractures and periosteal stripping on the vascular supply to epiphyseal plates. J. Bone Joint Surg., *47A:*551, 1965.

104. Yosipovitch, Z. H., and Palti, Y.: Alterations in blood pressure during leg-lengthening. A clinical and experimental investigation. J. Bone Joint Surg., *49A:*1352, 1967.

20 *The Lower Limb*

Paul P. Griffin, M.D.

TIBIAL TORSION

Torsion in the tibia may be directed either internally or externally. Its significance as a psychological or an anatomic problem is controversial, as are the methods of measurements and the effectiveness of treatment. Such controversy is brought about by the lack of a scientifically sound study that demonstrates the effectiveness of treatment, as well as the well-known fact that torsion of the tibia is seldom a problem in the adult.

Internal tibial torsion may be measured roentgenographically[17, 31] or by a tropometric method.[27, 50] These methods, although more accurate than clinical measurements, still are inaccurate to a certain degree. If the angle betwen the transmalleolar and transcondylar axis of the tibia is used to measure torsion, there is a progressive external rotation from birth to maturity, so that in the adult there is 20° of external torsion.[27, 31]

The patient with internal torsion is usually brought for evaluation because of toeing-in or because of a bowleg appearance. Many babies with internal tibial torsion have an external rotation "deformity" of the femur, in that the hip has excessive external rotation with internal rotation limited to 10° to 20°. This combination of external rotation of the thigh and internal torsion of the lower leg gives an appearance of bowing whether or not there is true tibia vara or genu varum.

In my experience there has seldom been a need for orthopaedic devices in treating internal torsion. From the number of children that I have seen who have worn various orthoses for months or years and still have had tibial torsion, I am inclined to believe that those patients in whom internal torsion does not spontaneously correct are not likely to improve with the devices presently used.

I have seen the appearance of medial torsion in young infants changed within 6 to 8 weeks by the use of a Denis Browne brace attached to shoes. In spite of the improved appearance, the relationship of the transcondylar to the transmalleolar axis was altered very little, and the correction obtained was through the ankle and knee joints where I think many infants have a medial rotation from their position in utero. The spontaneous correction of this torsion is delayed by sleeping and sitting and kneeling postures that hold the feet and knees in an internally rotated position.

In line with the present limited data that supports the need for treatment, splinting should be reserved for the 18- or 24-month-old child who has severe intoeing from internal tibial torsion but who does not have excessive external rotation of the hip. If a Denis Browne bar is used, its width should not exceed the width of the pelvis. A wider bar puts a valgus stress on the foot and knee. Tibial torsion may be familial,[6] and where there is a familial pattern it is not likely to correct with or without an external rotation brace, but in this group of patients I do treat the child when first evaluated, but with little evidence that it changes the torsion deformity.

Whereas internal torsion is more bothersome to parents, excessive external torsion is probably mechanically less desirable. External torsion gives an outtoe gait which increases stress on the feet and later may have some influence on running. Certainly, boys and girls with external torsion who participate in sports have more difficulty with shin splints than those with normal torsion or internal torsion.

GENU VALGUM

Physiologic Genu Valgum

Clinical Features. It is common for children between the ages of 2 and 6 years to have up to 15° of valgus deformity at the knee. This is usually but not always symmetrical. Children with as much as 15° of valgus deformity may complain of leg or foot pain and may fatigue easily. They seldom run well, and they are likely to be less active than their peers who have less valgus deformity. When the amount of valgus exceeds 15°, when it is asymmetric, or if the child is unusually short of stature, a growth abnormality should be suspected as a possible cause of the valgus and appropriate roentgenograms made of the knee.

Treatment. The natural history of physiologic genu valum is one of progressive improvement, beginning around 30 months of age, and most are corrected by 5 years of age, although a few go on until 7 or 8 years of age. Those children that have valgus deformity at 8 years of age seldom spontaneously correct. The valgus knee puts unusual stress on the medial side of the foot and may cause foot strain. In children with 15° of genu valgum I use a $^1/_8$- to $^3/_{16}$-inch medial heel wedge and occasionally an arch pad.

In a child with excessive genu valgum, that of 20° or so, particularly if the father or mother has genu valgum, I use a night brace to attempt to correct the deformity. The brace is a lateral straight single upright, without a knee joint, which is attached to a shoe. It has a thigh and calf band and a large knee pad that is used to pull the knee toward the upright. This is worn only at night.

The adolescent with genu valgum presents a special problem. Genu valgum is a functional as well as a cosmetic disability. It is rare to find an adolescent with genu valgum who can run well, and therefore most of these patients are not active in sports and do poorly in physical activities. A valgus knee also places stress on the patellofemoral joint and possibly contributes to chondromalacia.

When the genu valgum is great enough to produce approximately 10 cm. of space between the malleoli with the knees together or if it measures more than 15° to 20° when the child is 10 years old, surgical correction should be considered. There are several important observations to make before attempting to correct the deformity. One is to be sure that the distance between the malleoli is due to valgus deformity at the knee and not to fat thighs. The latter is a common finding in adolescent girls and must not be overlooked. By losing weight, improvement in the appearance is gained. A valgus deformity may be secondary to elongation of the distal medial condyle of the femur or to more rapid growth of the medial part of the proximal epiphysis of the tibia.

The correction should take place at the proper level, that is, at the site of deformity. If the deformity is in the tibia and correction is through the femur, the knee joint will be tilted laterally when the feet are together. The opposite is true when the deformity is in the femur and correction is obtained through the tibia. There is normally a slight valgus angulation between the shaft of the femur and the distal articular surface, which is necessary to keep the knee joint horizontal when the thighs are together, since the upper ends of the femora are separated by the pelvis. This necessary valgus angulation is greater in girls than boys and must be considered when looking at roentgenograms of the knees. On an average, girls have around 9° to 10° of valgus angulation of the distal femur, boys slightly less. Continued maturity, particularly in girls, causes further widening of the pelvis and influences the relationship of the knee to the horizontal plane.

In most patients with genu valgum the deformity is in the distal femur and therefore should be corrected through the femur. If the epiphyseal plate has sufficient growth potential, stapling of the medial part of the epiphysis with two or three staples gradually corrects the deformity (Fig. 20-1). Once cor-

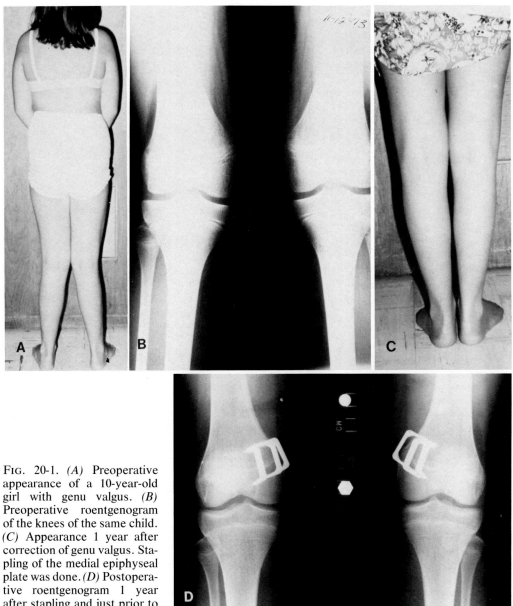

FIG. 20-1. *(A)* Preoperative appearance of a 10-year-old girl with genu valgus. *(B)* Preoperative roentgenogram of the knees of the same child. *(C)* Appearance 1 year after correction of genu valgus. Stapling of the medial epiphyseal plate was done. *(D)* Postoperative roentgenogram 1 year after stapling and just prior to staple removal.

rection is obtained, the staples should be removed. Timing is important. If done too late, correction will be inadequate. As a rule, surgery on girls should be done at a skeletal age of 10 years and on boys at a skeletal age of 11 years. The amount of correction that is obtained by stapling is mathematically related to the transverse width of the plate, the length of the leg distal to the plate, and the growth that occurs on the unstapled side of the plate. A simple way to decide if there is sufficient growth remaining to obtain correction is to trace the legs on a long, clear, x-ray film, divide the femur at the level of the femoral epiphysis, and visualize the distance of medial elongation

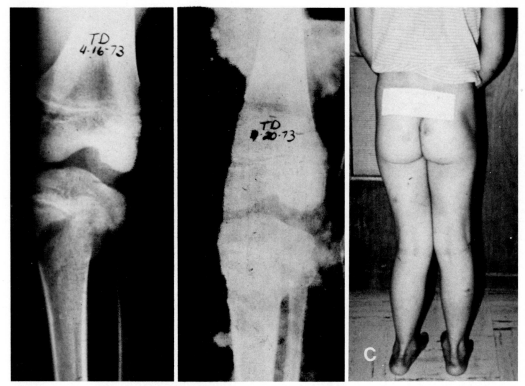

Fig. 20-2. *(A)* Fracture of the proximal tibia and fibula. *(B)* After reduction the medial side remains slightly open, in spite of manipulation. Note that the lateral joint space has opened. *(C)* Two years later genu valgum is evident.

necessary to straighten the extremity. An osteotomy of the distal femur can be done to correct the deformity when remaining growth potential is not sufficient.

When the deformity is in the tibia, the same principles apply. Stapling of the medial part of the proximal tibial epiphysis, if growth is sufficient to correct the deformity, is an effective method of treatment. If the remaining growth is insufficient to correct the deformity, an osteotomy of the tibia should be done after the epiphysis is closed.

Posttraumatic Genu Valgum

An injury to the distal femoral epiphysis or proximal tibial epiphysis may cause a valgus or varus deformity if growth of the epiphyseal plate is disturbed. Management of this is discussed under leg length inequality. However, there is a special situation that results in valgus deformity of the tibia after a fracture of the proximal metaphysis of the tibia. Valgus deformity may follow an undisplaced fracture, or a displaced fracture that is well reduced. (Fig. 20-2). Most fractures of the proximal tibial metaphysis open on the medial side, and great care should be taken to completely reduce the fragments and close any separation on the medial side. At times even maximum effort may be insufficient to completely reduce the fracture by manipulation. However, open reduction and anatomical reduction are likely to be followed by valgus deformity. Possibly the best solution to the situation is an osteotomy of the fibula. This allows better reduction of the tibia. The family should always be told of the possibility that a valgus deformity may develop.

The cause of this valgus growth pattern is uncertain. It is seen in children between 2 and 7 years of age who usually have genu

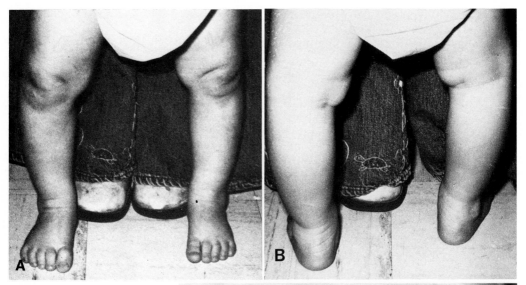

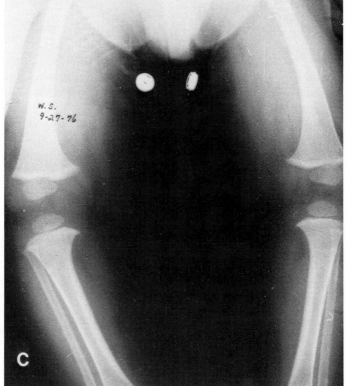

Fig. 20-3. *(A and B)* Physiologic genu varum. *(C)* Roentgenographic view of physiologic genu varum.

valgum. The natural growth pattern towards valgus may have some influence. After a fracture occurs, there is an increase in blood flow to the area. This stimulates growth. The fibula may tether growth on the lateral side or the vascularity may increase more on the medial side. Either causes increased growth on the medial part of the plate.

Management of the valgus is difficult. To immediately correct the valgus by osteot-

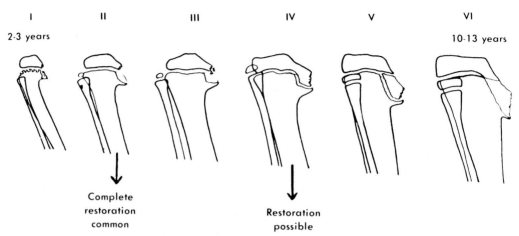

I   II   III   IV   V   VI

2-3 years   10-13 years

Complete
restoration
common

Restoration
possible

FIG. 20-4. The six stages of tibia vara, as related to age. (From Langenskiold, A.: Tibia vara. Acta Chir. Scand., *103*:9, 1952.)

omy of the tibia usually results in recurrence of the valgus. The medial side of the tibial epiphyseal plate may be stapled and correction obtained gradually, but in young children stapling of the medial epiphysis is technically difficult and must be done with great care. The staple is removed after correction has been obtained. I prefer to wait until the child is 8 or 9 years old and correct the deformity by a closing wedge osteotomy of the tibia through the proximal metaphysis, with an oblique osteotomy of the fibula. When the valgus deformity is too severe to postpone correction until 8 or 9 years of age, the osteotomy must overcorrect the valgus to allow for the tendency of the deformity to recur.

PHYSIOLOGIC GENU VARUM

In the infant and young child mild medial bowing of the lower extremities is normal. The bowing involves both the femur and the tibia. Gradual spontaneous correction is the natural course of genu varum, and the great majority are straight at 2 to 2 ¹/₂ years. Some of these children later develop genu valgum, which is also a temporary condition that begins to straighten at 4 years. Most are straight somewhere between 5 and 8 years of age. The presence of medial torsion exaggerates the bowed appearance.

Most parents seek medical help for their children with bowlegs after walking begins. Important in the history of the child is whether the deformity increased after walking began. If so, roentgenographic examination is probably warranted. The roentgenographic characteristics of physiologic genu varum are: (1) medial angulation of the upper one-third of the tibia and lower end of the femur; (2) a thickened medial cortex of the tibia and, to a lesser degree, the femur; (3) prominence of the medial metaphysis of the tibia and femur; (4) normal appearing epiphyseal plate, and (5) usually symmetric involvement (Fig. 20-3). The differential diagnosis includes rickets, metaphyseal dysplasia, and Blount's disease.

Treatment for physiologic bowlegs is not necessary, as the deformity improves spontaneously. Use of a Denis Browne bar may exaggerate the subsequent genu valgum that follows the correction of the bowleg. It is the responsibility of the orthopaedist to rule out other causes of genu varum that need specific treatment.

TIBIA VARA (BLOUNT'S DISEASE)

In 1937 Dr. Walter Blount reported on a series of 13 patients with bowed tibiae secondary to a growth disturbance of the medial portion of the proximal epiphysis of the tibia, and he reviewed 15 additional cases from the literature.[5] His excellent description of the tibia vara has resulted in its being commonly called "Blount's disease," even though the condition was reported in 1922 by Erlacher.[14]

Blount described an infantile type of tibia vara that begins between the first and third years of life and an adolescent type that has its onset after 9 years of age. The infantile type is the more common of the two. Both males and females are affected. Golding and coworkers[18] reported a male-to-female ratio of 17 to 11, whereas both Largenskiold[34] and Blount reported a predominance of females.

Infantile-type tibia vara usually occurs in obese children who have short stature and walk early. The course of the disease is usually progressive, with increasing varus of the proximal tibia, secondary joint changes that include ligamentous laxity, hypoplasia of the posterior medial plateau, which results in a flexion of the diaphysis on the proximal epiphyseal, and lateral shift of the tibia on the femur. There is in addition a medial torsion of the tibia. Rarely does mild Blount's disease remain static for some time and then progressively improve. Generally the deformity is progressive.

There are characteristic histological findings in the resting layer of epiphyseal cartilage in tibia vara.[34] These are: (1) islands of densely packed cells showing a greater degree of hypertrophy than could be expected from their topographical position, (2) islands of almost cellular fibrous cartilage, and (3) abnormal groups of capillary vessels.

Etiology

The infantile type of tibia vara is caused by a disturbance in growth and ossification of the posterior medial part of the proximal epiphysis of the tibia. It has not been clearly delineated as to why the growth disturbance occurs. There is no evidence that infection, trauma, or ischemia are contributing factors. It may be a response to abnormal stress from weightbearing on an already bowed leg. This is difficult to prove, but it is typically the case that heavy children whose legs are already bowed and who walk early are those most likely to develop Blount's disease.

Clinical Features

Clinically there is difficulty in differentiating the severe physiologic bowleg from Blount's disease. The diagnosis is made by the roentgenographic picture. Until there are definite changes in the medial metaphysis the physician cannot be certain whether the patient has Blount's disease. By repeated clinical and roentgenographic examinations the diagnosis can be made. Usually by age 2 years physiologic bowlegs will have shown improvement, while the deformity in Blount's disease will have increased and roentgenographic changes in the proximal tibia will be well developed.

On physical examination there is a sharp bowing just below the knee. A prominence is palpable on the medial tibial metaphysis. With the knee flexed 10° to 15° there may be significant instability of the tibia on the femur. The child walks with the knee flexed, and the varus may increase during the single support phase of gait.

Rickets, radiation change, multiple chondromatoses, traumatic epiphyseal disturbance, congenital bowing, in addition to the physiologic bowlegs, must be differentiated.

The diagnosis of tibia vara is a roentgenographic one. Langenskiold has separated the roentgenographic changes into six stages that are related to age. It is important that the orthopaedist treating tibia vara recognize these stages (Fig. 20-4).

Stage I. This stage is seen in children up to 3 years of age. There is an irregularity of the entire ossification of the metaphyses, with radiolucent zones separating islands of calcified tissue from the bony metaphysis. The medial part of the metaphysis protrudes and is beaked medially and distally.

Stage II. This is seen in children between $2^1/_2$ and 4 years of age. There is a sharp lateromedial depression in the ossification line of the medial one-third of the metaphysis that forms the characteristic beak. The upper portion of the beak is more radiolucent than the other parts of the metaphysis. The medial part of the bony epiphysis becomes more wedge-shaped and still is less developed than its lateral part.

Stage III. This occurs in children in the 4- to 6-year age group and is characterized by deepening of the depression filled by cartil-

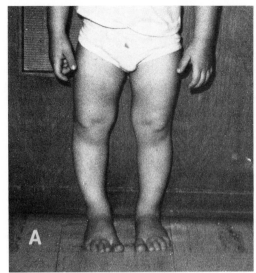

FIG. 20-5. *(A)* A 2-year-old with varus on weightbearing. *(B)* Roentgenogram of same patient at age 2 years, showing early Blount's disease. *(C)* At age 2½ years, the changes of Blount's disease have progressed. *(Legend continued on facing page.)*

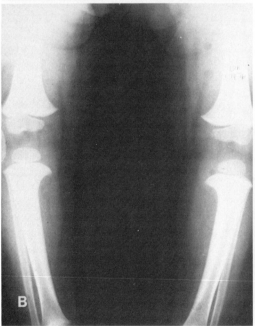

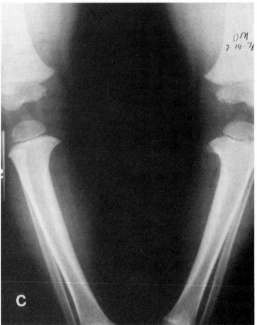

age in the metaphyseal beak, with the radiolucent area giving the appearance of a step in the metaphysis. The medial part of the bony epiphysis is still wedge-shaped and is less distinct, and small areas of calcification may be present beneath the medial border.

Stage IV. This may be seen in children between 5 and 10 years of age. The epiphyseal growth plate narrows and the bony

epiphysis enlarges. Consequently the step in the metaphysis increases in depth, and the bony epiphysis occupies the depression in the medial part of the metaphysis. There is a marked irregularity of the medial border of the bony epiphysis.

Stage V. This occurs in children between 9 and 11 years of age. A clear band traverses medially the lateral portion of the epiphyseal plate to the articular cartilage, separating the

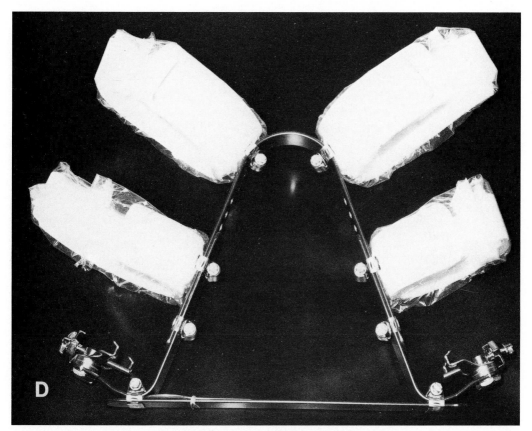

FIG. 20-5. *(Continued).* (D) The patient now wears this orthosis at night.

bony epiphysis into two portions and giving the appearance of a partial double epiphyseal plate. There is some irregularity of the triangular area of the bony epiphysis against the joint cartilage and the cartilage that covers the medial aspect. The articular surface of the medial part of the tibia is deformed, sloping medially and distally from the center condyle notch. As pointed out by Golding, the slope is also posteriorly as well as medially directed.

Stage VI. This is seen in children between 10 and 13 years of age. The branches of the medial part of the epiphyseal plate ossify and growth continues in its normal lateral part.

Treatment

In the 2- to 3-year-old child with Stage I or Stage II changes, specific treatment is not necessarily needed. These may be watched and periodically evaluated, or the physician may choose to prescribe a corrective orthosis for nighttime use. If the deformity has caused sufficient changes in the knee so that on weightbearing there is a definite increase in the varus of the knee but the roentgenographic changes are not severe enough to warrant surgical correction, an orthosis that exerts a corrective force on the knee should be used at night (Fig. 20-5). The varus and the medial torsion in patients who have shown progressive roentgenographic changes to Stage III or Stage IV can usually be corrected and the progressive course of the disease controlled by a dome osteotomy at the level of the distal tip of the tibial tubercle. The fibula should be osteotomized at a lower level but in the upper third of the diaphysis. Excessive overcorrection should be avoided, as the valgus obtained may remain. However, the os-

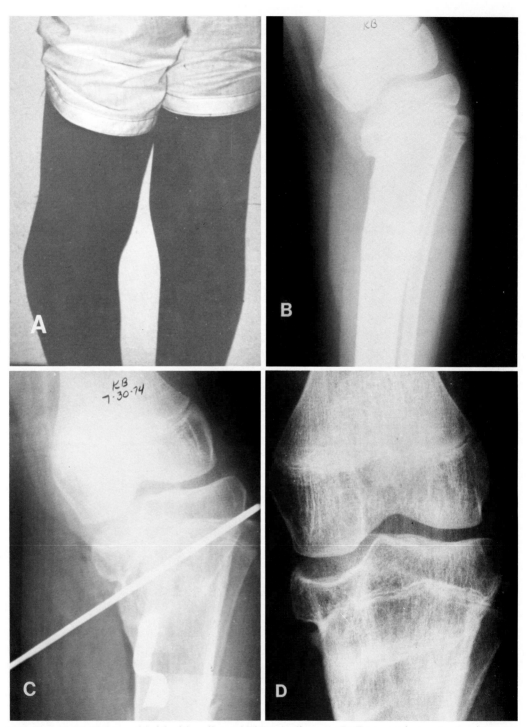

FIG. 20-6. *(A)* A 10-year-old girl with unilateral Blount's disease. *(B)* Two previous osteotomies were too far distal to the tubercle. The deformity is still severe (Stage IV). *(C)* A guide drill is placed parallel to the articular surface and as close as possible to the tubercle. *(D)* Roentgenogram taken after open-wedge osteotomy was performed. No further surgery was required.

teotomy should produce sufficient valgus to shift the stress of weightbearing onto the lateral plateau. In children over 9 years of age the medial epiphysis may be closed (Stage VI), and, if so, an epiphysiodesis of the lateral part of the proximal epiphysis of the tibia and the proximal epiphysis of the fibula should be done at the time of the osteotomy. Most patients under 8 years of age can be corrected and recurrence is not a problem. However, after 8 years of age recurrence requiring a second osteotomy is not uncommon.

Up to and including Stage IV in children under 8 years of age an adequate dome-shaped osteotomy of the proximal tibia is usually very effective. In patients with the changes of Stage V and over, a repeat osteotomy is likely to be needed if the child is 8 years old. Langenskiold has found that the neglected Stage VI patient over 8 years with excessive deformity of the medial plateau may need to have the medial plateau elevated and an epiphysiodesis of the tibia and fibula performed.[35] After this is healed, a dome osteotomy of the tibia, or an open wedge osteotomy and an oblique osteotomy of the fibula are needed to complete the correction. A common error in the management of the tibia vara is to make the osteotomy of the tibia too low. It must be made as close to the tubercle as possible to obtain adequate correction without excessive distortion of the contour of the tibia (Fig. 20-6). In older children the osteotomy may be made closer to the epiphyseal plate and a better correction obtained.

Adolescent Tibia Vara

The adolescent type of Blount's disease has its start usually when the child is older than 9 years. The roentgenographic appearance in the adolescent type is quite different. There is no steplike deformity of the epiphyseal plate, and the ossified portion of the epiphysis appears to be relatively normal. The overall appearance is of a prematurely closed medial portion of the growth plate. With tomograms there can be seen a line of bone that crosses the epiphyseal plate in some patients.

Treatment by dome osteotomy high on the tibia with an oblique osteotomy of the fibula

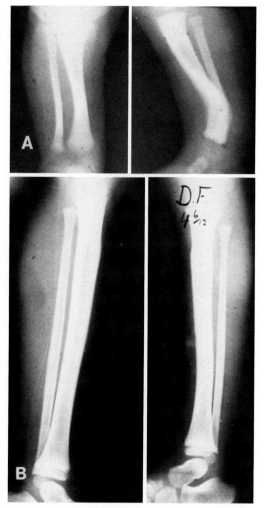

FIG. 20-7. *(A)* Posterior bowing of the tibia in a 3-month-old child. *(B)* The same child at age 4¹/₂ years. No treatment was given. Both tibiae are shown for comparison. Note that the fibula on the affected side is slightly shorter.

gives correction. However, the surgical correction should wait until the child is grown, since some of these correct spontaneously.

CONGENITAL ANGULAR DEFORMITIES OF THE TIBIA

Posterior Bowing

Congenital posterior bowing of the tibia occurs at the junction of the lower and middle thirds of the tibia. The bow is primarily

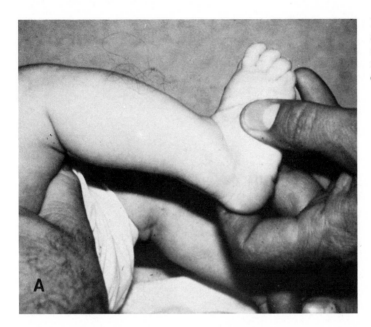

FIG. 20-8. *(A)* Anterior bow in a child with neurofibromatosis. The child's father also has neurofibromatosis. *(Legend continued on facing page.)*

posteriorly directed, but may be posteromedial. The fibula has a similar bow. Because the distal tibia is directed somewhat anteriorly in comparison to normal, the foot is in a calcaneous position. Plantar flexion is limited and the anterior muscles of the ankle and foot are shortened. This may be due to the foot and ankle resting in a dorsiflexed position in utero.

No treatment except passive stretching of the tight anterior musculature is required. The natural course is a progressive straightening of the tibia, and usually when the child reaches 4 years of age the tibia appears normal. Osteotomy is not indicated and should not be done. If the linear growth of the tibia or fibula shows inhibition, appropriate correction may be required later (Fig. 20-7).

Anterior Bowing

The congenital anteriorly bowed tibia occurs more frequently, is more serious, and has more variations in pathology at the area of bowing than does the posteriorly bowed tibia. The bowing is in the middle and lower thirds of the tibia, and almost always the fibula is similarly bowed and may have the same pathology.

Clinical Features

There are several types of anteriorly bowed tibiae. The first type occurs in association with a congenital absent fibula. In these patients the tibia is short, bowed, and has a thick sclerotic cortex. The primary problem in these children is the leg length inequality, and these are not considered further in this section.

Congenital pseudarthrosis of the tibia may generally describe the second and third types of anterior bowing. These two types are different in many ways, but both have the serious problem of pathologic fracture and pseudarthrosis at the apex of the bow. The fibula is similarly involved and may also fracture and develop nonunion alone or in combination with the tibia.

The second type of anterior bow presents as a narrowing of the tibia with sclerosis and partial or complete obliteration of the intramedullary canal. Surrounding the narrowed area of tibia is a thick fibrous tissue, which Aegerter[1] described as a hamartomatous proliferation of fibrous tissue. After the narrow segment fractures, the ends of the fragments become tapered.

The anterior bow with narrowing of the tibia (the second type) is associated with

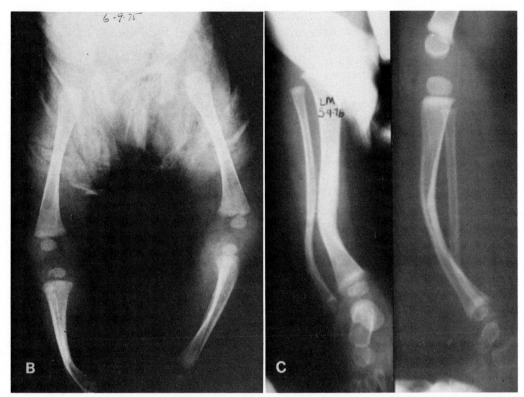

FIG. 20-8. *(Continued)*. *(B)* Roentgenogram of the same child at age 2 months. Note the narrow sclerotic segment of the tibia with the lateral anterior bow. *(C)* One year later. The tibia was protected first with a plaster cast and later with a foot-ankle-knee orthosis. Note the continued anterolateral bow and the narrow sclerotic segment, as seen on the lateral film. Similar changes are present in the fibula. The foot-ankle-knee orthosis protects the ankle joint from mediolateral stress, as well as giving protection to the tibia.

neurofibromatosis, although some authors have not described neurogenic material in the microscopic examination of specimens removed from the area of pseudarthrosis (Fig. 20-8). Green[22] did describe such changes. Others have reported a high incidence of associated neurofibromatosis in patients who developed pseudarthrosis of the tibia.[3, 13] Neurofibromatosis is not seen with the third type.

In the third type of bowing there is a cystic lesion of the apex of the bow. The tibia may be slightly narrow in the area of the lesion but usually there is no narrowing, and on occasion the width may be greater than normal. In the third type the bow is generally not as severe as it is in the tibia with the narrowed sclerotic segment. The lytic lesion contains material with the appearance of fibrous dysplasia, not neurogenic material.

Treatment

In all anteriorly bowed tibiae, the treatment is directed toward prevention of fracture. The leg should be protected with a long plaster cast from early infancy on, with the cast being changed as needed to accommodate growth. A long-leg brace with a molded cuff for the tibia can be used to protect the tibia when the child is large enough to be fitted with a brace.

Excision of the thick hamartomatous fibrous tissue from around the narrowed area of the tibia and bone grafting posteriorly along the concave side of the bow tend to strengthen the tibia and help prevent fracture. If there is a lytic area the graft should be applied on the concavity of the tibia. After it has been incorporated into the tibia the lytic area may be curetted and grafted. Great care should be used not to fracture the tibia at surgery. To curet and graft the lesion without previously strengthening the tibia by a posterior graft invites fracture, as the curettage decreases the strength of the tibia.

After a fracture has occurred there are many methods used in attempting to obtain union. In fact, there are so many techniques described, it is clear that none are highly successful. One of the basic procedures used in most techniques is excision of the relatively avascular, thick, hamartomatous fibrous tissue from around the bone fragment, excision of the sclerotic bone ends, and bone grafting (autogenous, if possible). Double onlay bone grafts with screw fixation; bypass bone grafts; intramedullary rods, and additional bone grafts; or compression clamps and bone grafts are some of the more frequently used techniques of treatment.[8, 37, 54]

The technique I prefer for treating the pseudarthrosis is excision of the fibrous material around the pseudarthrosis, removal of the sclerotic bone ends, posterior angulation of the fracture fragments (overcorrection of the anterior bow) and compression immobilization with a pin above and below, using the Charnley clamp. Onlay bone grafts are then placed on two sides of the tibia, and small chips and matchstick grafts are laid around the fracture. After the tibia heals, immobilization with a molded cuff and a long-leg brace is needed for a year or more. Additional grafting of the side should be done periodically if the bone begins to resorb.

In all of the techniques the greatest difficulty is in obtaining adequate internal fixation. The more distal the pseudarthrosis, the greater the difficulty. If the distal fragment is too small to safely accept a Steinmann pin for compression, a pin properly bent may be inserted in the intramedullary canal from the sole of the foot. This can replace the compression clamp and pins.

Regardless of the technique used, the prognosis for healing is guarded. Even if union is obtained, leg length discrepancy is likely to be present. The earlier the fracture occurs and the more distal the pseudarthrosis, the poorer the prognosis. Although primary amputation has been advised as the treatment of choice, I believe a reasonable attempt at obtaining union should be used in all cases, with even up to three or four attempts at bone grafting. Once it is obvious that even if union were to be obtained the leg would be unacceptably short and small, amputation is advised.

RECURRENT DISLOCATION AND SUBLUXATION OF THE PATELLA

Recurrent dislocation of the patella is a relatively uncommon condition, but occurs frequently enough that most orthopaedists have some experience with its management. The frequency of complete recurrent dislocation is far greater in girls than in boys.[7, 19, 36]

Etiology

There are multiple abnormal anatomic relationships that contribute to the development of recurrent dislocation of the patella.

Most patients have generalized relaxation of joint ligaments. Laxity of the medial capsule has to be a factor, for unless it is lax the patella cannot dislocate. Whether the medial capsule is lax as part of the elastic nature of the patient's ligaments or is lax because of repeated stress from the patella being pulled laterally by other forces is unclear, but both aspects are probably important.

The iliotibial band may be contracted or may have an abnormal attachment to the patella. A contracted iliotibial band or abnormal patellar attachment may play a role in displacing the patella laterally as the knee is flexed.

Both genu valgum and external torsion of the tibia encourage lateral dislocation of the patella.

A high-lying patella can more easily be displaced lateral to the lateral condyle when the tibia is externally rotated on the femur while slightly flexed and abducted and tension is produced by contracting the quadriceps muscle. These are the conditions that prevail when the patella dislocates in a patient who turns while dancing or twists while standing, and during running and changing direction. This is more likely to occur if the lateral condyle is small and the femoral groove is shallow.

All of these anatomic variations may play a role in the recurrent dislocation or subluxation of the patella. There are, however, instances when none of these can be identified with certainty, yet the patient has a history of dislocation or symptoms suggesting subluxation.

The normal excursion of the patella as the knee goes from full extension to flexion is first to strike the lateral condyle and then to move medially into the femoral sulcus. The medial facet of the patella does not contact the femoral surface until the knee is well flexed. If the lateral condyle is insufficient or the resultant dynamic force between the quadriceps and the patellar tendon insertion is directed too far laterally, the patella initially moves lateral to the lateral condyle and then moves medially back into the sulcus with further flexion of the knee. The medial return to the sulcus causes abnormal wear on the medial facet, which is the location of chondromalacia in most patellae.

The abnormality of patellar movement may be so slight that the lateral excursion of the patella is too limited for the patient to appreciate a displacement, or it may be such that it allows the patella to migrate laterally on flexion and then jump back medially over the condyle, or it may be severe enough for the patella to stay laterally displaced until the knee is again passively extended under the appropriate circumstances.

Clinical Features and Diagnosis

Recurrent dislocation may begin in the child as young as 5 or 6 years but usually does not manifest itself until adolescence, and, indeed, at times it is not manifested until the third decade of life. In many patients with recurrent dislocation the history is usually relatively simple. The patella frankly dislocates and may spontaneously reduce when the knee is extended either passively or actively.

With such a history diagnosis is no problem. There are, however, patients who complain that they feel the patella (or feel something) move laterally with certain motions of the knee. This is associated with

pain and rarely is followed by effusion in the joint. A more subtle patellofemoral abnormality may be present in which the patella is pulled laterally by pathologic forces but does not displace enough for the patient to appreciate any patellar displacement. Diagnosis is difficult in this type of patient. The symptoms may be confined to sudden pain while running or "giving way" of the knee when changing directions during walking or running.

In the patient whose patella frankly dislocates, physical examination usually shows a hypermobile patella that can be or can almost be dislocated by pushing it laterally. The patella is frequently higher than normal, and the patient is likely to have, in general, loose ligaments. The vastus medialis is flat and small and does not extend as far distally as normal. Varying degrees of genu valgum may be present.

The patient without a history of complete dislocation may have essentially the same physical findings, except that the patella is not quite as mobile. Patients with either type frequently have a positive so-called apprehension test. That test is done with the patient sitting on a table, the leg resting at 45° of flexion, and the quadriceps relaxed. A lateral-directed force is put on the patella. The fear of the pain that will result from displacement causes the patient to contract the quadriceps and to assume a facial expression showing apprehension of pain, with or without verbal comment.

A far more difficult diagnosis to make is that of mild subluxation when the patient does not feel a lateral displacement of the patella and when the only symptom is pain about the patella when the patient suddenly changes direction while walking or running or, occasionally, while rapidly ascending stairs. In these children, all physical findings may be normal or there may be some of the stigmata thought to be associated with recurrent dislocation of the patella. Chondromalacia with crepitus may or may not be present, although in most of these patients some degree of chondromalacia can be detected. A positive apprehension test is usually absent. The vastus medialis may be thin.

Routine roentgenograms taken in the classic manner may be normal, and they are usually normal in the patient with minimal subluxation. Occasionally the patella, as seen in the anteroposterior view, rests in a more lateral position than normal or if the patella dislocates as the knee flexes, it appears to rest in a lateral position on classic skyline roentgenograms. However, most patients with recurrent dislocation do not have lateral displacement of the patella on this view, as the film is routinely made, for if the knee is flexed and is not bearing weight the patella usually rides into the femoral sulcus and appears to be normal. The routine skyline view does not show the femoral surface that articulates with the patella.[36]

To be meaningful in showing the relationship of the patella to the femoral sulcus the skyline or tangential view should be made with the knee flexed 45°, the x-ray beam tilted 30° degrees off the horizontal, and the cassette held resting on the tibia with the x-ray beam perpendicular to the cassette. This is a technique that was used for years by Green[20] and others,[36] which Merchant has recently analyzed, redefined, and measured so as to make it more meaningful.[38] Merchant defined this as the patellofemoral congruence angle that should help the orthopaedist in diagnosing patellofemoral subluxation. The sulcus of the femur is bisected with a line that extends through the patella. The lowest point in the posterior surface of the patella is marked and a line is drawn through it from the point where the sulcus is bisected. The angle between the two lines is called the "congruence angle." (Fig. 20-9). Angles that are medial to the line of bisection are negative and those lateral to it are positive. The average angle is −6°, with a 11° standard deviation. Therefore, any angle less than +16° is within normal limits. In spite of carefully taken roentgenograms and measurement there will be patients whose history and physical findings are sufficient to make the diagnosis of subluxation or dislocation when the roentgenogram is normal.

Treatment

Well over 75 operative procedures for the treatment of congenital dislocation of the patella have been described. This alone attests to the complexity of the problem and to the ineffectiveness of the operative procedures.

The problems faced in treating subluxa-tion and dislocation of the patella are directed at prevention of recurrence without creating either a destructive force against the patellofemoral articulation or a growth disturbance of the proximal tibia that would cause recurvation.

Patients with the diagnosis of recurrent subluxation should initially perform isometric exercises to strengthen the quadriceps.

The first incident of dislocation of the patella should be treated by immobilization of the knee in extension for 4 weeks, followed by a program of isometric exercises. This may be successful in preventing recurrent dislocations. If conservative treatment does not relieve symptoms or prevent recurrent dislocations, surgical correction should be undertaken.

There are many recorded surgical approaches to the treatment of this problem. The most popular over the years has been the transfer of the insertion of the patellar tendon. If the tendon insertion is moved, it should not be moved distally. It should be moved medially only enough to have the patella articulate with the center of the femoral sulcus when the knee goes from extension to flexion. Excessive medial displacement can cause the patella to articulate too forcefully and too early in the flexion motion, so that there is a clicking sensation as the patella slides over the superior lip of the medial condyle when the knee flexes. This appears to be harmful to the medial facet of the patella. If, in addition, the insertion is transferred distally, the interarticular force between the femur and patella is increased, which may also cause further wear on the patellar articular surface. The normal knee rotates internally as the knee goes into the last few degrees of extension. When the patellar tendon is transferred medially this rotation probably does not take place.

In immature patients the tibial tubercle should not be injured by removal of a block of bone with the patellar tendon transfer, as this is likely to cause genu recurvatum.[7, 24, 36] However, the tendon insertion can be transferred along with a thin sliver of bone without injuring the tubercle. The tendon and bone are then inserted beneath an osteoperiosteal flap, using either sutures or a staple for fixation. It has been reported that even with this technique, recurvatum may

FIG. 20-9. Diagram showing plotting of the congruence angle. (From Merchant, C. C., *et al.*: Roentgenographic analysis of patellofemoral congruence. J. Bone Joint Surg., *56A:*1391, 1974.)

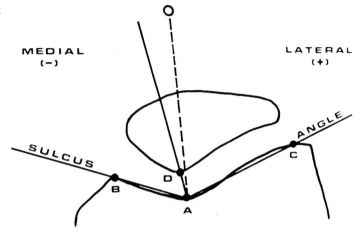

occur from excessive pull of the extensor mechanism, as the insertion of the tendon migrates distally with growth.[24, 36]

In my opinion, transfer of the patellar tendon alone is not sufficient treatment for recurrent subluxation or dislocation, and the location of the patellar tendon insertion is not the primary factor in subluxation and dislocation of the patella. I feel that the essential dynamic force in subluxation and dislocation of the patella is the action of the quadriceps muscle and the iliotibial band. If the quadriceps mechanism is properly aligned surgically, there is seldom a need to transfer the patellar tendon.

When treatment has been delayed and the articular surface has sustained extensive chondromalacia, patellectomy must be considered. If possible, it seems preferable to shave and drill the patella rather than to do a patellectomy, but excision is at times necessary.

The operative technique I prefer is the one described and used by Green.[20, 52] In this procedure the lateral influence of the iliotibial band on the patella is negated by dividing the lateral retinaculum and iliotibial band on the flat, completely freeing all fibers that seem to pull on the patella. By lenthening on the flat, two layers are identified that can be closed loosely to prevent herniation of the synovium. This technique of release is not essential, but the iliotibial band must be completely released from any attachment on the patella and the patellar ligament. The

medial retinaculum capsule is opened, the joint is inspected, and the medial capsule and retinaculum are reefed "pants over vest." The vastus medialis is advanced distally and laterally so that the distal lateral edge of the muscle is advanced to the distal lateral edge of the patella. The medial fibers should be left attached medially so that the dynamic force of the vastus medialis pulls the patella medially as the knee is extended and prevents lateral displacement. In older teenagers and young adults whose quadriceps patellar tendon angle is more than 30°, the insertion of the tendon may need to be moved medially, but only enough to decrease this angle to around 10°. In young children this should be avoided, as it may interfere with growth and may cause genu recurvatum.[24, 36] If necessary, the tendon can be transferred by removing it, with only a sliver of bone, and placing it beneath an osteoperiosteal flap.

If the patellar tendon is not transferred, flexion and extension of the knee in the side-lying position and with assistance is started 5 to 6 days postoperatively. A bivalved cast is used for 6 weeks and crutches are used for an additional 6 weeks, with partial weight-bearing being allowed. In those patients who have the tendon transferred medially, the beginning of the exercise program is delayed until 4 weeks after surgery.

The subluxating patella is treated the same as the dislocating patella. However, major emphasis is on releasing the lateral

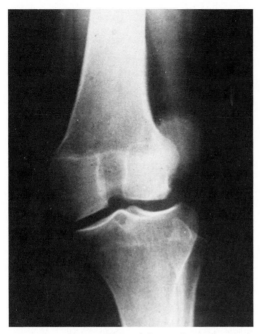

FIG. 20-10. Congenitally dislocated patella, moderately displaced. This could be reduced with full extension. The patient walked with the knee in flexion.

structures and transferring the vastus medialis laterally and distally. In an occasional teenage athlete with pain about the patella that occurs only when changing direction while running, but who has essentially normal appearing quadriceps, patellar, femoral and tibial relationships, I have limited the surgery to a release of the iliotibial band and lateral retinaculum from the patella, with relief of symptoms in most patients.

CONGENITAL DISLOCATION OF THE PATELLA

Congential dislocation of the patella is less common than the ordinary recurrent dislocation. Most of my patients have had associated anomalies of the musculoskeletal system or other systems.

The extent of the patellar dislocation may be such that the patella dislocates with each flexion of the knee and reduces with extension, or the patella may be so laterally displaced that it remains dislocated at all times. In the congenitally dislocated patella the primary anomaly is in the vastus lateralis and its fascia, and in the iliotibial band. The tightness in these two structures prevents the patella from staying in the femoral sulcus during flexion of the knee.

In the patient with a patella that dislocates each time the knee is flexed the complaint may be the recognition by the parent of a clicking sensation on flexion and extension of the knee. After a period of time this becomes painful and the child keeps the knee flexed so that the patella is perpetually dislocated, for it is the relocation motion that is painful. By keeping the knee flexed, a flexion contracture develops and the child walks with an unusual gait where the knee does not extend during weightbearing. Finding a laterally displaced patella upon palpation makes the diagnosis, which may be confirmed by a roentgenogram of the knee, if the patella has ossified. As seen in Figure 20-10, the tibia may be subluxed laterally on the femur as a result of the lateral tightness.

The contracture of the vastus lateralis may be so great that the patella is perpetually dislocated. When the patella stays dislocated in the newborn, the knee does not extend. Attempts at correcting the persistent flexion contracture by traction or casting will be unsuccessful. The small unossified patella is difficult to palpate, but when there is a high level of suspicion and a careful examination it can be palpated in a lateral position. The treatment is surgical release of the lateral retinaculum and the iliotibial band from the patella, excision of any fibrotic bands found in the vastus lateralis, extensive mobilization of the vastus lateralis from the lateral intermuscular septum, recession of the vastus from the patella and central slip of the quadriceps mechanism, and transfer of the vastus medialis distally and laterally, as described above. In older children, in addition, the patellar tendon may require medial transfer if, after the releases are performed, the patella rides laterally on flexion. Occasionally the patella is adherent to the periosteum and perichondrium over the lateral condyle. Great care is needed to free the patella without injury to its articular surface.

CONGENITAL DISLOCATION AND SUBLUXATION OF THE KNEE

Congenital dislocation of the knee is an uncommon anomaly seen with equal frequency in both sexes.[45] The dislocation may be either unilateral or bilateral. In the congenitally dislocated knee the tibia is displaced anteriorly. It is usually rotated in relation to the femur and may also have lateral displacement. There are associated congenital anomalies in 60 per cent of patients born with a congenital dislocation of the knee.

The diagnosis is made by the physical finding of anterior displacement of the tibia, with or without lateral displacement. Roentgenograms of the knee confirm the diagnosis. The condyles of the femur are prominent posteriorly and help to orient the rotation of the tibia to the femur. Usually the tibia is internally rotated and the femur frequently is capable of only limited internal rotation, making it difficult to correctly align the tibia and femur. The collateral ligaments of the knee are stretched, and it is difficult to know the appropriate plane for flexion-extension, as the mediolateral range of motion of the knee is usually as great or greater than the anteroposterior range. This finding may be present even after the dislocation is reduced.

Hyperextension is always present in the congenitally dislocated knee. However, hyperextension is frequently present in normal knees of a breech baby, as well as in those knees that are subluxated but not completely dislocated. It is important that these latter entities be differentiated from the dislocated knee, for the treatment and results vary significantly.

Etiology

Both congenital and environmental causes have been postulated.[30] There are cases in which there is a familial history, but the majority have no positive family history. The position in utero may influence the development of a dislocated knee when the fetus is in the breech position with the feet under the mandible, but the majority of the patients are not breech births. Fibrosis of the vastus lateralis or vastus intermedius is present in some cases. Those patients with fibrosis in the quadriceps muscle are likely to have lateral displacement of the patella in addition to dislocation of the knee.

For the knee to dislocate the posterior capsule has to be very loose and the cruciate ligaments either stretched, hypoplastic, or absent. These changes are possibly secondary to the dislocation, but they could be primary factors. Dislocation of the knee is a frequent finding in children with arthrogryposis multiplex congenita. In these children the muscle abnormality certainly must be an important factor in producing the dislocation.

Congenital *subluxation* of the knee is more common than dislocation. The difference can best be seen by roentgenographic examination, as the appearance of the subluxated knee on inspection is similar to that of the dislocated knee. The subluxated knee usually has up to 25° to 40° of flexion. The tibia may be moved manually, anteriorly and posteriorly, which easily causes subluxation and reduction of the knee (Fig. 20-11). The same etiologic factor that causes dislocation may also cause subluxation of the knee. It is important to make the correct diagnosis, for the treatment is different.

Treatment

Treatment should begin immediately after birth. If the roentgenogram shows subluxation, the affected knee is treated by passively flexing the knee as far as it will easily go. After manual pressure has been applied for 2 or 3 minutes the knee is held in this position by a plaster cast. The cast is changed at weekly intervals, and further flexion is obtained with each cast change until 90° of flexion is present. Further immobilization for 4 to 6 weeks, with the knee held in flexion with a bivalved cast or an orthosis that is removed several times each day, usually is sufficient to prevent recurrence of the subluxation. Great care must be taken to avoid the use of excessive force, for the distal femoral epiphysis can be displaced by this technique.

If there is uncertainty as to whether the knee is subluxated or dislocated, skin traction with the baby in the prone position and the traction directed so as to flex the knees may be used as the initial treatment (Fig.

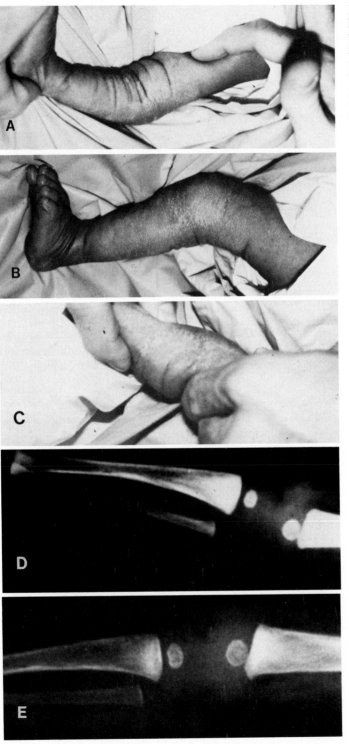

FIG. 20-11. Subluxation of the knee. *(A)* The knee in hyperextension. *(B)* The knee in flexion. *(C)* The tibia could be moved manually, anteriorly to the subluxed position and posteriorly to a position of reduction. *(D)* A lateral roentgenogram taken before traction was applied. *(E)* Lateral roentgenogram taken after treatment with traction followed by plaster immobilization in flexion.

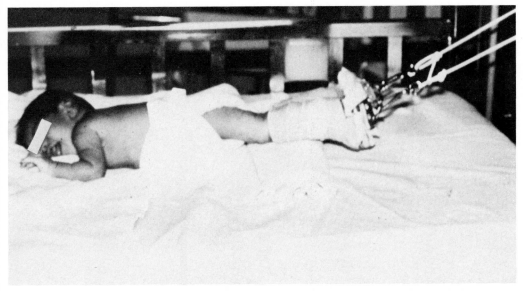

FIG. 20-12. This child has been placed in skin traction for reduction of subluxation.

20-12). Daily knee-flexion exercises can be performed on the baby by the therapist. These should be continued until the knees flex to 90°, after which a bivalved cast or orthosis is applied and the exercises continued for 4 to 6 more weeks. I prefer to use skin traction initially on my patients before putting the leg in plaster in managing congenital subluxation.

The dislocated knee should *not* be manipulated, but should be treated initially with skeletal traction. The technique used by Green[20] is to place a Kirschner wire in the distal femoral metaphysis, one through the distal tibia and one through the proximal tibia (Fig. 20-13). A weight placed on the femoral wire is directed forward and cephalad to counteract the distal force on the tibia. The proper rotational position is maintained by proper placing of the wires. After the tibia is pulled distally to clear the end of the femur the direction of the forces is changed to allow gradual flexion of the knee. If the rotational position is not corrected, the flexion obtained may be tangential or even perpendicular to the correct flexion-extension axis. It is necessary to have an infant on a Bradford frame or some similar device to obtain appropriate traction.

When it is apparent that traction is not sufficient to correct the deformity, open reduction is required. The operative procedure may vary in each patient, but certain basic features should be mentioned. The approach is best done through a long, anterior incision. After exposing the quadriceps, patella, anterior capsule, patellar tendon, and collateral ligaments, the quadriceps is the first structure that is corrected. If there is a discrete fibrous mass in the vastus lateralis or the vastus intermedius it should be excised. If the vastus lateralis and vastus intermedius form a fibrous mass that is adherent to the femur and that obliterates the suprapatellar pouch, the quadriceps should be lengthened by a V incision, with approximation of the V cephalad with a Y closure. The anterior capsule is then transversely divided. If the knee flexes to 80° or 90° no further dissection is needed. However, if flexion is still limited, the collateral ligaments should be freed so that they will slide posteriorly. The posterior capsule may need to be bluntly dissected from the femoral condyles and the iliotibial band divided. If, after the knee is reduced and flexed to 90°, there is anterior instability, the anterior cruciate may be moved forward on the tibia, but if the anterior cruciate is absent, I would not reconstruct it at this time, as with time the in-

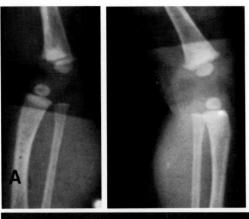

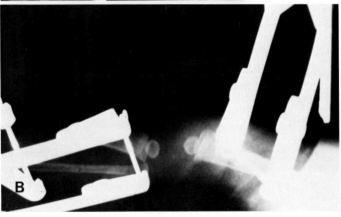

FIG. 20-13. *(A)* A severely subluxated knee. The normal knee is shown on the right for comparison. *(B)* The three-pin technique for reducing the severely subluxated or the truly dislocated knee.

stability may improve. If it does not improve, repair of the posterior capsule may be preferable to an attempt at cruciate reconstruction.

Prognosis

Those patients with knees that are subluxed and are reduced by simple traction or cast almost all do well. Those that have knees that are completely dislocated and need skeletal traction or open reduction do less well. It is uncommon to obtain more than 90° of motion, but the patient can usually expect sufficient function to live at least a sedentary life.

BIPARTITE PATELLA

The bipartite patella is a congenital anomaly with little clinical significance, except that frequently it must be differentiated from a fracture.

The patella usually arises from one center of ossification, but at times there are two or more centers. These centers usually fuse to form one bone but may remain separate, creating a bipartite or multiple-partite patella. The second or smaller ossified section of the patella is almost always in the upper outer section of the patella.

The diagnosis is made by roentgenographic examination, and unfortunately the roentgenogram is usually made following an injury. However, the distinguishing features of the congenital anomaly should separate it from an acute fracture. In the bipartite patella, the margins between the fragments are smooth and the edge is cortical bone, whereas in an acute fracture the edges are irregular and are cortical cancellous bone. Often the anomaly is bilateral and, when there is doubt, the opposite patella should also be examined.

DISCOID MENISCUS

A discoid meniscus is a condition in which the fibrocartilage structure of the knee is discoid in shape rather than semilunar. It occurs usually in the lateral compartment of the knee, but may occur in the medial compartment.[12, 39] Generally it is unilateral, but may be bilateral, and it occurs with equal frequency in males and females.

Etiology

The etiology of discoid meniscus is controversial. Ross, Tough and English thought it to be a congenital lesion resulting from arrest of the development of the meniscus in the embryo.[48] Kaplan was unable to find any evidence that the meniscus was ever discoid in shape during its development.[29] As no one had ever described a discoid-shaped meniscus in an embryo he believed there must be another explanation. His studies led him to believe the discoid-shaped meniscus was an acquired lesion resulting from the lateral femoral condyle repeatedly riding over the lateral meniscus during flexion and extension of the knee. According to Kaplan, in the discoid meniscus there is no attachment of the meniscus posteriorly to the tibia, and the ligament of Wrisberg is short. Whereas the normal lateral meniscus moves posteriorly with flexion and anteriorly with extension, the discoid meniscus is displaced posteriorly and medially by the short thick ligament of Wrisberg as the knee extends. The short ligament of Wrisberg does not allow the meniscus to move forward with the lateral condyle as the knee extends. On flexion of the knee the popliteal and coronary ligament pull the meniscus laterally. This medial and lateral movement of the meniscus beneath the pressure of the lateral condyle gradually deforms the cartilage into its discoid shape.

Clinical Features

The child with a discoid meniscus may present with the complaint of a "clunk" or "click" in the knee, or may have pain as the major complaint, or both. There may be a snapping in the knee that on observation gives the appearance of the tibia subluxating during flexion-extension, or the knee may give way while walking or running. Other patients have a dull ache that is intermittent, is aggravated by activity, but also is present at night and during inactive periods.

The physical findings are usually limited. Often the snap can be reproduced by flexing and extending the knee. If the meniscus is torn, pressure over the lateral compartment at the joint line may cause pain. A discoid meniscus may undergo cystic degeneration. The cyst is palpable along the joint line, usually just anterior to the lateral collateral ligament. If pain has been present for some time, there should be atrophy of the thigh muscle. Arthroscopy and arthrography are both helpful in confirming the diagnosis.

Treatment

No treatment is indicated in the nonpainful discoid meniscus. However, if the symptoms of a torn meniscus are present, or if a cyst is palpable over the lateral joint space, the meniscus should be removed. Meniscectomy of a discoid meniscus is more difficult to perform than removal of a torn semilunar meniscus. The meniscus is difficult to see as it displaces medially and posteriorly on extension and lateroposteriorly on flexion. A transverse incision over the lateral joint line is used to remove the meniscus. Care must be taken to protect both the popliteal artery, which lies close to the ligament of Wrisberg that connects the discoid meniscus to the medial femoral condyle, and the lateral inferior genicular artery that lies between the fibular collateral ligament and the synovium over the posterior lateral aspect of the meniscus. Postoperative care is the same as that for any other meniscectomy.

OSTEOCHONDRITIS DISSECANS

Osteochondritis is a lesion that affects the subchondral bone and articular surface of a joint. It is generally thought of as a disease of young adults but occurs not infrequently in children between 10 and 15 years of age. The youngest reported patient was 4 years old.[21]

The distal femur is the most common site of involvement, but it may also occur in the dome of the talus, the patella, the capitellum of the humerus, and in the femoral head. About 10 per cent of the patients have more than one lesion, with the involvement being usually symmetrical, but multiple lesions may be present without being symmetrical in distribution.

Alexander Pare described the removal of a loose body from a joint in 1558. In 1870 James Paget described this lesion and called it "joint necrosis," but Konig in 1887 gave the lesion the name by which it is now known. He believed that the lesion was due to trauma that resulted in "dissecting inflammation."

The mechanism that produces osteochondritis dissecans is almost certainly ischemic necrosis.[2] However, the etiology of the vascular incident that causes the ischemia is not known. No one has described the presence of a thrombosed vessel. It may well be that there is a multiple pathogenesis of the ischemia.

Etiology

Trauma, either directly or indirectly, with occlusion of the subchondral blood supply is generally thought to be the cause of osteochondritis dissecans.[10, 15, 49] Lesions similar to osteochondritis dissecans have been produced experimentally by Rehbein both by repeated hyperextension of the knee and by a direct force on the patella.[46]

Smillie separates this condition into juvenile and adult types. According to Smillie, the adult type is attributed to trauma brought about by a displacement of a meniscus or by instability of the joint. In the child, irregular ossification with isolation of a nidus of bone in the subchondral area creates the environment where minimal trauma causes the blood supply to the nidus to be interrupted.[49]

There is a hereditary or constitutional predisposition for development of osteochondritis dissecans. I have treated several patients and their cousins. Others have had similar experiences.[17, 41, 51] About 10 per cent of the patients have more than one lesion, which suggests a constitutional factor. Furthermore, the patients are more likely to have osteochondrosis of other areas, such as Osgood-Schlatter disease, osteochondrosis of the lower pole of the patella, and vertebral osteochondrosis. Six of 27 children in Green's series showed other osteochondritic lesions.[21]

I have observed an asymptomatic irregular ossification defect in the distal end of the femur in a 10-year-old boy progress to a symptomatic typical osteochondritis dissecans by the time he was 13 years old. It is my feeling that in the child the isolation of a nidus of ossified bone surrounded by cartilage in the subchondral area sets the stage for a fracture to occur at the interface between the bone and the nonossified cartilage. The cartilage may ossify and the necrotic nidus may be gradually incorporated. However, if the articular cartilage fractures, joint fluid will circulate into the fracture, preventing healing, and a loose body develops which eventually drops out of its bed.

Clinical Features

The major symptom in the child is pain, which is intermittent early in the course but later becomes constant. Strenuous activities increase the discomfort, not so much during the action, but rather after resting from vigorous activity. Mild swelling may be observed intermittently and the child may have an antalgic gait. Occasionally the joint is asymptomatic, or the symptoms may be too mild for the patient to seek help until the fragment separates, the loose body causes locking of the joint and swelling, and other signs of synovitis become more prominent.

The physical findings are usually minimal and depend upon the duration of symptoms and the joint affected. In the knee it is usually the case to find a full range of motion, no synovial thickening, and minimal thigh atrophy. When a loose body is present there may be a synovitis with effusion, and on occasion the loose body can be palpated. Pressure by palpation over the involved surface usually causes pain. The test described by Wilson is particularly helpful when the knee is affected. In this test the tibia is internally rotated on the femur with the knee flexed 90°. As the knee is extended, internal rotation is maintained and pain is experienced at around 30° of flexion, if the lesion is on the medial condyle. The pain is relieved by externally rotating the tibia.

The diagnosis is made by viewing the roentgenogram. Early, there is a radiolucent area with a small specule of bone (Fig. 20-14 A, B). Later the picture is one of a subchondral fragment of bone demarcated by a radiolucent line. The lesion in the knee may be seen on the routine anteroposterior roentgenogram in some patients. However, if it is located posterior to the most distal projection of the femur a tunnel view is needed for it to be seen. The usual position of the lesion is on the lateral portion of the medial condyle, but it occurs also on the lateral condyle.

Treatment

Green and Banks showed that in children conservative treatment gave an excellent prognosis for healing without residual deformity.[21] In children, when the diagnosis is made before the articular cartilage fractures, immobilization of the knee almost always leads to healing of the lesion in 16 to 20 weeks and in some patients even at 12 weeks. The immobilization is effected by means of a cylinder cast that extends from the upper thigh to just above the ankle (Fig. 20-14 C, D). The position in which the knee is immobilized is of utmost importance, for weightbearing between the tibia and femur should not exert pressure in the area of the lesion. Using a lateral roentgenogram of the knee, the position of flexion necessary to relieve the pressure exerted by the tibia on the lesion is determined and the plaster is applied with the knee held in that position. A follow-up roentgenogram is made after the cast is applied to be certain that the lesion is free of pressure. The lesion is usually located so that the knee has to be either in full extension to clear the posteriorly located lesion or in 40° to 45° of flexion to avoid the lesions that are more anteriorly located. If the knee has to be flexed the patient walks more comfortably with the heels of the shoes raised by adding appropriate lifts.

Almost without exception the knees of patients under 15 years of age heal if appropriate treatment is started before the defect separates. If the patient is skeletally mature or near maturity, healing after conservative treatment is not as likely. When the lesion has separated I prefer to remove the loose body and drill the bone in the base of the defect for medial condylar defects. However, when the defect is on the lateral condyle, the condyle should be replaced. Removal of a large posterior area of the lateral condyle causes instability of the knee and interferes with participation in sports. Smillie advocates replacement of the fragment and grafting of the bone, if necessary, to level the articular surface on both the medial and lateral defects. He uses small Smillie nails to hold the fragment in place. These need to be removed later. Kirschner wires, inserted so that they can be removed anteriorly without an incision, are preferable to Smillie nails.

After the fragment is removed and the base of the defect drilled, motion with minimal stress is started on the first or second postoperative day. The leg is suspended in a Thomas splint with a Pearson attachment so that the patient can passively flex and extend the knee. This is done every 30 minutes for 2 to 3 minutes during the day for about 7 to 10 days. Ambulation can begin on the seventh to tenth postoperative day with crutches and minimal weightbearing. Flexion and extension exercises are done from the side-lying position six to eight times a day for several minutes. This regimen is continued for about 10 to 12 weeks. Motion without stress is important for rapid healing of the defect. The results of surgical excision of the defect and drilling of the base are not as satisfactory as when healing of the lesion takes place with conservative treatment.

OSGOOD-SCHLATTER DISEASE

This syndrome, described first by Osgood in 1903, presents during adolescence as a swelling around the tibial tubercle and patellar tendon.[40]

Etiology

The etiology is controversial. Both Osgood and Schlatter, who described the entity a few months after Osgood, thought that the cause was trauma with partial avulsion of the tibial tubercle.[40] Woodfrey and Chandler[55] and Hughes,[25] however, presented evidence that the lesion is a result of traumatic tendonitis of the patellar tendon resulting in heterotopic bone formation in the tendon.

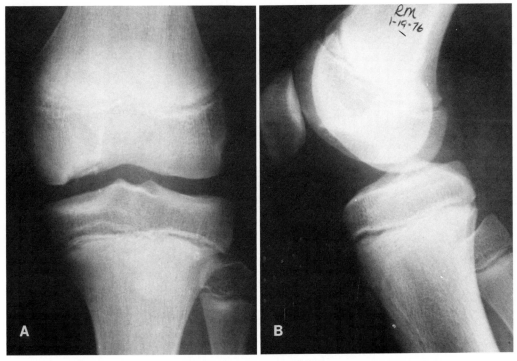

FIG. 20-14. *(A and B)* Anteroposterior and lateral views of the knee showing a typical osteochondritic lesion in a young adolescent. *(Legend continued on facing page.)*

Neither of these concepts can be confirmed or denied by present information. Codman, in his discussion of Osgood's paper, stated that he thought the cause was periostitis or new-bone formation from injury to the patellar tendon. The idea of traction on the tibial tubercle appeals to me as a reasonable etiologic factor, resulting in a traumatic epiphysitis. Certainly the mechanics of the quadriceps pull during the age at which there is rapid growth and widening of the epiphyses and apophyses support this view. If trauma to the patellar tendon were the cause, why does the age of these patients fall within such a limited range? The tendonitis that is present is secondary to the epiphysitis. Further evaluation is needed to elucidate the exact etiology.

Clinical Features and Diagnosis

The typical patient is a 11- to 15-year-old child, usually a boy, who is active in sports.

Pain is the presenting complaint. The pain occurs over the tibial tubercle when pressure is exerted and also when the quadriceps is stressed, as in ascending and descending stairs, running and jumping. There is soft-tissue swelling over the tibial tubercle. The remainder of the joint examination is negative.

The roentgenogram of the knee shows soft-tissue swelling anterior to the tubercle and thickening of the patellar tendon. In older patients there are bony changes in and around the patellar tendon insertion that have been divided into three types by Woolfrey.[55] In Type I the tibial tuberostity is prominent and irregular; in Type II the tibial tubercle is irregular and there is a small free fragment of bone anterior and superior to the tubercle; and in Type III there is a small regular tubercle with a small fragment of bone anterior and superior to the tubercle. These free fragments of bone are the result of heterotopic bone formation and are not fragments off the tubercle.

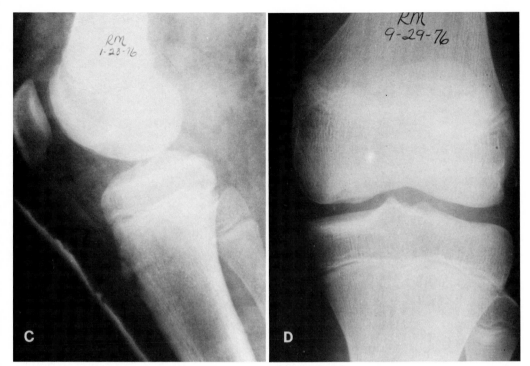

FIG. 20-14. *(Continued). (C)* This film, taken through the cast, shows the position of immobilization that removes weightbearing stress from the lesion. *(D)* After 18 weeks of immobilization, the lesion is healing.

Treatment

This is a self-limiting disease that spontaneously subsides with fusion of the tubercle at around 15 years of age. The longer the symptoms are present and the more severe the swelling, the more likely it is that there will be residual enlargement of the tubercle and heterotopic bone in the patellar tendon. When symptoms are severe enough to interfere with the patient's activities, I have recommended immobilization in a cylinder cast for 6 to 8 weeks. After removal of the cast, activity is limited to walking for another 2 to 3 weeks, and then full activity is resumed. The great majority of patients are able to return to full activity without further difficulty.

Operative treatment has been recommended for those patients with recurring symptoms following conservative therapy. I have had no occasion to use surgical therapy as immobilization has been an effective treatment.

POPLITEAL CYST

The popliteal cyst in children is a synovial cyst that arises from the semimembranous bursa, from beneath the medial head of the gastrocnemius, or from the joint capsule. Baker described a popliteal cyst arising as a herniation from the joint. This is a frequent finding in adults with rheumatoid or osteoarthritic arthritis, but it is not common in children.[4] Burleson and coworkers reported on 83 cysts occurring in the popliteal area of children of all age groups, which were treated by excision.[9] Of these, 46 arose from the semimembranous bursa, 26 from herniations of the joint, and eleven could not be accurately classified. The cyst is always found between the semimembranous bursa and the medial head of the gastrocnemius.

The typical popliteal cyst in the child, in my experience, arises from the semimembranous bursa. It is filled with a gelatinous fluid, and the lining of the cyst may be either fibrous tissue, synovial cells, inflammatory cells, or a mixture of the fibrous and synovial cell lining.

The popliteal cyst of childhood presents as a swelling of the medial side of the popliteal space just lateral to the semitendinosus. Tumors that are not located just lateral to the semitendinosus and between it and the medial head of the gastrocnemius should be looked upon as being something other than a typical Baker's cyst, for they are usually lesions of another type, such as fibroma, sarcoma, or a vascular anomaly. The cyst is usually asymptomatic, but it can cause discomfort if it enlarges excessively. In my experience, the massive cyst seen in adults that dissects downward and spreads beneath the posterior muscle does not occur in children, except in a rare rheumatoid arthritic joint. The cyst transilluminates, and this diagnostic test should always be done to prevent confusing it with a fibrous or vascular anomaly.

Observation of the asymptomatic nonenlarging cyst is appropriate in the child, as some cysts may regress and others may remain asymptomatic. In those that cause symptoms or that continue to enlarge, surgical excision should be done.

REFERENCES

1. Aegerter, E. E.: The possible relationship of neurofibromatosis, congenital pseudarthrosis and fibrous dysplasia. J. Bone Joint Surg., *32A:*618-626, 1950.
2. Aegerter E. E., and Kirkpatrick, J. A.: Orthopedic Diseases, ed. 4. Philadelphia, W. B. Saunders, 1975.
3. Andersen, K. S.: Congenital pseudarthrosis of tibia and neurofibromatosis. Acta Orthop. Scand., *47:*108-111, 1976.
4. Baker, W. M.: On the formation of synovial cysts in the leg in connection with disease of the knee joint. St. Bart. Hosp. Rep., *13:*245, 1877.
5. Blount, W. P.: Tibia vara: osteochondrosis: Deforman's tibiae. J. Bone Joint Surg., *19:*1, 1937.
6. Blumel, J., Eggers, G. W. N., and Evans, B.: Eight cases of hereditary bilateral medial tibial torsion in four generations. J. Bone Joint Surg., *39A:*1198, 1957.
7. Bowker, H. H., and Thompson, E. B.: Surgical treatment of recurrent dislocation of the patella. A study of 48 cases. J. Bone Joint Surg., *46A:*1451, 1964.
8. Boyd, H. B., and Sage, F. P.: Congenital pseudarthrosis of the tibia. J. Bone Joint Surg., *40A:*1245-1270, 1958.
9. Burleson, R. J., Bickel, W. H., and Dahlin, D.: Popliteal cyst: a clinicopathological survey. J. Bone Joint Surg., *38A:*1265, 1956.
10. Burrows, H. J.: Osteochondritis juvenilis. J. Bone Joint Surg., *41B:*455, 1958.
11. Campbell, W. C., and Crenshaw, A. H. (eds.): Campbell's Orthopaedics, ed. 5. St. Louis, C. V. Mosby, 1971.
12. Cave, E. F., and Staples, O. S.: Congenital discoid meniscus: a cause of internal derangement of the knee. Am. J. Surg., *54:*371, 1941.
13. Ducroquet, R., and Cottard, A.: Pseudarthrosis congenitale de jambe deformation osstua de la neurofibromatoses. J. Chir., *53:*483–502, 1939.
14. Erlacher, P. Deformerierende prozesse der epiphysengegend bei kindern. Arch. Orthop. Unfallchir., *20:*81, 1922.
15. Fairbank, H. A. T.: Osteochondritis dissecans. Br. J. Surg., *21:*67, 1933.
16. Fienman, N. L., and Yakovac, W. C. Neurofibromatosis in childhood. J. Pediatr., *76:*339-346, 1970.
17. Gardiner, T. B.: Osteochondritis dissecans in three members of one family. J. Bone Joint Surg., *37B:*139, 1955.
18. Golding, J. S. R., and McNeil-Smith, J. D. G.: Observations on the etiology of tibia vara. J. Bone Joint Surg., *45B:*320, 1963.
19. Goldthwait, J. E.: Dislocation of the patella. Trans. Am. Orthop. Assoc., *8:*327, 1897.
20. Green, W. T., Sr.: Personal communication, 1965.
21. Green, W. T., and Banks, H. B.: Osteochondritis dissecans in children. J. Bone Joint Surg., *35A:*26, 1953.
22. Green, W. T., and Rundall: Pseudarthrosis and neurofibromatosis. Arch. Surg., *46:*61, 1943.
23. Harrison, M. H. M.: The results of realignment operation on recurrent dislocation of the patella. Clin. Orthop., *18:*96, 1960.
24. Heywood, A. W. B.: Recurrent dislocation of the patella. A study of its pathology and treatment of 106 knees. J. Bone Joint Surg., *43B:*508, 1961.
25. Hughes, E. S. R.: Osgood Schlatter's disease. Surg. Gynecol. Obstet., *86:*323, 1948.
26. Hughston, J. C.: Subluxation of the patella J. Bone Joint Surg., *50A:*1003, 1968.
27. Hutter, C. G., Jr., and Scott, W.: Tibial torsion. J. Bone Joint Surg., *31A:*511, 1949.
28. Jones, J. B., Francis, K. C., and Mahoney, J. R.: Recurrent dislocating patella—a longterm followup study. Clin. Orthop., *20:*230, 1961.
29. Kaplan, E. B.: Discoid lateral meniscus of the knee joint: nature, mechanism and operative treatment. J. Bone Joint Surg., *39A:*77, 1957.
30. Katz, M. P., Grogone, B. J. J., and Sope, K. C.: The etiology and treatment of congenital dislocation of the knee. J. Bone Joint Surg., *49B:*112, 1967.
31. Khermosh, O., Lior, G., and Weissman, S. L.: Tibial torsion in children. Clin. Orthop., *79:*26, 1971.
32. Konig, F.: Ueber frei körper in den gelenken. Deutsche Zertschrift für Chir., *27:*90, 1887.

33. Lancourt, J. E., and Christini, J. A.: Patella alta and patella infera—their etiological role in patellar dislocation, chondromalacia and apophysitis of the tibial tubercle. J. Bone Joint Surg., *57A:*1112, 1975.

34. Langenskiold, A.: Tibia vara. Acta Chir. Scand. *103:*9, 1952.

35. Langenskiold, A. and Riska, E. B.: Tibia vara. J. Bone Joint Surg., *46A:*1405, 1964.

36. Macnab, I.: Recurrent dislocation of the patella. J. Bone Joint Surg., *34A:*957, 1952.

37. Masserman, R. L., Peterson, H. A., and Bianco, A. J.: Congenital pseudarthrosis of the tibia. Clin. Orthop., *99:*140-145, 1974.

38. Merchant, A. C., Mercer, R. L., Jacobsen, R. H., and Cool, C. R.: Roentgenographic analysis of patellofemoral congruence. J. Bone Joint Surg., *56A:*1391, 1974.

39. Murdock, G.: Congenital discoid medial semilunar cartilage. J. Bone Joint Surg., *38B:*564, 1956.

40. Osgood, R. B.: Lesions of the tibial tubercle occurring during adolescence. Boston Med. Surg. J., *148:*114, 1903.

41. Nielsen, N. A.: Osteochondritis dissecans, capituli humeri. Acta Orthop. Scand., *4:*307, 1933.

42. Paget, J.: On the production of some loose bodies in joints. St. Bartholomew Hosp. Rep., *6:*1, 1870.

43. Pare, A.: Oeuvres Completes, vol. 3. Paris, J. B. Balliere, 1841.

44. Phemister, D. B.: The causes of and the changes in loose bodies arising from articular surface of the joint. J. Bone Joint Surg., *61:*278, 1924.

45. Provenzano, K. W.: Congenital dislocation of the knee. N. Engl. J. Med., *236:*360, 1947.

46. Rehbein, F.: Die entstehung der osteochondritis dissecans. Arch. Klin. Chir., *265:*69, 1950.

47. Rosen, H., and Sandlick, H.: Measurement of tibiofibular torsion. J. Bone Joint Surg., *37A:*847, 1955.

48. Ross, J. A., Tough, I. C. K., and English, I. A.: Congenital discoid meniscus J. Bone Joint Surg., *40B:*262, 1958.

49. Smillie, I. S.: Osteochondritis dissecans. Baltimore, Williams & Wilkins, 1960.

50. Staheli, L. T., and Engel, G. M.: Tibial torsion: a method of assessment and a survey of normal children. Clin. Orthop., *86:*183, 1972.

51. Stougaard, J.: Familial occurrence of osteochondritis dissecans. J. Bone Joint Surg., *46B:*542, 1964.

52. Tachdjian, M.: Pediatric Orthopaedics, p. 723. Philadelphia, W. B. Saunders, 1972.

53. Tolon, S.: Torsion of the lower extremity. Proc. 12th Cong. of Int. Soc. Orthop. Surg. Traumatol., Amsterdam, Excerpta Medica, 1972.

54. Van Nes, C. P.: Congenital pseudarthrosis of the leg. J. Bone Joint Surg., *48A:*1467-1487, 1966.

55. Woolfrey, B. F., and Chandler, E. F.: Manifestation of Osgood-Schlatter's disease in late teenage and early adulthood. J. Bone Joint Surg., *42A:*327, 1960.

21 *The Foot*

Wood W. Lovell, M.D., Charles T. Price, M.D., and Peter L. Meehan, M.D.

STRUCTURE AND FUNCTION

The foot is in constant contact with the environment. It serves to propel the body and give information regarding our surroundings. Since we bear four times our body weight on each extremity at rest, the feet must be strong. The surfaces that we walk on vary, so the foot must be able to accommodate to these changes.

EMBRYOLOGY

Willis[21] points out that the human foot and leg are adaptations of the pelvic fin of an aquatic animal to terrestrial locomotion. The evolution from fin to foot is reviewed briefly in the embryology of the human fetus. For the first 6 months of intrauterine life the feet are inverted, the soles directed toward the abdomen. A more rapid growth of the scaphoid and cuneiform bones then occurs. The neck of the talus, which has been directed downward, has relatively delayed growth and turns inward and upward. The inner border of the talus grows upward. Lack of this change in growth rate leaves the foot in the equinovarus position.

Willis[21] further states that in the primitive foot there are five tarsal bones, plus an os tibiale and an os fibulare. Between the last two are the os intermedium proximally and the os centrale distally. Tarsals one, two and three become the cuneiforms. Tarsals four and five unite to form the cuboid. This occurs in the feet of all mammals. The os intermedium fuses with the posterior tubercule of the os tibiale to form the posterior process of the astragalus or, failing to fuse, persists as the anomalous os trigonum.

The os fibulare undergoes great posterior development to form the human heel. The os centrale becomes the scaphoid. The extension of the heel interrupts the tendons of the gastrocnemius and plantaris.

White[20] called attention to the torsion in the Achilles tendon and its surgical significance. Prior to this, Hoke had utilized this in developing his method of heelcord lengthening. Those fibers of the Achilles tendon that occupy a medial portion proximally twist laterally as they approach the calcaneus, so that they are then posterior to those fibers that originally occupied the lateral position. These are the fibers that originally inserted on the os tibiale.

ANATOMY

INTEGUMENT

The skin of the sole of the foot at the heel and over the metatarsal heads is equipped with a special tissue. In running and jumping, the feet must bear up to 10 times the body weight. Kuhns[14] emphasized that the elastic adipose tissue in these locations serves to cushion the stresses of weightbearing on the underlying bone and soft tissue. It is felt that part of the prolonged disability after os calcis fracture is related to rupture of the septae in the elastic adipose tissue.

BONY ARCHITECTURE

The bony architecture of the foot must accommodate the great variability in terrain over which we course throughout our lives. In contradistinction to the hand, the foot must be stable. The wedge-shaped mortise and tenon articulation between the talus and the tibia exemplifies this fact.

There are two arches in the foot. The longitudinal arch is keystoned medially by the neck of the talus. This is reinforced by the spring ligament between the sustentaculum tali and the navicular. The Y ligament of Bigelow between the calcaneus, navicular and cuboid supports it as well. The posterior tibial tendon, and indirectly the flexor hallucis longus, support the medial arch. The lateral longitudinal arch is keystoned by the cuboid. The transverse arc of the foot exists only at the level of the metatarsal bases. At the level of the metatarsal heads, there is no arch.

Acton[1] states that the weight borne by various positions of the foot varies according to the phase of gait and the position of the foot. In normal standing, weight is borne equally on the forefoot and hindfoot. The first metatarsal bears more weight than the lesser rays. If total weight is 24 units in normal stance, each foot would bear 12 units. The hindfoot of each would bear 6 units and the forefoot 6 units. In the forefoot, the weight would be borne in a ratio of 2:1:1:1:1 from the first to the fifth metatarsal.

According to Jones,[11] with the triceps surae relaxed, four-fifths of the load is borne by the hindfoot.

The slings affected by the tibial muscles and the peroneus longus tendon would seem to provide dynamic support for the longititudinal arch. They are, however, silent during stance phase of gait.[2] Dynamic support is provided more indirectly through the reflex contraction and shift of body weight. The plantar aponeurosis and short muscles act as tie rods for the longitudinal arch.

Ligamentous support for the ankle is symmetrical. There are discrete structures laterally, but medially they blend into a fan-shaped ligament. Laterally the three components, anterior and posterior, talofibular and calcanofibular, are under equal tension throughout a full range of motion. They radiate from the approximate axis of motion of the ankle. Medially, the axis of motion is 1 cm. distal to the medial malleolus. For this reason, the posterior talotibial ligament is a check rein to plantar flexion. Beneath the calcanotibial ligament is the middle portion of the tibiotalar ligament—a most important structure for stability of the ankle. Smith[14] has evaluated the subtalar region of the foot. He credits Jones[7] with redefining the area between the talocalcaneonavicular joint in front and the talocalcaneal joint behind into two parts. The sinus tarsi is the wide lateral part of this region. Jones refers to the narrower medial part as the canalis tarsi. This was the terminology used in older writings. Smith[18] found these ligaments in this area: (1) The inferior extensor retinaculum is a continuation of a retinaculum which lies in front of the ankle. This was fully described by Frazer[6] in 1920. Traced laterally, the retinaculum turns downwards around the lateral aspect of the neck of the talus, to which it is sometimes attached, and enters the sinus tarsi. Within the sinus, it divides into well-defined lateral intermediate and medial roots. The lateral root becomes incorporated into the deep fascia on the lateral aspect of the foot. The larger intermediate root descends vertically into the calcaneus. The slender medial root inclines into the canalis tarsi before being attached to the sulcus calcanei. (2) The cervical ligament lies in the anterior part of the sinus tarsi. Jones[11] used this term, and it is now accepted terminology. It is a broad flattened band which lies anterior to the intermediate route of the retinaculum. It is attached below to the dorsal surface of the calcaneus, medial to the extensor digitorum brevis, and extends medially and upwards to a tubercle on the inferolateral aspect of the neck of the talus. (3) The ligament of the canalis tarsi extends between the talus and the calcaneus. Other authors refer to this as the interosseous ligament. It is a broad band, flattened in the coronal plane, in which the fibers extend downward and laterally from the sulcus tali to the sulcus calcanei, crossing in its course either anterior or posterior to the medial route of the inferior extensor retinaculum.

The cervical ligament limits inversion; the ligament of the canalis tarsi limits eversion.

MUSCLES

There are ten tendons that span the ankle joint, when considering the plantaris and triceps surae as one. In order to prevent bowstringing of the tendons on the anterior aspect of the ankle, the thin crural fascia of the lower leg is reinforced by transverse bundles. This comprises the extensor retinaculum or the anterior annular ligament. Distally, there is a Y-shaped reinforcement. It attaches to the anterolateral surface of the calcaneus where it has three divisions, as previously noted. It spreads medially as two limbs blending into the medial malleolus of the tibia and into the plantar aponeurosis.

Since the triceps surae inserts into the tuberosity of the calcaneus 2 inches posterior to the axis of motion of the ankle, it is a powerful plantar flexor. The anterior tibial tendon is 2 inches from the axis of motion while the toe extensors are $1^1/_2$ inches from that point. Thus, they have ample leverage to act as ankle dorsiflexor muscles.

The muscles of the foot can be divided into extrinsic and intrinsic groups. There are similarities to the hand. The leg may be divided into four compartments. The anterior compartment containing the extensor digitorum longus, the extensor hallucis longus and the anterior tibial muscle is supplied by the deep portion of the peroneal nerve. They receive their vascularity from muscular branches of the tibial or anterior tibial artery. The lateral compartment of the leg contains the peroneus longus and peroneus brevis muscles. They are supplied by the superficial portion of the peroneal nerve and muscular branches of the peroneal artery. The superficial posterior compartment of the leg contains the gastrocnemius, the soleus and the popliteus muscles. They are innervated by the tibial nerve and receive their blood supply from sural branches of the popliteal artery. The deep posterior compartment contains the flexor hallucis longus, the extensor digitorum longus and the posterior tibial muscle. They, as well, are supplied by the tibial nerve and receive muscular branches from either the posterior tibial artery or the peroneal artery.

ANTERIOR COMPARTMENT

The extensor digitorum longus passes along a straight line from its origin on the proximal three-fourths of the anterior surface of the fibular shaft and in the interosseous membrane as well as along the lateral tibial condyle. The peroneus tertius is actually a part of the extensor digitorum longus. All tendons pass beneath the extensor retinaculum in the same canal. The peroneus tertius inserts on the dorsum of the base of the fourth or fifth metatarsals or on both sites. The extensor digitorum longus inserts onto the dorsal surface of middle and distal phalanges of the lateral four toes. It functions to extend the phalanges of the lateral four toes and acts as a secondary dorsiflexor of the foot. The peroneus tertius acts to dorsiflex the foot while everting it. The tibialis anterior arises from the proximal two-thirds of the lateral aspect of the tibia and interosseous membrane. As in the proximal muscles of the forearm, it also arises from investing fascia and adjoining planes. It inserts onto the medial and plantar surface of the first cuneiform and base of the first metatarsal. It dorsiflexes the foot and inverts it.

The extensor hallucis longus arises from the middle one-half of the anterior surface of the fibula crossing the anterior tibial artery proximal to the ankle and passes distally to insert into the base of the distal phalanx. It functions to extend the great toe and acts secondarily to dorsiflex the ankle.

The extensor digitorum brevis has no counterpart in the hand. It is an intrinsic muscle of the foot. It arises from the dorsal lateral surface of the calcaneus. It has three tendons that insert into the fibular borders of the extensor digitorum longus tendons to the second, third and fourth toes. The most medial belly of the extensor digitorum brevis is actually a separate muscle of the extensor hallucis brevis, which inserts into the dorsum of the base of the proximal phalanx of the great toe.

The lateral compartment contains the peroneus longus and peroneus brevis muscles. The peroneus longus arises from the lateral condyle of the tibia, the head and upper two-thirds of the lateral surface of the fibula, adjacent fascia, and intermuscular septae. It inserts into the lateral side of the first cuneiform and the base of the first metatarsal. It functions to plantar flex the foot while everting it.

The peroneus brevis arises from the lower two-thirds of the lateral surface of the fibula and the adjacent intermuscular septae. It inserts into the lateral side of the base of the fifth metatarsal. It functions to plantar flex and evert the foot.

As stated before, the posterior compartment of the leg is divided into deep and superficial compartments by the deep transverse fascia. This is a distinct sheet stretching from the tibia to the fibula. Each compartment has three extrinsic muscles to the foot. Those in the superficial compartment act as one.

The gastrocnemius arises from two heads: The medial head arises from the medial condyle, the adjacent part of the femur, and the capsule of the knee joint. The lateral head arises from the lateral condyle, the adjacent part of the femur, and the capsule of the knee joint. They insert into the calcaneus by means of a common tendon with the soleus. It functions to plantar flex the foot while secondarily flexing the knee and inverting the foot.

The soleus originates from the posterior surface of the head and upper one-third of the shaft of the fibula, the middle third of the medial border of the tibia, and the tendinous arch between the tibia and fibula. It inserts into the calcaneus by means of a common tendon with the gastrocnemius. It functions to plantar flex the foot and secondarily to invert the foot.

The plantaris crosses over from its origin on the lateral prolongation of the linea aspera of the femur and crosses distally between the gastrocnemius and the soleus to the medial side of the tendo Achilles, then inserts into the calcaneus. It is absent in 6 to 8 per cent of normal individuals. It functions to flex the leg and to rotate the tibia medially at the beginning of flexion. It serves as a secondary flexor of the ankle and invertor of the foot. The deep posterior compartment is comprised of the flexor hallucis longus, the

flexor digitorum longus and the posterior tibial muscles.

The flexor hallucis longus arises from the inferior two-thirds of the fibula and passes distally on the lower end of the tibia into a definite groove in the posterior aspect of the talus. It passes forward, turning around another pulley, the sustentaculum tali, to contribute a strong slip to the flexor digitorum longus before running between the two heads of the short flexor to insert into the base of the great toe. Its primary function is that of flexion of the great toe, while secondarily it aids in plantar flexion and inversion of the foot.

The flexor digitorum longus arises from the posterior aspect of the tibia between the popliteal line and the lower 3 inches of the tibia. Its primary function is that of flexion of the lateral four toes. Its secondary function is that of plantar flexion of the ankle and inversion of the foot. The flexor digitorum longus receives the total insertion of the quadratus plantae muscle. The point of attachment covers all but the medial side of the tendon.

The posterior tibial muscle arises from the entire posterior surface of the interosseous membrane, except its lower portion, and from the adjacent surfaces of the tibia and fibula. It inserts into the tuberosity of the navicular, the plantar surfaces of all cuneiform bones, the plantar surfaces of the base of the second, third and fourth metatarsal bones, the cuboid, as well as the sustentaculum tali. It functions to plantar flex and invert the foot.

The relationship of the tendons and neurovascular bundle with the medial malleolus is well known. It was recently pointed out by Ben-Menachem[3] that the blood supply to the foot in congenital anomalies is not constant. He demonstrated absence of either the dorsalis pedis or posterior tibial arteries in association with congenital abnormalities.

Acton[1] has written a comprehensive article on the surgical anatomy of the foot. The reader is encouraged to review this article.

After removing the skin and subcutaneous tissue from the sole of the foot, the plantar aponeurosis is visible. It arises from the medial process of the tuberosity of the calcaneus and sends forward strong longitudinal fibers that terminate in five bands, one on each toe. These five bands send a superficial slip to the skin crease at the base of each toe and a deep slip that splits to embrace each toe flexor tendon. The two halves of this deep slip attach to and contribute to the fibrous digital sheath and the transverse metatarsal ligaments. In addition to the central portion of the plantar aponeurosis, a medial portion invests the abductor hallucis and a lateral portion invests the abductor digiti quinti. A strong cord of the lateral portion acts as a tie rod from the lateral process of the calcaneus to the tuberosity of the fifth metatarsal.

The muscles of the sole of the foot can be considered four layers of intrinsics, with extrinsics added to the second and fourth layers.[10] The first layer includes the two abductors and a short flexor; the second, an accessory flexor and the lumbricals; the third, two short flexors and an adductor; and the fourth, the interosseii.

The first layer of muscles includes the abductor hallucis, the flexor digitorum brevis and the abductor digiti quinti. Both abductors insert, by a conjoined tendon shared by the respective short flexor, into the base of the proximal phalanx of the first and fifth digits. The flexor brevis arises from the medial tuberosity of the calcaneus, passes forward and divides into four tendons—exactly analogous to the tendons of the flexor sublimis in the hand.

The second layer is comprised of the flexor digitorum longus, the flexor hallucis longus, the quadratus plantae, and the lumbricals. The quadratus plantae arises from two pointed heads from the calcaneus and inserts on all but the medial side of the flexor digitorum longus. The lumbricals arise from the long flexor tendons and pass around the medial or hallux side of each lesser ray. Each lumbrical has a bipenniform origin from the two flexor tendons. The exception to this is the first lumbrical, which supplies the second toe. It arises only from the flexor tendon to the second toe.

The third layer consists of the flexor hallucis brevis, the flexor digiti quinti brevis and the adductor brevis. The flexor of the great toe arises from the cuboid and third cuneiform. The fifth toe flexor arises from the base of the fifth metatarsal. The flexor hallucis brevis inserts through a conjoined tendon shared with the abductor and the adductor hallucis. The flexor of the fifth toe inserts into the fifth digit by a conjoined tendon shared by the abductor.

The fourth layer consists of the interosseii. They differ from those of the hand in that the second instead of the third ray is the axis about which abduction and adduction take place in the foot. The four dorsal interosseii are bipenniform, filling the four intermetatarsal spaces. The three plantar ones are unipenniform, with their origins and insertions on the same ray. Mann and Inman[16] studied the phasic activity of the intrinsics of the foot by implanting electrodes in six intrinsics of the foot, including the short extensors, the three muscles of the first layer, the flexor hallucis brevis and one interosseous. They concluded that the intrinsic acts as a functional unit and plays an important role in the stabilization of the foot for propulsion.

Opinions vary as to the function of the interosseii and lumbricals. Spalteholz[19] felt that they only flexed the proximal phalanges of the lesser toes without extending the second and third phalanges, as in the hand. From this and the evidence presented by Forster,[5] Manter,[17] and Kelikian[12] concluded that the long extensors of the toes and the surface walked upon are the two factors that maintain extension of the interphalangeal joints of the toes. Acton's[1] dissections did not bear this out. He noted that in specimens from younger individuals it was possible to demonstrate extension of both interphalangeal joints by placing tension on either the interosseous or lumbrical muscles if gentle tension on the long flexor and extensor was maintained. He was also able to trace fibers from the lumbrical and interosseous tendons to the extensor hood.

The deep transverse metatarsal ligament in the foot joins the plantar plate of the metatarsophalangeal joints of all five rays. This description is at variance with the description in *Gray's Anatomy*[8] but corresponds to Cunningham's[4] description. The plantar plates are attached in a similar manner to the palmar plates in the hand.

The glenoid ligament of Cruveilhier is a term synonymous with plantar plate. The glenoid ligament of Cruveilhier corresponds to the volar, palmar or vaginal ligaments in the hand. These are pivotal to understanding the anatomy of this portion of the foot. With an understanding of all the structures that attach to the glenoid ligaments and their relationships, much of the anatomy will become clearer.

The following structures attach directly to the glenoid ligaments: (1) The deep transverse ligament of the sole (also called the transverse metatarsal ligament); (2) the extensor hood; (3) the plantar aponeurosis through its divergent bands; (4) the flexor tendon sheath; (5) the fan-like portions of the collateral ligaments of the metatarsophalangeal joints; and (6) the capsule of the metatarsophalangeal joints.

The distal two-thirds of the glenoid ligament is a dense, thick fibrocartilaginous structure forming a broad rectangular plate. In its proximal one-third, it is composed of a more pliable tissue which is continuous with the capsule of the metatarsophalangeal joint and attaches relatively loosely to the metatarsal neck. This latter portion begins to fold upon itself when the joint is flexed to a position midway between the extremes of flexion and extension. It is elongated when the joint is in extension.

The glenoid ligament of the metatarsophalangeal joint of the great toe differs from that of the corresponding joint in the thumb. In the great toe, this ligament contains two sesmoid bones, whereas in the thumb the sesmoids are within the substance of the conjoined tendons related to the respective sides of the joint.

These ligaments form the volar portion of the metatarsophalangeal capsular ligaments. Their grooved volar surfaces form the dorsal wall of the flexor tendon sheath. This permits the profundus tendon to glide on the plantar aspect of the metatarsophalangeal joint regardless of the degree of flexion. The extensor hood girdles the metatarsophalangeal joint (more properly, the proximal phalanx just distal to it) and is anchored into the glenoid ligament.

BIOMECHANICS

In evaluating the biomechanical aspects of the foot, definitions are essential to proper discussion. Rotation about a transverse axis will be termed *flexion* and *extension*. Rotation about a vertical axis when the foot is moving is termed *abduction-adduction* and when the leg is moving is termed *medial rotation-lateral rotation*. Rotation about an anteroposterior axis is *pronation* and *supination*. *Inversion* and *eversion* are used differently by various authors. We use it to refer to rotation about an anteroposterior axis of the talocalcaneonavicular joint.

Hicks[9] has demonstrated in studies of normal cadaver feet that all movements in the foot are rotations. Hinged joints have their motion predetermined. A ball and socket joint has its plane of movement determined by the direction of forces acting upon it. Different tendons, though they may run in oblique directions, always produce one of two movements—clockwise or counterclockwise rotation about an axis. Due to this, motion in the foot is of a compound nature. This holds true for other forces such as body weight. For example, a force that tends to produce abduction at the talocalcaneonavicular joint only succeeds in producing pronation: abduction and extension because this (or its opposite) is the only movement of which this joint is capable. This occurs because the axis of motion only permits this complex movement.

The talonavicular articulation, being of a ball and socket shape, might be expected to show a greater degree of freedom of movement. This may seem incompatible with the assertion that all joints are hinged joints. Hicks[9] explains that this joint is peculiar in being one-half of two different joint complexes. In conjunction with the talocalcaneal articulation, it forms the talocalcaneonavicular joint complex. In conjunction with the calcaneocuboid articular, it forms the midtarsal joint complex. The navicular, therefore, rotates on the talus about three different axes—about the talocalcaneonavicular axis when the talocalcaneonavicular complex is in action and about one or the other of the midtarsal axes when the midtarsal complex is in action. The motion remains a simple hinge movement in each case. He does state that action at all of these complexes may occur simultaneously.

The effect of forefoot twist in standing is interesting to analyze. The following table is helpful to understanding the interrelationships:

Table 21-1. Interrelationships of Joint Motion in Standing

Foot standing:				
Arch high	Supination-adduction-flexion	Supination	Flexion-pronation	Extension-pronation
				(i.e., pronation twist of forefoot)
Arch low	Pronation-abduction-extension	Pronation	Extension-supination	Flexion-supination
				(i.e., supination twist of forefoot)

Talocalcaneonavicular movement provides for rotation between the foot and leg, whereas the midtarsal joint provides for rotation between the anterior and posterior parts of the foot.

Lateral rotation of the leg results in supination of the foot.[15] This apparent double movement is nothing other than a simple hinge movement at the talocalcaneonavicular joint. It is difficult to visualize because the hinge is oblique. Thus, supination of the hindfoot in response to pronation of the forefoot results in raising of the medial arch. Kite[13] has called attention to the association of lateral torsion of the leg and flatfeet.

Several authors have called attention to the fact that the arrangement of axes of motion of the subtalar joint and a transverse tarsal joint play a role in increasing the stability of the foot when it is in supination. The axes of motion of the component joints of the transverse tarsal joint are divergent in the normal supinated foot, but coincide in a pronated foot. This permits an unstable hinge-like action in the midtarsal region of the pronated foot. Support of the longitudinal arch is not accomplished by muscle pull,[2] but by maintaining the tarsal bones in positions of overlapping girders of the arch. Pes planus develops through medial rotation of the bones, not by direct downward collapse.

EQUINOVARUS DEFORMITIES

CONGENITAL TALIPES EQUINOVARUS

INTRODUCTION

Congenital talipes equinovarus is a complex deformity involving all of the bones of the foot. The incidence in the United States and England is said to be one per one thousand live births. The sex ratio is approximately two males to one female. Wynne-Davies[87, 88, 89] reports that the incidence of the same deformity among first-degree relatives is between 20 and 30 times higher than the normal incidence in the white races. The authors are not aware of any studies relating to the incidence of congenital talipes equinovarus in the black race. It is more often unilateral than bilateral.

GENETIC IMPLICATIONS

The genetics of congenital idiopathic talipes equinovarus is not yet well defined. According to Wynne-Davies,[87, 88, 89] the inheritance pattern is multifactorial, the manifestation of which is dependent upon predisposing environmental influences as well as a genetic background for the anomaly. Under these circumstances, the predictability of occurrence within a family is less straightforward than a simple gene defect. Family studies have shown the incidence of congenital idiopathic talipes equinovarus is 20 to 30 times higher in first-degree relatives than in the general population, illustrating the genetic tendency. Such studies have also been helpful in counseling the parents of an affected child. For example, the risk to a future sibling of a child with congenital clubfoot and the normal parents is about 3 per cent, whereas if the parents are also affected, the risk may be as high as 25 per cent. Further studies are needed, however, to more clearly define the probability of recurrence within a family.

ETIOLOGY

The etiology of congenital talipes equinovarus remains an enigma, although many theories have been advanced. Scarpa[27, 34, 35, 70, 73] believed that the deformity was related to medial twisting of the navicular, cuboid and calcaneus bones in their relation to the talus. Adams[23] investigated a number of fetal and adult specimens and found that all soft-tissue abnormalities were secondary. He stated that the principal deformity was in the talus. The head and neck of the talus in his dissections were found to be attenuated and directed toward the plantar and medial aspects of the foot. Böhm[31, 32] felt that the congenital clubfoot was due to an arrest in development. He postulated that the foot in a normal embryo at the 5-week stage was in a position of equinovarus and that an arrest in development was responsible for persistence of the deformity at birth. Other theories that have been suggested include abnormal tendon insertions and dysplasia of peroneal muscles.[21, 63]

Settle[80] in his study to determine the gross anatomical abnormalities in congenital clubfoot found in 16 dissected infantile clubfeet that the tibiae were essentially normal, with the exception of a slight degree of internal torsion in four specimens. All of the tali were found to be severely distorted. The talus was reduced in size by approximately one-fourth and was plantar flexed at the ankle joint. The neck of the talus presented the most significant changes and was deviated medially and plantarward on the body. The navicular was dislocated medially and plantarward also in its relation to the head of the talus. The subtalar articular facet was also severely distorted. Only one articular surface was noted, and its axis was slanted medially.

The calcaneus was of normal shape but appeared slightly smaller than normal and was displaced into varus, equinus and internal rotation.

Settle[80] concluded by saying that congenital clubfoot appears to be a primary developmental deformity of the hind part of the foot and is present as early as the twelfth gestational week.

Irani and Sherman[49] dissected eleven extremities with equinovarus in stillborns and found no primary abnormalities of nerves, vessels, muscles or tendon insertions. In every specimen the neck of the talus was found to be short and distorted and the anterior portion of the talus was found to rotate in a medial and plantar direction. The deviation of the anterior end of the talus was felt to be the primary fault. The deviations were attributed to a defective cartilaginous anlage which was dependent upon a primary germ-plasm defect. Environmental factors very likely contribute to the deformity as well.

PATHOLOGY

The deformity in congenital idiopathic clubfoot is that of forefoot adduction combined with inversion and supination, as well as varus of the hindfoot with the calcaneus inverted under the talus. The talus is found to be in equinus. These changes, although present at birth, become pronounced with the passage of time due to soft-tissue contracture. The head of the talus is prominent at the dorsal lateral aspect of the foot. The navicular is medial to the head of the talus and may lie adjacent to the medial malleolus. The cuboid is also displaced medially in front of the calcaneus. The cuneiforms as well as the metatarsals contribute to the deformity as a result of the adduction deformity. The cavus deformity is related to contracture of the plantar aponeurosis as well as the abductor hallicus, the short toe flexors and the abductor digiti quinti. The plantar flexed position of the first metatarsal also aggravates the cavus deformity.

In unilateral congenital clubfoot, there is usually minimal shortening of the involved foot and extremity as well as a slight discrepancy in the calf. The shortening of the extremity may involve the femur, the tibia or the foot, and in some instances all of the bones of the extremity are involved. This discrepancy in the involved extremity and foot may be more noticeable in females.

CLINICAL FINDINGS

Generally, congenital clubfoot may be classified into two distinct groups.[24, 65] In the first group, commonly referred to as a normal or conventional congenital clubfoot, the foot presents the usual deformities. The foot is, however, much more supple than the second type. The second group, by contrast, is characterized as having a greater degree of stiffness, and the foot is very likely to show considerable difference in size. In the au-

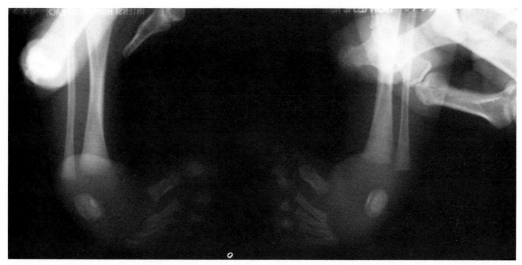

FIG. 21-1. Bilateral congenital clubfoot showing forefoot adduction and varus of the hindfoot. The ossification centers of the talus and calcaneus are superimposed, with a resultant talocalcaneal angle of zero.

thors' experience, the first type accounts for approximately 70 to 75 per cent of cases. In the second type, the calcaneus is smaller than normal, and because of the overlying adipose tissue it is difficult to palpate. There is often a transverse crease present in the region of the midfoot. This can be attributed to contracture of the plantar aponeurosis and the first layer of plantar muscles. The second type constitutes the recalcitrant type of deformity and is extremely difficult to correct by nonoperative means. The reduction in circumference of the calf is probably secondary to reduction in total muscle bulk.

Clinically, the foot in both types is held at a right angle to the ankle and long axis of the tibia. There is often very little prominence at the upper border of the heel. The talus is usually palpable at the dorsal lateral aspect of the foot and fills the sinus tarsi. The tubercule of the navicular is palpable medially. If an attempt is made to abduct the forefoot, resistance is encountered and the soft-tissue contractures are palpable on the medial aspect of the foot. Attempts at dorsiflexion of the foot demonstrate the marked contracture of the posterior soft tissues including the Achilles tendon and posterior capsule of the ankle. Finally, if the infant is supported and held erect, weight is borne on the dorsal lateral aspect of the foot rather than on the plantar aspect.

ROENTGENOGRAPHIC EXAMINATION

At birth, the primary centers of ossification include the talus and calcaneus and, in some instances, the cuboid. These structures can be demonstrated roentgenographically. The ossification center for the navicular appears at age 3 years in females and usually 1 year later in males. At the forefoot, the phalanges and metatarsals are ossified at birth (Fig. 21-1).

The technique of obtaining appropriate roentgenograms is of importance if the foot is to be assessed accurately. Beatson and Pierson[26] have described a method of obtaining anteroposterior and lateral roentgenograms that is simple and easily adapted to use. The child's hips are flexed 90° and the knees approximately 45° to 60°. The feet for the anteroposterior view are then held closely together and placed in 30° of plantar flexion on the cassette. The x-ray tube is then directed cranially from the vertical. The lateral view of the foot should be made with the foot plantar flexed 35° and the x-ray tube centered over the ankle and hindfoot. A stress lateral film following correction is also made, with the foot and ankle in extreme dorsiflexion. Lines drawn through the long axis of the talus as well as the inferior margin of the calcaneus should subtend an angle of 35° or greater if the deformity is corrected. Turco[83, 84] has emphasized the importance of the stress lateral roentgenogram in determining that the foot is satisfactorily corrected. The stress lateral view will also demonstrate overlap of the talus and calcaneus at their anterior ends.

In the anteroposterior view, similar lines are drawn through the long axes of the calcaneus and the talus and the resulting angle represents the talocalcaneal angle or Kite angle. The line through the talus should coincide with the first metatarsal and the line drawn through the calcaneus should coincide with the fifth metatarsal. The normal angle in the anteroposterior view varies between 20° and 35°. An angle greater than 35° indicates valgus and an angle less than 20° indicates varus of the hindfoot.

Simon[81] has developed the concept of analytical roentgenography of congenital clubfeet. He defines this term as an analytical method for roentgenographic evaluation of the four major deformities of clubfeet in whatever combination they may exist. The technique is based upon positioning the foot as close to the plantar grade or maximally corrected position as possible. If the foot is positioned properly, the degree of residual deformity following conservative treatment can be determined. In addition to the anteroposterior and lateral views of the foot, Simon[81] has suggested that the talo-first metatarsal angle (TMT angle) be determined. The normal TMT angle is zero to −20°. Measurements in a positive direction are abnormal. This angle is indicative of medial deviation of the foot at either the distal or proximal row of tarsal bones, or both. It is not helpful unless used in conjunction with the hindfoot talocalcaneal angle.

CLASSIFICATION OF IDIOPATHIC CONGENITAL TALIPES EQUINOVARUS

Congenital clubfeet do vary in severity.[24, 65] All such deformities have in common forefoot adduction, varus of the hindfoot, and equinus of the ankle and subtalar joint, as well as subluxation of the talonavicular joint.

The authors feel that aside from the congenital clubfoot that results from positional deformity, there are two major types of deformity. The most frequent type is the usual or conventional type. This accounts, as previously mentioned, for approximately 75 percent of the congenital clubfeet seen, and this group fortunately is much easier to correct by nonoperative means than the second type. The second type is extremely resistant to conservative measures and is characterized by a transverse crease (Fig. 21-2). The foot is short, rather stiff and seems to have a small calcaneus with associated contracture of the plantar structures. It has been the experience of the authors that this type of deformity virtually always requires surgical correction.

TREATMENT

Conservative Management

It should be possible to correct a very significant number of children with congenital clubfeet by conservative measures.[28] Success requires that the foot shows correction both clinically and roentgenographically. It would also imply that the foot is fully flexible, normal in appearance, painless and accepts conventional shoes.

A retrospective review was conducted in all patients treated at the Scottish Rite Hospital for idiopathic congenital clubfoot from 1950 to 1956 by Price and Lovell.[79] This time period was selected to allow at least a 20-year follow-up. During this period, 85 consecutive patients were treated before 4 months of age. Of this group, 63 patients were male and 22 patients were female, and all were Caucasian. Forty-nine patients had unilateral and 36 patients had bilateral clubfoot involvement, thus giving a total of 121 feet. The average age at initiation of treatment was 6 weeks. Thirty-eight patients with 54 clubfeet were lost to follow-up before the age of 10 years. Forty-seven patients with 67 affected feet were followed 10 years or longer. The average follow-up for this group was 17.8 years. Treatment consisted of weekly cast changes for 3 to 4 months and then biweekly changes. Recurrences were treated with further manipula-

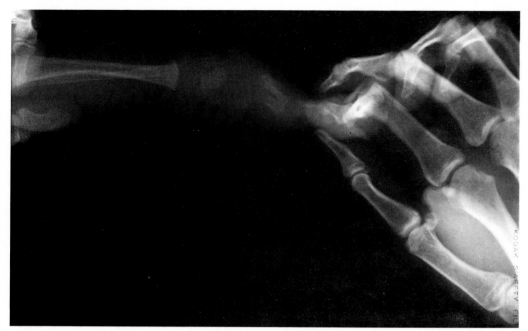

FIG. 21-2. Lateral roentogenogram of congenital clubfoot. Note the marked equinus of both the forefoot and the hindfoot. There is a transverse crease at the plantar aspect of the foot.

tions and cast application. The average total length of time in plaster casts was 20.4 months. Only three of the 67 clubfeet followed had operative procedures before the age of 10 years.

Results were classified as good, fair or poor by chart review. Approximately two-thirds qualified as a good result. Twelve feet were rated fair with slight residual deformity, slight over-correction, slight forefoot adduction or normal with tight heelcord. Twelve feet were poor with rockerbottom deformity, residual clubfoot or required triple arthrodesis.

In this series there was a striking difference in results according to sex. Only 31 per cent of females with clubfeet had a good result, while 76 per cent of males with clubfeet had a good result.

As a part of the study, an attempt was made to recall patients for clinical and roentgenographic examination. Twenty-two patients returned for follow-up at an average age of 23.6 years. There were 32 affected feet in this group. Sex, ratio, bilaterality, age at initial treatment, length of time in plaster, number of recurrences and percen-

tage of good results were found to be similar in all respects to the overall series. Using very strict criteria, 21 of 32 feet or approximately two-thirds had a good result by nonoperative means alone. An additional five patients or one-sixth had fair results and one-sixth had poor results.

The authors prefer the Kite method of nonoperative correction, although this method has now been modified.[51, 53, 56, 57, 58, 60, 61, 63, 78]

Treatment with serial casting should be initiated as early as possible. Early treatment suggests that treatment begin within the first few days of life, prior to development of secondary contractures. The earlier treatment is initiated, the greater the likelihood of success by nonoperative means.[64] The converse is also true. An effort should be made to achieve correction of the deformity within the first 3 months of life.[77]

Criteria for Correction. A corrected congenital clubfoot is one that is fully mobile with no restriction of motion at the subtalar joint with dorsiflexion of 15° to 20° degrees and with the heel in slight valgus. The forefoot can also be abducted slightly

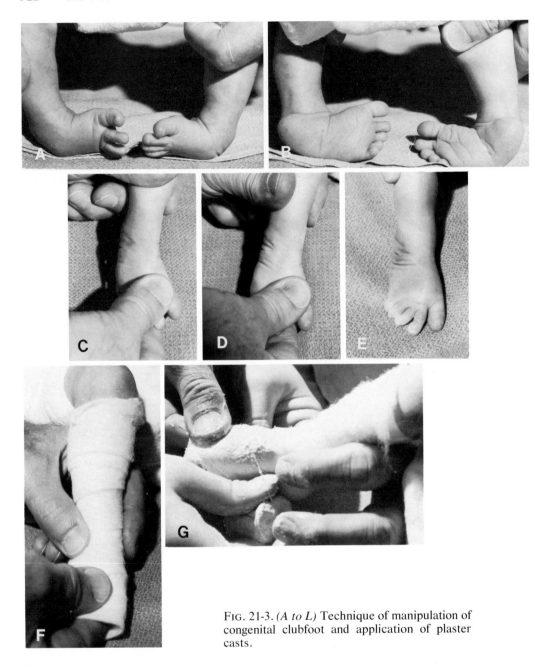

FIG. 21-3. *(A to L)* Technique of manipulation of congenital clubfoot and application of plaster casts.

beyond the midline and is quite supple. If there is unilateral involvement, its appearance should be similar to the contralateral foot.

Manipulation of Foot. The foot is manipulated prior to each change of cast.[62, 65] This is a very important procedure and should be done extremely carefully as well as gently in order not to injure the hyaline cartilage. It is this procedure which actually corrects the foot, and the plaster cast maintains the correction that follows each manipulation.

The technique of manipulation that the authors employ consists of grasping the forefoot between the thumb and index finger (Fig. 21-3). The leg is stabilized with the

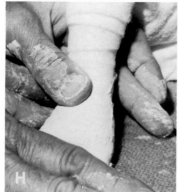

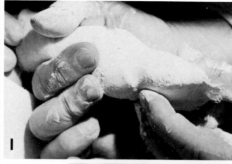

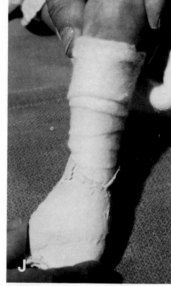

FIG. 21-3 *(Continued).*

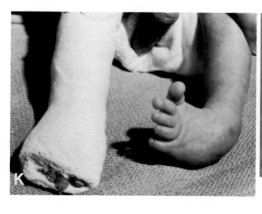

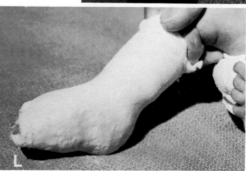

opposite hand. A distracting force is applied with elongation of the foot. This maneuver permits unlocking of the subtalar joint and eversion of the calcaneus. As the tarsus elongates due to the distraction force, slight pressure is applied at the sinus tarsi, and the head of the talus is displaced medially. The navicular is then gently displaced laterally to correct the talonavicular subluxation. This permits abduction of the forefoot in preparation for cast application.

Technique of Cast Application. In the newborn, a single 3-inch roll of plaster is adequate. The plaster is divided with a sharp

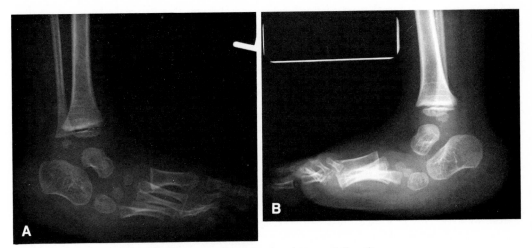

FIG. 21-4. *(A and B)* Rocker-bottom deformity.

knife and one-half of the roll is used for the foot in order to prepare a plaster slipper and the remainder of the roll of plaster serves to attach a slipper to the leg portion of the cast. The cast extends only to the knee and is changed weekly. Following manipulation in the manner described with the foot held in maximum correction, a single layer of sheet cotton is applied, extending from toes to the knee. The plaster is then applied in a circular manner about the forefoot and hindfoot by an assistant. A piece of plexiglass or some similar substance should be used to stabilize the foot during molding of the cast. Very careful molding of the cast follows in order that the correction that has resulted from manipulation be maintained. In order to correct the forefoot adduction deformity, it is particularly important to abduct the forefoot at the calcaneocuboid joint. A rocker-bottom deformity (Fig. 21-4) can be avoided if the forefoot is plantar flexed and the cast molded under the midtarsal joint. The foot is then everted, displaced posteriorly and dorsiflexed slightly. No attempt should be made to dorsiflex the foot above a right angle until the forefoot adduction and varus of the hindfoot is corrected. Following correction of these deformities clinically and with verification of position by appropriate roentgenograms (Fig. 21-5), the foot is manipulated gently in dorsiflexion to correct the equinus deformity. This is done with the knee extended and with uniform pressure applied by the cupped hand at the plantar aspect of the foot.

Following correction of all deformitites, a series of holding casts are necessary to permit the foot to accommodate to its newly corrected position. Generally, this requires a minimum of 2 or 3 months.

Retentive Splints. Retentive splints aid in maintenance of correction. Splintage should be combined with dedicated passive stretching of the foot by the parents. Straight last shoes are attached to a Denis Browne splint, turning the involved foot outward 10°. Splintage may be discontinued when the child is walking well, but passive stretching of the feet should be continued until the child is approximately 2 or 3 years of age and shows no tendency toward recurrence.

If there is recurrence of the deformity, the physician must make the decision as to whether additional casting or surgical correction is appropriate.

Operative Management

The attending physician, upon reaching an impasse in the nonoperative management, must make a decision as to what surgical procedure or procedures is indicated in order to correct the existing deformities. Often a combination of procedures may be necessary. Each foot must be evaluated carefully and dealt with in the appropriate manner. Many operative procedures have been described and all have merit.[24, 33, 35, 47, 52, 67, 68, 75] It is a mistake for the surgeon to attempt to adapt all feet to a particular operation. Bony procedures must not be done in the infant and young child, as damage to bone and articular cartilage will ensue. After analyzing the foot carefully in determining the extent of involvement of the various deformities, the appropriate surgical procedure must then be chosen.[52]

Forefoot Adduction. If the deformity is confined to the forefoot only, a Heyman, Herndon and Strong[46] procedure should be considered. Although the bases of the metatarsals may be exposed by vertical incisions, a curved incision extending from the base of the first metatarsal to the cuboid bone is preferred. The neurovascular structures are protected, and the intermetatarsal joints are released by capsulotomy and division of the ligaments. Injury to the articular cartilage and the growth plates must be avoided. Heyman, Herndon and Strong[46] have recommended that this procedure be limited to children under 7 years of age.

Tendon Transfer. Transfer of the anterior tibial tendon to the dorsum of the foot in the region of the fifth metatarsal base has been advocated by Garceau.[42, 43, 44] This procedure should not be done until correction of fixed structural deformity of the forefoot has been done. This can usually be accomplished with serial plaster casts with wedging of the forefoot in abduction. In the authors' experience, there is an occasional instance when this procedure is indicated. If the forefoot is flexible and tends to supinate during the swing phase of the gait, the authors have utilized the split anterior tibial transfer, moving the detached lateral one-half of the tendon to the second or third cuneiform. If the tendon is transferred too far laterally, overcorrection is possible. The second possible disadvantage of transferring the entire tendon is plantar flexion of the first metatarsal and clawing of the first toe due to the unopposed action of the peroneus longus muscle.

Transfer of the Posterior Tibial Tendon. Gartland advocated in the relapsed clubfoot transplantation of the posterior tibial tendon through the interosseous membrane anteriorly to the third cuneiform.

Fried[41] dissected the insertion of the tendon of the tibialis posterior in 56 recurrent clubfeet. The insertion was found to be abnormal in all instances. He felt that the abnormal contracture of this muscle contributed to the development of clubfoot. In view of this, the tendon was transferred after excision of the abnormal insertion to the third cuneiform. A posterior release consisting of lengthening of the Achilles tendon and posterior capsulotomy were performed at the same time to correct the equinus deformity.

The authors have not found it necessary to utilize the posterior tibial tendon transplant for recurrent clubfoot. It is difficult to accept the hypothesis that release and forward transplantation of this tendon will result in correction of the residual deformities.

Posterior Release. A posterior release alone is indicated in congenital clubfoot only after there has been complete correction of forefoot adduction and hindfoot varus both clinically and roentgenographically. If dorsiflexion is attempted before these deformities are corrected, a rocker-bottom deformity will follow.

All too often a posterior release is done when an impasse is reached, with persistence of forefoot adduction and hindfoot varus. A simple posterior release alone will not result in correction of these residual deformities. This is a very common error and very likely will result in increased stiffness in the foot because of adhesions secondary to lengthening of the Achilles tendon and posterior capsulotomy of the ankle and subtalar joints.

Posterior release consists of lengthening of the Achilles tendon by the Z-plasty method. It is necessary to lengthen the tendon in this manner in order to do an adequate posterior capsulotomy at the ankle and subtalar joints. The posterior deltoid ligament should be sectioned, as well as the posterior talofibular ligament and the calcaneofibular ligament. Sectioning of these structures enable correction of the equinus deformity of the talus and also permits the anterior end of the calcaneus and talus to ascend, with restoration of the normal talocalcaneal angle.

A long-leg plaster cast is applied, with the foot at a right angle, for 6 weeks. Upon removal of the cast, passive stretching of the foot is indicated, as well as application of a night splint.

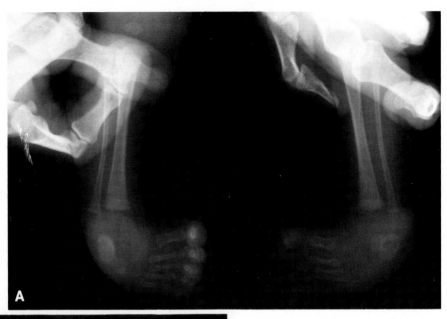

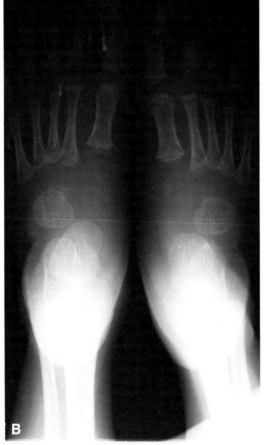

FIG. 21-5. Typical congenital clubfoot deformity showing forefoot adduction and varus of hindfoot bilaterally. (A) Before treatment. (B) After closed treatment. Note the restoration of the talocalcaneal angle and correction of the forefoot varus.

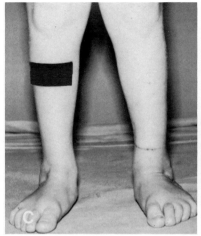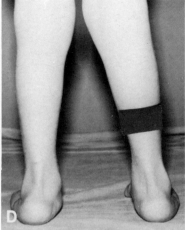

Fig. 21-5 *(Continued). (C and D)* Clinical photographs after correction of deformity on both sides.

Soft Tissue Release. Numerous authors have advocated a one-stage surgical release for correction of all residual elements of congenital talipes equinovarus.

Recently Turco[83, 84] has popularized this procedure, stating that in his experience a significant number of all clubfeet treated from birth had incomplete corrections and recurrent deformities requiring repeated manipulations and casts and finally one or more surgical procedures. He expressed disenchantment with the results of nonoperative treatment, saying that the one-stage posterior medial release corrects all existing deformities and results in a flexible plantargrade foot.

Turco[83, 84] described three groups of contractures in the congenital clubfoot, namely, posterior, medial and subtalar. In the recalcitrant clubfoot, all of the contractures must be released surgically. The posterior contractures involve the posterior capsule of the ankle and subtalar joints, the Achilles tendon, the posterior talofibular and the calcaneofibular ligaments. The medial contractures involve the deltoid and calcaneonavicular ligaments, the talonavicular joint capsule and the sheaths of the posterior tibial, flexor digitorum longus, and flexor hallucis longus tendons. The subtalar contractures involve the anterior talocalcaneal interosseous ligament and the bifurcated ligament.

All contractures must be released by meticulous dissection, avoiding injury to the articular cartilage of the joints as well as injury to the neurovascular structures. Anomalies of the blood supply to the foot may exist with absence of the anterior vessels. Absence of the anterior vessels has been reported by Ben-Menachem and Butler[29] following selective arteriography. If the posterior tibial artery is compromised in the dissection, a catastrophic result may occur.

The authors have found the posteromedial release as described by Turco[83, 84] to be quite satisfactory (Fig. 21-6). In most instances, the interosseous talocalcaneal ligament is not sectioned, as it is felt that this may result in excessive valgus deformity at the hindfoot. The posterior tibial tendon is not sacrificed but is lengthened in a Z-plasty fashion above the medial malleolus.

In many instances, the complete plantar release as described by Lucas[66] is also done. This procedure has been popularized by Westin[85] and consists of release of the abductor hallucis, the plantar aponeurosis, the short toe flexors and the abductor digiti quinti at their attachment to the calcaneus. These structures are released medially through the same incision. It appears that

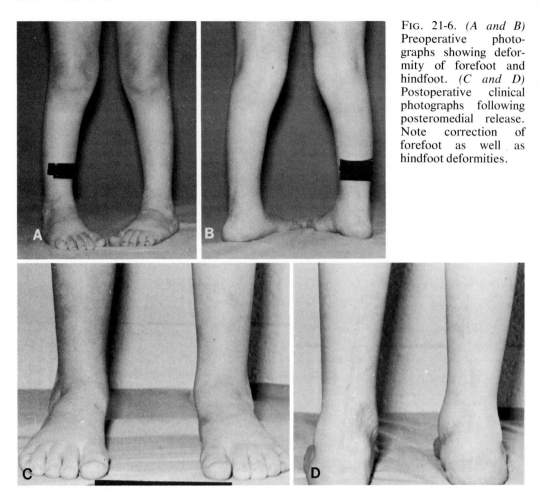

Fig. 21-6. *(A and B)* Preoperative photographs showing deformity of forefoot and hindfoot. *(C and D)* Postoperative clinical photographs following posteromedial release. Note correction of forefoot as well as hindfoot deformities.

the addition of the plantar release aids in elongation of the foot and correction of the forefoot adduction deformity.

Turco[83, 84] assessed 31 feet having the one-stage posteromedial release and followed the patients for 2 years or more. He found 27 feet to be excellent or good, three were considered to be fair results and one was considered a failure requiring additional surgery.

Barrett and Lovell[25] in an unpublished review studied 83 one-stage posteromedial releases performed at the Scottish Rite Hospital from 1975 to 1977. Thirty-two feet involving 22 patients with a diagnosis of idiopathic congenital talipes equinovarus were evaluated. Using very strict criteria, 11 feet in eight patients were graded excellent, 13 feet in nine patients were graded good, five feet in four patients were graded fair and three feet in two patients were graded poor.

The age at the time of surgery varied from 6 months to 7 years. The average age at time of surgery was 3 years. The average time of follow-up was 20.3 months. Ten patients had bilateral congenital clubfeet requiring bilateral posteromedial releases. Five patients had bilateral clubfeet and responded to cast correction on one side and unilateral posteromedial release was necessary on the opposite side. Seven patients had unilateral clubfeet and posteromedial releases.

The one-stage posteromedial release combined with the plantar release has not been done at the Scottish Rite hospital in patients under 4 months of age. Ideally, the procedure should be done after the age of 6 to 12 months. The use of magnification glasses and small instruments is a necessity when the procedure is done in a small foot.

The upper limit for age for the posteromedial release has been 7 years with the best results in children under 3 years of age.

Operations on Bone. *Osteotomy of the Metatarsals.* Berman and Gartland[30] suggested osteotomy of the bases of the metatarsals for structural adduction deformity of the forefoot. This procedure should be reserved for the child over 6 or 7 years of age. After exposure of the bases of the metatarsals, utilizing a transverse slightly curved incision or three longitudental incisions between the metatarsals, a dome-shaped osteotomy is done. The osteotomy of the first metatarsal is done just distal to the growth plate in order to avoid injury. Stout Kirschner wires are then used to transfix the first and fifth metatarsal bases. These may be cut subcutaneously and are removed 6 weeks later. The short-leg cast can usually be discontinued 6 weeks following surgery. Berman and Gartland[30] performed metatarsal osteotomy for the correction of rigid adduction of the forepart of the foot in 115 feet. Forty-four of the operations were done to correct resistant adduction of the forefoot associated with congenital clubfoot. In evaluating the end results, 84 per cent were classified as good and excellent and 16 per cent were classified as fair and poor.

Osteotomy of the Calcaneus. Dwyer[37, 38] noted that conservative measures often fail in a high number of children with talipes equinovarus. He expressed belief that the persistence of an inverted heel is the most important factor in preventing complete correction, in that relapse is encouraged by its presence.

In describing the deforming forces, Dwyer[37, 38] stated that in a clubfoot the heel is inverted and elevated so that the outer border of the foot receives most of the weight. As a result, the plantar fascia becomes contracted.

The operation advocated by Dwyer[37, 38] aims at correction of the varus of the heel, increasing its height and placing it directly under the line of weightbearing. Although the ideal age for this procedure is said to be 3 to 4 years, it can be done in older children.

Through a posterior incision, the Achilles tendon is exposed and divided in a sagittal plane, with the medial half dissected from its insertion at the calcaneus. The calcaneus is then divided with a broad osteotome more or less in the line of the flexor hallucis tendon. The distal fragment is tilted laterally and a bone graft taken from the proximal tibia is inserted in the interval, thus creating an opening wedge osteotomy.

Immobilization is recommended for 10 weeks, and normal activity returns rapidly with an improved gait.

In assessing his results in 56 feet in 48 patients, Dwyer[37, 38] stated that emphasis was placed on function rather than appearance. Twenty-seven of the 56 feet were regarded as a good result and 29 as a fair result.

The authors prefer a closing wedge laterally at the calcaneus, as described by Dwyer[37, 38] for pes cavus. This is a much simpler procedure and appears to correct the varus deformity of the hindfoot satisfactorily.

Wedge Resection of the Calcaneocuboid Joint. Evans[39] described an operation for the relapsed clubfoot. He stated that the essential deformity in clubfoot is in the midtarsal joint and that all other deformities are secondary. It would, therefore, appear that the essential lesion in a clubfoot is a congenital dislocation of the navicular on the talus, that the cuboid bone as well as the calcaneus is included with the dislocation, and that changes in the skeleton and soft tissue are secondary and adapted. Finally, the manipulative reduction must achieve replacement of the navicular on the talus. In doing so, the medial column of the foot is restored. Manipulation of a clubfoot invariably encounters resistance; the older the child the greater the resistance. The resistance, as previously mentioned, is secondary to contracted soft tissues and joint surfaces which are very likely incongruous. The elongated lateral column of the foot as well as the shape of the calcaneocuboid joint contributes to the resistance, according to Evans.[39] The aim of the operation is to secure a significant lateral rotation of the navicular to bring the first metatarsal into line with the talus and to correct equinus. Evans[39] correctly makes a strong point of applying serial plaster casts to correct the deformity as much as possible and increase the suppleness of the foot prior to operation.

The operation consists of Z-plasty lengthening of the tendon of the posterior tibial tendon and the tendo Achilles. A posterior capsulotomy at the ankle is also usually necessary, thus permitting correction of the equinus to a right angle or greater. The calcaneocuboid joint is then exposed through a lateral incision and an appropriate wedge or bone is excised at this joint. Evans[39] advises the use of two staples to hold the calcaneus and cuboid and to maintain apposition of their surfaces. Immobilization in a short cast is recommended for 5 months with walking permitted after 6 weeks.

In discussing the results, Evans[39] operated upon 30 feet between 1953 and 1956. The ages of the children ranged from 3 years to 14 years with the majority being between 4 and 8 years. He was impressed with the permanent correction of the deformity, finding that if the shape of the foot is satisfactory following removal of the plaster, it is likely to retain its correction. A second advantage according to Evans is that the operation can correct all elements of the deformity. Finally, the operation preserves the foot that is of good shape, accepts normal shoes and is plantargrade.

Abrams[22] in 1969 concluded, in reviewing the early results of the Evans operation in 31 feet, that 23 were good, seven fair, and one poor. His results, he felt, were comparable to the results of Evans.[39] He also agreed with Evans in that following fusion at the calcaneocuboid joint no subsequent loss of correction will occur. Abrams advised that the operation not be done before the age of 4 years or after the age of 9 years. It would seem that the ideal age is 6 years. If the procedure is done too early, overcorrection of the hindfoot may ensue, as wedge resection of the calcaneocuboid joint may remove too much cartilage.

Derotational Osteotomy of the Tibia and Fibula. Internal tibial torsion is extremely uncommon in congenital talipes equinovarus, in the authors' experience. In an occasional instance, derotational osteotomy of the proximal tibia and fibula may be indicated. It is important in the child who has corrected clubfeet and who toes inward to determine if the toeing inward is related to uncorrected forefoot adduction or to increased femoral anteversion. The intoeing is more likely to be the result of abnormal sitting with a resultant increase in femoral anteversion. Many children with congenital clubfeet that have been corrected tend to sit with feet tucked under their buttocks or in the reverse tailor position. In this instance, it is possible that a derotational osteotomy of the distal femur may occasionally be indicated in children over the age of 8 or 10 years.

Triple Arthrodesis. The Hoke[48] or Dunn[36] triple arthrodesis has been used as a salvage procedure by the authors (Fig. 21-7). It should only be done in children with a skeletal age of 12 years or older. This procedure is primarily indicated in the stiff, rigid and often painful foot that has not responded to serial casting or to other operative procedures. Often such children have been subjected to multiple soft-tissue as well as other operative procedures.

In the Hoke triple arthrodesis, an oblique incision 7 cm. in length is made overlying the midportion of the sinus tarsi. This incision is deepened to the floor of the sinus tarsi and the areolar tissue excised. The skin flaps must not be undermined in order to avoid skin loss. After exposure of the calcaneocuboid, subtalar and talonavicular joints, appropriate wedges are excised with correction of the deformities.

The joint surfaces are fish-scaled and a long-leg plaster cast applied with the foot held in the corrected position. Staples or strong Kirschner wires may also be used to maintain fixation of the involved joints in their properly corrected position. Total immobilization should be for a period of 3 months with a short-leg walking cast being applied at 6 weeks.

CONGENITAL METATARSUS VARUS

Congenital metatarsus varus is a relatively common condition and it appears to occur with increasing frequency. The deformity, although present at birth, may not be recognized until several months later or possibly after the child begins to walk.

A significant number of deformities related to congenital metatarsus varus, if untreated, will improve or correct completely.

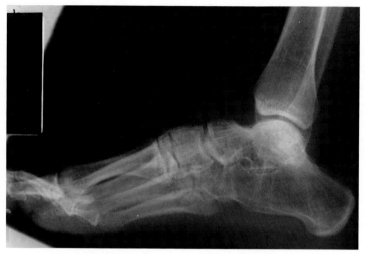

FIG. 21-7. Postoperative triple arthrodesis.

If the deformity persists or worsens, the child may be clumsy and may exhibit a toe-in gait. The adolescent and adult with this condition may complain of pain at the lateral border of the foot near the tarsometatarsal area. The shoe often irritates the prominence at the midportion of the foot laterally. It is possible that this deformity, if uncorrected, may also contribute to bunion formation with hallux valgus.

The incidence of congenital metatarsus varus is said to be one per thousand live births.[104] If one child in a family has the deformity, the chances of a second having a similar deformity is one in twenty.

Colonna[91] and Jacobs[93] noted the association of congenital hip dysplasia and congenital metatarsus varus. Jacobs[93] reviewed 300 consecutive cases of metatarsus varus and found 30 cases of dysplasia of the hip—an incidence of 10 per cent. A child with metatarsus varus deformity should, therefore, have a very careful evaluation of the hips.

CLINICAL APPEARANCE

Kite has suggested that congenital metatarsus varus, for descriptive purposes, represents a third of a congenital clubfoot.[95, 96, 97] McCormick and Blount[99] introduced the term "skewfoot" (Fig. 21-8).

The forefoot is adducted and supinated and the hindfoot is usually in a neutral position, although in a significant number of instances a valgus heel may be present.[99] The lateral border of the foot is convex and a prominence is noted at the tarsometatarsal area. The medial border of the foot is concave. There is an increased interval between the first and second toes with the great toe held in slight varus. Dorsiflexion of the foot and ankle is normal. If the forefoot is abducted passively and released, it returns to its original adducted and inverted position. An increase in the normal internal tibial torsion is also commonly seen in this condition.

The serpentine type of deformity as described by Peabody and Muro[101] is rare but has been reported by Kite. Such feet are difficult to correct conservatively because of a tendency to recur. They very often require surgical correction.

In the walking child with uncorrected metatarsus varus, a toe-in gait is noted. This may result in clumsiness with frequent falls. Abnormal shoe wear may be present, with the lateral portion of the shoe showing greater wear.

ROENTGENOGRAPHIC FINDINGS

Anteroposterior roentgenograms confirm the clinical findings, as outlined above, with

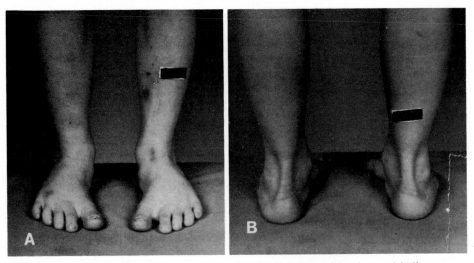

FIG. 21-8. *(A)* Congenital metatarsus varus showing forefoot adduction and hallux varus. Note the convex appearance of the lateral border. *(B)* The heels are in valgus.

forefoot adduction and apparent closeness and overlap of the lateral four metatarsals (Fig. 21-9). The talocalcaneal angle is increased if the heel is in a valgus position. The navicular, if ossified, is, in such an instance, subluxated laterally at the head of the talus. No abnormalities are usually present in the lateral film.

INCIDENCE

It would appear that congenital metatarsus varus is occurring with increasing frequency.[96, 102] At the Scottish Rite Hospital, Kite noted an average of one case per year from 1924 to 1938. For the following 5 years, the average number of cases was four each year. Since then the incidence has gradually increased, with the average for the past few years being 200 cases. A slightly greater preponderance has been noted in males.

TREATMENT

Conservative Treatment

Whereas correction of the congenital idiopathic clubfoot by serial plaster casts is not always successful, the converse is usually true, in our experience, with respect to congenital metatarsus varus. Treatment should be initiated as soon as possible. The foot is quite supple and secondary contracture of the forefoot can be avoided. If the deformity is a mild one, simple observation is in order or perhaps straight-last shoes may be used. Almost one-fourth of children seen with this deformity do not require treatment. McCauley, Lusskin and Bromley[98] expressed the belief that there is a significant tendency toward recurrence of the deformity following conservative management.

The authors have not found manipulation of the foot necessary prior to application of a plaster cast, although Kite,[95] McCormick and Blount,[99] as well as Ponseti and Becker,[102] have advocated manipulation in conjunction with serial plaster casts.

The technique of plaster of Paris cast application is similar to that used for congenital clubfoot. The plaster slipper is fashioned, abducting the forefoot with the point of fulcum at the tarsometatarsal joint. The plaster slipper is then joined to the leg component of the cast. If the heel is in valgus, the foot should be inverted slightly as the cast is continued to below the knee. The cast is changed weekly until the deformity is corrected. A holding cast should then be used for approximately 2 to 4 weeks. The period for correction varies from 4 to 10 or 12 weeks depending upon the severity of the defor-

FIG. 21-9. Anteroposterior roentgenogram of the feet in congenital metatarsus varus showing an increased talocalcaneal angle with supination and adduction of the forefoot. The increased space between the first and second toes can be seen.

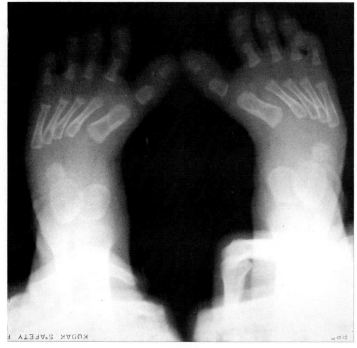

mity. Wedging of the cast in abduction is not advocated in the young infant. It may be advantageous in the older child.

Full correction implies that there is no deformity and the forefoot can be abducted fully both actively and passively. The convex appearance of the lateral border of the foot must be corrected and the prominence at the tarsometatarsal junction must be absent. It is not necessary to use retentive splints following correction. The abnormal internal tibial torsion associated with congenital metatarsus varus usually corrects spontaneously. A mild hallux varus deformity may persist for several years following cast correction and may be of concern to the parents. This deformity will eventually disappear with the wearing of shoes.

Surgical Treatment

In the child with congenital metatarsus varus over 4 years of age, surgical correction may be indicated. Serial plaster casts with wedging in abduction should first be utilized. If this fails, a tarsometatarsal and intermetatarsal release is an effective procedure for correction of the forefoot deformity.[92, 94] This operation should not be done in children over the age of 7 years. For the older child, osteotomy at the base of the metatarsals, as advocated by Berman and Gartland,[1] is occasionally necessary.

Thompson[103] concluded that the abductor hallucis muscle may contribute to a persistant hallux varus following correction of the metatarsus varus deformity. This muscle originates from the medial process of the tuberosity of the calcaneus, the plantar aponeurosis and the intermuscular septum. It inserts by a tendon, with the medial head of the flexor hallucis brevis to the medial side of the base of the first phalanx of the great toe. Thompson[103] advised resection of the entire abductor hallucis muscle to correct the hallux varus and also to reduce the metatarsus varus. He resected the abductor hallucis in 40 children with recurrent metatarsus varus.

Mitchell[100] has also suggested release of the abductor hallucis and advises that the procedure be restricted to the severe deformity that resists correction by serial plaster casts. He cautions that the child should be at

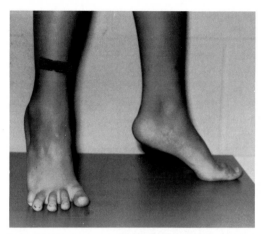

FIG. 21-10. A 5-year-old female with congenital contracture of the Achilles tendon, showing the weight borne on the forefeet during erect stance.

least 1 year of age. The operation as practiced by Mitchell consists of release of the abductor hallucis at its origin at the calcaneus. The foot should be held in plaster for 8 weeks following release with the forefoot abducted.

If the great toe exhibits an adducted position in the stance phase, division of the abductor hallucis tendon at its insertion is indicated, according to Mitchell.

CONGENITAL SHORT TENDO CALCANEUS (HABITUAL TOE WALKER)

This entity was first described by Hall, Salter and Bhalla[107] in 1967. It is not uncommon and predominates in boys. Children present as persistent toe walkers usually after the age of 3 years (Fig. 21-10). Most are able to lower the heels to the ground when standing, and heel-toe gait is possible but is usually awkward.

Examination reveals limited dorsiflexion ranging from mild restriction of motion to severe fixed equinus. Careful neurologic examination is entirely normal. Differential diagnosis includes cerebral palsy, diastematomyelia, spinal dysrhaphism, muscular dystrophy, spinal cord tumor, acute toe walking syndrome, functional toe walking in

an hyperactive child, and delayed maturation of the corticospinal tract.[105, 108, 109]

Griffin and coworkers[106] performed electromyographic gait analysis on a group of six children who were habitual toe-walkers. Electromyographic analysis demonstrated swing-phase activity of the gastrocnemius and soleus muscles during toe-toe gait in both toe-walkers and in normal children. However, on attempted heel-toe gait prolonged and increased activity of the tibialis anterior muscle was necessary in toe-walkers to overcome the force of the shortened tendo Achilles. Following treatment electromyographic studies returned to normal and no longer reflected the contracture of the triceps surae muscles.

Initial management should be nonoperative. Stretching exercises and manipulations have generally been unsuccessful. Serial stretching casts should be applied every 2 weeks for 6 to 8 weeks. It is not necessary to treat both feet simultaneously. Generally, casts alone restore a normal range of motion and gait pattern. However, if the ankle does not dorsiflex to neutral position despite a trial of nonoperative management, cautious sliding lengthening of the heel cord is indicated. The authors confirm Hall, Salter, and Bhalla's observations that tendo Achilles lengthening alone will restore dorsiflexion. In severe deformity posterior capsulotomy has occasionally been performed, but with little additional gain in range of motion. The results of surgery are generally rewarding. The postoperative regimen consists of long-leg casts for 6 weeks followed by night splinting for several months.

FLATFOOT DEFORMITIES

CONGENITAL VERTICAL TALUS

Congenital vertical talus is uncommon. The first clinical, anatomic, pathologic and roentgenographic study of this condition was published in 1914 by Henken.[118] Osmond-Clark,[126] in emphasizing its comparative rarity, stated that he had encountered the deformity in young children only on four occasions.

It is known by a variety of names to include "congenital convex pes planus," "congenital rigid rocker-bottom foot" and "congenital flatfoot with talonavicular dislocation." Lamy and Weismann[123] as well as Heyman and Herndon[119, 120] prefer the term "congenital vertical talus" because of its simplicity and its usefulness as a descriptive term which is easily recognized.

Although congenital vertical talus may occur as an isolated entity, in the experience of Coleman, Stelling and Jarrett,[111] it is very often seen in association with arthrogryposis multiplex congenita, myelodysplasia, mental retardation, or other congenital anomalies. We have seen it associated with Turner's syndrome and also in one instance with a congenital idiopathic clubfoot. Drennan and Sharrard[112] emphasized its frequent association with central nervous system abnormalities. Lamy and Weismann[123] also noted the high incidence of neurologic abnormalities in children with congenital vertical talus. Lloyd-Roberts and Spence[124] as well as Hark[116] found in their patients a preponderance of associated neurological abnormalities, particularly arthrogryposis.

The etiology of congenital vertical talus is unknown. Familial incidence involving mother and child has been observed by the authors. It is more common in males and very often is bilateral.

Silk and Wainwright[130] believe that this condition is due to disparity in growth between the muscles and bones of the leg.

Pathologic Anatomy

The pathologic abnormalities in congenital vertical talus are well known and have been described by several writers including Hughes,[122] Hark,[116] Coleman, Stelling and Jarrett.[111] The sustentaculum tali is hypoplastic and does not provide adequate support to the head of the talus.[128] Patterson, Fritz and Smith[129] were the first to report the histologic and anatomic findings in a 6-week-old white female infant who had bilateral congenital vertical talus and who succumbed to congenital heart disease. In the description of the dissection of the feet, they found abnormal tightness in the anterior tibial, extensor hallucis longus, extensor digitorum longus and peroneus longus muscle-tendon units. The muscles were grossly and histologically normal. The posterior tibial tendon and the peroneal tendons were anteriorly displaced and lying in grooves on the medial and lateral malleolus, respectively. The vertical position of the talus was described as one of equinus and the head of the talus was noted to be oval rather than spherical. Only two of the three normally present articulating facets on the superior surface of the calcaneus were present and these were found to be abnormal. The talonavicular and subtalar joints showed subluxation and the calcaneus occupied a position of equinus due to the contracture of the Achilles tendon.

Drennan and Sharrard[112] described the pathologic anatomy in a white female with myelomeningocele who died shortly after birth following closure of the myelomeningocele and spinal osteotomy. Their observations suggested that an imbalance between a weak tibialis posterior and strong dorsiflexors and evertors is the underlying cause of the deformity.

Clinical Findings

There is no mistaking the clinical appearance of a newborn infant with this condition. The plantar aspect of the foot is convex, thus giving it a rocker-bottom appearance. The head of the talus is palpable medially and at the sole. The talus is likely to be parallel to the long axis of the tibia and in marked equinus. The hindfoot is in valgus and equinus and the forefoot is abducted and dorsiflexed at the midtarsal joint. The foot is exceedingly rigid, and wearing of the shoes may be difficult. In an older child who is walking, the shoes become misshapen and callosities develop under the head of the talus. The gait is usually clumsy and quite awkward and there is very little push-off with the forefoot. The posterior aspect of the heel does not touch the ground. Pain usually develops at adolescence or shortly thereafter.

Sixteen children with congenital vertical talus have recently been reviewed at the Scottish Rite Hospital. Five of the cases had bilateral involvement, giving a total of 21 feet. Eight of the patients were male and eight were female. The age when seen varied from 4 weeks to 7 years.

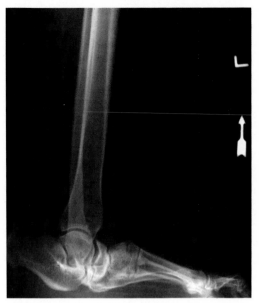

FIG. 21-11. Note the vertical position of the talus, the equinus position of calcaneus and the convexity of the plantar aspect of the foot.

ROENTGENOGRAPHIC FEATURES

The roentgenographic appearance of congenital vertical talus has been described by numerous authors.[110, 113, 116, 117, 119, 120, 121, 123, 127, 132] The talus occupies a vertical position and is often parallel with the long axis of the tibia (Fig. 21-11). The head of the talus lies medially and is palpable in the sole of the foot. The forefoot is dorsiflexed and the navicular, if ossified, is seen to lie on the neck of the talus. A marked lateral deviation of the calcaneus results in an increased talocalcaneal angle in the anteroposterior view. In the lateral view, notching of the neck of the talus results from the abnormal position of the navicular.

DIFFERENTIAL DIAGNOSIS

A severe flexible flatfoot may be confused with a vertical talus. It lacks the rigidity which is always present in congenital vertical talus. The rocker-bottom deformity is also absent in the flexible flatfoot, and the hindfoot can be passively corrected. Furthermore, the Achilles tendon does not show the severe degree of contracture that is seen in the congenital vertical talus.

A paralytic flatfoot may be associated with cerebral palsy, myelomeningocele and anterior poliomyelitis. No difficulty should be experienced in differentiating these conditions from a congenital vertical talus. Tarsal coalition usually results in a rigid flatfoot.

TREATMENT

Nonoperative Treatment

The authors believe that it is of utmost importance to initiate treatment as early as possible for congenital vertical talus. Soft tissue contractures occur rapidly, and delay in diagnosis and treatment results in increased rigidity and greater resistance to correction.

If the infant is seen within the first few days of life, it is possible by manipulation and corrective casts that an acceptable result may be obtained.

Manipulation of the foot is important in order to stretch the contracted soft tissues. The forefoot is placed in extreme equinus, thus aligning it with the hindfoot, and a distraction force is applied by grasping the foot between the thumb and the index finger. As the tarsus elongates, the forefoot is adducted and supinated. The hindfoot is inverted and an upward pressure is made under the head of the talus at the plantar aspect of the foot. The foot is held in this position as a plaster cast is applied. Careful molding of the cast is necessary, particularly at the midtarsal area, in order to correct the rocker-bottom deformity and to elevate the talus. The plaster slipper is then joined to the leg portion of the cast, which is extended to the knee with the foot maintained in a position of equinus and inversion.

The cast should be changed twice weekly until satisfactory correction of the deformity, both clinically and roentgenographically, is accomplished. If the foot cannot be corrected by conservative means, it is then necessary to proceed to surgical correction.

Tachdjian,[133] in discussing treatment, states that this should begin at birth. If closed reduction fails, he advises open reduction at 3 months of age. He emphasizes that if reduction is to be maintained, it is necessary to repair the capsule of the talonavicular joint inferiorly and medially as well as to tighten the posterior tibial tendon and the calcaneonavicular ligament.

Surgical Treatment

It is generally accepted that conservative measures, particularly in the older child, are usually not successful in the treatment of congenital vertical talus. In order to achieve lasting correction, the talonavicular dislocation must be reduced and maintained. Additionally, the talus must be elevated and the normal talocalcaneal relationship restored and held for an adequate period if recurrence is to be prevented.

Many different surgical techniques have been employed by various authors to achieve correction.[111] Osmond-Clark[126] advocated the reduction of the talonavicular and subtalar joints and maintenance of elevation of the talus by transplanting the distal end of the peroneus brevis tendon through the neck of the talus. A vertical tunnel is made in the neck of the talus, and the tendon of the peroneus brevis, after detaching it from the base of the fifth metatarsal, is passed through the tunnel and sutured back on to itself. He reported success in two children with bilateral deformity in utilizing this method.

Grice[114, 115] reported use of the anterior tibial tendon to the neck of the talus for support and advised that this procedure be combined with the extra-articular subtalar fusion.

Outland and Sherk[127] described a 3-year-old boy wtih congenital vertical talus who had been unsuccessfully treated with conservative measures for 2 years. Operative correction was achieved by lengthening the anterior structures, reducing of the talonavicular joint, followed by fixing with Kirschner wire to maintain reduction. Six weeks later, the pin was removed and the plaster immobilization continued for an additional 6 weeks. An extra-articular subtalar arthrodesis was then done, and this was followed by an Achilles tendon lengthening 3 months later.

Lamy and Weismann[123] advocated partial or total talectomy combined with lengthening of the tight peroneal and the extensor tendons.

Lloyd-Roberts and Spence[124] in assessing results in 28 feet in 22 patients treated at the Hospital for Sick Children by several nonoperative methods concluded that the deformity was neither corrected nor significantly improved in any instance.

Eyre-Brook[113] devised an operation consisting of lengthening of the extensor digitorum longus, the tibialis anterior and extensor hallucis longus tendons. The navicular is then reduced opposite the head of the talus. A wedge, based dorsally, is removed from the proximal part of the navicular and placed below the head of the talus to maintain the head in its proper position. Additionally, the spring ligament is reefed and the posterior tibial tendon is shortened. The extremity is immobilized with the foot in full plantar flexion and slight inversion. The cast is removed after 4 to 8 weeks, depending upon the age of the child.

Eyre-Brook[113] used this procedure in four cases, and the results 5 to 10 years after the operation disclosed that the stable reduction at the talonavicular joint was maintained.

Herndon and Heyman[119] reported open reduction of the deformity in six feet. The procedure consisted of division of the ligaments and capsular attachments of the subtalar and talonavicular joints. The navicular is then reduced after elevating the head of the talus. Lengthening of the peroneals and common toe extensors is advisable in older children. The forefoot is placed in marked equinus in order to align it with the calcaneus and to reduce the deformity at the midtarsal region. Two transfixing Kirschner wires have aided in maintaining reduction, with one driven through the base of the first metatarsal and the navicular into the body of the talus and the second passing from the plantar aspect of the foot through the calcaneus into the talus. Six weeks later, a heel cord lengthening and posterior capsulotomy is done. Plaster immobilization is advised for 4 months.

Coleman, Stelling and Jarrett[111] emphasized that from a pathologic and therapeutic standpoint, it appears that two major types of congenital vertical talus exist namely, Type I, in which the calcaneocuboid relationship is normal, and Type II, which is associated with a calcaneocuboid dislocation or subluxation.

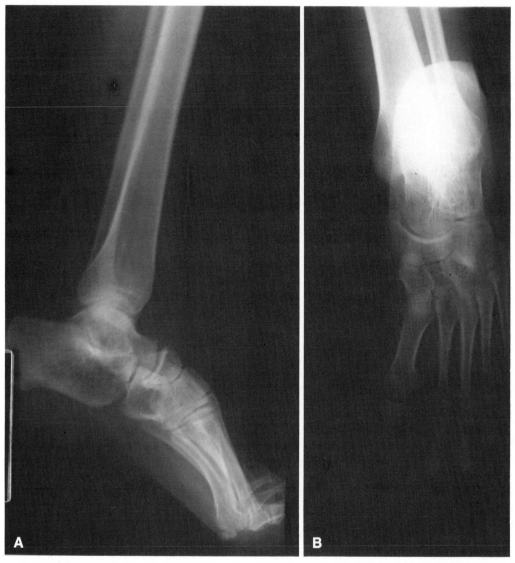

Fig. 21-12. Postoperative two-stage correction. *(A)* Note the normal talocalcaneal angle and proper relationship between the talus and the calcaneus. *(B)* The talus now presents a normal relationship to the long axis of the tibia.

These authors express disappointment with nonoperative treatment, and in their series none of the feet could be corrected by wedging casts or manipulation. They suggested preliminary casting of the foot into equinus with stretching of the extensor tendons as well as the skin on the dorsum of the foot.

Coleman, Stelling and Jarrett[111] advise that operative correction be performed in two stages following 4 to 6 weeks of plantar flexion wedging casts (Fig. 21-12). A dorsolateral incision centered over the sinus tarsus is made and the extensor digitorum longus, extensor hallucis longus and anterior tibial tendons are lengthened. A complete capsulotomy is done at the talonavicular and calcaneocuboid joints, permitting reduction of the talonavicular joint. Release of the talo-calcaneal interosseous ligament aids in reducing the talonavicular joint. The forefoot is placed in plantar flexion and the talonavicular joint is transfixed with a percutaneous Kirschner wire. Plantar flexion of the forefoot aids in aligning the foot properly because of the hindfoot being in a fixed equinus position. This also permits the posterior tibial and peroneus longus tendons to return to their normal position with improvement in the mechanics of the foot. In the child between $2\frac{1}{2}$ and 3 years of age, a talocalcaneal extra-articular bone block is done to provide stability to the subtalar joint and to maintain reduction and elevation of the talus. The procedure as described results in four accomplishments: (1) The talonavicular dislocation has been reduced and stabilized; (2) the talocalcaneal subluxation has been reduced and stabilized; (3) foot alignment has been corrected; (4) muscle balance of the foot has been restored.

Following suturing of the lengthened tendons, the wound is closed and a long-leg cast is applied with the knee in comfortable flexion and the foot and ankle in equinus. In 6 or 8 weeks the Kirschner wires are removed and the second stage follows. This consists of Achilles tendon lengthening, posterior capsulotomy, and the advancement of the posterior tibial tendon to the plantar surface of the navicular. The cast is removed 6 weeks later and a spring-loaded dropfoot brace is utilized for approximately 2 months.

These authors also recommend that in the child under the age of 1 year satisfactory reduction of the deformity and maintenance of the correction can be achieved in most instances without the use of the subtalar bone block.

In the Type II form, lesions with an abnormal calcaneocuboid joint require exposure of the calcaneocuboid joint and maintenance of the reduction with transfixion wire if some degree of recurrence of the deformity is to be prevented.

The authors prefer the operative correction of congenital vertical talus as described by Coleman, Stelling and Jarrett.[111] We would differ in that it is felt that a subtalar bone block is an essential part of the operative correction in all children. It has been our experience that the talus is not likely to retain its upright position unless the bone block is done (Fig. 21-12).

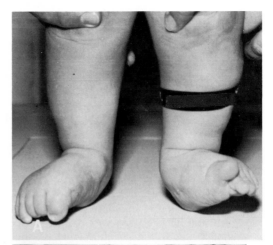

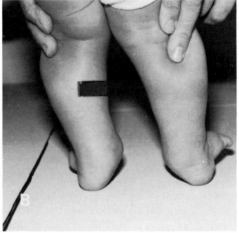

FIG. 21-13. *(A and B)* A 3-month-old child with flexible calcaneovalgus deformities of the feet.

Triple arthrodesis is necessary in a child of 12 years or more, and it may require possible excision of a portion of the head of the talus combined with lengthening of the Achilles tendon and the anterior structures. An axial pin traversing the talocalcaneal and ankle joint as well as a pin transfixing the talonavicular joint are usually necessary until the fusion is solid.

CALCANEOVALGUS FOOT

CLINICAL FEATURES

The calcaneovalgus foot is a relatively common finding in the newborn in its mild form (Fig. 21-13). The deformity is a flexible one, consisting of dorsiflexion of the fore-foot and hindfoot. In more severe defor-mities, the foot may be found lying against the anterior aspect of the tibia. Even in the milder form, the foot can be further dorsi-flexed without great resistance until it im-pinges upon the lower leg. In so doing, no luxation occurs at the talonavicular joint and the calcaneus accompanies the exten-sion of the forefoot. This is in contradis-tinction to the rare congenital vertical talus deformity, which shows severe abduction and extension of the forefoot in association with dislocation of the talonavicular joint and an equinus contracture of the cal-caneus. In severe calcaneovalgus deformi-ties, one finds an increased valgus position of the heel. In other cases the valgus is first demonstrable with maximum dorsiflexion of the foot. Abduction of the forefoot is usually of a mild degree. The foot can be returned to a more normal position without great difficulty. An important distinction between this foot and a congenital vertical talus foot is flexibility. The former is flex-ible and the latter is rigid.

Kite[135] has pointed out the association of this deformity and an external rotation con-tracture of the hips. He also emphasized the role that various sleeping patterns play in the persistance of these problems.[134] Children who sleep in a prone position with their hips flexed, abducted and externally rotated are those to whom he was referring. Wynne-Davies[137] has noted that the incidence of a calcaneovalgus foot is one per thousand live births. The sex ratio was 0.6 male to 1 female. She has found that the problem pre-dominates among the firstborn of young mothers. On the basis of her work, she con-cluded that the problem is partly genetic in origin. She was unable to delineate any clear pattern of inheritance. Wetzenstein[136] stud-ied 2,735 consecutive newborn infants and followed them for 2 years. He appraised clinically the degree of valgus of the hindfoot when the foot was maximally dorsiflexed. There were 147 patients with at least 20° of heel valgus, 333 with ten to fifteen degrees, 759 with zero to five degrees and 1,496 with no heel valgus. When seen at 2 years, 43 per cent of the 147 with at least 20° of heel valgus were considered to have flatfeet, while 23 percent of the group who were originally considered to have normal heel valgus were found to have flatfeet. He concluded that severe degrees of calcaneovalgus deformity have an increased likelihood of being asso-ciated with flatfootedness in later life.

TREATMENT

When examining a child with such a de-formity, one must be certain that active plantar flexion is possible. Various neuro-genic disorders such as myelomeningo-cele can result in posturing of the foot in a similar way. For a mild deformity that can be easily brought into plantar flexion, stretch-ing exercises are recommended. Kite[135] has advised that proper stretching is done by placing the heel in slight varus with one hand and plantar flexing and adducting the forefoot with the other. This is most easily accomplished with the thumb and index finger placed on the dorsal and plantar sur-faces of the foot, respectively. The external rotation contractures of the hips must also be stretched, if present. He further recom-mends that children be encouraged to sleep on their side in order to aid in the correction of the external rotation contracture of the hips.

For the more severe deformity, a series of short-leg casts applied by molding the foot into equinus at the ankle, varus at the hindfoot, and adduction at the midfoot are recommended. These are changed weekly in the young child and continued until the de-formity is corrected and active plantar flex-ion is present. Post-cast splinting is gener-ally unnecessary.

FLEXIBLE FLATFOOT

INTRODUCTION

Throughout the medical literature there has been much written about this relatively common problem. There have been many theories as to the etiology and to the proper treatment. Strikingly absent from the literature are long-term studies on those who have had no treatment and on those who have had various forms of con-servative treatment. There is a general feel-ing that exercises have limited value. Most of those who advocate surgery emphasize the importance of operating on symptomatic feet only. In order to properly assess the

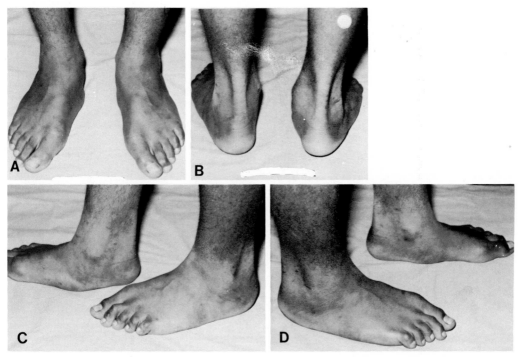

FIG. 21-14. *(A to D)* Clinical photographs of a 15-year-old male with severe flexible flatfeet.

need for treatment, one must have a clear understanding of the natural history of the problem without treatment. Helfet,[154] for example, has stated that the institution of shoe modifications in children increases the likelihood of symptoms later in life if these modifications are discontinued. However, there is no general agreement on this point.

CLINICAL FEATURES

The flexible flatfoot may be defined as a foot which assumes a pronated posture when weight is borne on the extremity. Abduction of the forefoot and valgus of the heel result in loss of the longitudinal arch (Fig. 21-14). When weight is relieved, it assumes a normal contour. Subtalar motion is normal to increased. Often such patients have associated generalized ligamentous laxity. As Inman has emphasized, the everted foot is mechanically weak. Much stress is put on the ligamentous support due to this posturing and the resultant medial shifting of the body weight. Normally, weight is borne over the lateral border of the foot and on the first and fifth metatarsal heads. Prolonged

posturing of the foot in the everted position may result in a heel cord contracture. The vast majority of patients with a flexible flatfoot deformity are asymptomatic with regard to their feet.

ROENTGENOGRAPHIC FEATURES

Roentgenograms may be made in the standing position in the anteroposterior as well as the lateral projections. The degree of heel valgus may be assessed on the anteroposterior film by measuring the Kite talocalcaneal angle. Divergence of the talus and calcaneus of more than 35° should be considered roentgenographic evidence of heel valgus. A lateral projection will demonstrate the location of the loss of the longitudinal arch (Fig. 21-15).

ASSOCIATION WITH CONGENITAL PES CALCANEOVALGUS

The significance of congenital pes calcaneovalgus in the origin of flexible flatfoot was addressed by Wetzenstein.[190] He quotes Erlacher, Gocht, Mau and Timmer as having

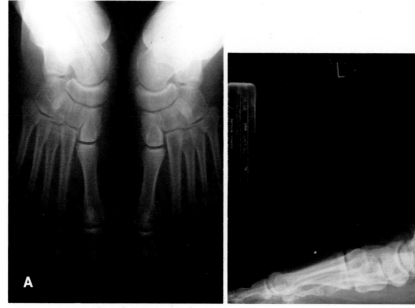

Fig. 21-15. A 13-year-old female with asymptomatic flexible flatfeet. *(A)* On this view can be seen a widened talocalcaneal angle. *(B)* Loss of the longitudinal arch is shown.

indicated that it can give rise to flatfeet. He reports that the calcaneovalgus deformity is seen in up to 30 per cent of live births and quotes reports citing incidences of up to 50 per cent. In 2,735 consecutive births, the degree of heel valgus was assessed. Those with heel valgus of greater than 20° were found in 147 cases. These children were followed for 2 years. At the end of that time, 43 per cent of the original 147 and 23 per cent of the previously normal group were judged to have a flexible flatfoot deformity. He concluded that those patients with severe valgus at birth have an increased risk of being flat-footed.

ETIOLOGY

Bone

There are several schools of thought as to the etiology of flatfeet. Harris and Beath[153] felt the problem related to weak support by the anterior portion of the calcaneus. They found it to be associated secondarily with a shortened Achilles tendon. With medial displacement of the head of the talus, or perhaps more accurately with lateral rotation of the calcaneus, the longitudinal arch can be maintained only by muscle and ligamentous support. Basmajian[139, 140] noted that there is little or no muscular activity in the normal foot when standing at rest. Harris and Beath's[153] thesis is that the function of the foot and its shape under the stress of weightbearing depend chiefly upon the design of the tarsal bones and their position in relation to each other. Support for the foot is provided both by passive factors (bone and ligament) and by active factors (muscle). These factors are reciprocal. In the strong foot, muscles are used to maintain balance, to adjust the foot to uneven ground, and to propel the body. In the weak foot, the muscles are called upon to maintain the normal shape of the foot at rest. Muscle cannot act unremittingly. The role of the os calcis in the production of the flatfoot was discussed by Percy Roberts[171] in 1916 in an address to the American Orthopaedic Association.

Other early investigators who felt that the os calcis in its relation to the talus was important in the development of the flexible flatfoot were Gleich,[171] Lord[171] and Chambers.[144] The rationale behind their operative procedures was that the weightbearing forces were directed medial to the foot. Surgery was designed to shift the center of weightbearing for the foot to a relatively more lateral position.

Chambers[144] during his studies at the Daniel Baugh Institute of Anatomy found that excessive heel valgus was associated with increased forefoot abduction. He found that the normal adolescent and adult foot had approximately 15° of what he termed abduction. Motion between the talus and calcaneus is what he was referring to. In the flexible flatfoot this ranged to 35°. He felt that excessive abduction resulted in the characteristic flattening of the longitudinal arch and that stretching of the ligaments is a sequel and not the primary cause of the problem.

Milch[174] states that the term *balance* as applied to the foot structure does not refer to muscle activity but to the arrangement of the bones and ligaments which furnish a stable base upon which weight can be borne with the least demand for muscular exertion.

Muscle

Electromyographic studies of the foot have been utilized in recent years to elucidate the role of muscle in support of the longitudinal arch of the normal foot and flatfoot. Basmajian[139, 140] quotes Duchenne, who 100 years ago stated that by faradization of the peroneus longus muscle in flatfooted children he was able to produce the progressive formation of a normal plantar arch. Morton[140] felt that the structural stability of the foot was not dependent on muscles. He felt that appreciable muscle exertion was needed only when the center of gravity moved beyond the margins of structural stability. Only a slight controlling action by the muscles is required when the center of gravity remains between those margins. In 1952 he further showed that static foot strains are relatively low in intensity, following well within the capabilities of ligaments. His calculations showed that only acute, heavy, but transient forces, such as those in the take-off phase of walking, require the dynamic action of muscle.

In 1941, R. L. Jones,[140] using the method of palpation in the living and direct observation in the cadaver, concluded that not more than 15 to 20 per cent of the total tension stress on the foot is borne by the posterior tibial and peroneal muscles. A much greater part of this stress is borne by the plantar ligaments of the foot and to some extent by the short plantar muscles.

W. Jones[140] felt that maintenance of the normal arch of the foot resulted from the dual control exerted by passive elasticity of the ligaments and the active contractility of muscles. He concluded that the plantar aponeurosis and the plantar tarsal ligaments hold the anterior and posterior pillars of the arch together and that actively contracting intrinsic muscles between the aponeurosis and the tarsal ligaments also play an important role. Basmajian[139] in 1954 from electromyographic studies concluded that the tibialis anterior, peroneus longus, and intrinsic muscles of the foot played no role in the normal static support of the longitudinal arch of the foot. Smith[188] in 1954, using skin electrodes, confirmed this work.

In 1963, Basmajian[140] also concluded that after simultaneous study of the tibialis anterior, tibialis posterior, peroneus longus, flexor hallucis longus, abductor hallucis and flexor digitorum brevis in 20 subjects only heavy loading elicits muscle activity. In the relaxed standing position, the longitudinal arch is supported by bone and ligament. With loads of 400 pounds or more, the muscles do come into play, but even then muscles form a dynamic reserve.

Anatomical studies by J. H. Hicks[155, 156] on the function of the plantar aponeurosis are interesting. He likens the human foot to a truss which is a triangular structure composed of two rods and a tie. In the foot the tie is the plantar aponeurosis and there are five rods radiating from a common posterior rod. The plantar aponeurosis resists the deforming effect of body weight, and in its absence the foot loses its normal shape. The height of the triangle or truss increases when the base shortens. The shortening of the plantar aponeurosis is brought about by a windlass mechanism. The drum of the windlass is the metatarsal head; the cable which is wound around the drum is the plantar ligament of the metatarsophalangeal joint to which the plantar aponeurosis is firmly attached; and the handle, which winds the cable, is the proximal phalanx.

In 1954, Hicks[156] pointed out that when standing, passive extension of the great toe results in: (1) elevation of the longitudinal arch, (2) inversion of the hindfoot, (3) lateral rotation of the leg, and (4) tightening of the plantar aponeurosis. Elevation of the arch was accomplished without muscle forces.

It would be well to review the movements of the foot. Hicks,[155, 156] Sheppard,[185] Fick[178] (1911) and Manter[178] (1941) have demonstrated that the joint complex that makes up the hindfoot acts as a hinge. As in the cases of inversion and eversion, abduction and adduction are complex movements in the foot and involve motion in all of the peritalar joints. Inversion and adduction are always combined in supination. Eversion and abduction are always combined in pronation. The peritalar and midtarsal joints are thus oblique hinge joints.

Inman[158] has shown that with eversion of the heel, as in pronation of the foot, all the articulations in the midfoot become unlocked and maximal motion in the talonavicular and calcaneocuboid joints occurs. If the heel is inverted and the forefoot is held firmly fixed, thus producing a twist in the foot, something happens to convert the entire foot into a rigid structure. Zadek[193] (1935) pointed out that loss of the longitudinal arch of the foot is secondary to abduction of the foot and heel valgus. A low longitudinal arch in a foot without abduction is often found in a strong stable foot that is symptom free. Rose[178] felt that it was the limiting of extension at the midfoot of the joints of the metatarsals that was the main determinant of the posture that the foot assumed when standing, together with the relative lengths of the metatarsals. He stated that the posture of the foot is not dependent on muscle.

Jack[159] based his work on two premises. Firstly, he felt that severe degrees of flatfootedness were disabling. Secondly, he felt that the medial longitudinal arch of the foot and, therefore, the posture of the foot depended upon the intrinsic structure of the bones and joints and the integrity of the plantar ligaments. Muscles are concerned solely with balance and protection of the ligaments from abnormal stress. They can lift the arch but cannot maintain it where there is a bony or ligamentous defect.

The strong arguments that have evolved against the longitudinal arch being supported by muscle have not always been accepted. While presenting the third H. O. Thomas Memorial Lecture in Liverpool, Sir Arthur Keith (1928)[162] said, "There is no need in Liverpool to insist that the longitudinal arch of the foot is dependent on properly and automatically balanced action of muscles in the leg and foot. Hugh Owen Thomas perceived this truth imperfectly but Sir Robert Jones has always taught it to his pupils with emphasis." Haraldsson[152] felt the etiology was an imbalance in the strength of muscles and ligaments of the foot and the weight to be carried. He quotes Niederecker (1950, 1959) as stressing the role of muscle anomalies in the causation of the condition and discussed a statically unfavorable insertion of the tibialis anterior and peroneus tertius as well as the occurrence of a peroneus quartus muscle. Hoke[152] (1931) based his procedure on a concept of muscle weakness as being the primary etiological factor. Other thoughts on etiology have been voiced in the past. Stracker (1953)[152] believed that neurogenic factors are responsible. Priester (1958)[152] postulated an endocrine disorder. Böhm (1930)[152] was said to have been concerned with inhibition of the normal development of the ankle.

TREATMENT

Conservative Treatment

This is a difficult subject. Clearly, it can be assumed from the literature that conservative treatment is fundamental in the management of these patients. However, there is a great deal of controversy as to the definition of conservative management. Fremont Chandler[145] recommended exercises consisting of heel cord stretching and toe flexor strengthening. He felt that molded foot plates or prolonged use of plaster were rarely indicated. Yet some would question this mode of treatment. Shaffer (1951)[152] and Hackenbrock (1961)[152] believed that some cases of flatfootedness in children spontaneously resolve without any form of treatment.

Various shoe modifications have been utilized in the management of this problem. Scaphoid pads, heel wedges, sole wedges, Thomas heels, extended medial counters,

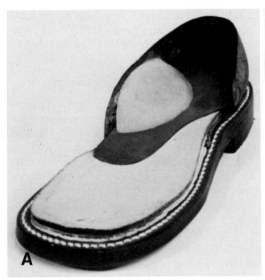
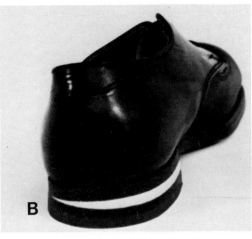

FIG. 21-16. *(A)* A 3/16-inch scaphoid pad with an extended medial counter. *(B)* Shoes with a 1/8-inch medial heel wedge.

and others have been recommended and used by various authors in varying combinations.

Rose[177] felt that the scaphoid pad was unphysiologic. He considered that the heel valgus was the essential element to control and that the scaphoid pad was ineffectual in accomplishing this end. He recommended medial heel and sole wedges.

LeLièvre[169] agreed that arch supports were unsound. He said that with upward pressure on the plantar aspect of the tarsal navicular, the sole of the foot is then sheared between two antagonistic parallel forces. The infrascaphoid pressure is exerted upward from below, and just posterior to it the weight of the body is thrown on the medial border of the foot because of the valgus position of the os calcis. The result is stretching of the plantar musculature.

Lowman[172] and Milch[173] felt that exercises and shoe modifications were futile.

Helfet,[154] too, disagreed with the use of arch supports. He felt that once a child is used to shoe modifications that it is difficult for them to give them up. Heel wedges, in his opinion, only lead to early wearing out of the shoes. He introduced heel seats and reported having used them in over 500 children. After $2^1/_2$ years of use, he found that an arch had formed. He did not report specific numbers but left the impression that success was rather uniform. Rose[178] reported on the meniscus that Schwartz designed to control heel valgus.

The authors' treatment plan recognizes the difficulty in making the diagnosis of flatfootedness in a child before 18 to 24 months. The generalized ligamentous laxity of children must be kept in mind. One must be certain that the foot represents a flexible type of flatfoot and does not represent a prehallux syndrome.[164] Exercises are not felt to be useful. In the presence of heel cord contracture, stretching exercises are indicated. Avoidance of improper sitting when it results in external rotation of the foot and ankle is important. This position accentuates the forefoot abduction and heel valgus posture of the foot. Shoe modifications are instituted only in those with moderate to severe deformities. Parents should be counseled that the shoes being utilized are proper shoes but will not correct the deformity. The shoes should fit the heel well and provide adequate room for the forefoot. Various shoe modifications have been used. In the young child, a $^3/_{16}$-inch scaphoid pad may be combined with a $^1/_8$-inch medial heel wedge (Fig. 21-16). If shoe wear is excessive an extended medial counter may be added. In the older child and in the younger child with more severe deformity, the Helfet heel seat, Schwartz meniscus or the UCB heel cup may be utilized for better control of heel valgus. Modified shoes can prolong shoe life for the patient with severe deformity.

Surgical Treatment

When surgery is contemplated for this condition there are several factors to observe. Jones[161] stated that pronated feet are a common occurrence in early childhood at which time joint flexibility is greater than in later ages. The feet may well share in this laxity and to such structural immaturity the pronated feet of this age group may reasonably be attributed. Rose[178, 179] stated, "In most patients symptoms are absent, trivial or experienced only during times of exceptional stress and are then relieved by appropriate shoe modifications." Legg[167] advocated in 1907 that not all cases of flatfeet will become symptomatic. Crego[146] also cautions that few patients with flexible flatfeet are symptomatic. Golding-Bird (1889)[150] when reporting his surgical procedure advised his colleagues that surgery should be done only for the symptomatic foot. Leonard[170] reported that of 1,446 flatfeet seen over a 10-year period in his clinic 25 were judged to be symptomatic enough to warrant surgical intervention.

The various types of surgical procedures advocated may be divided into three broad categories. Depending on the basic pathology perceived, procedures were designed to repair abnormal (1) ligaments, (2) tendons or (3) bone. Milch[173] and Schoolfield[181, 182] reinforced or advanced the deltoid ligament. Jones[161] advocated reinforcement of incompetent plantar fascia by separating the inner half of the heel cord and attaching it to the neck of the first metatarsal. Phelps[57] (1891) shortened all the structures on the medial aspect of the foot.

In 1905, Painter[176] reported resection of the peroneal tendons for severe rigid feet. Reyerson (1909)[180] transferred the peroneii to the first cuneiform and reported that the results were similar to peroneal tendon section. Gocht (1905)[152] advocated medialization of the Achilles tendon, and Hubscher

(1910)[152] shortened the flexor hallucis longus to which was sewn the posterior tibial tendon. Transfer of the anterior tibial tendon to the navicular was first done by Muller[152] in 1903. Lowman (1923)[172] and Young (1939)[192] incorporated this concept into their procedures. Zadek[193] stated that Achilles tendon lengthening alone was reported by Hoffer (1893), Kohler (1893), Hertle (1910), Els (1913) and Friebe (1920). He also reported that Wilson and Patterson in 1905 placed the extensor hallucis longus into a canal made in the navicular. Zadek also stated that Momberg (1912) used fascia lata, and later Fischer and Barron used peroneal tendon as a free graft and passed them from the navicular to the tibia. Thus, they acted as a passive force designed to elevate the arch.

Bony procedures have been many. Excision of the navicular was recommended by Golding-Bird (1878),[155] and later by Davy (1889).[147] Legg (1907)[167] reported 13 cases in which there had been 100 per cent relief of pain, 1 to 5 years postoperatively. Talectomy was also advocated by Weinhechner, Vogt, Morestin and Eiselsberg.[57]

Subtalar arthodesis has been done by several on the premise that heel valgus was the primary problem. Soule (1921),[187] Leavitt (1943),[166] Rugtvit (1964),[179] Haraldsson (1964)[152] have reported on the use of this procedure in the management of the flexible flatfoot. Some have used Grice's[151] original procedure and others have utilized variations of it. Variations of the Grice have been reported by Dennyson,[148] Seymour[184] and Brown.[141]

Chambers[144] blocked the subtalar joint by raising a flap of bone in the sinus tarsi using a tibial bone graft—the basis of his operation being that the anterior lip of the body of the talus does not make contact with the floor of the sinus tarsi unless the posterior talocalcaneal facets fail to conform to what was called "the ideal pattern of normalcy." LeLièvre puts bone in the sinus tarsi. He does not necessarily attempt to obtain a fusion but wants to prevent heel valgus. Zadek[193] does a transverse wedge resection based medially of the subtalar joint. Haraldsson[152] reported a series of 54 feet on whom surgery was done before age 12 years. Surgery was done between ages 4 and 11 years. Surgery was done on the younger children because he felt that to be most effective surgery must be done before the onset of symptoms—the premise being that pathologic displacement of the foot bones will, if untreated, result in structural changes in the skeleton and soft tissues with fixation of the distortion and increasing symptoms. A series by Brenning (1960)[152] was quoted where one-half of 58 feet in 6- and 7-year-old patients had symptoms. Fifty of his patients had greater than 1 year follow-up; 34 had greater than 2 years follow-up. Twenty-one of 30 patients with preoperative symptoms were relieved of their symptoms by surgery. Overall he reported 40 with good results, 10 who were considered improved, and four who had a poor result.

Supramalleolar tibial osteotomies have been done in the past for severe flatfeet. Trendelenberg[57] (1889) used such a procedure for correction of deformity secondary to Pott's disease. Hahn[57] (1889) and Meyer[57] (1890) utilized it for the symptomatic rigid flatfoot.

Calcaneal osteotomy was first done by Gleich (1893).[171] Whether he actually did the operation on living patients or just in the postmortem room is not clear. Zadek[193] credits Oblalinski (1895) for popularizing the operation. The procedure consisted of an oblique osteotomy of the calcaneus with the posterior fragment being displaced anteriorly. Lord[171] and Koutsogiannis[165] modified the original procedure by displacing the posterior fragment both anteriorly and medially.

Baker[138] and Silver[186] have advocated calcaneal osteotomies for valgus deformities in the cerebral palsied patient. Evans[149] has proposed a lateral opening wedge osteotomy to correct severe valgus deformity.

Osteotomy of the neck of the talus of the closing wedge type was proposed by Sir William Stokes.[57] Couchoix[57] and Wachter[57] also utilized this procedure. Perthes[57] (1913) did a closing wedge osteotomy of the navicular and used the bone removed in doing an opening wedge osteotomy of the calcaneus. Wilms[57] (1914) concurred with this approach.

Radical wedge resections have been done. Legg[167] stated that Larabrie removed the whole of the navicular, the head of the talus, a portion of the internal cuneiform and a corner of the cuboid in very severe flatfeet.

Talonavicular fusions have been done in combination with other procedures for this problem. Soule (1921)[189] recognized that to correct forefoot abduction and heel valgus was to correct the depressed arch. Lowman (1923)[172] combined this with transfer of the anterior tibial tendon to the navicular. Ogston (1884)[175] was an early advocate of this procedure. Naviculocuneiform fusion has been utilized by many surgeons. Hoke (1931)[157] combined this with fusion of the navicular to the middle cuneiform. Jack[159] reported in 1953 the results in 46 feet in 25 patients aged 11 to 14 with flatfeet 15 months to 5 years postoperatively. At the time, there were 54 per cent excellent, 28 per cent good and 18 per cent poor results. Seymour[184] reassessed 17 of 25 patients 16 to 19 years postoperatively and found 31 per cent excellent, 19 per cent good and 50 per cent unsatisfactory results. Tarsal degenerative changes developed in many. Butte[142] reviewed 72 patients who had had the Hoke procedure and found 50 per cent satisfactory and 50 per cent unsatisfactory results.

Surgeons frequently combined procedures, such as Haraldsson did in doing a Grice extra-articular arthrodesis together with a transfer of the anterior tibial tendon to the navicular. Caldwell[143] credits Durham in 1935 for devising a procedure that consists of: (1) division of the posterior tibial tendon at its insertion into the navicular; (2) elevation of a ligamentous capsular flap from the medial aspect of the foot; (3) naviculocuneiform fusion; and (4) insertion of a ligamentous flap into the sustentaculum and reattachment of the posterior tibial tendon. Caldwell reported that this procedure had been done in 76 feet of 38 patients. He found 58 of 76 or 76 per cent with excellent results, 14 of 76 or 18 per cent with good, and four of 76 or 5 per cent with poor results. Crego[146] reports the late results of various operative procedures in children. He estimated that surgery was done in one in 35 or 40 patients with flatfeet. All surgery had been done in patients less than 15 years old. He reiterated that this was a common problem and that most patients were asymptomatic with it. Indications for surgery were

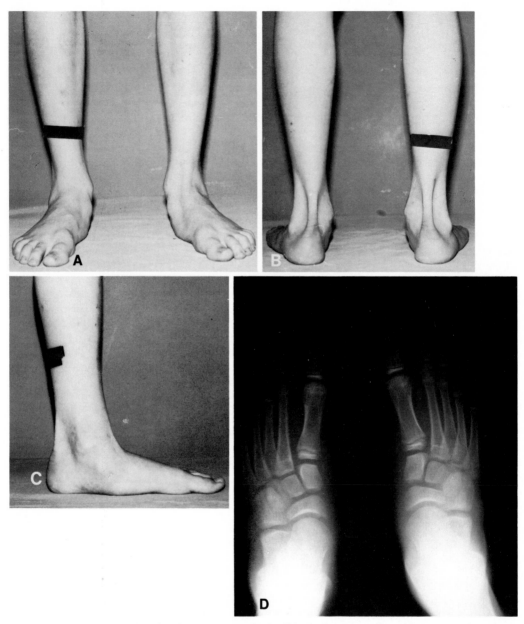

FIG. 21-17. A 12-year-old male with symptomatic flexible flatfeet not relieved by appropriate shoes and modifications. *(A, B, C)* Clinical photographs. *(D)* Roentgenogram showing the talocalcaneal angle.

those feet that were flat and pronated with painful rocker-bottom deformities. He reviewed 102 feet (of 53 children) that had undergone 111 surgical procedures. Eighty-five feet were considered to have been flex-ible flatfeet. Accessory naviculars were found in 11.

Fusion between the talonavicular and naviculocuneiform joints was done 15 times between 1927 and 1935. Satisfactory results

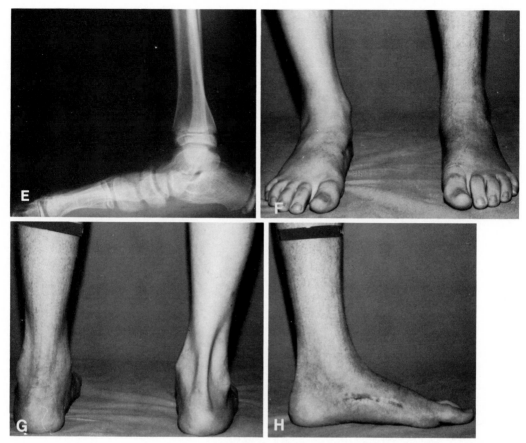

FIG. 21-17 *(Continued)*. *(E)* Note the loss of the longitudinal arch. *(F to H)* Appearance of the feet following reconstructive surgery. *(Continued on overleaf)*

were obtained in 73 per cent. The Hoke procedure was done in nine with only two satisfactory results. Subtalar and talonavicular fusion was done in 24 feet between 1934 and 1944, with 78 per cent satisfactory results. A modified Hoke procedure, consisting of talonavicular, naviculocuneiform and sustentaculum tali and neck of talus fusion, was done 27 times with 48 per cent satisfactory results. The Hoke triple arthrodesis was done in 26 feet with 77 per cent acceptable results. He emphasized the need for subtalar fusion when symptoms are present. The authors favor a surgical procedure which is a modification of the Hoke and Miller procedures. It is indicated for the adolescent when there is pain in the foot not relieved by

proper shoes, rapid abnormal shoe wear and deformity. Surgery should be delayed until the skeletal age of 10 years.

In the adolescent child who has a painful flexible flatfoot, there is loss of the longitudinal arch with a tight heel cord and a lax spring ligament. The posterior tibial tendon is also elongated and stretched. The surgical procedure preferred is as follows (Fig. 21-17):

1. An incision approximately 3 inches in length is made along the medial border of the foot extending from the base of the first metatarsal to the navicular.

2. The anterior tibial tendon at its insertion into the base of the first metatarsal and first cuneiform is identified.

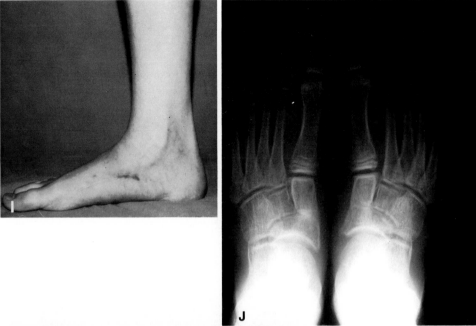

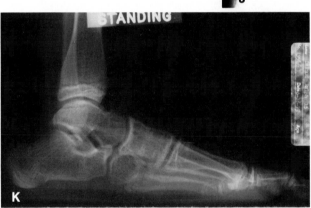

Fig. 21-17 *(Continued)*. *(I)* Appearance of the feet following reconstructive surgery. *(J)* Note the formal talocalcaneal angle and naviculocuneiform fusion. *(K)* Note the restoration of the longitudinal arch and the navicular cuneiform fusion.

3. The posterior tibial tendon at its insertion into the navicular in the plantar aspect of the foot is identified.

4. An osteoperiosteal flap is then developed, with the flap beginning at the insertion of the anterior tibial tendon, and reflected posteriorly. The flap, which is ½ inch in width, extends from the posterior tibial insertion at the navicular to the anterior tibial tendon.

5. The capsule at the naviculocuneiform joint is incised and the cartilage from the joint surface parallel to the bone is removed.

Removal of a wedge with the base positioned medially should not be attempted.

6. The tubercle or prominence of the navicular should be excised and saved.

7. A dorsally based osteotomy is done with an opening wedge dorsally at the first cuneiform. The inferior aspect of the cuneiform should be intact so that an opening wedge dorsally is formed.

8. The tubercle of the navicular is then wedged into the greenstick opening osteotomy of the first cuneiform. This, in effect, tends to elevate the arch.

9. The osteoperiosteal flap that has been created is passed under the anterior tibial tendon and sutured to itself with the sutures pulled toward the plantar aspect of the foot. This should be done with the foot in slight supination.

10. The spring ligament and the posterior tibial tendon plantar expansion are tightened with sutures into the osteoperiosteal flap.

11. A transfixion wire is used across the naviculocuneiform joint with the foot in slight supination and slight varus with the ankle in slight equinus.

12. A cautious heel cord lengthening may in some instances be necessary.

13. The wound is closed and the extremity placed in a short-leg cast in the position described.

14. Total immobilization must continue for 3 months. A short-leg walking cast should be used for the final 6 weeks.

This procedure tends to do the following:

1. It elevates the depressed equinus position of the talus.

2. It tightens the soft tissue on the plantarmedial aspect of the foot, creating dorsiflexion at the talonavicular joint, and elevates the arch.

3. It increases the supination of the first metatarsal-first cuneiform joint by tightening the anterior tibial and placing the posterior tibial insertion more distally.

4. It increases the lever arm (by fusion of the naviculocuneiform joint) on which the posterior tibial-anterior tibial tendons can work.

5. It shortens the medial column of the foot.

6. It corrects the abnormal talcalcaneal angle.

7. It corrects the talonavicular subluxation.

If there is excessive heel valgus present, the authors recommend a Hoke triple arthrodesis. The skeletal age of 12 years must be attained before such a procedure may be performed. Subtalar fusion alone is of concern since the peritalar joint complex acts as a unit. To restrict motion in one joint is likely to lead to premature degenerative changes in the others. The ability of a Grice extra-articular arthrodesis to withstand the stress placed upon it by an otherwise healthy individual is also a matter of concern.

TARSAL COALITION

Tarsal coalition was formerly known as peroneal spastic flatfoot, having first been described by Jones[213] in 1897. Blockley,[196] Cowell,[201] Harris,[208, 209] Harris and Beath,[200] Lapidus[217] and Webster and Roberts[231] have used this term also. Mitchell[220] prefers the term *spasmodic flatfoot.*

By definition, this condition represents a congenital synostosis or failure of segmentation between two or more tarsal bones. The resulting deformity almost always produces a rigid flatfoot. It has been known to exist for over two centuries, having first been described in 1750.[197]

Slomann[225, 226, 227] made an important contribution to the recognition of calcanonavicular coalition when he emphasized the need of oblique roentgenograms. Badgley[194] in 1927 discussed the treatment of this type of coalition and related it to the cause of peroneal spastic flatfoot. Harris and Beath[210] in 1948 identified the talocalcaneal coalition as another cause of peroneal spastic flatfoot.

CLASSIFICATION

Tarsal coalition may exist in the following types: calcanonavicular, talocalcaneal, talonavicular, navicularcuneiform, calcaneocuboid, cubonavicular, block coalition.

In all of the above types, the coalition may be fibrous, cartilaginous or osseous.[207, 210] The fibrous type may show only minimal restriction of inversion and eversion, whereas the cartilaginous and osseous types demonstrate no subtalar movement.

The incidence of this condition is unknown. Harris and Beath[210] in their examination of 3,600 Canadian Army males found an incidence of 2 per cent. The incidence of flexible flatfoot in this group was 6 per cent.

The calcanonavicular coalition is the most common type, with the talocalcaneal type being second in frequency of occurrence.[198, 199, 201, 209, 211, 212]

Clark and Lovell[199] reviewed 94 tarsal coalitions representing 70 patients with 24 patients having bilateral involvement. Sixty of the 94 tarsal coalitions were of the calcanonavicular type, 31 of the talocalcaneal type, two of the talonavicular

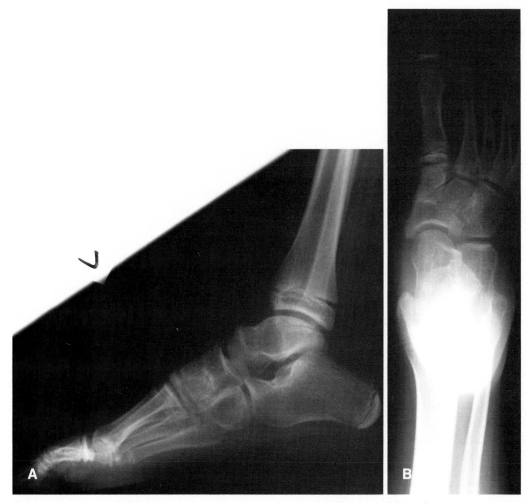

FIG. 21-18. *(A and B)* Roentgenogram showing navicular cuneiform coalition of the osseous type. This is a very rare coalition.

type and one of the naviculocuneiform type. The average age was 13.8 years and there were 40 males and 30 females.

It is of interest that in the series described above, tarsal coalition was seen in Legg-Perthes disease, Blount's disease, cerebral palsy, dysplasia epiphysalis multiplex, idiopathic scoliosis, slipped capital femoral epiphysis and Scheuermann's disease.

Tarsal coalition associated with a ball and socket ankle joint was noted by Lamb.[215] The authors have seen one such case, symptomatic and necessitating treatment.

Naviculocuneiform coalition has been re-ported in only two instances.[205, 218] Figure 21-18 illustrates such a coalition recently seen because of a painful foot. Calcaneocuboid coalition, reported by Wagoner,[229] is rare and has not been seen by the authors. Mahaffey[219] has described this condition also. In the case reported by Veneruso,[228] there was complete absence of a metatarsal and toe. It apparently does not restrict subtalar motion although it may be associated with pain. Cubonavicular coalition is also of infrequent occurrence.[202, 203, 230] Lapidus[217] described a case of bilateral congenital talonavicular fusion. The authors have seen one such case associated with a talocalcaneal coalition and a ball and socket ankle joint.

ETIOLOGY AND GENETIC ASPECTS

Etiology of tarsal coalition remains unknown. Harris and Beath[210] attributed this condition to the presence of an accessory bone which unites to adjacent tarsal bones. Badgley[194] stated that abnormal growth changes in the foot might possibly be a factor. Jack[212] suggested that coalition was due to an error in differentiation which may result in a complete bony fusion at one extreme or to a small accessory bone at the other.

An autosomal dominant transmission is said to occur in this condition. Wray and Herndon[232] reported three cases of calcanonavicular coalition in three successive generations of a family involving males. They concluded that some examples of calcanonavicular coalition are caused by a specific gene mutation that behaves as an autosomal dominant with reduced penetrance. Webster and Roberts[231] reported talocalcaneal coalition occurring in two sisters. Massive familial tarsal synostosis has been noted by Bersante and Samilson.[195]

CLINICAL FEATURES

The majority of patients with tarsal coalition at some time develop pain in the involved foot, and this usually follows injury or excessive activity.[196, 198, 200, 206, 223] The pain is described as being in the region of the sinus tarsi near the talonavicular joint or throughout the foot. The complaints are often aggravated by increased activity and may prevent further participation in athletics.

Symptoms are unlikely to appear until the second decade of life and are related to rapid ossification of the fibrous or cartilaginous coalition.[200] The increased activity associated with the early teens draws attention to the condition. Generally the involved foot presents with pes planus and limited or absent subtalar motion. Very often peroneal spasm may be noted, as well as spasm of the anterior tibial and common toe extensors.

Simmons[224] has reported tarsal coalition accompanying pes cavus, and the authors have seen one such child.

The etiology of the pain in tarsal coalition has been debated. It has been suggested that the restriction of motion at the involved joints results in pain purely on a mechanical basis. Osteoarthritis may occur with narrowing of the talonavicular joint. The spasm of the peroneals and other tendons is probably secondary or possibly a reflex protective reaction to pain.

Outland and Murphy[222, 223] called attention to the anatomic relationship between the calcaneus and navicular. These bones are held by the plantar calcanonavicular ligament. The subtalar and the midtarsal joints, as a result, work synchronously. With forward movement of the calcaneus on the talus, the navicular glides over the head of the talus. If subtalar motion is eliminated as the result of a tarsal coalition, a reactive bone spur forms at the dorsal lateral aspect of the head of the talus.[200] Furthermore, if the restriction of motion is complete, alteration of the shape of the talar head may occur and eventually there may be degenerative arthritis with narrowing and irregularity of the talonavicular joint.

ROENTGENOGRAPHIC FINDINGS

A calcanonavicular coalition is seldom demonstrated in routine anteroposterior and lateral views of the foot.[227] It is best seen in a 45° oblique projection as described by Slomann (Fig. 21-19).[226]

The width of the calcanonavicular coalition extending from the anterior process of the calcaneus to the navicular may vary, with the average width being 1 cm. The osseous coalition is readily identified. The presence of a fissure associated with irregularity and sclerosis is indicative of a cartilaginous or fibrous coalition. Another finding in the calcanonavicular coalition is hypoplasia and smallness of the head of the talus.[200]

An axial view of the calcaneus as described by Harris and Beath[210] is essential to demonstrate talocalcaneal coalition (Fig. 21-20). These authors recommended a 45° angle axial view of the calcaneus. Conway and Cowell[200] have suggested if there is dif-

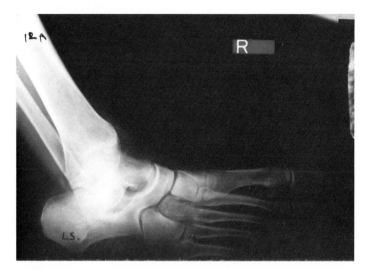

FIG. 21-19. An oblique film demonstrates a very large osseous calcanonavicular coalition.

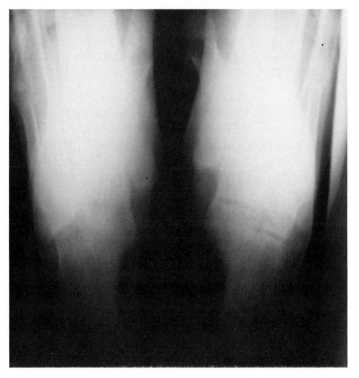

FIG. 21-20. Harris axial view demonstrating osseous coalition on the left and a normal medial facet on the right. This represents a left talocalcaneal coalition.

ficulty in obtaining adequate visualization of the posterior and medial facets with this method, a lateral standing film of the foot should be made in order to determine the proper angle for the axial view. A line is drawn through the joint spaces of the poste-

rior and middle facets and the angle which this line forms with the horizontal is used as the x-ray beam angle for the axial view.

The middle facet talocalcaneal coalition occurs at the sustentaculum tali. If the coalition is osseous, the middle facet is com-

Fig. 21-21. Axial view showing obliquity of the medial facet, hypoplasia of the sustentaculum tali and narrowing of the joint are pathognomonic of a cartilaginous talocalcaneal coalition. Contrast this to the transverse joint on the left with normally developed sustentaculum.

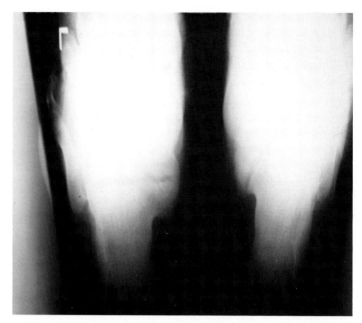

Fig. 21-22. Secondary signs of tarsal coalition are demonstrated in the lateral view of the foot and ankle. These include a broadened lateral process of the talus, narrowing of the posterior facet and beaking of the head of the talus.

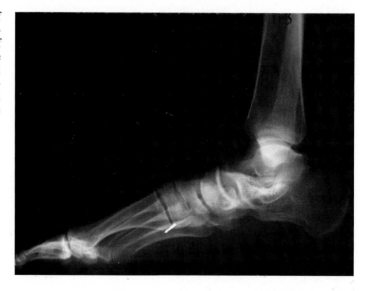

pletely obliterated. In the fibrous or cartilaginous coalition at this site, the joint is narrowed and irregular. The plane of the articulation between the talus and calcaneus is oblique rather than horizontal and the sustentaculum tali is hypoplastic (Fig. 21-21). Secondary signs as described by Cowell[201] include narrowing of the posterior subtalar joint, osteophyte formation of the talus and broadening of the lateral process of the talus at the sulcus calcaneus (Fig. 21-22).

Conway and Cowell[200] described in 1969 anterior facet involvement resulting in a talocalcaneal coalition. They recommended that if the Harris view is negative for middle facet involvement, tomograms in the lateral projection should be secured to demonstrate the anterior facet. Anatomically the anterior facet does not lie in the same plane as the middle and posterior facets and, therefore, the routine axial view does not demonstrate this facet.

The authors have also noticed that peroneal spastic flatfoot may be associated with infections such as tuberculosis, rheumatoid arthritis, osteoid osteoma of the talus and osteochondritis dissecans of the head of the talus. Cowell[201] has reported osteochondral fractures involving the under surface of the talar head as an additional cause of peroneal spastic flatfoot.

TREATMENT

The treatment of a child with tarsal coalition must be individualized. If there is little discomfort, nothing other than restriction of excessive activities may be necessary. A pair of stout shoes with a long medial counter, Thomas heels and $1/8$-inch medial heel wedge may also be helpful in relieving symptoms.[199] A short-leg walking cast may be used for a period of 4 to 6 weeks in the more painful cases associated with peroneal muscle spasm. If pain is not relieved by the above measures, the authors have followed the recommendation of Cowell[200, 201] in the cartilaginous calcocanonavicular coalition and have performed an arthroplasty utilizing the extensor digitorium brevis muscle. Cowell emphasized that this procedure must be done before degenerative changes occur in a young patient. It is accompanied by resection of the coalition. A lateral Ollier incision is used, and after identifying the coalition it is removed as a rectangular block of bone and the entire origin of the extensor digitorium brevis muscle is placed in the defect and tied over a button, medially. A cast is applied with the foot in a neutral position for 10 days. It is then removed and range of motion exercises instituted. Weightbearing should be delayed until motion in the subtalar joint is essentially normal. The purpose of the arthroplasty is to relieve pain and restore motion. Mitchell and Gibson[221] have also advised excision of the calcanonavicular coalition. A triple arthrodesis is indicated in all types of calcanonavicular

coalition if pain is not relieved by conservative measures or if degenerative changes are present.

All talocalcaneal coalitions that fail to respond to nonoperative means as described above should have a triple arthrodesis of the Hoke type.

ACCESSORY NAVICULAR

The accessory navicular is a supernumerary bone in the human foot. It may be found either attached to or fused with the medial border of the navicular. In relationship to the navicular its usual position is posterior and inferior. The tendon of the posterior tibial muscle attaches to it instad of its usual attachment to the navicular.

Kidner[233] credits Bauhin in 1605 for first describing the accessory navicular. In early writings it was considered a sesamoid bone by some authors and a nonunion of a navicular fracture by others.

The accessory navicular appears in many lower mammals either as a part of a fully formed sixth ray or a remnant of such.

Zadek[234] stated that a separate cartilaginous center for the tuberosity of the navicular may be found in the fetus. He reports that the accessory navicular is present as a separate bone in approximately 10 per cent of humans and that it persists as a separate bone in 2 per cent.

Zadek[234] followed 14 patients into adult life who were seen as children with accessory naviculars. Fusion to the navicular occurred in five; partial fusion occurred in three cases; and failure to fuse in six cases.

Microscopic studies[234] were carried out on removed surgical specimens demonstrated that the accessory navicular and navicular are joined by a layer of soft tissue. This soft-tissue plate consisted of hyaline cartilage, dense fibrocartilage or a mixture of the two. The plate varied in thickness and frequently showed active ossification on each side. In no case studied was a well-developed freely movable joint found with smooth hyaline articular cartilage capping each bone and with the two articulating bones bound together by a synovial lined fibrous capsule, such as would be found in a true joint. Found in several specimens was

FIG. 21-23. A 15-year-old asymptomatic female with bilateral accessory naviculars.

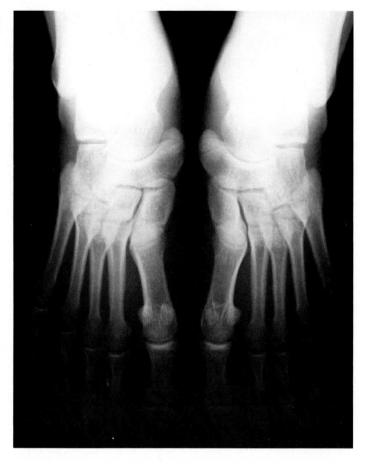

evidence of trauma in the form of hemorrhages, organizing fibrous tissue containing giant cells, and callus-like reparative tissue. This would help to explain the acute symptoms and localized pain seen in some patients.

CLINICAL SIGNS AND SYMPTOMS

Patients present in late childhood and early adolescence with pain localized over the medial aspect of the foot and along the posterior tibial tendon. These symptoms are aggravated by activity and relieved by rest. Frequently soft-tissue swelling and erythema are encountered over the prominence medially. On standing there may be a loss of the longitudinal arch. The presence of an accessory navicular is not constantly related to loss of the longitudinal arch of the foot on weightbearing.

Roentgenograms confirm the clinical impression of accessory navicular. The anteroposterior and lateral oblique views define the accessory navicular (Fig. 21-23).

TREATMENT

Nonoperative Treatment

Shoe modifications designed to support the longitudinal arch are successful in relieving symptoms in most patients. Inserts or fixed modifications can be applied to athletic shoes to allow the patient to continue to participate in activities of choice.

Surgical Treatment

Those patients not relieved by shoe modifications or those whose medial prominence is such that proper fitting is not possible are surgical candidates.

The Kidner procedure[233] is the procedure of choice and may be done in the growing child since it does not interfere with the normal growth of the foot. The authors have been pleased with results obtained.

PES CAVUS

Pes cavus when translated means "hollow foot" and commonly refers to any exaggeration of the normal longitudinal arch. In the past, a variety of confusing synonyms have been used. These include: "bolt feet" (Andry 1741),[237] bowed feet, nondeforming clubfoot (Shaffer, 1885), claw-cavus foot, claw foot, pes arcuatus, talipes plantaris, and talipes cavus.

To be as specific as possible *pes cavus* should be used only to refer to fixed equinus of the forefoot on the hindfoot. In this context true *pes cavus* may occur as an isolated deformity but is often associated with other deformities such as equinus, varus, adductus, or calcaneous.

ETIOLOGY AND PATHOGENESIS

As noted by F. C. Dwyer[255] the confusing and conflicting theories of development and treatment display "a story of repeated failure to comprehend the basic pathogenesis and mechanics of the deformity which remains a mystery to this day, comparable only with problems such as scoliosis."

ETIOLOGY

The etiology of *pes cavus* can be broken into four major categories: neuromuscular, congenital, idiopathic, and other causes (see below). Pes cavus is a frequent sign of underlying neurologic disease. The most common neuromuscular cause is Charcot-Marie-Tooth disease followed in frequency by spinal dysrhaphism.[239, 254, 255, 262, 266, 272] James and Lassman have emphasized that progressive cavovarus of the foot may be associated with spina bifida occulta.

Etiology of Pes Cavus

Neuromuscular
  Charcot-Marie-Tooth
  Spinal dysraphism
  Roussy-Levy syndrome
  Freidreich's ataxia
  Cerebral palsy
  Poliomyelitis
  Spinal muscular atrophy
  Syringomyelia
  Diastematomyelia
  Primary cerebellar disease
  Guillian-Barré
  Interstitial hypertrophic neuritis of childhood
  Mollaret's spinocerebellar degeneration
  Multiple sclerosis
  Traumatic peroneal palsy
  Spinal cord tumor
Congenital
  Residual of clubfoot
  Arthrogryposis
Idiopathic
Other causes
  Traumatic
  Infections
  Ledeerhose disease (plantar fibromatosis)

Abnormal gait and deformity of the foot may be the presenting complaint for extrinsic lesions of the cauda equina. External cutaneous manifestations such as excess hair, nevus, sacral dimples or sacral lipoma may help establish the diagnosis. James and Lassman further reported improvement in the foot abnormalities of 66 per cent of the patients undergoing laminectomy and correction of the lesion. Brewerton, Sandifer, and Sweetman[239] established a Pes Cavus Clinic at the Royal National Orthopaedic Hospital. In their initial group of 77 patients, 44 percent had roentgenographic evidence of a neural arch defect, and 75 per cent were found to have underlying neurologic disease on the basis of the examination, electromyography, or nerve conduction studies.

Other than neuromuscular origin, cavus feet are also seen as a residual of clubfoot or arthrogryposis. Idiopathic pes cavus is probably an uncommon entity.

PATHOGENESIS

Numerous theories have been elaborated to explain the pathogenesis of pes cavus (Table 21-2). These causes may be subdi-

Table 21-2. Theories of Pathogenesis

Intrinsic Muscle Imbalance

Duchenne (1867)	Weakness of short muscles of hallux and interossei
Sherman (1905)	Paralysis of interossei and lumbricales
Mills (1924)	Paralysis of small muscles of foot supplied by lateral plantar nerve
Lambrinudi (1927) Stamm (1948)	Lumbrical and interosseus imbalance
Garceau and Brahms (1956)	Overactivity of superficial plantar muscles

Extrinsic Muscle Imbalance

Barwell (1865)	Weak gastroc with overactive posterior tibials
Fisher (1889)	Weak extensor digitorum longus with weakness of anterior tibials in severe cases.
Golding-Bird (1883)	Weak peronei causing overactive anterior tibials and posterior tibials
Tubby (1896)	Overactive peroneus longus
Steindler (1917)	Weak gastroc and anterior tibial with overactive peroneus longus and toe flexors
Hibbs (1919)	Overactive long extensors acting against contracted calf and plantar fascia
Royle (1927)	Weakness of gastroc-soleus and overactive posterior tibial
Ollerenshaw (1927)	Overactive extensor digitorum longus
Altakoff (1931)	Overaction of calf muscles
Lowman	Strong extensor digitorum longus and peroneus longus with weak anterior tibial
Cole (1940)	Normal extensor digitorum longus with weak anterior tibial
Scheer & Crego (1946)	Weak gastrocnemius and soleus
Bentzon	Overactive peroneus longus
Karlholm and Nilsonne (1968)	Relatively strong posterior tibial

Combination of Extrinsic and Intrinsic Muscle Imbalance

Ducroauet (1910)	Paresis of flexor hallucis brevis with overaction of extensor hallucis longus
Little (1938)	Insufficient interossei with weak extensor digitorum longus
Dickson and Diveley (1939)	Overaction of intrinsics caused by short tendo Achilles
Irwin (1958)	Several varieties of intrinsic-extrinsic imbalance lead to clawing
Chuinard (1973)	Imbalance of extensors, plantar flexors, or intrinsics cause deformity
Kirmisson (1906)	Primitive laxity of dorsal ligaments of foot
Tubby (1912)	Rheumatoid arthritis of tarsal joints
Rugh (1927)	Primary contracture of plantar fascia
Gilroy (1929)	Congenital abnormality
Saunders (1935)	Loss of synergic muscle control and ill-fitting shoes

vided into four categories: (1) intrinsic muscle imbalance (2) extrinsic muscle imbalance (3) combination of imbalance involving intrinsic and extrinsic muscles and (4) non-muscular causes.

Intrinsic Muscle Imbalance

Intrinsic muscle weakness as a cause of pes cavus was first proposed by Duchenne (1867),[251] who felt that clawing of the foot was similar to clawhand. However, the intrinsic muscles of the foot are not anatomically the same as those in the hand.[247, 277, 284] The interossei of the foot insert mainly into the base of the proximal phalanx and do not send a slip to the extensor hood for interphalangeal joint extension as noted in the hand. Although electromyographic studies

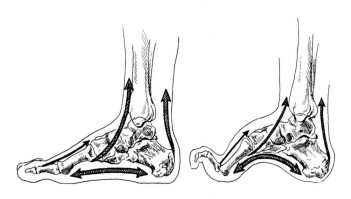

FIG. 21-24. The normal muscular balance of the foot is demonstrated on the left. A right triangle of muscle forces is generated by the gastrocnemius soleus group posteriorly, the plantar muscles distally, and the tibialis anticus anteriorly. Weakness, as demonstrated in the diagram on the right, causes imbalance in the foot with resultant pes cavus. (Redrawn from Chuinard, E., and Baskin, M.: Clawfoot deformity. J. Bone Joint Surg., *55A*:351-362, 1973.)

of the cavus foot have shown definite abnormalities in the intrinsic muscles and short toe flexors, interpretation of these findings has been difficult.[287]

Coonrad, Irwin, Gucker and Wray[246] postulated intrinsic overactivity rather than weakness as a cause of pes cavus. This was based on an observation of cavovarus in polio patients who had preservation of intrinsic and short toe flexors but an otherwise flail leg. Levik (1921)[280] had previously demonstrated the arch raising effect of the short toe flexors.

Extrinsic Muscle Imbalance

Extrinsic muscle imbalance has also been widely held as a cause of pes cavus. Golding-Bird (1883)[265] proposed that weakness of the peroneus longus was etiologic. Since then, Bentzon,[238] Steindler,[305] and others have felt that the condition was due to overactivity of the peroneus longus. Dwyer[245, 255] pointed out that peroneal spasticity and overactivity produced flatfoot, not pes cavus. What is often regarded as overaction of the peroneus longus is actually secondary contracture after the metatarsals become flexed. Hibbs[268] attributed clawing and depression of the metatarsal head to overactive long extensors working against the contracted gastrocnemius and plantar fascia. Other theories of extrinsic imbalance have also been proposed.[244, 256, 276, 289, 292, 299]

Combination of Intrinsics and Extrinsics

The combination of intrinsic and extrinsic imbalance has been proposed by Irwin (1953),[271] who identified four possible pathogenetic mechanisms. Chuinard[242] also favors a variety of possible mechanisms. He described the muscles of the ankle and foot as a right triangle (Fig. 21-24). The base consists of short flexors, abductors, and long toe flexors. The hypotenuse consists of extensor hallucis longus and anterior tibial muscles. The right angle is completed by the triceps surae. Imbalance in any portion of the triangle results in deformity.

Nonmuscular Causes

Postulated nonmuscular causes of pes cavus include improper shoe wear, primary abnormality of bone, and weight of bed clothes during protracted illness.[263, 282, 293, 294, 298] Rugh and Little postulated primary contracture of the plantar fascia. A tight plantar fascia is a uniquely consistent finding in the cavus foot, and contracture of this structure also accounts for the frequent associated finding of varus. However, is contracture a primary or a secondary development? The primary contracture theory does not account for metatarsophalangeal joint dorsiflexion, since the plantar fascia inserts into the base of the proximal phalanges and contracture should produce MP flexion.

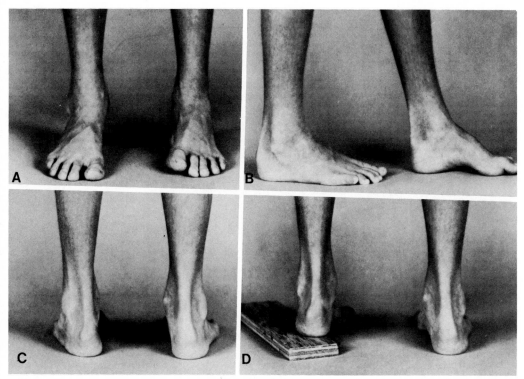

FIG. 21-25. (*A through D*) The typical appearance of a cavovarus foot is demonstrated in the standing position. The great toe is clawed, and the longitudinal arch is raised with apparent flexion and supination of the forefoot. The heel is in varus. In (*D*) is shown Coleman's block test. In this patient the heel varus corrects when the hindfoot is elevated, evidence that the primary deformities in the first and second metatarsals and can be corrected by a dorsal wedge osteotomy through the base of the metatarsals combined with a plantar release.

In summary, numerous etiologic theories have been presented. There is so much synergism in the foot that it is impossible to assess the function of any one isolated component. The authors believe that the cavus foot generally results from an imbalance between the intrinsic and extrinsic muscle groups, although no one pathomechanical process accounts for all of the varieties of pes cavus.

EVALUATION

Since it is difficult to make any generalizations about the pathogenesis, treatment must be individualized and is determined primarily by careful clinical analysis of each patient. Examination begins with the inspection of the forefoot, hindfoot, and toes. Each component of the deformity should be pas-

sively tested to see if the foot is supple and can be realigned. If passive realignment is not possible, each soft tissue and skeletal structure should be carefully assessed to determine which elements prevent realignment. The plantar muscles and fascia are generally contracted and should be assessed with the first metatarsophalangeal joint flexed and extended. The position of the forefoot on the hindfoot is always one of flexion and may include further flexion of the first metatarsal, causing pronation of the forefoot. The hindfoot may be in neutral position if pure pes cavus is present but it is frequently in varus or calcaneus position. Coleman[245] has described a rather simple test for hindfoot flexibility in the cavovarus foot (Fig. 21-25). In this test the patient stands with the heel and lateral border of the foot on a 1-inch block with the forefoot on the floor.

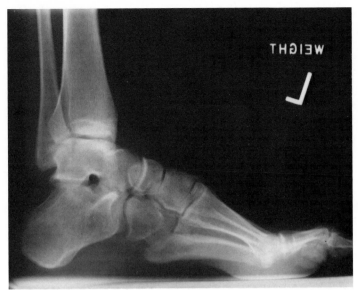

FIG. 21-26. Lateral weight-bearing film showing cavus deformity with a higher arch, calcaneus position of the hindfoot, plantar flexion of the first metatarsal and flexion deformity of the great toe. Note the open subtalar joint.

If the heel varus corrects, the problem is isolated to the forefoot. If varus persists, both hindfoot and forefoot are rigid. The toes should be observed for clawtoe deformity and metatarsal head depression. One should observe whether passive elevation of the metatarsal heads allows correction of the clawtoe deformity. A thorough muscle evaluation should be performed with particular attention to the triceps surae, the long toe extensors, and the tibialis anterior.

Roentgenograms of the feet should include a weightbearing lateral view (Fig. 21-26). The degree of pes cavus can be measured by the angle formed by lines drawn through the center of the longitudinal axes of the calcaneus and the first metatarsal, as described by Hibbs.[268] An assessment of the degree of calcaneus is provided by the posterior angle between the long axes of the tibia and the calcaneus. This is normally 120° or 130°.[242] An angle greater than 130° demonstrates calcaneal deformity. Scheer and Crego[299] noted that the Tuber angle measures 50 to 70° in pes cavus and only 22 to 45° in the normal foot (Fig. 21-27).

In addition, every evaluation should include a thorough family history, thorough neurologic examination, roentgenograms of the entire spine, nerve conduction and electromyographic studies. Myelography should be performed when indicated, particularly in the presence of stigmata of spinal dysrhaphism.

TREATMENT

Initial management should include a period of observation to determine whether the deformity is static or progressive. During this period of observation, stretching exercises of the plantar fascia, short plantar muscles and Achilles tendon, should be initiated. Support of the metatarsals with a metatarsal bar may provide symptomatic relief. If the deformity is progressive, nonoperative management is rarely effective. Appropriate tendon transfers to balance a paralytic foot are discussed in the chapter on neuromuscular disorders.

To correct existing deformity, soft-tissue procedures are indicated only in the presence of mild or supple pes cavus. In children, soft-tissue procedures should be performed to retard progression of the deformity until skeletal maturity has been reached. In adolescents, soft-tissue procedures such as transfer of the long extensor tendons are occasionally indicated to prevent recurrence.

Procedures on bone are indicated in the adolescent and mature foot when the defor-

FIG. 21-27. *(A)* Lateral view of a normal foot showing a normal Tuber angle. *(B)* Abnormal Tuber angle in pes cavus.

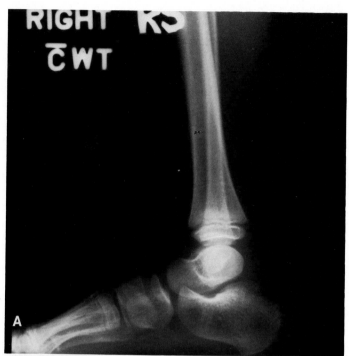

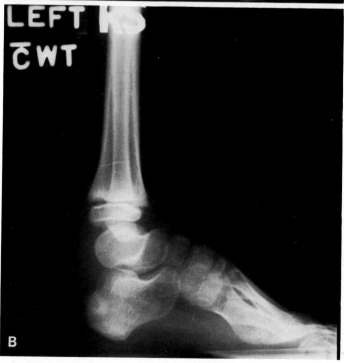

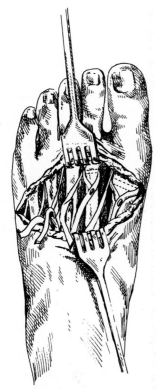

FIG. 21-28. A technique of transfer of the long extensors to the head of the metatarsals. (Redrawn from Chuinard, E., and Baskin, M.: Clawfoot deformity. J. Bone Joint Surg., *55A*: 360, 1973)

mity is fixed. Isolated deformities such as forefoot flexion (true pes cavus) or heel varus are best treated by specific procedures for each deformity. Triple arthrodesis is preferred when deformity is severe, complex, or secondary to progressive neuromuscular disorder.

SOFT-TISSUE PROCEDURES

Tendo Achilles Lengthening

When moderate pes cavus is believed secondary to limited active and passive dorsiflexion of the ankle, stretching exercises may eliminate this problem. If the tendo Achilles does not respond to stretching exercises, cautious surgical lengthening is indicated and is usually combined with posterior capsulotomy.

Plantar Fasciotomy

Release of the plantar fascia and short flexor muscles from the calcaneus was popularized by Steindler.[305] Plantar release as a solitary procedure should be used only for relatively supple deformity in younger patients who do not have clawing of the toes, calcaneus of the heel, or varus. Steindler and others (Hibbs) warned against simultaneous plantar release and tendo Achilles lengthening since tension against the os calcis is necessary to stretch the plantar structures. Numerous variations of plantar fasciotomy have been reported.[270, 293, 294, 303] The authors prefer the technique of Lucas.

Postoperative stretching casts are used for 8 weeks, followed by night casts and passive stretching exercises for 12 to 18 months. Long-term experience with plantar fasciotomy alone has not been very rewarding, although it remains a useful adjunctive procedure.

More extensive plantar releases have been described[36, 69] and include sectioning of the posterior tibial tendon, the bifurcated Y-ligament (calcaneocuboid and calcaneonavicular ligaments), and the spring ligament. In general, these extensive releases have not been widely employed.

Extensor Tendon Transfer

Transplantation of the long extensor tendons to the metatarsal heads for claw toes and pes cavus was first described by Sherman[301] in 1905 and later by Forbes[257] in 1913. Ducroquet (1910) described transferring the extensor hallucis longus to the neck of the first metatarsal. Robert Jones[275] in 1917 described the same procedure, which today is known as the Jones procedure. Stuart in 1924 modified the procedure by adding fusion of the interphalangeal joint. Other modifications have since been described[244, 259, 267, 268, 280] (Fig. 21-28). The rationale for this type of transfer is that it removes the deforming force causing clawing and metatarsal head depression. The transferred tendon then can actively elevate the metatarsal head. Interphalangeal fusion gives the long flexor tendons a better lever arm to flex the metatarsophalangeal joint.

Results with this procedure have generally been good when used in combination with other procedures.[242, 259, 285] However,

FIG. 21-29. Crescentric osteotomy of the calcaneus to correct calcaneocavus deformity. (Redrawn from Samilson, R.L.: Crescentic osteotomy of the calcaneus. *In* Bateman, J.E. (ed.): Foot Science. p. 20. Philadelphia, W. B. Sunders, 1976)

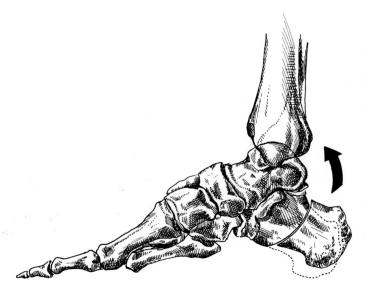

Lambrinudi[279] felt that interphalangeal fusion alone was adequate. He stated that transferring the extensor tendons is not physiologic since the muscles are not strong and the metatarsals are relatively fixed. The authors feel that interphalangeal fusion and extensor transfer is a satisfactory procedure for the relief of claw toes. This procedure is usually combined with plantar release. Best results are obtained when the forefoot is supple and clawing corrects on passive elevation of the metatarsal heads.

Other Soft-Tissue Procedures

Transfer of the anterior tibial tendon either to the head of the first metatarsal[258] or to the calcaneus[271] has been described. In Fowler's procedure, transfer is combined with a plantar-based opening wedge osteotomy of the medial cuneiform. Lateral transfer of the anterior tendon to the cuneiforms is not recommended in cavovarus deformity because the action of the peroneus longus as a flexor of the first metatarsal is enhanced.[255, 306]

Selective neurectomy of the motor branches of the medial and lateral plantar nerves has been advocated by Coonrad and coworkers[246] and Garceau and Brahms.[261] This procedure may be indicated in the child with functioning intrinsics and an otherwise flail foot.

PROCEDURES IN BONE

Wedge Osteotomy of the Calcaneus (Dwyer)

Dwyer[254] described plantar fasciotomy and closing lateral wedge osteotomy of the calcaneus for pes cavus. This is based on the theory that inversion of the heel causes the gastrocnemius-soleus muscle group to become active invertors. This force along with plantar fascia contracture leads to structural varus and cavus. Osteotomy to realign the hindfoot theoretically contributes to gradual stretching of the plantar structures. However, Dwyer himself reported good and excellent results in only 64 per cent of 170 assessed after calcaneal osteotomy. Many of these feet had also required supplementary operations.

The authors share the opinion of others[250, 304] that the Dwyer osteotomy corrects heel varus but has limited usefulness for forefoot cavus.

Crescentic Osteotomy of the Calcaneus

For the correction of calcaneocavus deformity crescentic osteotomy of the calcaneus has been described.[296, 297] This is crescentic in two planes (like a shallow bowl) with the convexity in the posterior direction (Fig. 21-29). In this manner the posterior fragment can be displaced craniad and into valgus. After correction the osteotomy is fixed with Steinmann pins and immobilized for 3 months. Results of this method have not been published and the authors have had no personal experience with the procedure.

Tarsal Wedge Osteotomy

Steindler[305] in 1921 recommended a dorsally based tarsal wedge osteotomy through the cuboid and the neck of the talus. Saunders (1935)[298] proposed a more distal osteotomy at the level of the naviculocuneiform joint. This consists of excision of a dorsally based wedge of bone through the cuboid and naviculocuneiform joints. Other tarsal osteotomies have also been described.[236, 258, 273]

Tarsal osteotomy corrects pes cavus when the forefoot is flexed on the hindfoot. However, circulation to the toes may be jeopardized, the foot is shortened, and pseudarthrosis may result. In the authors' experience this has not been a satisfactory procedure.

Procedures on the Metatarsals

McElvenny and Caldwell[286] advocated correction of the cavus foot by elevating and supinating the first metatarsal. Fusion of the first metatarsocuneiform joint maintained the correction. If necessary, the naviculo-cuneiform joint was included also in the arthrodesis. They found the procedure to be excellent in the passively correctable pes cavus and a valuable adjunct to triple arthrodesis in rigid cavus.

The authors agree that first metatarsal osteotomy is successful when deformity is confined to the forefoot and have used Coleman's "block test" to determine hindfoot flexibility (see Fig. 21-25). If the hindfoot varus is supple and the first metatarsal is supinating the forefoot, metatarsal osteotomy is performed. This is accomplished by removing a dorsally based wedge from the proximal first and second metatarsals (Fig. 21-30). The osteotomy is closed and fixed with smooth Steinmann pins and the leg is immobilized in a short-leg cast with the heel in valgus position.

In rigid pes cavus proximal osteotomies through the base of all the metatarsals has

been advocated.[260, 261] Generally, this has not been an accepted procedure, as correction takes place distal to the deformity.

Triple Arthrodesis

G. G. Davis (1913)[248] first described "horizontal transverse section" of the foot for cavus. Hoke in 1921 described arthrodesis of the subtalar and talonavicular joints. In 1923 Ryerson[295] included the calcaneocuboid joint and thus introduced the triple arthrodesis. Since that time numerous authors have reported variations and results of resection arthrodesis procedures. Satisfactory and lasting results have been reported by a number of authors.

Scheer and Crego[299] recommended a two-stage correction for severe pes cavus. At the first stage the subtalar joint was approached posteriorly and a wedge of bone was removed. Four weeks later through a sinus tarsae incision a complete triple arthrodesis was performed, coupled with plantar fasciotomy to raise the forefoot. At follow-up an average of $2^3/4$ years later 24 of 27 patients were doing satisfactorily.

The authors prefer the method of Hoke as popularized by Kite. In a review of 104 triple arthrodesis procedures performed for a variety of conditions at the Scottish Rite Hospital between 1943 and 1974, 75 per cent had satisfactory correction. The nonunion rate was 9 per cent. Excision of wedges from the calcaneus rather than the talus has virtually eliminated avascular necrosis of the talus. Triple arthrodesis should be performed when deformity is severe, complex, or secondary to a progressive neuromuscular disorder.

OSTEOCHONDROSES

The term *osteochondroses* refers to a group of conditions occurring in the juvenile age period. They are characterized by similar roentgenographic findings of increased density and fragmentation of an epiphyseal or apophyseal center. The lesions were all originally attributed to some form of avascular necrosis. Current evidence indicates that some are due to true osteonecrosis, while others are abnormalities of enchon-

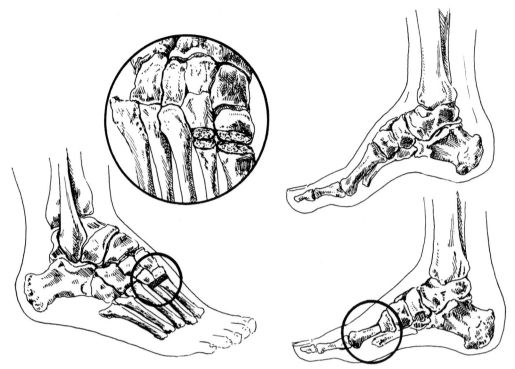

FIG. 21-30. Dorsal wedge osteotomy of the first and second metatarsals. This osteotomy may be performed through a single dorsal incision or through a medial and dorsal incision if plantar structures are released simultaneously. Care must be taken to avoid damage to the dorsalis pedis artery.

dral ossification. Each anatomic location is identified by its own eponym.

FREIBERG'S INFARCTION (OSTEOCHONDRITIS OF THE METATARSAL HEAD)

Freiberg[309, 310] presented a comprehensive description of this entity in 1914. He described an anterior form of metatarsalgia in which the pain was confined to the second metatarsal head and was associated with a "crushed in" roentgenographic appearance of the metatarsal head (Fig. 21-31).

The lesion is due to avascular necrosis of the metatarsal head. It generally involves the second metatarsal head but occasionally involves one of the lateral toes. Repetitive trauma from the stress of weightbearing may be etiologic.[308, 312] Freiberg's infarction is more commonly seen in individuals in whom the first metatarsal is shorter than the second. Maximum incidence is in the second decade of life, usually in adolescents.

The patient presents with pain localized under the second metatarsal head. There is usually local swelling and limitation of motion at the second metatarsophalangeal joint. Roentgenograms show the irregularity and flattening of the metatarsal head. Early in the disease there is a sclerotic appearance. Later in the disease the lesion is osteolytic, with hypertrophy of the metatarsal head. Early in the disease there is a sclerotic appearance. Later in the disease the lesion is osteolytic, with hypertrophy of the metatarsal shaft.

Treatment in the adolescent should be nonoperative. Initial management consists of a low-heel shoe with a metatarsal bar or metatarsal pad. If pain is severe or persis-

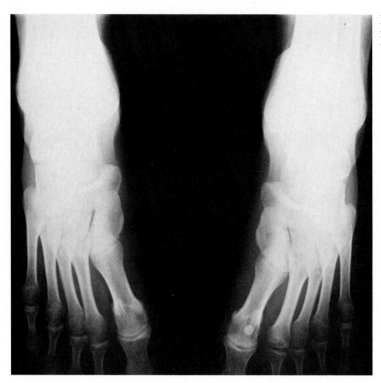

Fig. 21-31. Freiberg's infraction, left second metatarsal.

tent, the foot should be immobilized in a short-leg walking cast for 3 to 4 weeks. After maturity symptoms usually recur, necessitating resection of the second metatarsal head.[311]

KÖHLER'S DISEASE (OSTEOCHONDRITIS OF THE TARSAL NAVICULAR)

Köhler's disease is described as avascular necrosis of the tarsal navicular.[316] It is thought that repetitive compressive forces on the immature ossific nucleus leads to fragmentation and loss of blood supply. The navicular is the last tarsal bone to ossify and occupies a position at the apex of the longitudinal arch of the foot where it is at constant stress during weightbearing.[317] Some support for this theory is found in the fact that Köhler's disease is more common when navicular ossification is delayed beyond normal.[314] The process is also more common in boys, since the navicular ossifies later in boys than in girls. However, in many pa-

tients the roentgenographic findings of increased density and fragmentation of the navicular may represent a normal variant of ossification.[313] This variant is occasionally present on the opposite asymptomatic side and is sometimes familial.

Clinically, the child presents with pain and swelling in the region of the navicular. The average age of onset in girls is 4 years and in boys is 5 years. The onset may be precipitated by an incident of minor trauma following which the child is noted to limp and complain of pain. Two roentgenographic variations are seen (Fig. 21-32). A thin wafer of bone may be present with patchy increased density, giving the suggestion of collapse. In others, the navicular appears to have normal shape with minimal fragmentation and uniform increase in density.

The course is always benign and self-limited. Waugh[317] demonstrated that the navicular receives its blood supply peripherally from a circumferential leash of vessels. Revascularization is rapid, while surrounding reactive tissue and cartilage

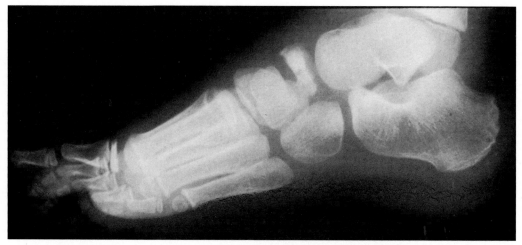

FIG. 21-32. Köhler's disease, showing increased density and collapse of the navicular.

prevent deformity. Treatment is symptomatic.[315] Arch supports and restriction of activities usually suffice. In more presistent or painful cases a short-leg walking cast may be applied for 4 weeks with good results. Ossification is usually complete and normal within 2 years of presentation.

SEVER'S DISEASE
(CALCANEAL APOPHYSITIS)

Sever's disease is a self-limited apophysitis of the os calcis at the insertion of the Achilles tendon.[320, 321, 322] It is associated with pain and tenderness over the posterior aspect of the calcaneus. The condition is aggravated by activity. Increased density and partial fragmentation of the calcaneal apophysis may be noted roentgenographically, but this does not represent avascular necrosis. The heel of the opposite asymptomatic foot may have a similar roentgenographic appearance (Fig. 21-33).

The condition is most common in 6- to 10-year-old males, and treatment is symptomatic. Mild restriction of activities or elevation of the heel of the shoe generally affords prompt relief. Heel cord stretching exercises should be instituted to prevent recurrence. In severe cases a short-leg walking cast may be indicated for 4 weeks' duration.

OSTEOCHONDRITIS DISSECANS
OF THE TALUS

This is an uncommon entity characterized by an avascular osteochondral fragment that separates from the underlying bone. Characteristically, the fragment is located at the superior medial aspect of the dome of the talus.[332, 334] Berndt and Harty [326] demonstrated that a transchondral fracture is produced in this area when compression is applied to he ankle when it is in the position of internal rotation, dorsiflexion, and inversion. Repetitive trauma with ischemic changes in the subchondral bone has been implicated in the etiology of osteochondritis dissecans of the talus just as it has been implicated in osteochondritis affecting other joints.[326, 327, 328, 333, 336] This process is more common in boys and there is often a history of repetitive trauma. However, several authors have noted a familial tendency.[330, 337] Cases of multiple joint involvement have been reported.[331]

Clinically, the patient is usually an adolescent who complains of diffuse discomfort and swelling in the ankle joint.[329, 335] If one suspects osteochondritis of the talus, anteroposterior roentgenograms of the ankle mortise should be obtained in varying degrees of plantar flexion.

If the fragment is not displaced and there

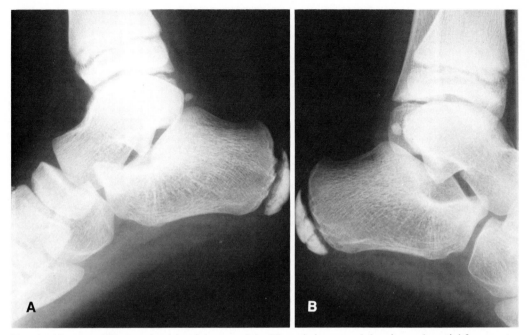

Fɪɢ. 21-33. *(A and B)* Apophysitis of the os calcis. There is increased density and partial fragmentation of the apophysis.

is no history of locking, treatment consists of immobilization in a short-leg cast.[327] Weightbearing should not be permitted. Under the age of 16 years healing of the fragment usually occurs in 3 months. If after 3 to 4 months of immobilization there is no roentgenographic or clinical evidence of improvement, surgical intervention is indicated.

At surgery a transmalleolar approach provides optimal visualization of the lesion. It is best to perform an oblique osteotomy of the medial malleolus after predrilling and partial insertion of a malleolar screw to facilitate later replacement of the malleolus. If the fragment is small or completely detached it should be removed and its bed curetted. If the articular cartilage is not severely damaged and the fragment is large enough, it should be preserved by pinning the fragment with smooth Kirschner wires. These wires should penetrate the opposite cortex of the talus so that they can be removed after the fragment has united with the underlying bone. Postoperatively the leg should be immobilized in a short-leg cast until union is complete.

FOREFOOT DEFORMITIES

CONGENITAL DEFORMITIES

Congenital malformations of the forefoot and toes are not uncommon in childhood. Most of the deformities have a familial tendency. In general, toe deformities in children are unresponsive to nonoperative treatment. Some do not progress or cause symptoms in later life. With advancing age, however, the abnormality becomes more fixed while shoes become less accommodating. More severe deformity produces pressure symptoms in adulthood and should be surgically corrected. Examination during weightbearing is essential to help separate significant from insignificant deformity.

Cᴏɴɢᴇɴɪᴛᴀʟ Cʟᴇꜰᴛ Fᴏᴏᴛ (Lᴏʙsᴛᴇʀ Cʟᴀw)

Congenital cleft foot is a rare deformity consisting of various combinations of deficiency of the central three metatarsals and phalanges. The first and fifth rays are often present and the phalanges.[10] The first and fifth rays are often present and the phalanges of these rays deviate toward the midline cleft (Fig. 21-34). The hindfoot is usually normal.

Cleft foot is generally accompanied by cleft hand or other digital anomalies. Typically this deformity is bilateral and familial, being inherited as an autosomal dominant trait with incomplete pentrance.[338, 343, 344, 345] Other associated abnormalities such as cleft lip and palate, deafness, and genitourinary tract anomalies have also been noted.[340, 344] Because of the coincident development of genitourinary tract and limb buds during embryogenesis, intravenous pyelogram is indicated in the evaluation of any child with congenial cleft foot.

Surgical correction is not necessary for function but may be indicated for cosmesis or to facilitate shoe wear. Several types of correction have been described, dependent upon the extent of the deficit.[339, 342, 345, 348] Surgery generally consists of excision of bony remnants, creation of skin flaps to allow closure of the cleft and metatarsal osteotomies to narrow the feet. The split forefoot and toes are surgically syndactylized to maintain correction.

SYNDACTYLY

Syndactyly of the toes as an isolated deformity does not limit function and rarely becomes symptomatic.[352, 359] Correction to improve cosmesis is inadvisable. Occasionally surgery is indicated when multiple digits are webbed or if osseous structures are incompletely separated.

Surgical separation is accomplished by the same technique as that used for syndactyly of the fingers. Skin grafting is required.

MACRODACTYLY

Gigantism of one or more toes is a rare abnormality but creates a problem in shoe fitting and cosmesis (Fig. 21-35). Any child with localized gigantism should be evaluated to rule out the possibility of neurofibromatosis.[350, 353]

Surgical correction is indicated when hypertrophy interferes with adequate shoe wear. To reduce the size of forefoot or toes, total or partial osteoectomy with resection of an adequate amount of soft tissue should

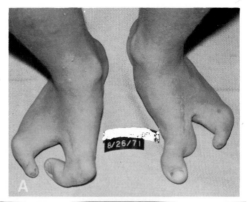

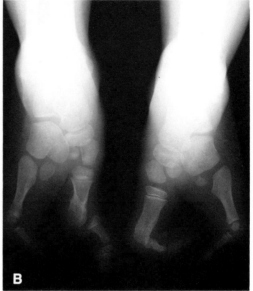

FIG. 21-34. A 9-year-old male with a cleft foot. (*A*) Clinical photograph. (*B*) Roentgenographic views.

be performed.[360] Correction should be accomplished in two or three stages if necessary and should be carefully planned in advance. Epiphysiodesis is helpful in preventing longitudinal growth, but does not limit circumferential growth.

POLYDACTYLY

Polydactyly is a common malformation that varies widely in extent and is frequently associated with other anomalies. Duplication of the toes occurs more often in Blacks than in Caucasians. The familial occurrence

FIG. 21-35. *(A and B)* Macrodactyly.

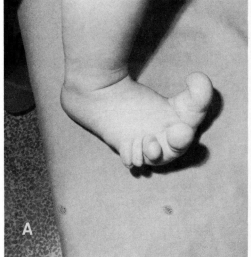

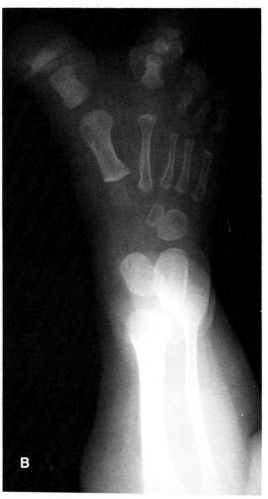

of polydactyly is not unusual. Venn-Watson (1976)[361] presented an excellent report on polydactyly of the foot based on a study of 72 patients.

The fibular side of the foot is involved most often.[356] The most common deformity is duplication of the fifth toe with a Y-shaped metatarsal or a fifth metatarsal with a broad head (Fig. 21-36). Duplications of the hallux, which are less common, are often associated with a short-block first metatarsal.

Treatment consists of surgical excision of the most peripheral toe. If the accessory digit is entirely fleshy, a silk ligature about the base can be applied in the nursery and will accomplish the desired result.

When the duplication involves osseous structures, amputation of the accessory digits should be accomplished between the age of 10 and 15 months. Redundant skin and soft tissue should be excised to reduce the forefoot to normal dimensions. Duplicated metatarsals or bony protrusions of the common metatarsal should be removed. A wide metatarsal head should be narrowed surgically. Accessory tendons should be sutured to the adjacent tendon. The capsule and ligaments of the metatarsophalangeal joint must be carefully reconstructed to prevent varus or valgus deformity of the remaining toe. Polydactyly should be treated early to allow maximum time for remodeling of the foot. Excellent results can be antici-

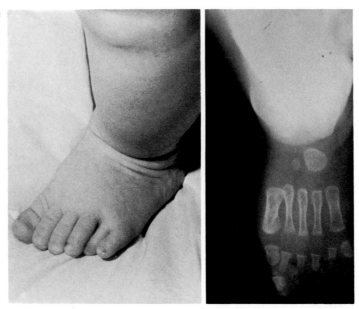

FIG. 21-36. Duplication of the fifth toe in which the proximal phalanx shares a broad fifth metatarsal head.

pated, except for a duplicated hallux with a short first metatarsal.

CONGENITAL HALLUX VARUS

Congenital hallux varus consists of medial angulation of the great toe at the metatarsophalangeal joint.[370, 371] This condition is due to an extra toe anlage in the medial part of the foot which undergoes a developmental arrest and pulls the great toe into varus.[367] The anlage is frequently evident as a supernumerary bone but may exist as a tight fibrous band. Frequently the first metatarsal is broad and short. The lateral toes may also be pulled into varus. This congenital malformation, bilateral in 20 per cent of patients, should be differentiated from medial deviation of the great toe associated with hallux varus or metatarsus primus varus.[365, 368]

Nonoperative treatment is ineffective. Several authors have described operative procedures, which are best performed between 1 and 2 years of age.[363, 364, 366, 367, 369] Correction must include resection of the tethering band or bone, capsulotomy of the metatarsophalangeal joint, and syndactylization of the first to the second toe to prevent recurrence. McElvenny, in addition, used the tendon of the extensor hallus brevis

to reinforce the lateral capsule. Farmer designed a rotational skin flap in order to lengthen the tight medial soft tissues. After any surgical correction the joints should be held in the proper position with a Kirschner wire and cast for 3 weeks and a cast alone for 3 more weeks.

ADOLESCENT BUNION

Introduction

Although an uncommon problem for the surgeon dealing with children, this is a subject of some debate. There are several terms which are used to describe this problem, including *metatarsus primus varus, metatarsus primus adductus, hallux valgus* and *adolescent bunion*. Its etiology and treatment remain a topic where many disagree. Currently the popularly held concept of metatarsus primus varus being the etiology is not accepted by all. In the early literature, it seems to have been assumed that bunion deformities resulted from improper footwear. It was reasoned that since the problem was seen primarily in the female and since the female often utilized shoes that were more stylish than they were physiologic, the cause of the bunion deformity was improper footwear.[379] The concept of abnormal deviation of the first metatarsal has many proponents. Reidle was credited by Kleinberg[389] as being the first to suggest this as the primary problem. One of the earliest references in the English literature to metatarsus primus varus is by Truslow.[401] There have been many authors since who feel that it is etiologically related to adolescent bunion. Lapidus,[391] Kleinberg,[389] Mitchell,[382, 394] Durman,[375] Hardy and Clapham,[381] Carr and Boyd[374] and Bonney and McNab[373] are among those who share this view. Obliquity of the first cuneiform-metatarsal joint was observed by Truslow,[401] Lapidus,[391] Kleinberg,[389] Durman[375] and Berntsen.[372] Hallux valgus was felt to be primary by Ewald[378] and Piggott.[396] Hiss[384] felt that muscle imbalance was primary.

Phylogenetically, the increased intermetatarsal angle is similar to that of other primates who utilize their feet for climbing. Hiss,[384] Lapidus,[391] and Truslow[401] have referred to this in their writings. During evolution, the foot had adapted itself from a grasping device to a supporting structure. In so doing, the human foot had to lose some of its mobility. The hallux straightened and the lesser toes diminished. The hallux of primates resembles the human thumb in its greater range of motion and the larger angle formed by the first and second metatarsals.

Etiology

In an excellent article, Inman[385] made several interesting observations. He makes reference to the work of Wells,[402] who studied the feet of South African natives. He found abduction of the first metatarsal in association with hallux valgus. Engle and Morton[377] found hallux valgus in the West African population. These groups did not wear shoes. Lam Sim-Fook and Hodgson[390] found that 2 per cent of nonshoewearing Chinese displayed definite hallux valgus. Inman[385] also describes mechanically the reasons why a pronated foot may develop a hallux valgus deformity. Hiss[384] reviewed 1,812 cases involving 3,092 bunions. He noted that 60 per cent of his patients had what he termed everted feet, 32 per cent had a loss of what was called the spring arch, and

82 per cent had what was described as malposition of the arch bones.

Metatarsus Primus Varus. Support for the theory that metatarsus primus varus is the etiology of adolescent bunion deformity has come from several sources. Durman[375] studied 374 feet of 178 adult patients who stated that they had no foot problems. Nine of these patients were found to have significant bunion deformities. In 356 normal feet, the first intermetatarsal angle varied from zero to 16° and the metatarsophalangeal joint angle varied from zero to 20°. He concluded that the ideal normal foot is one in which the first and second metatarsals are parallel and the great toe extends directly forward in the long axis of the first metatarsal. The average normal foot had a metatarsophalangeal angle of 20° and an intermetatarsal angle of 10°.

He then measured 18 feet with hallux valgus. The intermetatarsal angle ranged from 10° to 18° and the metatarsophalangeal angle 22° to 56°. Another group was evaluated, consisting of 886 patients. In this group, there were 80 females and 102 males under 19 years of age. Twenty females and three males were found to have hallux valgus. Among the four hallux valgus feet in males, two had intermetatarsal angles of 10° or more. In the female group, of the 27 feet, 18 or 66 per cent had intermetatarsal angles of 10° or more.

There have been other detailed studies of feet with hallux valgus. Hardy and Clapham[381] studied several variables in the foot with hallux valgus. The intermetatarsal angle of 252 controlled feet was noted to range from zero to 17° with a mean of 8.5°. In 177 feet examined due to complaints referable to them, the angle ranged from 4° to 27° with a mean of 13°. This widening of the intermetatarsal angle between these two groups was said to have been statistically significant. Also of interest was that 46 per cent of the 177 had the onset of their symptoms before age 20 years. Thirty per cent of these were symptomatic before age 15 years.

Another group was examined, consisting of 125 controls. There were 73 males and 52 females. The first intermetatarsal angle was 1.3° greater in the female. This was a statistically significant difference.

Long First Metatarsal. An interesting facet to the work of Hardy and Clapham[381] was the finding that those patients with a high degree of hallux valgus and a low intermetatarsal angle had first metatarsals longer than the second. This difference was significant when compared to those who had a high degree of hallux valgus associated with a widened first intermetatarsal angle.

Cuneiform Variation. Abnormality of the first cuneiform has been discussed by many authors. In a group of Durham's,[375] 28 of 31 hallux valgus feet in adolescents were felt to have cuneiform abnormality. Of his original group of 886 patients, he found 11 per cent of normals with cuneiform variation and in 47 per cent of those with hallux valgus. Ewald[378] in 1912 noted obliquity of the distal articulation of the first cuneiform in hallux valgus. Berntsen[372] in 1930 supported this observation when he reported cuneiform deformity in 67 percent of hallux valgus feet while noting this in only 6 percent of normal feet. Others have reported similar findings.[378]

In light of Inman's[385] observations, one wonders whether these variations are on the basis of rotation of the medial cunieform with pronation of the foot.

Os Intermetatarseum. The presence of the rare os intermetatarseum[390] has been described as a possible cause of metatarsus primus varus in some patients.

Associated Disease. Certain generalized diseases have been associated with hallux valgus. Neuromuscular disease including cerebral palsy, poliomyelitis, myelodysplasia may have concomitant bunion deformity. Adolescent bunion is also seen with such diverse and unrelated conditions as Sprengel's deformity, multiple osteochondromatosis, hemihypertrophy, juvenile rheumatoid arthritis and otopalatal-digital syndrome.[400]

Family History

A familial incidence has been found. Johnston[386] studied one family through seven generations and concluded that hallux valgus was an autosomal dominant with incomplete penetrance. A family history was found in 63 per cent by Hardy and Clapham[38] and in 58 per cent by Mitchell.[382,394] Bonney and McNab[373] noted an increased incidence of an early onset of symptoms in those with a positive family history.

Anatomy

Haines and McDougall[380] give an excellent description of the anatomy of hallux valgus. Of particular interest was the discussion of the nature of the medial prominence. They credit Lane in 1887 for considering the medial prominence a part of the metatarsal that had originally articulated with a proximal phalanx of the great toe, and not a new growth. This area had lost contact with the articular cartilage of the proximal phalanx as it deviated laterally. The cartilage became soft and inelastic, losing its white color. Anderson in 1881 presented a cadaver preparation in which the great toe formed a right angle with the long axis of the first metatarsal. He found tissue destruction rather than new formation in the region of the medial prominence. Work by Payr in 1894 and Hewbach in 1897 supported Lane's theory. Stein in 1938 stated that the medial prominence was not an extosis.

In mild cases the cartilage over the eminence is well preserved but late; the eminence may even lose its cortical layer, exposing an uneven surface of spongy bone.

The sagittal groove was ascribed to pressure of the margin of the phalanx by Clarke in 1900 and Jordan and Brodsky in 1951. Hanes and McDougall[380] feel it more likely that it is formed by degeneration of the cartilage where cartilage-to-cartilage contact had been lost. The weakness of the bony trabeculae deep to the groove and their arrangement parallel to the surface suggests that the groove is a region of minimal pressure and is a fossa nudata due to lack of adequate stimulation rather than an erosion due to access.

Clinical Features

Patients may present as an adolescent with painful feet. On examination, a prominent first metatarsal head with lateral deviation of the great toe is observed. When standing, these deformities are increased and there is a widening of the forefoot. Secondary problems are related to hammer toe deformities and painful PIP joints, inflam-

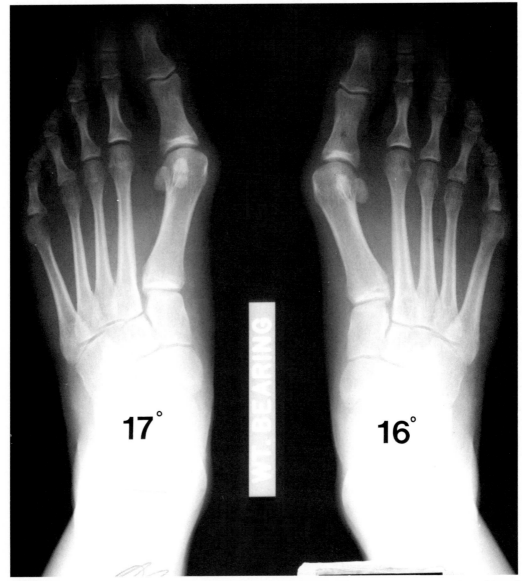

FIG. 21-37. Roentgenograms of the feet of a symptomatic 14-year-old female. Note the widened first intermetatarsal angle.

mation of the bursa overlying the first metatarsal head, and metatarsalgia involving the lesser metatarsals.

Symptomatic adolescent hallux valgus is different than that seen in the adult in several ways: (1) the degree of valgus of the great toe is usually less; (2) there are no arthritic changes in the metatarsophalangeal joint; (3) the bursa overlying the medial prominence is not chronically thickened; and (4) frequently, epiphyseal plates are still viable

and further longitudinal growth is possible.[400]

Roentgenographic Features

Films are made with the patient standing in order to allow standard measurement of the first intermetatarsal angle. Intermetatarsal angles in excess of 10° are considered to be increased and to represent metatarsus primus varus (Fig. 21-37). The sesamoid bones are observed on standing antero-

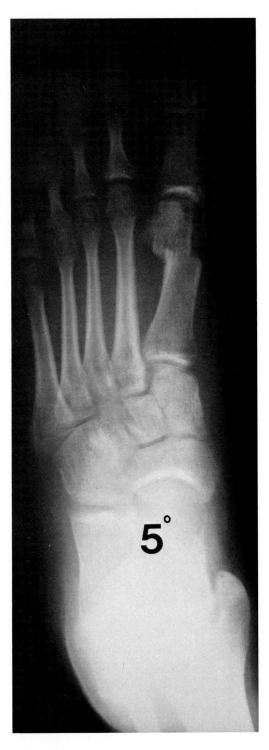

posterior roentgenogram to be laterally
displaced, although, as Inman[385] has pointed
out, this may only represent rotation of the
first metatarsal. In advanced problems, the
congruity of the metatarsophalangeal joint
may become interrupted.

Treatment

Conservative management of the symptomatic foot includes foot wear that properly
fits the width of the forefoot. This may
necessitate the purchasing of a shoe with a
wider forefoot than hindfoot sections. One
might also consider the use of a scaphoid
pad if there is a loss of the longitudinal arch,
and heel wedges if there is excessive heel
valgus.

Surgical Treatment. Indications for surgery include pain, failure to respond to
proper shoes, difficulty obtaining proper
shoes, and cosmesis.

Surgical procedures should be individualized. Those patients with metatarsus
primus varus should have this corrected by
metatarsal osteotomy. This can be done at
the base,[389, 391, 398, 401] mid-shaft,[403] or distally.[372, 382, 394, 395] Those who do not have
metatarsus primus varus may need lesser
procedures.[379, 392, 397, 399] Resection[388] or interposition[393] arthroplasty would not be
often indicated in the adolescent, as degenerative changes are unlikely to be severe
enough to warrant these procedures. Arthrodesis of the metatarsophalangeal is
rarely to be considered in the adolescent.
Ellis[376] has recommended stapling of the
lateral portion of the first metatarsal growth
plate. This would not seem to be a good
choice in view of the difficulty with epiphyseal stapling done in more accessible areas.
The Joplin[387] procedure is a complicated
one, but one which has given its proponents
satisfactory results.

The authors favor either the Mitch-
ell[373, 382, 394] or Wilson[403] procedures. The
reader is referred to the original descriptions
of the operative technique for details. These
procedures have proven themselves reliable
(Fig. 21-38, 21-39). Postoperative care can
be facilitated by the use of a toe spica cast.

This is applied over the forefoot to include
the great toe, utilizing one roll of 2-inch
plaster.

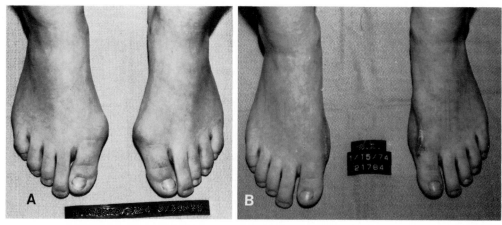

FIG. 21-39. Adolescent bunion, pre- and postoperatively. *(A)* Preoperative, *(B)* postoperative.

Complications. One must not underestimate these procedures. Bonney and McNab[373] reviewed the operative results in 54 adolescents. Twelve were in need of further surgery. In 34 of 54 feet operated upon, the metatarsus primus varus returned to its original state or to a larger intermetatarsal angle than before surgery. When permanent correction was obtained, the results were better. They concluded that primary failure may result from: (1) simple failure to swing the first metatarsal toward the second, (2) obtaining a "false" correction by soft-tissue compensation with subsequent swinging out of the first metatarsal on removal of plaster; (3) producing correction by swinging the proximal end of the first metatarsal medialward instead of having the distal end lateralward. Failure of maintenance of the initial correction was felt to be related to: (1) too early weightbearing; (2) inadequate immobilization during the critical period; (3) osteotomy of the first metatarsal distal to a growing epiphysis with further bone growth occuring in a varus direction with consequent early recurrence of the deformity. In 14 feet that had good primary correction by osteotomy distal to the first metatarsal growth plate, 10 had recurrence. In 20 feet operated upon after the growth plate had closed that showed good results, nine recurred. Other causes of failure, as cited by Bonney and McNab, include: (1) operative production of an ele-

vated or a depressed first metatarsal; (2) long continued postoperative stiffness of the first metatarsophalangeal joint; (3) careless trimming of the medial prominence with a consequent increase of the hallux valgus; (4) failure to obtain correction of the hallux valgus due to unrelieved soft tissue contracture; and (5) overcorrection of the metatarsus primus varus combined with trimming of the medial prominence leading to medial subluxation of the first metatarsophalangeal joint.

CONGENITAL SHORT FIRST METATARSAL (METATARSUS ATAVICUS)

Congenital short first metatarsal is presented here only to point out that the condition is a variation of normal.[404] In 1927, Morton[406] described metatarsus atavicus (congenital short first metatarsal) as a specific cause of metatarsalgia. More recently Viladot[408] revived the concept of first ray insufficiency due to short first metatarsal. Theoretically, metatarsalgia is due to increased weightbearing by the second metatarsal. The forefoot pronates so that more weight is borne on the first metatarsal. This pronation lowers the longitudinal arch and contributes to the metatarsalgia.

However, Harris and Beath[405] questioned this hypothesis and stated that the short first metatarsal can bear its share of weight simply by increased flexion at the metatarsotarsal joint. In a foot survey of the Canadian Army Harris and Beath roentgenographically examined over 7,000 individual feet. They found that approximately 40 per cent of these individuals had a short first metatarsal. In this group there was no increased incidence of pes planus, callus formation, thickening of the second metatarsal, or foot symptoms due to strenuous activity.

CONGENITAL OVERRIDING OF THE FIFTH TOE

This is a familial problem in which the fifth toe is in varus and overlaps the fourth toe. The capsule of the metatarsophalangeal joint is contracted, the extensor tendon is shortened, and there is a contracted band of skin between the fourth and fifth toes. The condition causes symptoms in approximately half of the feet involved.

Nonoperative treatment consisting of passive stretching of the little toe into plantar flexion and abduction is generally unsuccessful but may be used preoperatively or in infancy to decrease contracture. Splinting and taping have likewise been unsuccessful. If symptoms warrant, operative correction is indicated. Several procedures have been described for the correction of the overriding fifth toe.

Lantzounis (1940)[416] recommended severing the extensor digitorum longus of the fifth toe and suturing it to the head of the fifth metatarsal. Lapidus (1942)[417] described a procedure in which the long extensor tendon of the fifth toe is severed proximally at the middle of the fifth metatarsal. The distal end of the tendon is drawn down to a second incision on the dorsal medial aspect of the fifth toe. Capsulotomy of the metatarsophalangeal joint is performed. Then the stump of the tendon is rerouted under the plantar aspect of the proximal phalanx and sutured to the abductor digiti quniti tendon under enough tension to correct the deformity.

Several procedures have been suggested for release of the extensor tendon and tight dorsal structures with plastic elongation of the skin fold that is created when the deformity is corrected. Goodwin and Swisher[411] recommended Y-advancement with capsulotomy and Z-lengthening of the long extensor tendon. Stamm[424] described a similar procedure but used V-Y advancement for the skin. Wilson[427] and Sharrard[423] also advocate the V-Y advancement in children. DuVries[410] described a similar procedure to Stamm's except "dog-ears" are excised after correction of the deformity. Scrase,[422] however, was dissatisfied with plastic elongation of the skin contracture and noted recurrence in a few cases.

Cockin (1968)[409] described an operation devised by R. W. Butler. This consists of a radical release of the metatarsophalangeal joint through a racket-shaped incision around the base of the fifth toe. There are both dorsal and plantar handles to the racket. Dorsal and plantar capsulotomies are performed with release of the extensor tendon. Lasting full correction of the deformity was obtained in 91 per cent of 70 procedures. Tachdjian has also found this procedure satisfactory.[17]

McFarland (1950)[419] resected the base of the proximal phalanx and produced a surgical syndactly between the fourth and fifth toes. Scrase[422] used this procedure in 42 patients with 39 good results. Leonard and Rising,[418] Kelikian[414] and Tachdjian[425] have also advocated McFarland's procedure.

Proximal phalangectomy has been proposed by Ruiz-Mora[421] and others (Fig. 21-40).[420, 426] Ruiz-Mora described a plantar approach with excision of an elliptical segment of skin. The flexor tendons are severed and allowed to retract. Janecki and Wilde[413] recently reported results of 31 Ruiz-Mora procedures in patients followed for an average of 3 1/2 years. All patients had complete correction of the deformity and relief of symptoms. However, 23 per cent developed a painful prominent fifth metatarsal head or a bunionette deformity, and in 32 per cent symptomatic hammertoe deformity of the fourth toe developed. Based on their observation Janecki and Wilde recommended resection of only the head and neck of the proximal phalanx. Sharrard[423] advised against excision of the proximal phalanx in children because of its effect on the growth of the little toe.

The authors feel that congenital overriding of the fifth toe is often asymptomatic and requires no treatment. When symptoms occur surgery is indicated. Surgical correction is generally successful and the proce-

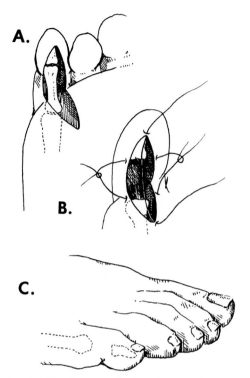

A.

B.

C.

Fig. 21-40. Two methods of correcting congenital overriding of the fifth toe. *(A, B, and C)* The Ruiz-Mora procedure, as described by Janecki and Wilde. (Redrawn from Janecki, C.J., and Wilde, A.H.: Results of phlangectomy of the fifth toe. J. Bone Joint Surg., *58A*: 1005, 1976 and redrawn from Kelikian, H.: Hallus Valgus, Allied Deformities of the Forefoot and Metatarsalgia. p. 328. Philadelphia, W. B. Saunders, 1965)

dures most widely used are those described by Ruiz-Mora[421] and McFarland.[419]

CONGENITAL CURLY TOES

This is the most common congenital deformity of the lesser toes. Usually mild, bilateral, and symmetrical, the abnormality consists of plantar flexion, varus deviation and supination of the lateral two, three or four toes. The terminal pulp may lie under the adjacent medial toe, resulting in abnormal pressure and callus formation under the adjacent medial metatarsal head.

The deformity, frequently familial, is present at birth and remains supple until

adolescence. In infancy Giannestras[428] recommends strapping the deformity between adjacent toes. However, Sweetnam[433] noted that 25 per cent of 50 affected feet improved whether treated or untreated and the remainder did not respond to nonoperative methods. At an average age of 13 years none of Sweetnam's[433] patients were symptomatic. Therefore, most patients require no treatment. When the curly toe impinges on its adjacent toe, symptoms are likely to ensue after maturity, especially in women who wear tight shoes. For these unusually advanced deformities surgical intervention is indicated.

Sharrard[431] recommends transfer of the flexor digitorum longus to the lateral aspect of the extensor hood, as described by Girdlestone and Taylor.[434] This procedure can be performed at any age after 1 year. In older children when the deformity is more rigid, Sharrard[431] recommends green-stick osteotomy of the middle phalanx of the toe as an adjunct to the tendon transfer.

Kelikian[429] recommended surgical syndactaly of the curly toe to a normal adjacent toe. In older adolescents and adults he recommends partial proximal phalangectomy and syndactaly. Trethowan[435] advocated excision of the proximal interphalangeal joint with division of the extensor tendon. DuVries[432] recommended wedge excision of the bone and joint at the apex of the curvature.

Giannestras described a simpler procedure for children between the ages 2 and 12 years. He attributed this procedure to Eric Price of Melbourne, Australia. It consists of simple tenotomy of both flexor tendons through a longitudinal plantar incision. Pollard and Morrison[430] recently reported results of flexor tenotomy of 56 toes in 20 children. All maintained full passive range of motion and had cosmetic improvement with no disability at follow-up. They compared these results to 63 Girdlestone-Taylor procedures.[434] After the latter procedure 58 per cent had a stiff metatarsophalangeal joint and less than satisfactory cosmetic improvement.

In the authors' experience surgical correction in childhood is only rarely indicated, but flexor tenotomy is preferred

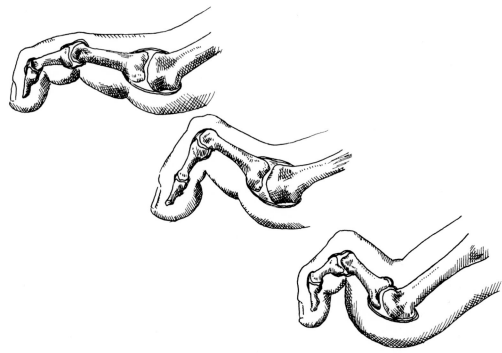

FIG. 21-41. *(Top left to bottom right)* A mallet toe with flexion deformity at the distal interphalangeal joint, a hammer toe with flexion contracture at the proximal interphalangeal joint, and a claw toe with flexion contractures of both interphalangeal joints and an extension contracture of the metatarsophalangeal joint. (Redrawn from Chuinard, E., and Baskin, M.: Clawfoot deformity. J. Bone Joint Surg., *55A*:356, 1973)

when the deformity is passively correctable. In adolescents with rigid deformity, resection arthrodesis of the PIP joint is performed.

CONGENITAL MALLET TOE

This congenital deformity consists of marked flexion at the distal interphalangeal joint, resulting from failure of development of the intrinsic extensor mechanism (Fig. 21-41). Only one or two toes are affected. The web space between the affected toes and normal adjacent toes is frequently shallow. Mallet toe is asymptomatic in childhood but develops a painful callus on the distal end of the toe in adolescence. An attempt should be made to differentiate this from the acquired mallet toe, which is rarely seen in childhood and results from ill-fitting shoes. Acquired deformity generally results in ham-

mer toe rather than mallet toe. Surgical correction, best performed after the age of 12 years, consists of resection arthrodesis of the distal interphalangeal joint.

ACQUIRED FOREFOOT DEFORMITIES

Acquired deformities of the forefoot are more common in adults than in children. The role in shoe wear in production or prevention of deformity is controversial. Only Sim-Fook and Hodgson have compared the feet of shod and unshod members of the same population. The relative incidence of various deformities reported by Sim-Fook and Hodgson are shown in Table 21-3. There is little doubt that restrictive, ill-fitting shoes can cause deformity and pain. However, many disorders have a familial tendency and suggest a genetic predisposition.

Table 21-3. Incidence of Foot Deformities in the Chinese Population[445]

Deformity	Incidence in shoe-wearing group (%)	Incidence in unshod group (%)
Hallux valgux	33	1.9
Hallux rigidus	17	10.3
Overlapping fifth toe	14.4	3.7
Hammer toe	11	4.7
Flat foot	10.1	7.5
Short first metatarsal	7.0	16.8
Metatarsus lactus	7.0	38
Metatarsus primus varus	6.0	24.3
Hypermobile metatarsus	0.9	13.1

ADOLESCENT HALLUX RIGIDUS

Hallux rigidus is characterized by painful limitation of dorsiflexion of the metatarsophalangeal joint of the great toe. This is common in adults secondary to arthritis (usually traumatic) of the metatarsophalangeal joint. In adolescents the problem is more complex.

Clinical Features

Adolescent hallux rigidus presents between the ages of 12 and 20 years. Women are predominantly affected (70 to 90 per cent of cases) and the condition may be bilateral or unilateral. Symptoms are of gradual onset and consists of pain at toe-off and on attempted toe walking. Early in the course of development, examination shows spasm in the short toe flexors with limited active and passive dorsiflexion. However, passive dorsiflexion has been noted to be normal under anesthesia. With progression, there is capsular swelling, contracture and finally development of rigidity and degenerative changes, narrowing and the presence of osteophytes at the metatarsophalangeal joint. The interphalangeal joint may be hypermobile. Shoe wear is excessive at the lateral heel and sole and under the distal phalanx of the great toe.

Etiologic Factors

The true etiology of hallux rigidus remains unknown. Bonney and MacNab noted that 50 per cent of adolescent patients with hallux rigidus had a positive family history but only 10 per cent of adults had a positive family history for hallux rigidus.

Usually the foot is long and slender with an elongated first metatarsal. Nilsonne[458] categorized 497 normal feet and found that the first metatarsal was longer than the second in 34.4 per cent, equal in length in 13.4 per cent, and shorter in 52.2 per cent. In adolescent hallux rigidus the first metatarsal was longer than the second metatarsal in 81.2 per cent of Nilsonne's patients. A similar occurrence has been noted by[460] Watson-Jones,[463] and others [442, 443, 455] feel that the disorder is exacerbated by abnormal shoe wear. The long first ray is difficult to fit without cramping and may contribute to repetitive trauma. When hallux rigidus is unilateral, it usually affects the larger foot and is frequently relieved by proper shoeing.

Another frequent finding is that the foot is pronated with an elevated first metatarsal.[442, 443, 450, 453] Jack observed that hallux rigidus often precedes pes planus, and that pronation worsens as symptoms develop. Bingold and Collins proposed that a hypermobile first metatarsal leads to an abnormal gait. As the first metatarsal elevates, increased weight is borne by the head of the second metatarsal. This leads to thickening of the second metatarsal, which can be appreciated roentgenographically. The foot also pronates and excessive weight is shifted from the first metatarsal head distally toward the metatarsophalangeal joint. Pronated flat feet and hallux rigidus are often seen together, but the exact etiologic relationship is still in question.

Treatment

Nonoperative treatment is frequently successful when initiated early in the development of hallux rigidus. Properly fitted shoes alone may suffice. There should be adequate length and breadth for the toes. A shoe with a rigid sole plate gives symptomatic relief. Giannestras,[446] on the advice of F. R. Thompson, recommends intermittent home traction using a Chinese finger-trap for suspension. When these methods fail or the process is advanced, operative intervention is indicated.

Resection of the base of the proximal phalanx (Keller procedure) or head of the first metatarsal (Mayo procedure) has been advocated.[443, 451, 454, 456, 460] Results have not been uniformly successful, and resection arthroplasty is to be avoided during growth.

First metatarsophalangeal arthrodesis has been increasingly recommended more frequently.[443, 447, 449, 457] This treatment, however, is unacceptable to most patients, particularly women who prefer variable heel heights.

Extension osteotomy of the base of the proximal phalanx[452] or head of the first metatarsal[455, 462] converts the full range of plantar flexion to a functional range of dorsiflexion and plantar flexion. These procedures provide physiologic correction, although long-term effects are not known. Prior to cessation of growth the procedure should be performed through the neck of the first metatarsal to avoid injury to the growth plate of the proximal phalanx.

Other operative procedures have been suggested but have not been widely employed.[444, 460, 463]

HAMMER TOE

Hammer toe deformity was originally described by Blum (1883)[464] to include dorsiflexion of the metatarsophalangeal joint and plantar flexion of the proximal interphalangeal joint (Fig. 21-41). This deformity may be congenital or acquired.

More often hammer toe deformity of the second toe is acquired and associated with hallux valgus. Hallux valgus and overlapping second toe should be corrected at the same time. If the metatarsophalangeal joint of the second toe is not subluxed or dislocated, resection arthrodesis of the proximal interphalangeal joint as described by Jones[472] should be performed. When the metatarsophalangeal joint is subluxed or dislocated, Giannestras[469] recommends proximal interphalangeal arthrodesis combined with resection of the base of the proximal phalanx. These more severe deformities may also be treated by resection of the base of the proximal phalanx and surgical syndactalization, as described by Kelikian.[474]

Hammering of the third and fourth toes is less common but is treated the same as deformity of the second toe.

Other procedures have been proposed for correction of hammer toe.[465, 476, 478, 488] Proximal phalangectomy has been advocated for severe deformity. This is, however, unnecessary and leaves a short useless toe. Cahil and Connor,[466] in a long-term follow-up of 74 patients with proximal phalangectomy reported that 50 per cent of the patients had objectively poor results and 25 per cent were dissatisfied.

CLAW TOES

In true clawing of the toes the metatarsophalangeal joints are extended and both interphalangeal joints are flexed. In contrast to hammer toe which may involve only one or two toes, claw toe deformity usually affects all the lesser toes and may involve the great toe. It is not seen before the age of 3 and is unusual before the age of 7 years. Claw toes are rarely symptomatic before the age of 10 years.

Clawing is usually associated with pes cavus and frequently is a manifestation of underlying neurologic disease. The theories regarding pathogenesis of clawing parallel those of pes cavus. DuVries[492] clearly demonstrated in cadavers that clawing results from simultaneous tension on long flexor *and* long extensor tendons.

In children, before the deformity becomes fixed, treatment should be directed toward the underlying disease. When varus or valgus are present tendon transfer should be performed to restore balance to the foot. Other soft-tissue procedures may be indicated to retard the development of pes cavus (see pes cavus and Chapter 8).

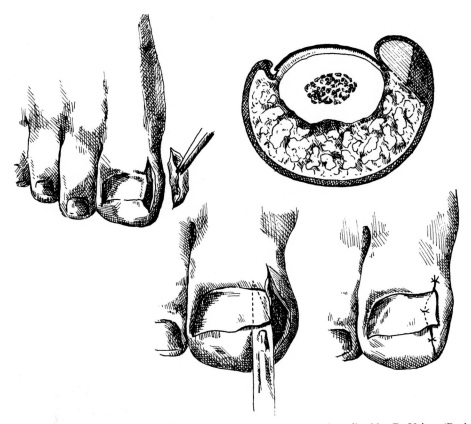

FIG. 21-42. Excision of hypertrophic nail lip and underlying fat, as described by DuVries. (Redrawn from DuVries, H.L.: Disorder of the skin and toenails. *In* Inman, V.T. (ed.): DuVries' Surgery of the Foot. ed. 3. pp. 212, 213. St. Louis, C. V. Mosby, 1973)

Several soft-tissue procedures have been described for supple claw toes. Forrester-Brown (1938)[493] described transfer of the flexor sublimus tendons into the extensor tendon for clawing of the great toe. Taylor[503] credited Girdlestone with the transfer of the flexor profundus tendon into the dorsal expansions of the extensor tendons. Taylor reported 50 good results in 68 patients. Pyper[500] however, reported only 50 per cent good results using the same procedure. Parrish[499] described a dynamic correction for claw toes. The long flexor tendon is released distally and split longitudinally. The split tendon is then passed along each side of the midportion of the proximal phalanx. The halves are sutured together over the dorsum of the phalanx to create a sling, which flexes the metatarsophalangeal joint. Parrish reported 40 good results in 46 procedures. The authors have not had experience with these procedures and prefer extensor tendon release or transfer to the metatarsal neck, combined with capsulotomy of deformed joints.

In general, soft-tissue procedures on the toes are not warranted in children who have supple deformity, and the procedures are ineffective in those with rigid deformity.

Rigid claw toes generally are seen in older children. After allied deformities are corrected, clawing should be relieved by resection arthrodesis of the proximal interphalangeal joint and transfer of the long extensor tendon to the metatarsal neck. Other procedures have also been described for fixed clawing.[491, 494, 495, 496, 498] The authors have had no experience with these other procedures and have had satisfactory results after PIP joint arthrodesis and extensor tendon transfer.

ABNORMALITIES OF SKIN AND NAILS

VERRUCA PLANTARIS (PLANTAR WARTS)

Plantar warts are common lesions seen in children and adolescents. This condition should be distinguished from plantar keratosis. Generally, verrucae do not occur directly under the metatarsal heads and are painful to lateral pinch, whereas plantar keratosis is painful to direct pressure but not to pinch. A typical verruca is also circumscribed with either an oval or circular outline.

Plantar warts are histologically similar to warts found on other parts of the body except that the pressure of weightbearing causes them to become flattened. The etiology is viral.

Several modes of treatment have been advocated including oral Vitamin A, injection, irradiation therapy, psychotherapy, cautory, curettage, cryotherapy and surgical excision. By whatever method, an attempt should be made to remove the lesion from the foot without scarring. Small lesions can be padded or ignored and occasionally resolve spontaneously. Larger, persistent or painful lesions should be treated.

Caustic or keratolytic agents are poorly tolerated by children and should not be used. The simplest method of treatment involves the application of liquid nitrogen. When applying the liquid nitrogen one must be certain to freeze the central core of the lesion.

If the lesion recurs, curettage should be performed. To do this the foot is prepared and draped in a surgical field. Local Xylocaine is used as an anthestic. The keratonized surface of the wart should be pared down with a #15 blade. The natural cleavage plane between the verruca and normal skin is then identified. A small, sharp curet is inserted into this plane and the verruca may be enucleated with gentle pressure. After the lesion has been removed, the edges are trimmed slightly and a sterile dressing is applied. This gentle removal heals rapidly and seldom results in recurrence or scarring.

INGROWN TOENAILS

Ingrown toenail is generally initiated by improper shoe pressure or improper nail cutting. Nail trimming should normally be done transversely to prevent the corners from growing into the pulp. Once penetration of an edge of the nail has begun, mechanical irritation causes hypertrophy of the nail fold, with subsequent infection and formation of granulation tissue. The great toe becomes progressively swollen, tender and reddened.

Initial treatment should be directed at preserving the nail. This consists of elevation, soaks and antibiotics. Gently inserting a few strands of cotton in the nail groove and underneath the tip of the nail may permit the nail to grow out beyond the tip of the nail groove.

When infection is advanced, removal of the nail should be performed for control of the infection. No attempt should be made to perform definitive surgery on an infected toe. After the infection has subsided, the nail should be allowed to grow back.

If ingrowing recurs or if the nail is stunted and irregular, additional surgical procedures may be necessary. The simplest method of surgery involves eliptical excision of the hypertrophied nail lip and underlying fat, as described by DuVries[518] (Fig. 21-42). The lateral margin of the nail is then elevated and the skin edge is sutured underneath the free nail margin (Fig. 21-42).

BIBLIOGRAPHY

Structure and Function

1. Acton, R. K.: Surgical anatomy of the foot. J. Bone Joint Surg., *49A:*555-567, 1967.
2. Basmajian, J. V., and Stecko, G.: The role of muscles in arch support of the foot; an electromyographic study. J. Bone Joint Surg., *45A:*1184-1190, 1963.
3. Ben-Menachem, Y., and Butler, J. E.: Arteriography of the foot in congenital deformities. J. Bone Joint Surg., *56A:* 1625–1630, 1974.
4. Cunningham, D. J.: Text-Book of Anatomy. London, Oxford University Press, 1953.
5. Forster, A.: Considerations sur l'attitudes des orteils chey l'homme. Arch. Anat. Histol. Embryol., *7:*247–261, 1927.

6. Frazer, J. E.: The Anatomy of the Human Skeleton. London, Churchill, 1920.
7. Gardner, E., Gray, D. L., and O'Rahally, R.: The prenatal development of the skeleton and joints of the human foot. J. Bone Joint Surg., *41A:*847–876, 1959.
8. Gray, H.: Anatomy of the Human Body, ed. 27. Edited by Charles Mayo Goss
9. Hicks, J. H.: The mechanics of the foot. J. Anat. *87:*345–357, 1953.
10. Hollinshead, W. H.: Anatomy for Surgeons, vol. 3. New York, Hoeber, 1958.
11. Jones, F. W.: Structure and Function as Seen in the Foot. London, Bailliere, Tindall and Cox, 1944.
12. Kelekian, H.: Hallux Valgus, Allied Deformities of the Foot and Metatarsalgia. Philadelphia, W. B. Saunders, 1965.
13. Kite, J. H.: Flat feet and lateral rotation of legs in young children. J. Int. Coll. Surg., *25:*77–84, 1956.
14. Kuhns, J. G.: Changes in elastic adipose tissue. J. Bone Joint Surg., *31A:*541–547, 1949.
15. Lovett, R. W., and Cotton, F. J.: Some practical points in the anatomy of the foot. Boston Med. Surg. J., *139:*101–107, 1898.
16. Mann, R., and Inman, V. T.: Phasic activity of intrinsic muscles of the foot. J. Bone Joint Surg., *46A:*469–481, 1964.
17. Manter, J. T.: Variations of the interosseous muscles of the human foot. Anat. Rec. *93:*117–124, 1945.
18. Smith, J. W.: The ligamentous structures in the canalis and sinus tarsi, J. Anat., *92:*616–620, 1958.
19. Spalteholz, W.: Hand Atlas of Human Anatomy, 7th English ed. Translated by L. F. Borkev, Philadelphia, J. B. Lippincott Company
20. White, J. W.: Torsion of the achilles tendon, its surgical significance. Arch. Surg., *46:*784–787, 1943.
21. Willis, T. A.: Orthopaedic anatomy of the foot and ankle. A.A.O.S. Instr. Course Lect., J. W. Edwards, 1947.

Congenital Talipes Equinovarus

22. Abrams, R. C.: Relapsed club foot. The early results of an evaluation of Dillwyn Evans operation. J. Bone Joint Surg., *51A:*270, 1969.
23. Adams, W.: Club Foot, Its Causes, Pathology and Treatment. London, Churchill, 1866.
24. Attenborough, C. G.: Severe congenital talipes equinovarus. J. Bone Joint Surg., *48B:*31-39, 1966.
25. Barrett, J. P., and Lovell, W. W.: Soft tissue release for congenital talipes equinovarus. In preparation.
26. Beatson, R. R., and Pearson, J. R.: A method of assessing correction in club feet. J. Bone Joint Surg., *48B:*40, 1966.
27. Bechtol, C. O., and Mossman, H. W.: Club foot. Embryological study and associated muscle abnormalities. J. Bone Joint Surg., *32A:*827, 1950.
28. Bell J. F., and Grice, D. S.: Treatment of congenital talipes equinovarus with modified Denis Browne splint. J. Bone Joint Surg., *26:*799, 1944.

29. Ben-Menachem, Y., and Butler, J. E.: Arteriography of the foot in congenital deformities. J. Bone Joint Surg., *56A:*1625, 1974.
30. Berman, A., and Gartland, J. J.: Metatarsal osteotomy for the correction of adduction of the forepart of the foot in children. J. Bone Joint Surg., *53A:*498, 1971.
31. Böhm, M.: The embryologic origin of club foot. J. Bone Joint Surg., *11:*229-250, April, 1929.
32. ——: Das menschliche bein. Deutsch. Orthop., *9.* Stuttgart, Enke, 1935.
33. Bost, F. C., Schottstaedt, E. R., and Larsen, L. J.: Plantar dissection. An operation to release the soft tissues in recurrent or recalcitrant talipes equinovarus. J. Bone Joint Surg., *42A:*151, 1960.
34. Brockman, E. P.: Congenital Clubfoot (Talipes Equinovarus). Bristol, Wright and Sons, Ltd. and New York, Wood and Co., 1930.
35. ——: Modern methods of treatment of club foot. Br. Med. J., *2:*512, 1937.
36. Dunn, N.: Stabilizing operations in the treatment of paralytic deformities of the foot. Proc. R. Soc. Med., *15:*15, 1922.
37. Dwyer, F. C.: Osteotomy of the calcaneus for pes cavus. J. Bone Joint Surg., *41B:*80, 1959.
38. ——: The treatment of relapsed clubfoot by the insertion of a wedge into the calcaneus. J. Bone Joint Surg., *45B:*67, 1963.
39. Evans, D.: Relapsed club foot. J. Bone Joint Surg., *43B:*722, 1961.
40. Flincheum, D.: Pathological anatomy in talipes equinovarus. J. Bone Joint Surg., *35A:*111-114, 1953.
41. Fried, A.: Recurrent congenital club foot. The role of the M. tibialis posterior in etiology and treatment. J. Bone Joint Surg., *41A:*243, 1959.
42. Garceau, G. J.: Anterior tibial transposition in recurrent congenital clubfoot. J. Bone Joint Surg., *22:*932, 1940.
43. Garceau, G. J., and Manning, K. R.: Transposition of the anterior tibial tendon in the treatment of recurrent congenital clubfoot. J. Bone Joint Surg., *29:*1004, 1947.
44. Garceau, G. J., and Palmer, R. M.: Transfer of the anterior tibial tendon for recurrent clubfoot. A long-term follow-up. J. Bone Joint Surg., *49A:*207, 1967.
45. Garland, J. J.: Posterior tibial transplant in the surgical treatment of recurrent club foot. A preliminary report. J. Bone Joint Surg., *46A:*1217, 1964.
46. Heyman, C. H., Herndon, C. H., and Strong, J. M.: Mobilization of the tarsometatarsal and intermetatarsal joints for the correction of resistant adduction of the forepart of the foot in congenital clubfoot or congenital metatarsus varus. J. Bone Joint Surg., *40A:*299, 1958.
47. Hirsch, C.: Observations on early operative treatment of congenital club foot. Bull. Hosp. Joint Dis., *21:*175, 1960.
48. Hoke, M.: An operation for stabilizing paralytic feet. Am. J. Orthop. Surg., *3:*494, 1921.
49. Irani, R. N., and Sherman, M. S.: The pathological anatomy of club foot. J. Bone Joint Surg., *45A:*45-52, 1963.
50. Kendrick, R. E., Sharma, N. K., Hassler, W. L.

and Herndon, C. H.: Tarsometatarsal mobilization for resistant adduction of the forepart of the foot. J. Bone Joint Surg., *52A:*61, 1970.

51. Kite, J. H.: Non-operative treatment of congenital club feet. South. Med. J., *23:*337, 1930.

52. ———: The surgical treatment of congenital club feet. Surg. Gynecol. Obstet., *61:*190, 1935.

53. ———: Principles involved in the treatment of club foot. J. Bone Joint Surg., *21:*595, 1939.

54. ———: Congenital metatarsus varus. Report of 300 cases. J. Bone Joint Surg., *32A:*500, 1950.

55. ———: Congenital metatarsus varus. A.A.O.S. Instruc. Course Lect. Ann Arbor, J. W. Edwards, 1950.

56. ———: Some suggestions on the treatment of clubfoot by casts. J. Bone Joint Surg., *45A:*406, 1963.

57. ———: Conservative treatment of the resistant recurrent clubfoot. Clin. Orthop., *34:*25, 1964.

58. ———: The Clubfoot. New York, Grune & Stratton, 1964.

59. ———: Congenital metatarsus varus. J. Bone Joint Surg., *49A:*388, 1967.

60. ———: Errors and complications in treating foot conditions in children. Clin. Orthop., *53:*31, 1967.

61. ———: Conservative treatment of the resistant recurrent clubfoot. Clin. Orthop., *70:*93, 1970.

62. Larsen, E. H.: Congenital clubfoot. J. Bone Joint Surg., *45B:*620, 1963.

63. Lipmann, K. A. W.: The Kite method in the treatment of clubfoot. J. Bone Joint Surg., *33B:*463, 1951.

64. Lloyd-Roberts, G. C.: Congenital club foot. J. Bone Joint Surg., *46B:*369, 1964.

65. Lovell, W. W., and Hancock, C. I.: Treatment of congenital talipes equinovarus. Clin. Orthop., *70:*79, 1970.

66. Lucas, L. S.: Surgical procedures in treatment of chronic clubfoot. West. J. Surg., *56:*542, 1948.

67. McCauley, J. C., Jr.: Surgical treatment of clubfoot. Surg. Clin. North Am., *31:*561, 1951.

68. ———: Treatment of clubfoot. A.A.O.S. Instruc. Course Lect., *16:*93, 1959.

69. ———: Triple arthrodesis for congenital talipes equinovarus deformities. Clin. Orthop., *34:*25, 1964.

70. ———: Clubfoot. History of the development and the concepts of pathogenesis and treatment. Clin. Orthop., *44:*51, 1966.

71. McCauley, J., Jr., Lusskin, K., and Bromley, J.: Recurrence in congenital metatarsus varus. J. Bone Joint Surg., *46A:*525, 1964.

72. McCormick, D. W., and Blount, W. P.: Metatarsus adductus. "Skewfoot." J.A.M.A., *141:*449, 1949.

73. Orofino, C. F.: The etiology of congenital clubfoot. Acta Orthop. Scand., *29:*59, 1959.

74. Peabody, C. W., and Muro, F.: Congenital metatarsus varus. J. Bone Joint Surg., *15:*171, 1933.

75. Polo, G. V., and Lechtman, C. P.: Surgical treatment of congenital talipes equinovarus adductus. Clin. Orthop., *70:*87, 1970.

76. Ponseti, I. V., and Becker, J. R.: Congenital metatarsus adductus, The results of treatment. J. Bone Joint Surg., *48A:*702, 1966.

77. Ponseti, I. V., and Smoley, E. M.: Congenital clubfoot: The results of treatment. J. Bone Joint Surg., *45A:*261-275, 1963.

78. Preston, E. T., and Fell, T. W. Jr.: Congenital idiopathic clubfeet. Clin. Orthop., *122:*102, 1977.

79. Price, C. T., and Lovell, W. W.: Non-operative treatment of congenital clubfoot. In preparation.

80. Settle, F. W.: The anatomy of congenital talipes equinovarus Sixteen dissected specimens. J. Bone Joint Surg., *45A:*1341-1354, 1963.

81. Simon, G. W.: Analytical radiography of club feet. J. Bone Joint Surg., *59B:*485, 1977.

82. Stewart, S. F.: Club foot: Its incidence, cause and treatment. An anatomical-physiological study. J. Bone Joint Surg., *33A:*577-590, 1951.

83. Turco, V. J.: Surgical correction of the resistant clubfoot. One-stage posteromedial release with internal fixation. A preliminary report. J. Bone Joint Surg., *53A:*477, 1971.

84. ———: Surgical correction of the resistant congenital clubfoot—One-stage release with internal fixation. The American Academy of Orthopaedic Surgeons Film Library.

85. Westin, G. W.: Personal communication,

86. Wiley, A. M.: Club foot. An anatomical and experimental study of muscle growth. J. Bone Joint Surg., *46B:*464, 1964.

87. Wynne-Davies, R.: Family studies and the course of congenital club foot. J. Bone Joint Surg., *46B:*445-463, 1964.

88. ———: Talipes equinovarus. J. Bone Joint Surg., *46B:*464-476, 1964.

89. ———: Heritable Disorders in Orthopaedic Practice. London, Blackwell, 1973.

Congenital Metatarsus Varus

90. Berman, A., and Gartland, J. J.: Metatarsal osteotomy for the correction of adduction of the forepart of the foot in children. J. Bone Joint Surg., *53A:*498, 1971.

91. Colonna, P. C.: Care of the infant with congenital subluxation of the hip. J.A.M.A., *166:*715, 1958.

92. Heyman, C. H., Herndon, C. H., and Strong, J. M.: Mobilization of the tarsometatarsal and intermetatarsal joints for the correction of resistant adduction of the forepart of the foot in congenital clubfoot or congenital metatarsus varus. J. Bone Joint Surg., *40A:*299, 1958.

93. Jacobs, J. E.: Metatarsus varus and hip dysplasia. Clin. Orthop., *16:*19, 203, 1960.

94. Kendrick, R. E., Shorman, N. K., Hassler, W. L., and Herndon, C. H.: Tarsometatarsal mobilization for resistant adduction of the forepart of the foot. J. Bone Joint Surg., *52A:*61, 1970.

95. Kite, J. H.: Congenital metatarsus varus. A.A.O.S. Instruc. Course Lect. Ann Arbor. J. W. Edwards, 1950.

96. ———: Congenital metatarsus varus: Report of 300 cases. J. Bone Joint Surg., *32A:*500, 1950.

97. ———:Congenital metatarsus varus. J. Bone Joint Surg., *49A:*388, 1967.

98. McCauley, J., Jr., Lusskin, R., and Bromley, J.: Recurrence in congenital metatarsus varus. J. Bone Joint Surg., *46A:*525, 1964.

99. McCormick, D. W., and Blount, W. P.: Metatar-

sus adductovarus. "Skewfoot." J.A.M.A. *141:* 449, 1949.

100. Mitchell, G.: Personal communication,

101. Peabody, C. W., and Muro, F.: Congenital metatarsus varus. J. Bone Joint Surg., *15:*171, 1933.

102. Ponseti, I. V., and Becker, J. R.: Congenital metatarsus adductus: The results of treatment. J. Bone Joint Surg., *48A:*702, 1966.

103. Thompson, S. A.: Hallux varus and metatarsus varus—a five-year study. Clin. Orthop., *16:*109, 1960.

104. Wynne-Davies, R.: Family studies and the cause of congenital clubfoot—talipes equinovarus, talipes calcaneovalgus and metatarsus varus. J. Bone Joint Surg., *46B:*445, 1954.

Congenital Short Tendo Calcaneus

105. Buie, W. B. B.: Acute toe walking syndrome. Med. J. Aust., *2:*752, 1975.

106. Griffin, P. P., Wheelhouse, W. W., Shiavi, R., Bass, W.: Habitual toe walkers; a clinical and electromyographic gait analysis. J. Bone Joint Surg., *59A:*97-101, 1977.

107. Hall, J. E., and Salter, R. B., and Bhalla, S. K.: Congenital Short Tendo Calcaneus.

108. Sharrand, W. J. W.: Pediatric Orthopedics and Fractures. Oxford, Blackwell, 1971.

109. Tachdjian, M. O.: Pediatric Orthopedics. Philadelphia, W. B. Saunders, 1972.

Congenital Vertical Talus

110. Coleman, S. S., Martin, A. F., and Jarrett, J.: Congenital vertical talus: Pathogenesis and treatment. J. Bone Joint Surg., *48A:*1442, 1966.

111. Coleman, S. S., Stelling, F. H., III, and Jarrett, J.: Congenital vertical talus: Pathomechanics and treatment. Clin. Orthop., *70:*62, 1970.

112. Drennan, J. C., and Sharrard, W. J. W.: The pathologic anatomy of convex pes valgus. J. Bone Joint Surg., *53B:*455, 1971.

113. Eyre-Brook, A.: Congenital vertical talus. J. Bone Joint Surg., *49B:*618, 1967.

114. Grice, D. S.: The role of subtalar fusion in the treatment of valgus deformities of the feet. Ann Arbor, J. W. Edwards Publishers, Inc., *16:*127, 1950.

115. ———: Extra-articular arthrodesis of the subastragalar joints for correction of paralytic flatfeet in children. J. Bone Joint Surg., *34A:*927, 1952.

116. Hark, F. W.: Rocker-foot due to congenital subluxation of the talus. J. Bone Joint Surg., *34A:*344, 1950.

117. Harrold, A. J.: Congenital vertical talus in infancy. J. Bone Joint Surg., *49B:*634, 1967.

118. Henken, R.: Contribution à l'étude des formes osseuses du pied plat valgus congénital. Paris, Thèse de Lyon, 1914.

119. Herndon, C. H., and Heyman, C. H.: Problems in the recognition and treatment of congenital convex pes planus. J. Bone Joint Surg., *45A:*413, 1963.

120. Heyman, C. H.: The diagnosis and treatment of congenital convex pes valgus or vertical talus. St. Louis, C. V. Mosby Company, *16:*117, 1959.

121. Hughes, J. R.: Symposium on congenital vertical talus. J. Bone Joint Surg., *39B:*580, 1957.

122. ———: Pathologic anatomy and pathogenesis of congenital vertical talus and its practical significance. J. Bone Joint Surg., *52B:*777, 1970.

123. Lamy, L., and Weismann, L.: Congenital convex pes valgus. J. Bone Joint Surg., *21:*79, 1939.

124. Lloyd-Roberts, G. C., and Spence, A. J.: Congenital vertical talus. J. Bone Joint Surg., *40B:*33, 1958.

125. Mead, N. C., and Anast, G.: Vertital talus, congenital talonavicular dislocation. Clin. Orthop., *21:*198, 1961.

126. Osmond-Clark, H.: Congenital vertical talus. J. Bone Joint Surg., *38B:*334, 1956.

127. Outland, T., and Sherk, H. H.: Congenital vertical talus. Clin. Orthop., *16:*214, 1960.

128. Parrish, T. F.: Congenital convex pes valgus accompanied by previously undescribed anatomic derangements. South. Med. J., *60:*983, 1967.

129. Patterson, W. R., Fitz, D. A., and Smith, W. S.: The pathologic anatomy of congenital convex pes valgus. J. Bone Joint Surg., *50B:*456, 1968.

130. Silk, F. F., and Wainwright, D.: The recognition and treatment of congenital flat foot in infancy. J. Bone Joint Surg., *49B:*628, 1967.

131. Storen, H.: On the closed and open correction of congenital convex pes valgus with a vertical astragalus. Acta Orthop. Scand., *36:* 352, 1965.

132. ———: Congenital convex pes valgus with vertical talus. Acta Orthop. Scand., Suppl. 94, 1967.

133. Tachdjian, M. O.: Congenital convex pes valgus. Orthop. Clin. North Am., *3:*131, 1972.

The Calcaneovalgus Foot

134. Kite, J. H.: The treatment of flatfeet in small children. Postgrad. Med., *15:*75–78, 1954.

135. ———: Flatfeet and lateral rotation of legs in young children, J. International Coll. Surg., *25:*77–84, 1956.

136. Wetzenstein, H.: The significance of congenital pes calcaneovalgus in the origin of pes planovalgus in childhood. Acta Orthop. Scand., *30:*64–72, 1960.

137. Wynne-Davies, R.: Family studies and the cause of congenital clubfoot, talipes equinovarus, talipes calcaneovalgus and metatarsus adductus. J. Bone Joint Surg., *46B:*445–463, 1964.

Flexible Flatfoot

138. Baker, L. D., and Hill, L. M.: Foot alignment in the cerebral palsy patient. J. Bone Joint Surg., *46A:*1–15, 1964.

139. Basmajian, J. V., and Bentzon, J. W.: An electromyographic study of certain muscles of the leg and foot in the standing position. Surg. Gynecol. and Obstet., *98:*662–666, 1954.

140. Basmajian, J. V., and Stecko, G.: The role of muscles in arch support of the foot. J. Bone Joint Surg., *45A:*1184–1190, 1963.

141. Brown, A.: A simple method of fusion of the subtalar joint in children. J. Bone Joint Surg., *50B:*369–371, 1968.

142. Butte, F. L.: Naviculo-cuneiform arthrodesis for flatfoot. J. Bone Joint Surg., *19:*496–502, 1937.

143. Caldwell, G. D.: Surgical correction of relaxed flatfoot by the Durham flatfoot plasty. Clin. Orthop., *2:*221–226, 1953.

144. Chambers, E. F. S.: An operation for the correction of flexible flatfeet of adolescents. West. J. Surg., *54:*77–86, 1946.

145. Chandler, F. A.: Children's feet, normal and presenting common abnormalities. Am. J. Dis. Child., *63:*1136–1146, 1942.

146. Crego, C. H., and Ford, L. T.: An end-result study of various operative procedures for corrective flatfeet in children. J. Bone Joint Surg., *34A:*183–195, 1952.

147. Davy, R.: On excision of the scaphoid bone for the relief of confirmed flatfoot. Lancet, *1:*675–677, 1889.

148. Dennyson, W. G., and Fulford, G. E.: Subtalar arthrodesis by cancellous grafts and metallic internal fixation. J. Bone Joint Surg., *58B:*507–510, 1976.

149. Evans, D.: Calcaneo-valgus deformity. J. Bone Joint Surg., *57B:*270–278, 1975.

150. Golding-Bird, C. H.: Operations on the tarsus in confirmed flatfoot. Lancet, *1:*677–678, 1889.

151. Grice, D. S.: An extra-articular arthrodesis of the subastragalar joint for correction of paralytic flatfeet in children. J. Bone Joint Surg., *34A:*927–940, 1952.

152. Haraldsson, S.: Pes plano-valgus staticus juvenilis and its operative treatment. Acta Orthop. Scand., *35:*234–256, 2964/65.

153. Harris, R. I. and Beath, T.: Hypermobile flatfoot with short tendo Achilles. J. Bone Joint Surg., *30A:*116–140, 1948.

154. Helfet, A.: A new way of treating flatfeet in children. Lancet, *1:*262–264, 1956.

155. Hicks, J. H.: The function of the plantar aponeurosis. J. Anat., *85:*414–415, 1951.

156. ———: The mechanics of the foot. II. The plantar aponeurosis and the arch. J. Anat., *88:*25–30, 1954.

157. Hoke, M.: An operation for the correction of extremely relaxed flatfeet. J. Bone Joint Surg., *13:*773–783, 1931.

158. Inman, V. T.: The human foot. Manitoba Med. Rev., *46:*513–515, 1966.

159. Jack, E. A.: Naviculo-cuneiform fusion in the treatment of flatfoot. J. Bone Joint Surg., *35B:*75–82, 1953.

160. Johnston, T. B.; Davies, D. V. and Davies, F.: Gray's Anatomy, ed. 32, pp 544-545 and 672-688. Toronto, Longmans Green, 1958.

161. Jones, B. S.: Flatfoot. J. Bone Joint Surg., *57B:*279-282, 1975.

162. Keith, A.: The history of the human foot and its bearing on orthopaedic practice. J. Bone Joint Surg., *11:*10-32, 1929.

163. Kidner, F. C.: The prehallux (accessory scaphoid) and its relation to flatfoot. J. Bone Joint Surg., *11:*831-837, 1929.

164. ———: The prehallux in relation to flatfoot, J.A.M.A., *101:*1539-1542, 1933.

165. Koutsogiannis, E.: Treatment of mobile flatfoot by displacement osteotomy of the calcaneous. J. Bone Joint Surg., *53B:*96-100, 1971.

166. Leavitt, D. G.: Subastragaloid arthrodesis for the os calcis type of flatfoot. Am. J. Surg., *59:*501-508, 1943.

167. Legg, A. T.: Treatment of rigid flatfoot. Excision of scaphoid. Boston Med. Surg. J., *156*(23):741-743, 1907.

168. ———: The treatment of congenital flatfoot by tendon transplantation. Am. J. Orthop. Surg., *10:*584-586, 1912-13.

169. LeLièvre, J.: Current concepts and correction in the valgus foot. Clin. Orthop., *70:*43-55, 1970.

170. Leonard, M. H., *et al.:* Lateral transfer of the posterior tibial tendon in certain selected cases of pes planus (Kidner operation). Clin. Orthop., *40:*139-144, 1965.

171. Lord, J. P.: Correction of extreme flatfoot. J.A.M.A., 81:1502-1506, 1923.

172. Lowman, C. L.: An operative method for correction of certain forms of flatfoot. J.A.M.A., *81:*1500-1502, 1923.

173. Milch, H.: Reinforcement of the deltoid ligament for pronated flatfoot. Surg. Gynecol. Obstet. *74:*876-881, 1942.

174. Miller, O. L.: A plastic flatfoot operation. J. Bone Joint Surg., *9:*84-91, 1927.

175. Ogston, A.: On flatfoot and its cure by operation. Br. Med. J., *9:*110-111, 1884.

176. Painter, C. F.: Peroneal resection as a means of correction in rigid valgus. Boston Med. Surg. J., *153:*164-166, 1905.

177. Rose, G. K.: Correction of the pronated foot. J. Bone Joint Surg., *40B:*674-683, 1958.

178. ———: Correction of the pronated foot. J. Bone Joint Surg., *44B:*642-647, 1962.

179. Rugtveit, A.: Extra-articular subtalar arthrodesis, according to Green-Grice in flatfeet. Acta Orthop. Scand., *34:*367-373, 1964.

180. Ryerson, Ed. W.: Tendon transplantation in flatfoot. Am. J. Orthop. Sug., *7:*505-507, 1909-10.

181. Schoolfield, B. I.: An operation for the cure of flatfoot. Ann. Surg., *110:*437-446, 1936.

182. ———: Operative treatment of flatfoot. Surg. Gynecol. Obstet., *94:*136-140, 1952.

183. Seymour, N.: The late results of naviculocuneiform fusion. *49B:*558-559, 1967.

184. Seymour, N., and Evans, D. K.: A modification of the Grice subtalar arthrodesis. J. Bone Joint Surg., *50B:*372-375, 1968.

185. Shephard, E.: Tarsal movements. J. Bone Joint Surg., *33B:*258-263, 1951.

186. Silver, C. M., Simon, S. D., Spindell, E., Litchman, H. M., and Scala, M.: Calcaneal osteotomy for valgus and varus deformities of the foot in cerebral palsy. J. Bone Joint Surg., *49A:*232-246, 1967.

187. Smith, J. B., and Westin, G. W.: Follow-up notes on articles previously published, subtalar extra-articular arthrodesis. J. Bone Joint Surg., *50A:*1027-1035, 1968.

188. Smith, J. W.: Muscular control of the arches of the foot in standing, an electromyographic assessment. J. Anat., *88:*152-163, 1954.

189. Soule, R. I.: Value of bone pin arthrodesis in the treatment of flatfoot. J.A.M.A., *77:*1871-1874, 1921.

190. Wetzenstein, H.: The significance of congenital pes calcaneo-valgus in the origin of pes plano-

valgus in childhood. Acta Orthop. Scand., *30:*64-72, 1960.

191. Wynne-Davies, R.: Family studies and the cause of congenital clubfoot, talipes equinovarus, talipes calcaneo-valgus and metatarsus adductus. J. Bone Joint Surg., *46B:*445-463, 1964.

192. Young, C. S.: Operative treatment of pes planus. Surg. Gynecol. Obstet., *68:*1099-1101, 1939.

193. Zadek, I.: Transverse-wedge arthrodesis for the relief of pain in rigid flatfoot. J. Bone Joint Surg., *17:*453-467, 1935.

Tarsal Coalition

194. Badgley, C. E.: Coalition of the calcaneus and the navicular. Arch. Surg., *15:*75, 1927.

195. Bersante, F. A., and Samilson, R. L.: Massive familial tarsae synostosis. J. Bone Joint Surg., *39A:*1187, 1957.

196. Blockley, N. J.: Peroneal spastic flat foot. J. Bone Joint Surg., *37B:*191, 1955.

197. Buffon, G.-L.: Histore naturelle avee las description du cabinet du roy. Tome, *3:*47, 1750.

198. Chambers, C. H.: Congenital anomalies of the tarsae navicular with particular reference to calcaneo-navicular coalition. Br. J. Radiol., *23:*580, 1950.

199. Clark, N. T., and Lovell, W. W.: Tarsal coalition. In preparation.

200. Conway, H. R., and Cowell, H. R.: Tarsal coalition: clinical significance and roentgenographic demonstration. Radiology, *92:*799, 1969.

201. Cowell, H. R.: Talocalcaneal coalition and new causes of peroneal spastic flatfoot. Clin. Orthop., *85:*16, 1972.

202. Del Sel, J. M., and Grand, N. E.: Cubo-navicular synostosis. A rare tarsal anomaly. J. Bone Joint Surg., *18:*479, 1936.

203. ———: Cubo-navicular synostosis. A rare tarsal anomaly. J. Bone Joint Surg., *41B:*149, 1959.

204. Glessner, J. R., Jr., and Davis, G. L.: Bilateral calcaneonavicular coalition occurring in twin boys. A case report. Clin. Orthop., *47:*173, 1966.

205. Gregersen, H. N.: Naviculocuneiform coalition. J. Bone Joint Surg., *59A:*128, 1977.

206. Hark, F. W.: Congenital anomalies of the tarsal bones. Clin. Orthop., *16:*425, 1960.

207. Harris, R. I.: Rigid valgus due to talocalcaneal bridge. J. Bone Joint Surg., *37A:*169, 1955.

208. ———: Peroneal spastic flatfoot. A.A.O.S. Instruc. Course Lect., *15:*116, 1958.

209. ———: Retrospect: Peroneal spastic flatfoot (rigid valgus foot). J. Bone Joint Surg., *47A:*1657, 1965.

210. Harris, R. I., and Beath, T.: Etiology of peroneal spastic flatfoot. J. Bone Joint Surg., *30B:*624, 1948.

211. Heikel, H. V. A.: Coalito calcaneo-navicularis and calcaneus secondarius. A clinical and radiographic study of twenty-three patients. Acta Orthop. Scand., *32:*72, 1962.

212. Jack, E. A.: Bone abnormalities of the tarsus in relation to peroneal spastic flat foot. J. Bone Joint Surg., *36B:*530, 1954.

213. Jones, R.: Peroneal spasm and its treatment. Report of meeting of Liverpool Medical Institution held 22nd April, 1897. Liverpool Med. Chir. J., *17:*442, 1897.

214. ———: The soldier's foot and the treatment of common deformities of the foot. Br. Med. J., *1:*709, 1916.

215. Lamb, D.: The ball and socket ankle joint—a congenital abnormality. J. Bone Joint Surg., *40B:*240, 1958.

216. Lapidus, P. W.: Bilateral congenital talonavicular fusion. Report of a case. J. Bone Joint Surg., *20:*775, 1938.

217. ———: Spastic flat foot. J. Bone Joint Surg., *28:*126, 1946.

218. Lusby, H. L. J.: Navicular-cuneiform synostosis. J. Bone Joint Surg., *41B:*150, 1959.

219. Mahaffey, H. W.: Bilateral congenital calcaneocuboid synostosis. J. Bone Joint Surg., *27:*164, 1945.

220. Mitchell, G.: Spasmodic flatfoot. Clin. Orthop., *70:*73, 1970.

221. Mitchell, G. P., and Gibson, J. M. C.: Excision of calcaneo-navicular bar for painful spasmodic flat foot. J. Bone Joint Surg., *49B:*281, 1967.

222. Outland, T., and Murphy, I. D.: Rotation of tarsal anomalies to spastic and rigid flat feet. Clin. Orthop., *1:*217, 1953.

223. ———: The patho-mechanics of peroneal spastic flat foot. Clin. Orthop., *16:*64, 1960.

224. Simmons, E. H.: Tibialis spastic varus foot with tarsal coalition. J. Bone Joint Surg., *47B:*533, 1965.

225. Slomann, H. C.: On coalition calcaneonavicularis. J. Orthop. Surg., *3:*586, 1921.

226. ———: On coalition calcaneonavicular coalition by roentgen examination. Acta Radiol., *5:*304, 1926.

227. ———: On the demonstration and analysis of calcaneonavicular coalition by roentgen examination. Acta Radiol., *5:*304, 1926.

228. Venerusa, L. C.: Unilateral congenital calcaneocuboid synostosis with complete absence of a metatarsal and toe. A case report. J. Bone Joint Surg., *27:*718, 1945.

229. Wagoner, G. W.: A case of bilateral congenital fusion of the calcanei and cuboids. J. Bone Joint Surg., *10:*220, 1928.

230. Waugh, W.: Partial cubo-navicular coalition as a cause of peroneal spastic flat foot. J. Bone Joint Surg., *39B:*520, 1957.

231. Webster, F. S., and Roberts, W. M.: Tarsal anomalies and peroneal spastic flatfoot. J.A.M.A., *146:*1099, 1951.

232. Wray, J. B., and Herndon, C. N.: Hereditary transmission of congenital coalition of the calcaneus to the navicular. J. Bone Joint Surg., *45A:*365, 1963.

Accessory Navicular

233. Kidner, F.: The pre-hallux (accessory scaphoid) in its relation to flat-foot. J. Bone Joint Surg., *11:*831–837, 1929.

234. Zadek, I., and Gold, A.: The accessory tarsal scaphoid. J. Bone Joint Surg., *30A:*957–968, 1948.

Pes Cavus

235. Adelaar, R. S., Donnelly, E. A., Meunier, P. A., Stelling, F. H., *et al.*: A long term study of triple arthrodesis in children. Orthop. Clin. North Am., 7:895–908, 1976.
236. Alvik, I.: Operative treatment of pes cavus. Acta Orthop. Scand., 23:137–141, 1954.
237. Andrey, N.: Orthopaedia. London, A. Millar, 1743.
238. Bentzon, P. G. K.: Pes cavus and the M. peroneus longus. Acta Orthop. Scand., 4:50-53, 1933.
239. Brewerton, D. A., Sandifer, P. H., and Sweetnam, D. R.: "Idiopathic" pes cavus. Br. Med. J., 62:659–661, 1963.
240. Brewster, A. H., and Larson, C. B.: Cavus feet. J. Bone Joint Surg., 22:361-368, 1940.
241. Brockway, A.: Surgical correction of talipes cavus deformities. J. Bone Joint Surg., 22:81–91, 1940.
242. Chuinard, E. G., and Baskin, M.: Claw foot deformity. J. Bone Joint Surg., 55A:351–362, 1973.
243. Clawson, D. K.: Claw toes following tibial fracture. C.O.R.R., 103:47-48, 1974.
244. Cole, W. H.: The treatment of claw foot. J. Bone Joint Surg., 22:895–908, 1940.
245. Coleman, S. S., and Chestnut, W. J.: A simple test for hindfoot flexibility in the cavovarus foot. C.O.R.R., 123:60–63, 1977.
246. Coonrad, R. W., Irwin, C. E., Gucker, T., and Wray, J. B.: The importance of plantar muscles in paralytic varus feet. J. Bone Joint Surg., 38A:563–566, 1956.
247. Cralley, J., Fitch, K., and McGonagle, W.: Lumbrical muscles and contracted toes. Anat. Ang., 138:348–353, 1975.
248. Davis, G. G.: The treatment of hollow foot (pes cavus). Am. J. Orthop. Surg., 11:231, 1913.
249. Dickson, F. D., and Diveley, R. L.: Operation for correction of mild claw foot. J.A.M.A., 87:1275-1277, 1926.
250. Dekel, S., Weissman, S. L. (Tel-Aviv): Osteotomy of the calcaneus and concomitant plantar stripping with talipes cavo-varus. J. Bone Joint Surg., 55B:802–808, 1973.
251. Duchenne, G. B.: Physiologie des Mouvements. Paris, Baillaire, 1867.
252. Dunn, N.: Calcaneo-cavus and its treatment. J. Orthop. Surg., 1:711, 1919.
253. DuVries, H. L.: Surgery of the Foot, ed. 3. St. Louis, C. V. Mosby, 1973.
254. Dwyer, F. C.: Osteotomy of the calcaneum for pes cavus. J. Bone Joint Surg., 41B:80-86, 1959.
255. ———: The present status of the problem of pes cavus. C.O.R.R. 106:254–275, 1975.
256. Fisher, R. L., and Shaffer, S. R.: An evaluation of calcaneal osteotomy in congenital clubfoot and other disorders. C.O.R.R., 70:141–147, 1970.
257. Forbes, A. M.: Claw foot and how to relieve it. Surg. Gynecol. Obstet., 26:81, 1913.
258. Fowler, S. B., Brooks, A. L., and Parrish, T. F.: The cavo-varus foot. J. Bone Joint Surg., 41A:757., 1959.
259. Frank, G. R., and Johnson, W. M.: The extensor shift procedure in the correction of clawtoe deformities in children. South. Med. J. 59:889–896, 1966.
260. Garceau, G. J.: Pes cavus. A.A.O.S. Instruc. Course Lect., 18:184–186, 1961.
261. Garceau, G. J., and Brahms, M. A.: A preliminary study of selective plantar muscle deviation for pes cavus. J. Bone Joint Surg., 38A:553–562, 1956.
262. Giannestras, N. J.: Foot Disorders: Medical and Surgical Management, Ed. 2, pp. 178–181, 506–514, Philadelphia, Lea & Febiger, 1976.
263. Gilroy, E.: Pes cavus, clinical study with special reference to its etiology. Edinb. Med. J., 36:749, 1929.
264. Girdlestone, G. R.: The Journal of the Chartered Society of Physiotherapy, 32:167, 1947.
265. Golding, Bird, C. H.: Pes valgus, acquisitius, pes pronatus acquisitus, pes cavus. Guy's Hosp. Rep., 41:439-473, 1883.
266. Heron, J. R.: Neurological syndromes associated with pes cavus. Proc. R. Soc. Med., 62:270–271, 1969
267. Heyman, C. H.: Operative treatment of claw foot. J. Bone Joint Surg., 14:335-337, 1932.
268. Hibbs, R. A.: An operation for "claw foot" J.A.M.A., 73:1583–1585, 1919.
269. Hill, N. A., Wilson, H. J., Chevres, F., and Sweterlitch, P. R.: Triple arthrodesis in the young child. C.O.R.R., 70:187–190, 1970.
270. Howard, R. J.: Operative treatment of early cavus feet. South. Med. J., 64:558, 1971.
271. Irwin, C. E.: The calcaneus foot. Ann Arbor, J. W. Edwards Publishers, Inc., 15:135–143, 1958.
272. James, C. C., and Lassman, L. P.: The diagnosis and treatment of progressive lesions in spina bifida occulta. J. Bone Joint Surg., 44B:828, 1962.
273. Japas, C. C.: Surgical treatment of pes cavus by tarsal V-osteotomy. J. Bone Joint Surg., 50A:927, 1968.
274. Jones, A. R.: Discussion on the treatment of pes cavus. Proc. R. Soc. Med., 20:41, 1926.
275. Jones, R.: Notes on Military Orthopedics. New York, Hoeber, 1917.
276. Karlholm, S., and Nilsonne, U.: Operative treatment of the foot deformity in Charcot-Marie-Tooth disease. Acta Orthop. Scand., 39:101–106, 1968.
277. Kelikian, H.: Hallus Valgus, Allied Deformities of the Forefoot and Metatarsalgia, p. 305–326. Philadelphia, W. B. Saunders, 1965.
278. Kirk, Ar. A., Kunkle, H. M., and Waine, H. J.: Ledge tenodesis of the extensor hallucis longus. J. Bone Joint Surg., 53A:774–776, 1971.
279. Lambrinudi, C.: An operation for claw toes. Proc. R. Soc. Med., 21:239, 1927.
280. Levick, G. M.: The action of the intrinsic muscles of the foot and their treatment by electricity. Br. Med. J. 1:381–382, 1921.
281. Levitt, R. L., Canale, S. T., Cook, A. J., and Gartland, J. J.: The role of foot surgery in progressive neuromuscular disorders in children. J. Bone Joint Surg., 55A:1396–1410, 973.
282. Little, N. J.: Claw foot. Med. J. Aust., 2:495, 1938.
283. Makin, M.: The surgical management of Fried-

reich's ataxia. J. Bone Joint Surg., *35A:*425–436, 1953.

284. Mann, R., and Inman, V. T.: Phasic activity of intrinsic muscles of the foot. J. Bone Joint Surg., *46A:*469–481, 1964.

285. M'Banali, E. I.: Results of modified Robert Jones operation for clawed hallux. Br. J. Surg., *62:*647–650, 1975.

286. McElvenny, R. T., and Caldwell, G. D.: A new operation for correction of cavus foot. Clin. Orthop., *11:*85–92, 1958.

287. Meary, R.: "Le Pied Creux Essential" Symposium. Rev. Chir. Orthop., *53:*389–467, 1967.

288. Mills, P.: Etiology and treatment of claw foot. J. Bone Joint Surg., *6:*142, 1924.

289. Ollerenshaw, R.: Claw foot. Proc. R. Soc. Med., *20:*1126, 1927.

290. Parrish, T. F.: Dynamic correction of clawtoes. Orthop. Clin. North Am., *4:*97–102, 1973.

291. Patterson, R. L., Parrish, F. F., and Hathaway, E. N.: Stabilizing operations on the foot. J. Bone Joint Surg., *32A* 1–26, 1950.

292. Royle, N. D.: A new conception in the etiology of claw foot and associated talipes equinus. J. Bone Joint Surg., *6:*664, 1924.

293. Rugh, J. T.: An operation for the correction of plantar and adduction contracture of the foot arch. J. Bone Joint Surg., *6:*664, 1924.

294. ———: The etiology of cavus and a new operation for its correction. Bull N. Y. Acad. Med., *3:*423–434, 1927.

295. Ryerson, E.: Arthrodesing operations on feet. J. Bone Joint Surg., *5:*458-471, 1923.

296. Samilson, R. L.: Crescentic osteotomy of the calcaneus for calcaneocavus feet. *In* Bateman, J. E. (ed.): Foot Science. Philadelphia, W. B. Saunders, 1976.

297. Samilson, R. L., Specht, E. E., DuVries, H. L. *In* Inman, V. T. (ed): Surgery of the foot, ed. 3., p. 271. St. Louis, C. V. Mosby, 1973.

298. Saunders, J. T.: Etiology and treatment of claw foot. Arch Surg., *30:*179–198, 1935.

299. Scheer, G. E., and Crego, C. H.: A two-state stabilization procedure for correction of calcaneocavus J. Bone Joint Surg., *38A:*1247–1253, 1956.

300. Sharrard, W. J. S., and Smith, T. W. D.: Tenodesis of the flexor hallucis longus for paralytic clawing of the hallux in childhood. J. Bone Joint Surg., *58A:*224–226, 1976.

301. Sherman, H. M.: The operative treatment of pes cavus. Am. J. Orthop. Surg., *2:*374–380, 1905.

302. Siffert, R. S., Forster, R. I., and Nachamie, B.: Beak triple arthrodesis for correction of severe cavus deformity. C.O.R.R., *45:*101–106, 1966.

303. Spitzy, H.: Operative correction of claw foot. Surg. Gynecol. Obstet., *45:*813–815, 1927.

304. Stauffer, R. N., Nelson, G. E., and Bianco, A. J.: Calcaneal osteotomy in treatment of cavovarus foot. Mayo Clin. Proc., *45:*624—*635, 1970.*

305. Steindler, A.: Operative treatment of pes cavus. Surg. Gynecol. Obstet., *24:*612-615, 1917.

306. Tachdjian, M. O., Pediatric Orthopaedics, pp. 1378–1397. Philadelphia, W. B. Saunders, 1972.

307. Wilson, F. C., Fay, G. F., Lamotte, P. and Wil-liams, J. C.: Triple arthrodesis. A study of factors affecting fusion after three hundred and one procedures. J. Bone Joint Surg., *47A:*340–348, 1965.

Freiberg's Infraction

308. Braddock, G. T. F.: Experimental epiphyseal injury and Freiberg's disease. J. Bone Joint Surg., *41:*154, 1959.

309. Freiberg, A. H.: Infraction of the second metatarsal bone: a typical injury. Surg. Gynecol. Obstet., *19:*191, 1914.

310. Freiberg, A. H.: The so-called infraction of the second metatarsal bone. J. Bone Joint Surg., *8:*257, 1926.

311. Margo, M. K.: Surgical treatment of conditions of the fore part of the foot. J. Bone Joint Surg., *49A:*1665–1674, 1967.

312. Smillie, I. S.: Freiberg's infraction (Kohler's second disease). J. Bone Joint Surg., *37:*580, 1955.

Köhler's Disease

313. Brailsford, J. F.: Osteochondritis of the adult tarsal navicular. J. Bone Joint Surg., *21:*111–120, 1939.

314. Karp, M. G.: Kohler's disease of the tarsal scaphoid. J. Bone Joint Surg., *19:*84–96, 1937.

315. Kidner, F. C., and Muro, F.: Kohler's disease of the tarsal scaphoid or os naviculare pedis retardation. J.A.M.A., *83:*1650, 1924.

316. Kohler, A.: Uber enine haufige bisher anscheinend unbekannte Erkrankung einzelner kindlicher Knochen. Munch. Med. Wochen., *55:*1, 923, 1908.

Sever's Disease

318. Dickinson, P. H., Coutts, M. B., Woodward, E. P., and Handler, D.: Tendo-achilles bursitis. J. Bone Joint Surg., *48A:*77–81, 1966.

319. Keck, S. W., and Kelly, P. J.: Bursitis of the posterior part of the heel. J. Bone Joint Surg., *47A:*267–273, 1965.

320. Pappas, A. M.: The osteochondroses. Pediatr. Clin. North Am., *14:*549–570, 1967.

321. Sever, J. W.: Apophysitis of the os calcis. N. Y. Med. J., *95:*1025, 1912.

322. ———: Apophysitis of the os calcis. Am. J. Orthop., *15:*659, 1917.

323. Sharrard, W. J. W.: Paediatric Orthopaedics and Fractures, pp. 400–401. Oxford, Blackwell, 1971.

324. Smyth, F. S., Jr.: Local affections of the bones and soft tissues of the foot pp. 377–378. Surgery of the Foot, ed. 3. St. Louis, C. V. Mosby, 1973.

325. Tachdjian, M. O.: Pediatric Orthopedics, pp. 406–408. Philadelphia W. B. Saunders, 1972.

Osteochondritis Dissecans of the Talus

326. Berndt, A. L., and Harty, M.: Transchondral fractures (osteochondritis dissecans) of the talus. J. Bone Joint Surg., *41A:*988–1020, 1959.

327. Cameron, B. M.: Osteochondritis dissecans of the

ankle joint. J. Bone Joint Surg., *38A:*857–861, 1956.

328. Davis, M. W.: Bilateral talar osteochondritis dissecans with lax ankle ligaments. J. Bone Joint Surg., *52A:*168–170, 1970.

329. Fairbank, H. A. T.: Osteochondritis dissecans. Br. J. Surg., *21:*67–82, 1933.

330. Gardiner, T. B.: Osteochondritis dissecans in three members of one family. J. Bone Joint Surg., *37B:*139, 1955.

331. Green, W. T., and Banks, H. H.: Osteochondritis dissecans in children. J. Bone Joint Surg., *35A:*26–47, 1953.

332. Mukherjee, S. K., and Young, A. B.: Dome fracture of the talus. J. Bone Joint Surg., *55B:*319–326, 1973.

333. Marks, K. L.: Flake fracture of the talus progressing to osteochondritis dissecans. J. Bone Joint Surg., *34B:*90–92, 1952.

334. Ray, R. B. and Coughlin, E. J., Jr.: Osteochondritis of the talus. J. Bone Joint Surg., *29:*697–706, 1947.

335. Smyth, F. S.: Local affections of the bones and soft tissues of the foot. *In* Surgery of the Foot. St. Louis, C. V. Mosby, 1973.

336. Vaughan, C. E., and Stapleton, J. G.: Osteochondritis dissecans of the ankle. Radiology, *49:*72–78, 1947.

337. Wagoner, G., and Cohn, B. N. E.: Osteochondritis dissecans. Arch. Surg., *23:*1–25, 1931.

Congenital Cleft Foot

338. Barsky, J.: Cleft hand: Classification, incidence and treatment, J. Bone Joint Surg., *46A:*1707–1720, 1964.

339. Cowan, R.: Surgical problems associated with congenital malformations of the forefoot. Can. J. Surg., *8:*29–40, 1965.

340. Leiter, E., and Lipson, J.: Genitourinary tract anomalies in lobster claw syndrome. J. Urol., *115:*339–341, 1976.

341. McFarland, B.: Congenital deformities of the spine and limbs. *In* Platt, H. (ed.): Modern Trends in Orthopaedics. New York, Hoeber, 1950.

342. Maisels, D. O.: Lobster claw deformities of the hands and feet. Br. J. Plast. Surg., *23:*269–282, 1970.

343. Meyerding, H. W., and Upshaw, J. E.: Heredofamilial cleft foot deformity. Am. J. Surg., *74:*889–892, 1947.

344. Mosavy, S. H., and Vakhshuri, P.: Split hands and feet. South African Med. J., *49:*1842–1844, 1975.

345. Phillips, R. S.: Congenital split foot (lobster claw) and triphalangeal thumb. J. Bone Joint Surg., *53B:*247–257, 1971.

346. Stiles, K. A., and Pickard, I. S.: Hereditary malformations of the hands and feet. J. Hered., *34:*340–344, 1943.

347. Walker, J. C., and Clodius, L.: The syndrome of cleft lip, cleft palate and lobster claw deformities of hands and feet. Plast. Reconstruct. Surg., *32:*627–636, 1963.

348. Weissman, S. L., and Plaschkes, Y.: Surgical correction of lobster-claw feet. Plast. Reconstruct. Surg., *49:*89–92, 1972.

Syndactyly, Macrodactyly, Polydactyly

349. Anderson, K. S., and Rousing, H.: Diplopedia. Acta Orthop. Scand., *42:*291–295, 1971.

350. Charters, A. D.: Local gigantism. J. Bone Joint Surg., *39B:*542–547, 1957.

351. Cobey, M. C., and Cobey, J. C.: A true prehallux. J. Bone Joint Surg., *48A:*953–954, 1966.

352. Cowan, R. J.: Surgical problems associated with congenital malformations of the forefoot. Can. J. Surg., *8:*29–40, 1965.

353. Diamond. L. S., and Gould, V. E.: Macrodactyly of the foot. South. Med. J., *67:*645–650, 1974.

354. Jaeger, M., and Refior, H. J.: The congenital triangular deformity of the tubular bones of hand and foot. C.O.R.R., *81:*139–150, 1971.

355. Karchinov, K.: Congenital diplopodia with hypoplasia or aplasia of the tibia. J. Bone Joint Surg., *55B:*604–611, 1973.

356. Kelikian, H.: Deformities of the Lesser Toes in Hallux Valgus, Allied Deformities of the Forefoot and Metatarsalgia. Philadelphia, W. B. Saunders Co., 1965.

357. Rechnagel, K.: Megalodactylism. Acta Orthop. Scand., *38:*57–66, 1967.

358. Smith, R. J.: Osteotomy for delta-phalanx deformity. C.O.R.R., *123:*91–94, 1977.

359. Specht, E. E.: Minor congenital deformities and anomalies of the toes. *In* Inman, V. (ed.): Surgery of the Foot. St. Louis, C. V. Mosby, 1973.

360. Tsuge, K.: Treatment of macrodactyly. Plast. Reconstruct. J., *39:*590–599, 1967.

361. Venn-Watson, E. A.: Problems in polydactyly of the foot. Orthop. Clin. North Am., *7:*909–927, 1976.

362. Watson, H. K., and Boyes, J. H.: Congenital angular deformity of the digits. J. Bone Joint Surg., *49A:*333, 1967.

Congenital Hallux Varus

363. Farmer, A. W.: Congenital hallux varus. Am. J. Surg., *95:*274–278, 1958.

364. Haas, S. L.: An operation for the correction of hallux varus. J. Bone Joint Surg., *20:*705–708, 1938.

365. Hawkins, F. B.: Acquired hallux varus, cause, prevention & correction. C.O.R.R., *76:*169–176, 1971.

366. Horwitz, M. T.: Unusual hallux varus deformity and its surgical correction. J. Bone Joint Surg., *19:*828–829, 1937.

367. McElvenny, R. T.: Hallux varus. Q. Bull. Northwest. Med. School, *15:*277–280, 1941.

368. Miller, J. W.: Acquired hallux varus: A preventable and correctable disorder. J. Bone Joint Surg., *57A:*183–187, 1975.

369. Myginal, H. B.: Surgical treatment of congenital hallux varus. Nord. Med., *49:*914–916, 1953.

370. Sloane, D.: Congenital hallux varus. J. Bone Joint Surg., *17:*209-211, 1935.

371. Thomson, S. A.: Hallux varus and metatarsus varus. C.O.R.R., *16:*109–118, 1960.

Adolescent Bunion

372. Berntsen, A.: De l'hallux valgus, contribution à son etiologie et à son traitement. Rev. Orthop., *17:*101–111, 1930.
373. Bonney, G., and McNab, I.: Hallux valgus and hallux rigidus. J. Bone Joint Surg., *34B:*366–385, 1952.
374. Carr, C. R., and Boyd, B.: Correctional osteotomy for metatarsus primus varus and hallux valgus. J. Bone Joint Surg., *50A:*1353–1367, 1968.
375. Durman, D. C.: Metatarsus primus varus and hallux valgus. Arch Surg., *74:*128–135, 1957.
376. Ellis, V. H.: A method of correcting metatarsus primus varus. J. Bone Joint Surg., *33B:*415–417, 1951.
377. Engle, E. T., and Morton, D. S.: Notes on foot disorders among natives of the Belgian Congo. J. Bone Joint Surg., *13:*311–318, 1931.
378. Ewald, P.: Die atiologie des hallux valgus, Deutsch. Z. Chir., *114:*90–103, 1912.
379. Fuld, J. E.: Surgical treatment of hallux valgus and its complications. Am. Med., *25:*536–539, 1919.
380. Haines, R. W., and McDougall, A.: The anatomy of hallux valgus. J. Bone Joint Surg., *36B:*272–293, 1954.
381. Hardy, R. H., and Clapham, J. C. R.: Observations on hallux valgus. J. Bone Joint Surg., *33B:*376–391, 1951.
382. Hawkins, F. B., Mitchell, L., and Hedrick, D. W.: Correction of hallux valgus by metatarsal osteotomy. J. Bone Joint Surg., *27:*387–394, 1945.
383. Henderson, R. S.: Os intermetatarsium and a possible relationship to hallux valgus. J. Bone Joint Surg., *45B:*117–121, 1963.
384. Hiss, J. M.: Hallux valgus: Its course and simplified treatment. Am. J. Surg., *11:*51–57, 1931.
385. Inman, V. T.: Hallux valgus: A review of etiologic factors, Orthop. Clin. North Am., *5*(1):59–66, 1974.
386. Johnston, O.: Further studies of the inheritance of hand and foot anomalies. Clin. Orthop., *8:*146–160, 1956.
387. Joplin, R. J.: Sling procedure for correction of splay-foot, metatarsus primus varus and hallux valgus. J. Bone Joint Surg., *32A:*779–785, 1950.
388. Keller, W. L.: The surgical treatment of hallux valgus and bunion. N.Y. Med. J., *80:*741–742, 1904.
389. Kleinberg, S.: The operative care of hallux valgus and bunions. Am. J. Surg., *15:*75–81, 1932.
390. Lam, S., and Hodgson, A.R.: A comparison of foot forms among the non-shoe and shoe-wearing Chinese population. J. Bone Joint Surg., *40A:*1058–1062, 1958.
391. Lapidus, P. W.: Operative correction of metatarsus varus primus in hallux valgus. Surg. Obstet. Gynecol., *58:*183–191, 1934.
392. McBride, E. D.: A conservative operation for bunions. J. Bone Joint Surg., *10:*735–739, 1928.
393. Mayo, C. H.: The surgical treatment of bunions. Ann. Surg., *48:*300–302, 1908.
394. Mitchell, L., *et al.:* Osteotomy-bunionectomy for hallux valgus. J. Bone Joint Surg., *40A:*41–58, 1958.
395. Peabody, C. W.: The surgical cure of hallux valgus. J. Bone Joint Surg., *13:*273–282, 1931.
396. Piggott, H. H.: The natural history of hallux valgus in adolescence and early adult life. J. Bone Joint Surg., *42B:*749–760, 1960.
397. Silver, D.: Hallux valgus. J. Bone Joint Surg., *5:*225–232, 1923.
398. Simmonds, F. A., and Menelaus, M.D.: Hallux valgus in adolescents. J. Bone Joint Surg., *42B:*761–768, 1960.
399. Stanley, L. L.: Bunions. J. Bone Joint Surg., *17:*961–968, 1935.
400. Trott, A.: Hallux valgus in the adolescent. A.A.O.S. Instruc. Course Lect., *21:*262–268, 1972.
401. Truslow, W.: Metatarsus primus varus or hallux valgus? J. Bone Joint Surg., *7:*98–108, 1925.
402. Wells, L. H.: The foot of the South African native. Am. J. Phys. Anthrop., *15:*185–289, 1931.
403. Wilson, J. N.: Oblique displacement osteotomy for hallux valgus. J. Bone Joint Surg., *45B:*552–556, 1963.

Congenital Short First Metatarsal

404. Giannestras, N. J.: Foot Disorders. Philadelphia, Lea & Febiger, 1973.
405. Harris, R. I., and Beath, T.: The short first metatarsal. J. Bone Joint Surg., *31A:*553–565, 1949.
406. Morton, D. J.: Metatarsus atavicus. J. Bone Joint Surg., *9:*531–544, 1927.
407. Nilsonne, H.: Hallux rigidus and its treatment. Acta Orthop. Scand., *1:*295–303, 1930.
408. Viladot, A.: Metatarsalgia due to biomechanical alterations of the forefoot. Orthop. Clin. North Am., *4:*165–178, 1973.

Congenital Overriding of the Fifth Toe

409. Cockin, J.: Butler's operations for an overriding fifth toe. J. Bone Joint Surg., *50B:*78–81, 1960.
410. DuVries, H. L.: DuVries' Surgery of the Foot, ed. 3 pp. 545–547, St. Louis, C. V. Mosby, 1973.
411. Goodwin, F. C., and Swisher, F. M.: The treatment of congenital hyperextension of the fifth toe. J. Bone Joint Surg., *25:*193–196, 1943.
412. Jahss, M. H., Diaphysectomy for severe acquired overlapping fifth toe, pp. 211–221. *In* Bateman, J. E. (ed.): Foot Science. Philadelphia, W. B. Saunders, 1976.
413. Janecki, C. J., and Wilde, A. H.: Results of phalangectomy of the fifth toe for hammertoe, the Ruiz-Mora procedure. J. Bone Joint Surg., *58A:*1005–1007, 1076.
414. Kelikian, H.: Hallux Valgus, Allied Deformities of the Forefoot and Metatarsalgia. Philadelphia, W. B. Saunders, 1965.
415. Kelikian, H., Clayton, L., and Loseff, H.: Surgical syndactylia of the toes. Clin. Orthop., *19:*208, 1961.
416. Lantzounis, L. A.: Congenital subluxation of the fifth toe and its correction by a periosteocap-

sulotomy and tendon transplanation. J. Bone Joint Surg., *22:*147–150, 1940.

417. Lapidus, P. C.: Transplantation of the extensor tendon for correction of the overlapping fifth toe. J. Bone Joint Surg., *24:*555–559, 1942.

418. Leonard, M. H., and Rising, E. E.: Syndactylization to maintain correction of overlapping fifififi fifififi Clin. Orthop., *43:*241–243, 1965.

419. McFarland, B.: Congenital deformities of the spine and limbs p. 107. *In* Platt, H. (ed.): Modern Trends in Orthopaedics. London, Butterworth, 1950.

420. Michele, A. A., and Krueger, F. J.: Operative correction for hammertoe. Milit. Surg., *103:*52–53, 1948.

421. Ruiz-Mora, J.: Plastic correction of overriding fifth toe. Orthopaedic Letters Club, *6,* 1954.

422. Scrase, W. H.: The treatment of dorsal adduction deformity of the fifth toe. J. Bone Joint Surg., *36B:*146, 1954.

423. Sharrard, W. J.W.: The surgery of deformed toes in children. Br. J. Clin. Prac., *17:*263–272, 1963.

424. Stamm, T. T.: Br. Surg. Prac., *4,* 161, 1918.

425. Tachdjian, M. O.: Pediatric Orthopedics, pp. 1416–1422. Philadelphia, W. B. Saunders, 1972.

426. Thompson, C. T.: Surgical treatment of disorders of the fore part of the foot. J. Bone Joint Surg., *46A:*1117–1128, 1964.

427. Wilson, J. N.: V-Y Correction for Varus Deformity of the Fifth Toe. Br. J. Surg., *41:*133–135, 1953.

Congenital Curly Toes

428. Giannestras, N. J.: Foot Disorders, p. 102–107. Philadelphia, Lea & Febiger, 1973.

429. Kelikian, H.: Hallux Valgus, Allied Deformities of the Forefoot and Metatarsalgia, p. 330. Philadelphia, W.B. Saunders, 1965.

430. Pollard, J. P. and Morrison, P.J.M.: Flexor tenotomy in the treatment of curly toes. Proc. R. Soc. Med., *68:*480–481, 1975.

431. Sharrard, W. J. W.: The surgery of deformed toes in children. Br. J. Clin. Prac., *17:*263–270, 1963.

432. Specht, E. E.: DuVries' Surgery of the Foot, Inman, V. T. (ed.) St. Louis, C.V. Mosby, 1973.

433. Sweetnam, R.: Congenital curly toes, an investigation into the value of treatment. Lancet, *2:*398–400, 1958.

434. Taylor, R. G.: The treatment of claw toes by multiple transfers of the flexor with extensor tendons. J. Bone Joint Surg., *33B:*539–542, 1951.

435. Trethowan, W. H.: The treatment of hammer toe. Lancet, *1:*1257–1258, 1312–1313, 1925.

Toe Deformity

436. Engle, E. T., and Morton, D. J.: Notes on foot disorders among natives of the belgian congo. J. Bone Joint Surg., *13:*311–318, 1931.

437. James, C. S.: Footprints and feet of natives of the solomon islands. Lancet, *2:*1390–1393, 1939.

438. Sharrard, W. J. W.: The surgery of deformed toes in children. Br. J. Clin. Prac., *17:*263–270, 1963.

439. Sim-Fook, L., and Hodgson, A. R.: A comparison of foot forms among the non-shoe and shoe-wearing Chinese population. J. Bone Joint Surg., *40A:*1058-1062, 1958.

440. Stewart, S. F.: Footgear—it's history, uses and abuses. C.O.R.R., *88:*119–130, 1972.

441. Well, L. H.: The foot of the south african native. Am. J. Phys. Anthrop., *15:*185–289, 1931.

Adolescent Hallux Rigidus

442. Bingold, A. C., and Collins, D. H.: Hallux rigidus. J. Bone Joint Surg., *32B:*214–222, 1950.

443. Boney, G., and MacNab, I.: Hallux valgus and hallux rigidus. J. Bone Joint Surg., *34B:*366–385, 1952.

444. Cochrane, W. A.: An operation for hallux rigidus. Br. Med. J., *1:*1095–1096, 1927.

445. Davies-Colley, N.: On contraction of the metatarsophalangeal joint of the great toe (hallux flexus). Trans. Clin. Soc. London, *20:*165, 1887.

446. Giannestras, N. J.: Foot Disorders, p. 400–402. Philadelphia, Lea & Febiger, 1973.

447. Glissan, D. J.: Hallux valgus and hallux rigidus. Med. J. Aust, *2:*585–588, 1946.

448. Gudas, C. J.: An etiology of hallux rigidus. J. Foot Surg., *10:*113–124, 1971.

449. Harrison, M. H. M., and Harvey, F. J.: Arthrodesis of the first metatarsophalangeal joint for hallux valgus and rigidus. J. Bone Joint Surg., *45A:*471–480, 1963.

450. Jack, E. A.: The aetiology of hallux rigidus. Br. J. Surg., *27:*492–497, 1940.

451. Jansen, M.: Hallux valgus rigidus and mallens. J. Orthop. Surg., *3:*98–90, 1921.

452. Kessel, L., and Bonney, G.: Hallux rigidus in the adolescent. J. Bone Joint Surg., *40B:*668–673, 1958.

453. Lambrinudi, C.: Metatarsus primus elevatus. Proc. R. Soc. Med., *31:*1273, 1938.

454. Lloyd, E. I.: The prognosis of hallux valgus and hallux rigidus. Lancet, *2:*263, 1935.

455. McMurray, T. P.: Treatment of hallux valgus and rigidus. Br. Med. J., *2:*218–220, 1936.

456. Monberg, A.: On the treatment of hallux rigidus. Acta Orthop. Scand., *6:*239–247, 1935.

457. Moynihan, F. J.: Arthrodesis of the metatarsophalangeal joint of the great toe. J. Bone Joint Surg., *49B:*544–551, 1967.

458. Nilsonne, H.: Hallux rigidus and its treatment. Acta Orthop. Scand., *1:*295–303, 1930.

459. Sharrard, W. J. W.: The surgery of deformed toes in children. Br. J. Clin. Prac., *17:*263–270, 1963.

460. Strombeck, J. P.: Hallux rigidus und seine behandlung. Acta Chir. Scand., *73:*53–83, 1934.

461. Viladot, A. Metatarsalgia due to biomechanical alterations of the forefoot. Orthop. Clin. North Am. *4:*165–178, 1973.

462. Watermann, H.: Die Arthritis Deformans des Grosszehengrundgelenkes als selbstandiges Krankheitsbild. Z. Orthop. Chir., *48:*346–355, 1927.

463. Watson-Jones, R.: Treatment of hallux rigidus (Reply letter to Mr. Cochrane). Br. Med. J., *1:*1165–1166, 1927.

Hammer Toe

464. Blum, A.: De l'orteil en marteau. Bull. Mem. Soc. Chir. Paris, *9:*738–745, 1883.
465. Brahams, M. A.: Common foot problems. J. Bone Joint Surg., *49A:*1653–1664, 1967.
466. Cahill, B. R., and Connor, D. E.: A long-term follow-up on proximal phalangectomy for hammer toes. Clin. Orthop., *86:*191–192, 1972.
467. DuVries, H. L.: Hammer toe, mallet toe and claw toe, pp. 241–249. *In* Inman, Verne T. (ed): DuVries' Surgery of the Foot. St. Louis, C. V. Mosby Company, 1973.
468. Ely, L. W.: Hammer toe. Surg. Clin. North Am., *6:*433, 435.
469. Giannestras, N. J.: Foot Disorders: Medical and Surgical Management, pp. 410–415. Philadelphia Lea & Febiger, 1973.
470. Glassman, F., Wolin, I., and Sideman, S.: Phalangectomy for toe deformities. Surg. Clin. North Am., *29:*275–280, 1949.
471. Jahss, M. H.: Operation for advanced hammer toe. Orthop. Rev., *4:*57–58, 1975.
472. Jones, R.: Notes on Military Orthopaedics, pp. 38–57. New York, Hoeber, 1917.
473. Kelikian, H. Clayton, L., and Loseff, H.: Surgical syndactylia of the toes. Clin. Orthop., *19:*208, 1961.
474. Kelikian, H.: Hallux Valgus, Allied Deformities of the Forefoot and Metatarsalia. Philadelphia W. B. Saunders, 1965.
475. Lapidus, P. W.: Operation for correction of hammer toe. J. Bone Joint Surg., *21:*977–982, 1939.
476. McConnell, B. E.: Hammer toe surgery. South. Med. J. *68:*595, 1975.
477. McFarland, B.: Congenital Deformities of the Spine and Limbs. In Platt, H. (ed.): Modern Trends in Orthopaedics. London, Butterworth, 1950.
478. Margo, M. K.: Surgical treatment of conditions of the fore part of the foot J. Bone Joint Surg., *49A:*1665–1674, 1976.
479. Merrill, W. J.: Conservative operative treatment of hammer toe. Am. J. Orthop., *10:*262–263, 1912.
480. Michele, A. A., and Krueger, F. J.: Operative correction for hammer toe. Milit. Surg., *103:*52–53, 1948.
481. O'Neill, B. J.: An arthroplastic operation for hammer toe. J.A.M.A. *57:*12–7, 1911.
482. Sehig, S.: Hammertoe: A new procedure for its correction. Surg. Gynecol. Obstet., *72:*101, 1941.
483. Sharrard, W. J. W.: The surgery of deformed toes in children. Br. J. Clin. Prac., *17:*263–272, 1963.
484. Soule, R. E.: Operation for the correction of hammer toe. N. Y. Med. J., *91:*649–650, 1910.
485. Tachdjian, M. O.: Pediatric Orthopedics, pp. 1410–1411. Philadelphia, W. B. Saunders, 1972.
486. Taylor, R. G.: An operative procedure for the treatment of hammer toe and claw toe. J. Bone Joint Surg., *22:*608–609, 1940.
487. _____: The treatment of claw toes by multiple transfers of the flexor into extensor tendons. J. Bone Joint Surg., *33B:*539–542, 1951.
488. Trethowan, W. H.: The treatment of hammer toe. Lancet, *1:*1257–1258, 1312–1313, 1925.
489. Young, C. S.: An operation for the correction of hammer toe and claw toe. J. Bone Joint Surg., *20:*715–719, 1938.

Claw Toes

490. Brockway, A.: Surgical correction of talipes cavus deformities. J. Bone Joint Surg., *22:*81–91, 1940.
491. Dickson, F. D., and Dively, R. S.: Functional Disorders of the Foot, pp. 244-249. Philadelphia, J.B. Lippincott, 1944.
492. DuVries, H. L.: DuVries Surgery of the Foot, pp. 241–249. St. Louis, C. V. Mosby., 1973.
493. Forrester-Brown, M. F.: Tendon transplantation for clawing of the great toe. J. Bone Joint Surg., *20:*57–60, 1938.
494. Frank, G. R., and Johnson, W. M.: The extensor shift procedure in the correction of clawtoe deformities in children. South. Med. J., *59:*889-896, 1966.
495. Heyman, C. H.: Operative treatment of claw foot. J. Bone Joint Surg., *14:*335–337, 1932.
496. Hibbs, R. A.: An operation for "claw foot." J.A.M.A., *73:*1583–1585, 1919.
497. Jahss, M. H. Operation for advanced hammertoe. Orthop. Rev., *4:*57–58, 1975.
498. Lambrinudi, C.: An operation for claw toes. Proc. R. Soc. Med., *21:*239, 1927.
499. Parrish, T. F.: Dynamic correction of clawtoes. Orthop. Clin. North Am., *4:*97–102, 1973.
500. Pyper, J. B.: The flexor-extensor transplant operation for clawtoes. J. Bone Joint Surg., *40B:*528–533, 1958.
501. Sharrard, W. J. W.: The surgery of deformed toes in children. Br. J. Clin. Prac., *17:*262–272, 1963.
502. Tachdjian, M. O.: Pediatric Orthopedics, p. 1415. Philadelphia, W. B. Saunders, 1972.
503. Taylor, R. G.: The treatment of claw toes by multiple transfers of the flexor into extensor tendons. J. Bone Joint Surg., *33B:*539–542, 1951.

Plantar Warts

504. Brahms, M. A.: Common foot problems. J. Bone Joint surg., *49A:*1653–1664, 1967.
505. Branson, E. C., and Rhea, R. L.: Plantar warts: cure by injection. New Engl. J. Med., *248:*631–632, 1953.
506. Dingman, R. O., and Grabb, W. C.: The intractable plantar wart. J. Michigan Med. Soc., *61:*297–299, 1962.
507. Duthie, D. A., and McCollum, D. I.: Treatment of plantar warts with elastoplast and podophyllin. Br. Med. J., *2:*216–218, 1951.
508. DuVries, H. L.: New approach to the treatment of intractable verruca plantaris (plantar warts). J.A.M.A., *152:*1202–1203, 1953.
509. _____: Disorders of skin and toenails. *In* Surgery of the Foot, ed.3. St. Louis, C. V. Mosby, 1973.
510. Haggart, G. E.: The conservative and surgical treatment of plantar warts. Surg. Clin. North Am., *14:*1211–1218, 1934.
511. Margo, M. K.: Surgical treatment of conditions of the fore part of the foot. J. Bone Joint Surg., *49A:*1665–1674, 1967.

512. May, H.: The surgical treatment of intractable plantar warts. Surg. Clin. North Am., *31:*607–616, 1951.
513. Reeves, R. J., and Jackson, M. T.: Roentgen therapy of plantar warts. Am. J. Roentgenol., *76:*977–978, 1956.
514. Robinson, D. W.: Treatment of complication of plantar warts. Arch. Surg., *66:*434–439, 1953.
515. Tachdjian, M. O.: Pediatric Orthopedics, pp. 1440–1442. Philadelphia. W. B. Saunders, 1972.

Ingrown Toenail

516. Bose, R.: A technique for excision of nail fold for ingrowing toenail. Surg. Gynecol. Obstet., *132:*511–512, 1971.
517. Brahms, M. A.: Common foot problems. J. Bone Joint Surg., *49A:*1653–1664, 1967.
518. DuVries, H. L.: Disorders of skin and toenails. *In* Surgery of the Foot., ed. 3. St. Louis, C. V. Mosby, 1973.
519. Heifetz, C. J.: Ingrown toe-nail. Am. J. Surg., *38:*298–313, 1937.
520. ———: Operative management of ingrown toenail. J. Missouri Med. Assoc., *42:*213–316, 1945.
521. Ilfeld, F. W., and August, W.: Treatment of ingrown toenail with plastic insert. Orthop. Clin. North Am., *5:*95–97, 1974.
522. Kopell, H. P., *et al.:* Ingrown toenail: new concept. N. Y. J. Med., *66:*1215–1217, 1966.
523. Margo, M. K.: Surgical treatment of conditions of the fore part of the foot. J. Bone and Joint Surg., *49A:* 1665–1674, 1967.
524. Mogenson, P.: Ingrowing toenail. Acta Orthop. Scand., *42:*94–101, 1971.
525. O'Donoghue, D. H.: Treatment of ingrown toe nail. Am. J. Surg., *50:*519–522, 1940.
526. Sharrard, W. J. W.: Pediatric Orthopedics and Fractures, pp. 920–921. Oxford, Blackwell, 1971.
527. Tachdjian, M. O.: Pediatric Orthopedics, pp. 1440–1442. Philadelphia, W. B. Saunders, 1972.

22 *The Amputee*

Robert E. Tooms, M.D.

While the number of juvenile amputees is relatively small, this group comprises a significant segment of the pediatric population with major orthopaedic problems. The prosthetic and surgical management of these children, although similar in many respects to that of the adult amputee, may be extremely complex. Experience has proved that the child amputee is best managed in a specialized setting, separate and apart from the standard adult amputee clinic or the usual crippled children's clinic dealing with a variety of orthopaedic disabilities.[11, 23, 124]

By definition, the child amputee is skeletally immature and the epiphyses of his long bones are still open.[53] Not only are the limbs of a growing child increasing in length and in circumference, but the metabolism of all his tissues is progressing at a remarkably high rate, and he is rapidly maturing from a neuromuscular developmental standpoint.[3] This growth factor, or biologic dynamism, possessed by the child is the cardinal difference between child and adult amputees. Apart from these physiologic differences, it is further apparent that, in contrast to the adult, the child is emotionally immature, variably dependent upon others for his basic needs, and subject to the wishes of his parents and others in decision making.[10] All of these factors may at times enhance the effectiveness of prosthetic and surgical care of the child amputee, or they may be detrimental to the ultimate success of the treatment program, if not recognized and properly managed.

The rapidly growing child requires frequent adjustments of his prosthesis. Because he grows taller, length adjustment of the prosthesis is necessary at frequent intervals. Because his stump enlarges and changes in configuration, socket modification or replacement is also needed quite often. To maintain good cosmesis and ensure proper fit of clothing and footwear, prosthetic feet and other components must be frequently altered or replaced. Children engage in extremely vigorous play activities, often in environments hostile to the plastic, metal, and leather used in prosthetic fabrication. The child amputee is no different from his normal peers in this respect, and desirably so. In short, rapid growth plus hard usage require that there are almost constant maintainance and frequent replacement of prosthetic devices used by children. Lambert has reported that children followed at the University of Illinois required a new lower limb prosthesis annually up to the age of 5 years, biennially from 5 to 12 years, and then one every 3 to 4 years until age 21 years.[100] The above facts are perhaps obvious, but are cited to point out the need for the child amputee to be re-evaluated by all members of the clinic team on a regular and frequent basis. Experience has shown that such clinic visits should be made once every 3 to 4 months for optimal care.

Limb deficiencies in children have been divided into two broad catagories based on etiology: congenital and acquired. Since 1968 annual surveys of specialized child amputee clinics in the United States have consistently shown that approximately 60 per

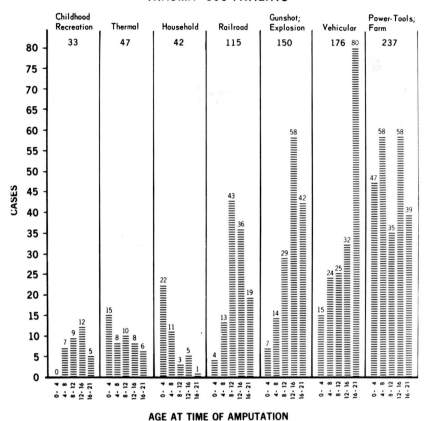

FIG. 22-1. Etiology of acquired amputations due to trauma. (From Northwestern University Medical School Prosthetic-Orthotic Program, Juvenile Amputee Course Manual.)

cent of childhood amputations are congenital in origin and 40 per cent are acquired.[81] A survey of prosthetic facilities across the country revealed significantly higher numbers of acquired limb deficiencies.[39] This discrepancy presumably indicates the more complex congenital limb deficiencies are referred to specialized child amputee clinics for care, while the more conventional acquired amputation problems can be satisfactorily treated by clinicians in less specialized settings.

ACQUIRED AMPUTATIONS

ETIOLOGY

Acquired limb deficiencies in children are secondary to trauma or disease, with trauma being responsible for limb loss approximately twice as often as disease.[6, 101] In the many traumatic incidents resulting in amputation, power tools and machinery are the worst offenders, followed closely be vehicular accidents, gunshot wounds and explosions, and railroad accidents, in that order. Smaller, but significant, numbers are due to household accidents, thermal injuries, and injuries sustained in connection with childhood recreational activities (Fig. 22-1). As might be expected, vehicular accidents, gunshot wounds, and power tool injuries are the commonest causes of limb loss in the older child (those of 12–21 years). In the toddler (ages 1–4 years) accidents with power tools such as lawn mowers and other household accidents are·the most frequent causes of amputation.

Malignant tumors account for more than half the amputations performed for disease processes, with the largest number of cases occurring in the 12 to 21 year age group. Vascular malformations, neurogenic disorders, and a large variety of miscellaneous disorders are responsible for the remainder of amputations in this category (Fig. 22-2).

In more than 90 per cent of acquired amputations only one limb is involved, and it is the lower limb which is involved in 60 per cent of cases. Males outnumber females in incidence of acquired limb loss by three to two, a statistic probably attesting to the more hazardous work and recreational activities in which males engage.

SURGICAL PRINCIPLES

The well-established surgical principles for amputation surgery in the adult are just as applicable to amputations performed in children.[3, 12, 53, 100] The cardinal dictum is to conserve all limb length possible, consistent with appropriate treatment for the condition necessitating the amputation. The biologic dynamism, or growth factor, present in the child may permit surgical techniques not successful in the adult. Skin grafts, firm traction, and wound closure under tension may be *judiciously* utilized in the child to conserve limb length without compromising wound healing or subsequent prosthetic use.[3, 31, 64, 75]

In other ways, however, the growth factor may prove disadvantageous following amputations in children. One such disadvantage is relative loss of stump length due to epiphyseal loss.[3, 100] Loss of stump length is most marked in above-knee amputations where the distal femoral epiphysis, accounting for approximately 70 per cent of the length growth of the femur, is sacrificed. When a standard mid-thigh amputation is performed in a 5-year-old child, the above-knee stump present at age 16 will be quite short and a considerably less than optimal lever for prosthetic use (Fig. 22-3). This complication points up the second major surgical dictum in amputation surgery in the child: Wherever possible, always perform a disarticulation rather than a supraepiphyseal or transdiaphyseal amputation in a growing child. Aside from the highly desirable preservation of epiphyseal growth, dis-

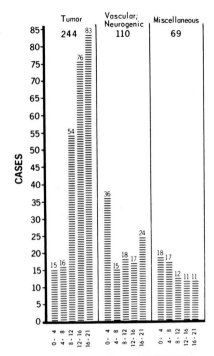

FIG. 22-2. Etiology of acquired amputations due to disease. (From Northwestern University Medical School Prosthetic-Orthotic Program, Juvenile Amputee Course Manual.)

articulation provides a sturdy end-bearing stump and a long lever arm to enhance prosthetic use. In the growing child prominent condyles or malleoli resulting from disarticulation undergo atrophy with the passage of time, eliminating the cosmetic objection to this type of surgery.[3, 12, 53, 100] Furthermore, disarticulation precludes subsequent development of terminal overgrowth of bone, a complication discussed below.

COMPLICATIONS

Terminal Overgrowth

The most frequent complication of amputation surgery in children is terminal overgrowth. This is an appositional growth of bone at the transected end of a long bone in the skeletally immature individual, being

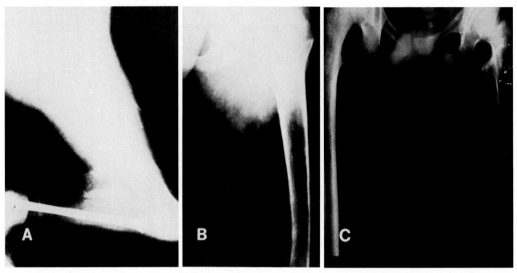

FIG. 22-3. *(A)* Roentgenogram of a left lower limb illustrating tibial hemimelia with severe soft-tissue webbing in the popliteal area. *(B)* This limb deficiency was treated by means of an amputation through the distal third of the femur. *(C)* At skeletal maturity there is marked shortening of the femur on the amputated side due to loss of the distal femoral epiphysis, with a resultant very short amputation stump.

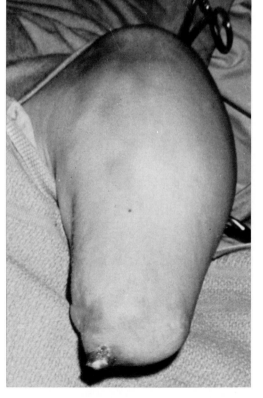

seen most commonly in the humerus, fibula, tibia, and femur, in that order.[3] Although terminal overgrowth does not occur following disarticulation, it is in no way related to epiphyseal bone growth, and previous attempts to prevent this problem by epiphysiodesis have not been successful.[168] In this condition the appositional growth of new bone exceeds the growth of the overlying soft tissues and, if untreated, the bone end may actually penetrate the skin (Fig. 22-4). Many surgical techniques have been devised in an attempt to prevent terminal overgrowth, but the best method at present remains stump revision with appropriate resection of the bony overgrowth.[2, 140] This has been necessary in 8 to 12 per cent of most large reported series of acquired amputations in children.[2, 3, 6, 11, 12, 53] Once this condition occurs, recurrences are common

FIG. 22-4. Terminal overgrowth of the humerus in a posttraumatic above-elbow amputation. The bony overgrowth has actually penetrated the soft tissues at the end of the amputation stump.

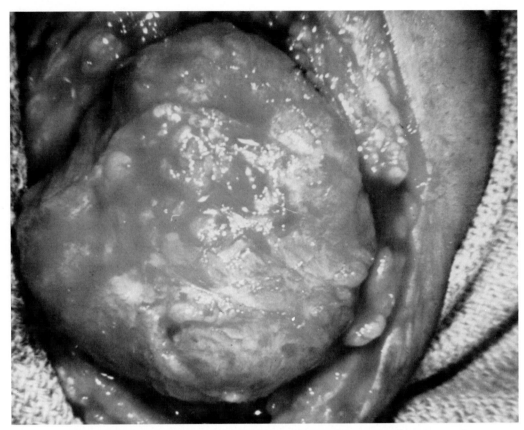

FIG. 22-5. This large bursa developed over the end of the humerus in an acquired above-elbow amputation. Surgical excision of the bursa as well as the underlying bony overgrowth is necessary to eradicate the problem.

and may necessitate repeated stump revisions at 2- to 3-year intervals until skeletal maturity. Newer techniques utilizing intramedullary implants of silicone rubber[156, 157] or porous polyethylene[122] to prevent terminal overgrowth appear promising and may eventually prove to be effective. It was formerly believed that terminal overgrowth did not occur in congenital limb deficiencies, but it is now known that the condition does occur in a small percentage of this category of amputations. Aitken[2] has postulated that such cases may represent true instances of intrauterine amputation.[58, 71, 99]

Bursa Formation

Bursa formation may occur over any bony prominence subjected to recurrent pressure from a prosthetic socket, but is most commonly seen overlying an area of terminal overgrowth (Fig. 22-5). Conservative treatment of these lesions by aspiration, corticosteroid injection, or stump wrapping has not been more than temporarily effective. Bursae are best managed by surgical excision of the bursal tissue, combined with appropriate resection of the underlying bone.[3, 6, 12] Surgery must be followed by socket adjustment or fitting with a new socket, as indicated.

Bony Spurs

These frequently form at the margin of transected bone in amputation stumps and are due to periosteal stimulation at the time of surgery. These spurs should be clearly

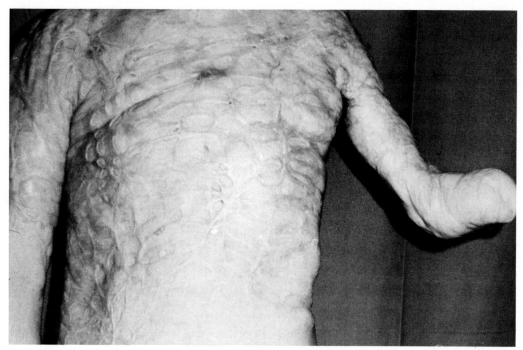

FIG. 22-6. Massive scarring and extensive skin grafting secondary to thermal burns present a very difficult prosthetic fitting problem in this child with a below-elbow amputation.

distinguished from terminal overgrowth, since they are rarely an indication for stump revision.[3]

Stump Scarring

Extensive stump scarring from trauma or skin grafts is amazingly well tolerated by the child (Fig. 22-6). High tissue metabolism, exuberent vascularity, and tissue plasticity present in children permit prosthetic use in stumps that would quickly break down in the adult. Stump revision to higher levels is seldom indicated because of stump scarring or skin grafts unless other significant problems such as terminal overgrowth are coexistant.[3] However, prosthetic modification is often required to disperse weightbearing forces and diminish shear at the stump-socket interface.[64]

Neuromas

These form in amputation stumps, as elsewhere, wherever a peripheral nerve is transected. A variety of surgical techniques has been employed to prevent neuroma formation, without significant success. High, sharp transection of nerves at the time of amputation so the cut ends lie in normal tissue well away from the amputation site remains the most effective way to prevent painful neuroma formation. In a large series of acquired childhood amputations Aitken found that slightly less than 4 per cent required surgical treatment for neuromas, most being satisfactorily managed by socket adjustments.[3] Neuromas are not present in congenital limb deficiencies.

Phantom Limb

Phantom limb sensation always occurs following acquired amputations in children, as it does in adults. However, if the amputation is performed on a child under the age of 10 years the phantom sensation is rapidly lost.[100] This is in contrast to teenagers and adults whose phantom limb may persist indefinitely. *Painful phantom limb* does not occur in growing children, but has been reported in the teenager. Neither phantom limb sensation nor painful phantom limbs occur in children with congenital limb deficiencies.[100]

PROSTHETIC MANAGEMENT

Although prosthetic devices used for the child amputee are remarkably similar to those used for adults, they are also strikingly different in many respects. While it is quite obvious that the components used in fabricating a prosthesis for a child must be varied according to the age and size of the child, it is sometimes not so obvious that the length of the lever arms and, therefore, the resultant forces generated are radically different in a small child as compared to an adult. It is, therefore, extremely important that established prosthetic principles be closely observed in fabricating a prosthesis for a child. Light-weight materials should be used in small amounts in prostheses for infants and both the strength and weight increased as the child grows older and subjects his prosthesis to harder use.[163]

Upper Limb Prosthetic Fitting

Prosthetic fitting and training should be coordinated with the normal development of motor skills in the growing child. It is unreasonable to expect a 1-year-old infant to effectively utilize the complex harnessing and cable systems employed in an adult above-elbow prosthesis. At this age a child possesses neither the kinesthetic motor skills necessary to use the prosthesis actively, nor a sufficiently long attention span to permit productive training sessions. Selection of prosthetic components compatible with the child's motor development and short frequent training sessions of sufficient simplicity are mandatory if child, parents, physician, and therapist are all to avoid frustration and achieve successful prosthetic use.

As a general rule, prosthetic fitting of the upper limb can be successfully initiated when the child has achieved adequate sitting balance. This will usually be at an approximate age of 6 months. The terminal device is passive in this initial prosthesis and is not activated by cable control until the child exhibits interest in attempting to insert objects into the passive terminal device. This will occur in most children at some time during the second year of life, but may be later in those children with higher levels of amputation. In an above-elbow or higher level prosthesis, the elbow lock may be activated by means of a pull-tab (used by the mouth or the sound opposite hand) incorporated into the prosthesis at the time of terminal device activation. However, a remotely controlled elbow lock should not be employed until the child develops sufficient coordination to utilize this device successfully. This will usually be in the third year of life.

The primary purpose of the normal human upper limb is the appropriate placement of the hand in space. Likewise, the primary purpose of an upper limb prosthesis is to enable the wearer to position his terminal device in an appropriate position to achieve useful prehension. Prehensile activities in the infant are of the two-handed clasping variety, with subsequent progression to the more functional one-handed grasp, and then to finger-tip prehension as motor skills develop.[10] For this reason, many centers prefer to use a plastic mitten or plastisol-covered wafer as the initial terminal device for infants, feeling that this allows the child to utilize two-handed clasping activities more advantageously. Others feel the small plastisol-covered hook (No. 12-P) is equally effective in affording two-handed grasp and, in addition, in assisting the child to pull up to the standing position (Fig. 22-7). Also, the hook can be cable activated at the appropriate time without the expense of purchasing a new terminal device. Another terminal device suitable for initial fitting of infants and small children is the innovative Child Amputee Prosthetic Project (CAPP) terminal device (Fig. 22-8). Early experiences with this unique design indicate a significant improvement in both cosmesis and function over older devices of similar size. As the child grows older and larger the original terminal device is progressively replaced with larger terminal devices (10-P, 99, and 88) and finally with the adult-size 5X hook (Fig. 22-7). As adolescence is approached, consideration is given to the use of a prosthetic hand. Presently available prosthetic hands

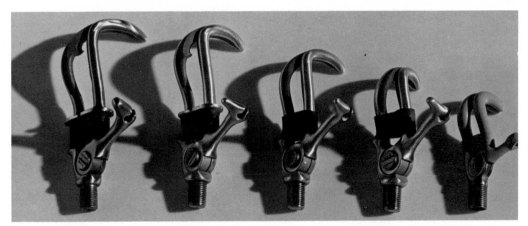

FIG. 22-7. Dorrance prosthetic hook terminal devices. From left to right are numbers 5-XA, 88, 99, 10, and 12-P.

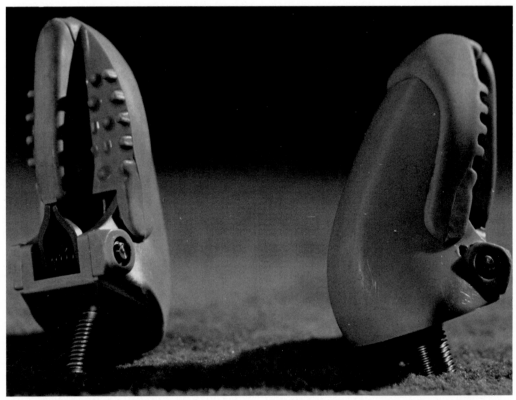

FIG. 22-8. The CAPP prosthetic terminal device is an innovative design originated at the Child Amputee Prosthetic Project at the University of California at Los Angeles. The large gripping surfaces provide the infant or small child with excellent friction for holding objects and are easily replaced as they become worn.

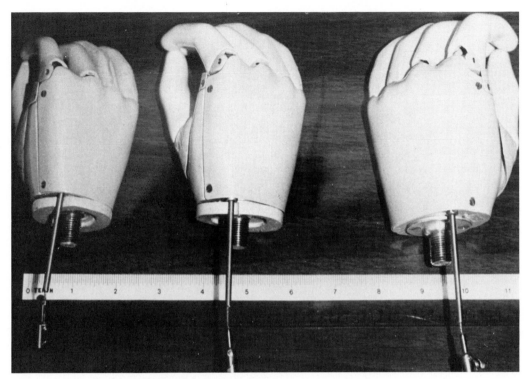

Fig. 22-9. Dorrance prosthetic hand terminal devices. From left to right are sizes No. 2, No. 3, and No. 4. (Photo courtesy of Hosmer-Dorrance Company.)

come in a variety of sizes (Dorrance #2, #3, and #4) and are extremely functional (Fig. 22-9). Hands are considerably heavier than hooks and their weight is disadvantageously positioned at the end of the prosthetic lever arm. This may prevent use of a hand in short below-elbow amputations and in higher level amputations where available forces for elbow flexion are minimal. Furthermore, the high initial cost of the hand, the most costly maintenance, and the necessity for frequent replacement of the cosmetic glove are economic deterrents to use of the hand in cases where funds are limited. Quite often, however, the psychological benefits of wearing a prosthetic hand outweigh the economic considerations and some of the minor functional deficiencies of the devices.

Prosthetic wrist units are usually of the manually controlled friction variety and provide passive substitution for pronation and supination in the prosthesis. Oval wrist units are cosmetically more pleasing than the standard round units. In the infant the

CAPP wrist unit constructed of Delrin plastic has the advantage of lightness. Wrist flexion units should be considered in bilateral upper limb amputees to provide better prosthetic function for activities close to the face. Younger amputees will rarely use the flexion feature, however.

Elbow hinges are used with most types of prostheses for amputations distal to the elbow. The hinges are part of the suspension system, attaching to a triceps pad or half cuff. Flexible hinges are used in almost all cases to take advantage of any residual pronation and supination in the stump. Wrist disarticulation amputees retain 100 per cent of pronation and supination unless the distal radioulnar joint has been damaged. Patients with shorter amputation levels retain progressively less pronation and supination. Whatever the level, only 50 per cent or less of the available stump pronation and supination is actually transmitted through the prosthesis. In some infants, in very short stumps, and in certain older children using

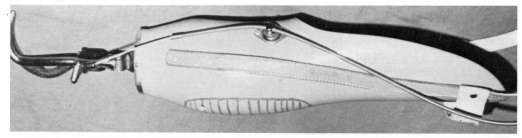

FIG. 22-10. The lined area on this wrist-disarticulation prosthesis indicates the channel fabricated for the distal ulna. This allows the bulbus end of the amputation stump to enter this socket more easily.

their prostheses for heavy lifting, rigid elbow hinges may be more effective for prosthetic suspension.

Outside elbow-locking mechanisms are used for the elbow disarticulation amputee where humeral rotation is readily transmitted through the socket and where length is a significant consideration. In the above-elbow and shoulder disarticulation amputee a more sturdy inside elbow-locking mechanism is used with a manually controlled turntable, which provides passive substitution for humeral rotation.

A variety of passive prosthetic shoulder joints is available for the shoulder-disarticulation-type amputation and the forequarter amputation, each with its advantages and disadvantages. Newer research models have been introduced that incorporate universal or flexion-abduction joints.

Harnessing provides suspension of the prosthesis and, combined with the Bowden cable system, utilizes body motion for terminal device and elbow operation and for control of the elbow-lock mechanism. A figure-of-eight harness is most often employed with both above- and below-elbow prostheses, but a shoulder saddle and chest strap may be required in patients who have skin problems or who for other reasons cannot comfortably wear a figure-of-eight harness. Harnessing for shoulder disarticulation and forequarter prostheses is highly individualized. Body-powered prostheses for these higher amputation levels are inefficient and externally powered prostheses are highly desirable for such patients. (Externally powered prostheses are discussed in detail in the section on congenital limb

deficiencies). Teflon lining is frequently used in the cable housing to diminish friction and increase the longevity of the cable. This is especially beneficial to small children and high level amputees.

The following are brief descriptions of the various prostheses used for the major levels of upper limb amputations in children:

Wrist Disarticulation. The double wall socket of this prosthesis is fabricated with a channel for the distal ulna in order to allow the bulbous end of the stump to enter the socket more readily (Fig. 22-10). Flexible elbow hinges are necessary to take advantage of the full pronation and supination normally present in these stumps. Harnessing is by means of a standard below-elbow figure-of-eight harness with a single-control Bowden cable.

Below-Elbow Amputations. Long and medium length stumps are fitted with a socket of standard double-wall construction with slight preflexion of the socket. Short stumps and especially very short below-elbow stumps present problems of socket suspension and retention of the stump in the socket when the elbow is flexed above 90°. These stumps are fitted in one of three ways, the most standard of which is with a markedly preflexed socket, the so-called banana arm. This allows positioning of the terminal device near the face with only limited elbow flexion, but is cosmetically objectionable to some. A second choice is to use a split socket with step-up hinges (Fig. 22-11). These hinges provide approximately 10° of forearm flexion for each 5° of stump flexion. Durability of these joints is poor and live lift is markedly decreased. This type of fitting is used

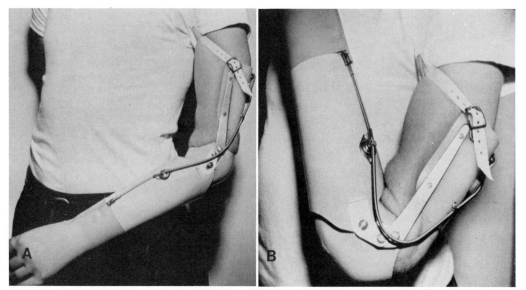

FIG. 22-11. *(A)* The split-socket prosthesis is designed for the very short below-elbow amputation. *(B)* Step-up elbow hinges provide 10° of forearm flexion for each 5° of stump flexion. (From The child with an acquired amputation, with the permission of the National Academy of Sciences, Washington, D.C.)

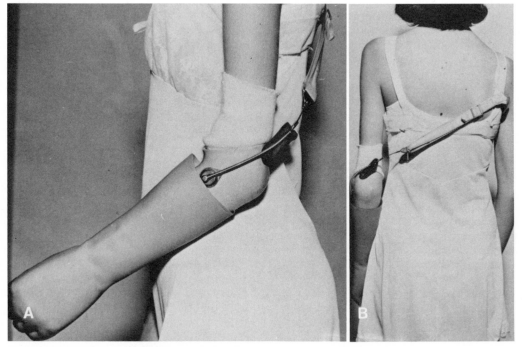

FIG. 22-12. *(A)* The modified Muenster prosthesis incorporates a self-suspending socket for the very short below-elbow amputation stump. *(B)* Harnessing for the Muenster prosthesis is of the simplified "figure-of-nine" variety. (From The child with an acquired amputation, with the permission of the National Academy of Sciences, Washington, D.C.)

primarily in bilateral cases. Standard below-elbow figure-of-eight harnessing is used with both of the above fittings. The third choice is the highly successful modified Muenster prosthesis.[51, 61] This design originated with Drs. Hepp and Kuhn in Muenster, Germany, and consists of a self-suspending socket fitted with the elbow in 35° of flexion (Fig. 22-12). Further flexion is possible to only 90 or 100°. The excellent cosmesis plus the outstanding live lift and axial loading capabilities provided by this prosthesis have made it quite successful in many clinics.[47, 57] A further advantage is harnessing with a solitary axillary loop, the so-called figure-of-nine harness. The primary disadvantage of the Muenster prosthesis is limted elbow flexion, which precludes its use in bilateral cases. Neither the snug fit of this socket in the growing child nor excessive clothing wear because of the low takeoff of the terminal device control cable has been a significant problem in our personal series of Muenster fittings, but these have been reported as troublesome problems in some clinics.[56, 133]

Elbow Disarticulation. The socket is constructed with a large anterior biceps window to allow easier insertion of the bulbous stump end, and the entire trim line of the socket brim is level with the axilla (Fig. 22-13). These modifications from the standard fitting allow for growth accommodation, provide better ventilation, and make the prosthesis more easily donned and doffed. An outside elbow lock must be used at this level. Harnessing is with a standard *below-elbow* figure-of-eight harness to which is attached an elbow-lock control strap. A standard *above-elbow* dual control Bowden cable provides elbow flexion and terminal device operation.

Above-Elbow Amputations. The socket is of standard double-wall construction with a standard trimline. An inside elbow joint is used. A standard above-elbow figure-of-eight harness with a dual control Bowden cable is the harness of choice (Fig. 22-14). An across-the-back strap is used almost routinely to take advantage of biscapular motion as well as humeral flexion in the control system and to prevent upward sliding of the control attachment straps. In attaching the cable, the location and length of the forearm lift loop must be varied to coincide with the size of the child for maximum efficiency. For short stumps, the use of anterior and posterior wings on the socket enhances rotational stability, and a spring-lift assist for the forearm is advantageous.

Shoulder Disarticulation. The distal portions of this prosthesis are the same as those used for the above-elbow amputee. The humeral section is flattened on the medial side to allow room for bulky clothing in cold weather. Selection of the shoulder joint is variable, but we have used the passive abduction joint most often (Fig. 22-15). Harnessing for body powered prostheses is the greatest problem at this level and, where available, external power is preferable. When body power is used, harnessing must be individualized and must take into account both the excursion and force that can be generated by a specific control motion. In larger children, the control motion for elbow flexion and terminal device operation is scapular abduction with chest strap suspension. Elbow-lock control is usually achieved by means of shoulder elevation, with the anchor point for the control strap being a waist belt. In younger children, because of limited excursion in scapular abduction, shoulder elevation is normally used as the control motion for elbow flexion and terminal device operation, the anchor point being provided by a perineal strap. With this system, trunk rotation is usually used for elbow-lock control motion. As one may well imagine, body gyration is often quite marked in using a body powered prosthesis at this amputation level, and prosthetic rejection and non-use is frequent. Externally powered prostheses, as will be discussed in the section on congenital limb deficiencies, have done much to improve prosthetic function and acceptance at this level of limb loss.

Forequarter Amputations. All components in the prosthesis for this level of amputation are the same as those used in the shoulder disarticulation prosthesis up to the socket. Socket suspension may be difficult and often requires an extension of the socket behind the neck and over the opposite shoulder (Fig. 22-16). Effective control motions of sufficient force and excursion are extremely difficult to find in children, and truly func-

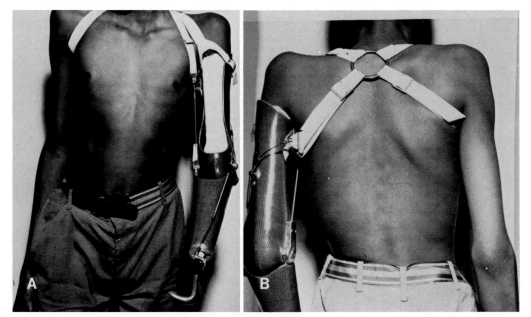

FIG. 22-13. (A) The elbow disarticulation prosthesis incorporates a large anterior biceps window to allow easy insertion of the bulbus stump. (B) An outside elbow lock is placed on the medial side of the socket at the elbow joint level and harnessing is of the "figure-of-eight" variety. (From The child with an acquired amputation, with the permission of the National Academy of Sciences, Washington, D.C.)

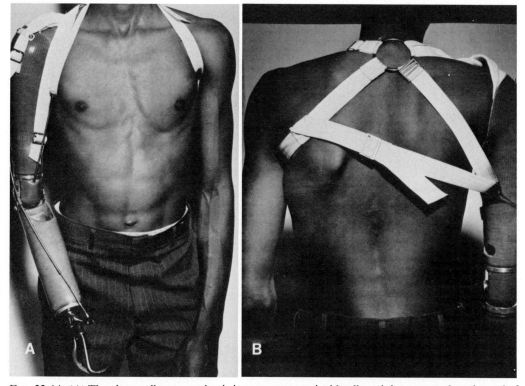

FIG. 22-14. (A) The above-elbow prosthesis incorporates an inside elbow joint mounted on the end of the socket by means of a turntable, which provides substitution for humeral rotation. (B) Harnessing is of the above-elbow "figure-of-eight" type with an across-the-back strap to take advantage of bis-capular motion as well as humeral flexion in the control system. (From The child with an acquired amputation, with the permission of the National Academy of Sciences, Washington, D.C.)

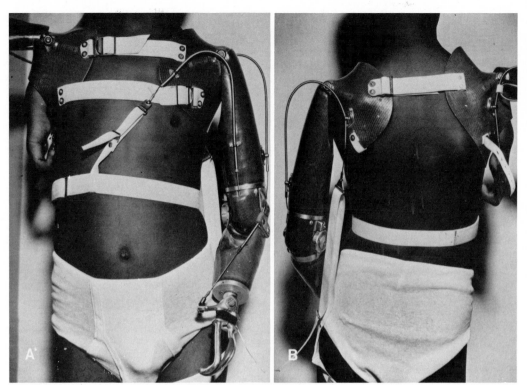

FIG. 22-15. *(A)* This young boy is fitted with a fairly typical shoulder disarticulation prosthesis on the left side. The inside elbow lock is controlled by means of a waist band. *(B)* Elbow flexion and terminal device operation are provided by shoulder elevation with the central strap being anchored to a perineal loop. Body powered prostheses for this level of amputation necessitate a great deal of body gyration in order to achieve the desired prosthetic function. (From The child with an acquired amputation, with the permission of the National Academy of Sciences, Washington, D.C.)

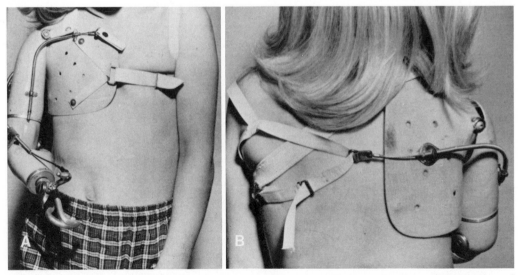

FIG. 22-16. *(A)* Elbow-lock control in this forequarter prosthesis is by means of a pull strap activated by the opposite hand or the mouth. *(B)* Elbow flexion and terminal device operation are achieved by harnessing the opposite shoulder for control motion. (From The child with an acquired amputation, with the permission of the National Academy of Sciences, Washington, D.C.)

tional operation requires the use of external power. Terminal device operation and elbow flexion of a limited degree can be obtained by harnessing the opposite shoulder for control motion. Elbow-lock control is achieved by using chin nudges or mouth straps.

Lower Limb Prosthetic Fitting

In the lower limb, as in the upper limb, prosthetic fitting and training should be coordinated with the normal development of motor skills in the growing child.[10, 11, 12, 32, 48] The average infant develops sitting balance at approximately 6 months of age and begins crawling on all fours at about the same time. Between 8 and 12 months of age he learns to pull himself up and stand with support. Independent ambulation is usually achieved at approximately 12 months of age. Initial ambulation is carried out with the feet widely spread to achieve a more stable base of support, the lower limbs are usually externally rotated at the hip to enhance knee stability (by rotating the knee axis of motion away from the line of progression), and the arms are typically held away from the trunk to enhance balance. With continuing neuromuscular maturation the child's gait progressively improves, but it is not until approximately 5 years that his gait really reaches the heel-strike, mid-stance, and toe-off gait typical of the adult.

From the foregoing synopsis of lower limb functional development it is evident that lower limb prosthetic fitting need not be attempted until the child amputee begins pulling himself up to the erect position between 8 and 12 months of age. It is only at this point that having two lower limbs of equal length becomes necessary. In bilateral lower limb deficiencies the age of fitting will be a more arbitrary decision based on the time when a normal child would be expected to stand. In the above-knee amputee, stabilizing the prosthetic knee by means of locking mechanisms will be necessary until the child demonstrates adequate control of the prosthetic knee joint. Knee stability is conveniently obtained by attaching an adjustable strap-and-buckle device across the anterior aspect of the knee joint. Finally, it should be obvious that very young lower limb amputees cannot be expected to walk with the normal heel-strike, mid-stance, toe-off gait seen in older amputees, and training efforts expended to achieve this type of prosthetic gait prior to age 5 or 6 years will be fruitless.

The normal human lower limb is designed to provide weightbearing stability and locomotion. In the prosthetic lower limb, stance phase stability is achieved by proper prosthetic alignment and locomotion is attained by proper sequential body and stump motion acting on prosthetic levers and joints.[10] The young child is not concerned with the appearance of his gait, but only with progression from one point to another with the greatest expediency. Children will walk in some manner with the most malaligned and malfunctioning prostheses imaginable, provided there is minimal stability and adequate suspension. Judicious selection of prosthetic components, skillful prosthetic fabrication, and intelligent training combined with frequent follow-up by all members of the clinic team are necessary to achieve excellent prosthetic gait in the child.

The following are brief descriptions of the various prostheses used for the major levels of lower limb amputations in children:

Syme's-Type Ankle Disarticulation. This level of amputation is a true ankle disarticulation combined with a Syme's-type soft-tissue closure.[38, 70, 120] This provides an end-bearing stump and yet preserves epiphyses and avoids bone transection. In young children the stump is not often bulbous and with growth of the child the malleoli atrophy and an excellent cosmetic prosthesis can be fabricated.[3, 53, 100] In such instances, a hard (unlined) plastic laminate socket comparable to a long below-knee (BK) socket is used, incorporating end-bearing features and utilizing supracondylar strap suspension (Fig. 22-17A). A solid ankle-cushion heel (SACH) prosthetic foot is used at this level, as it is for almost all lower limb amputation levels in the child. In older children, fitting with either an expandable socket or a socket with a removable medial window may be necessary to accomodate bulbous distal ends (Fig. 22-17B). These sockets are usually self-suspending.

Below-Knee Amputations. The patellar

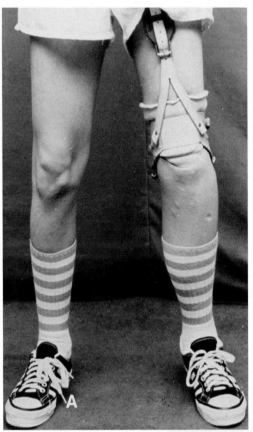

Fig. 22-17. *(A)* A cosmetically acceptable Syme prosthesis can be fabricated after the bulbus stump end has atrophied with growth of the child. *(B)* In most instances the Syme prosthesis will have a medial opening window to allow entrance of the bulbus distal end of the stump into the prosthetic socket.

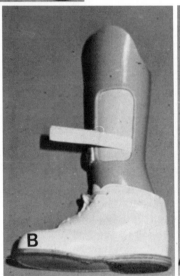
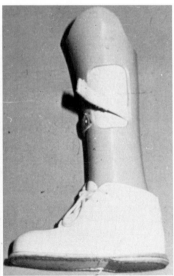

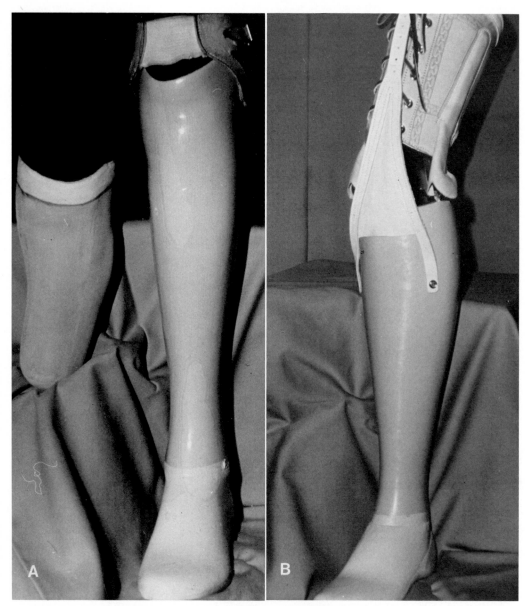

FIG. 22-18. (A) The patellar tendon-bearing (PTB) prosthesis is standard for the below-knee amputation and may be unlined or may incorporate a soft insert. (B) Side joints and a thigh corset added to the PTB prosthesis provide additional stability for very short or extremely tapered stumps or for those individuals with ligamentous laxity of the knee.

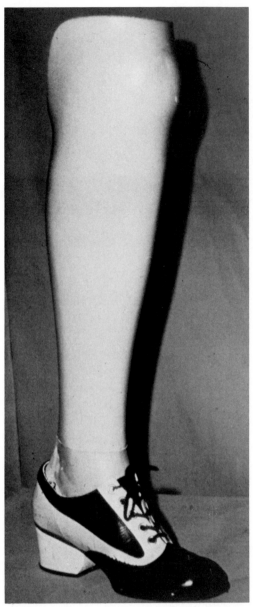

with ligamentous laxity of the knee, or markedly scarred stumps (Fig. 22-18B). The so-called PTB variants are often helpful in the prosthetic management of certain stump problems, or may be preferred by the older child for cosmetic reasons or by virtue of their self-suspending characteristics. Where mediolateral socket instability from a variety of causes is a problem, or where there is genu recurvatum, the patellar tendon-supracondylar (PTS) prosthesis is valuable (Fig. 22-19). The cosmesis of this prosthesis is excellent when the amputee is standing, but there is often an objectionable anterior gap between socket and stump when the amputee is seated. This has been a cause for rejection of this type of fitting in a number of patients. The supracondylar wedge (of several varieties) method of suspension provides good cosmesis and suspension plus mediolateral socket stability for the older amputee with minimal stump changes due to growth (Fig. 22-20).

Knee Disarticulation. The bulbous stump produced by amputation at this level in the older child and adult is not so pronounced in the very young child, and the condyles tend to atrophy with age, as mentioned with the Syme's-type ankle disarticulation. Younger children can usually be fitted with a solid plastic socket of either quadrilateral contour or "plug-fit," incorporating end-bearing (Fig. 22-21) Supplementary suspension with a Silesian belt may be necessary where the femoral condyles are quite atrophic. Outside knee joints must be used at this level, precluding the advantage of swing phase frictional knee control. In the older child with prominent condyles the socket may incorporate a removable panel or leather lacer opening to permit donning and doffing, or an expandable socket may be utilized in some cases. The four-bar linkage knee (Fig. 22-22) may be used in larger children, and it does

tendon-bearing (PTB) prosthesis is the standard prosthesis for this amputation level (Fig. 22-18A). The hard socket is generally preferred, but soft inserts may be used if desired. A SACH foot is standard and suspension is achieved by a supracondylar strap. Side joints and leather thigh lacers may occasionally be indicated for infants, very short or extremely tapered stumps, patients

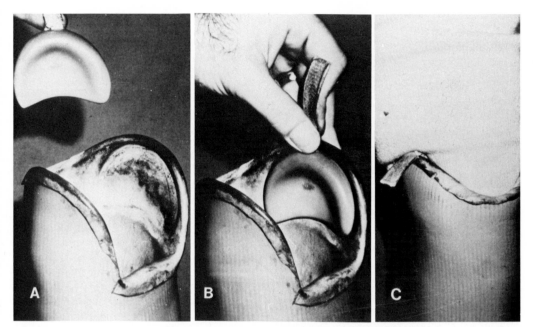

FIG. 22-20. *(A)* Suspension of the below-knee prosthesis may be accomplished by means of a removable wedge. *(B)* This wedge fits into a recess fabricated in the medial brim of the socket. *(C)* When in place, the wedge fits snugly over the medial epicondyle of the femur and provides stable suspension and excellent cosmesis.

allow swing phase frictional or hydraulic knee control while properly positioning the knee axis of rotation in relation to the sound limb. A SACH foot is used with all knee disarticulation prostheses.

Above-Knee Amputations. The prosthetic socket used for the above-knee amputation is of total contact plastic laminate, and is quadrilateral in contour. An inside knee mechanism of the single axis, constant friction variety is standard in younger children (Fig. 22-23). In the infant, knee stability should be provided by a locking mechanism until the child demonstrates adequate control of the prosthetic knee. This is best accomplished by means of a strap-and-buckle device attached across the anterior aspect of the prosthetic knee joint. Gradual loosening of this device allows progressive knee flexion at the discretion of the therapist as the child develops knee control. The very active teenager may utilize a hydraulic or pneumatic swing phase knee control sufficiently well to justify the cost of this component. Prosthetic suspension is most often achieved by a Silesian bandage or by a hip joint with pelvic belt in the younger child. Suction suspension can be successfully incorporated into the prosthesis when the child is old enough to independently don and doff the prosthesis, and it affords benefits of secure suspension and increased cosmesis. A SACH foot is prescribed for above-knee amputees unless the additional knee stability afforded by an articulated wooden foot is needed with extremely short stumps.

Hip Disarticulation. Prosthetic components at this level are the same as those used in the above-knee prosthesis except, of course, for a thigh section used in lieu of the AK socket. The socket is a plastic laminate pelvic "bucket" encasing the amputated side and extending around the pelvis on the sound side. Front opening with Velcro closures is provided for easy donning and doffing (Fig. 22-24). The hip joint is placed inferior and anterior to the axis of rotation of the anatomical hip joint to provide excellent prosthetic stability in mid-stance. SACH feet are usually used in children, but an ar-

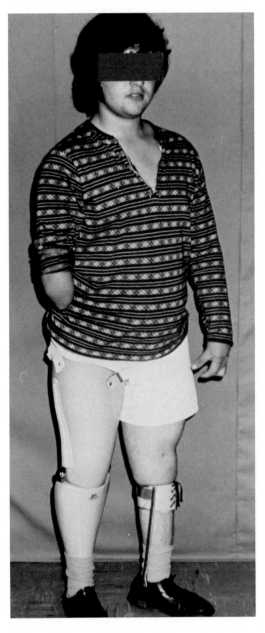

ticulated wooden foot may be selected to enhance knee stability.

Hemipelvectomy. The prosthesis used at this level is identical to the hip disarticulation prosthesis, with appropriate modifications made in the socket to accomodate the anatomical loss.

FIG. 22-21. The older child with a knee disarticulation can often be fit with a solid plastic laminate socket, since the femoral condyles tend to atrophy with age. This end-bearing prosthesis is suspended by means of a Silesian belt.

Immediate Postsurgical Prosthetic Fitting

The technique of immediate postsurgical prosthetic fitting is as applicable for the juvenile amputee as it is for the adult.[28, 32, 139, 141] Rapid stump maturation, early ambulation and resumption of normal activities, and a diminution of the psychological impact of limb loss are highly desirable benefits accrued by children from this technique. The only significant problem which has been observed in our experience is the tendency for the young child to attempt unprotected weightbearing too early. Appropriate supervision of ambulation and proper gait training will minimize this problem. It has been frequently reported that the very young child will often not fully appreciate the loss of a limb until the time of first cast change.

LIMB LOSS FROM MALIGNANCY

A separate section on prosthetic fitting following limb loss from malignancy seems appropriate in order to strongly emphasize the need to proceed promptly with prosthetic care in these children. In the past, the prevalent attitude of both physicians and lay administrators of state-sponsored crippled children's services was to delay prosthetic fitting of such children for 12 to 18 months in order to minimize the cost of fitting prostheses on children who would die from early metastases and not utilize them. Since most amputations for malignancy are in the lower limb, failure to provide prompt prosthetic substitution condemns the unfortunate victim to a level of limited ambulation and prevents resumption of normal school, social, and recreational activities at a time when the psychological benefit of these normal activities is so badly needed.

During the past decade a number of reports in the literature has shown conclusively that at least two-thirds of patients with limb loss from malignancy will use their

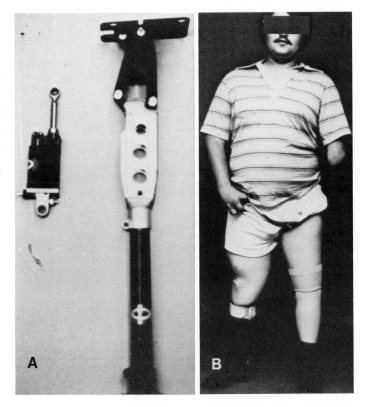

FIG. 22-22. *(A)* The four-bar linkage prosthetic knee allows incorporation of swing phase control of the knee while properly positioning the knee axis of rotation in relation to the sound limb. *(B)* Cosmesis is achieved by placing a foam rubber covering over the endoskeletal knee mechanism and shank.

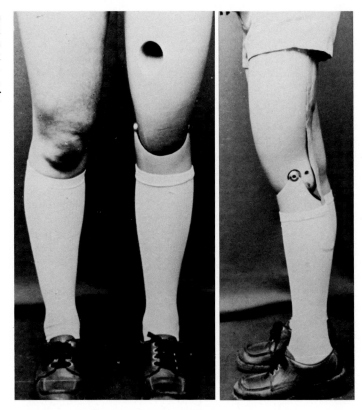

FIG. 22-23. The above-knee prosthesis has a quadrilateral socket and an inside knee joint, which provides constant or variable swing phase control. In this prosthesis suspension is provided by means of suction.

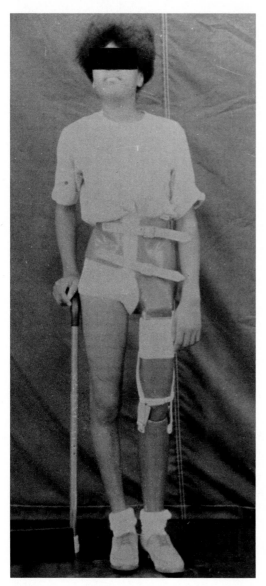

FIG. 22-24. The socket of the hip disarticulation prosthesis encases the amputated side and extends around the pelvis on the sound side. The hip joint is located inferior and anterior to the axis of rotation of the anatomical hip joint in order to provide stance phase stability.

findings and responded appropriately by authorizing early prosthetic fitting for children with limb loss due to malignancy, and the benefits have been apparent. However, there are still too many states which forbid early prosthetic care of these children. Our efforts to change these regulations must not cease until there is universal agreement to permit early prosthetic fitting if there is no evidence of metastasis and if the stump is suitable for fitting.

CONGENITAL LIMB DEFICIENCIES

Numerous surveys of the child amputee population have indicated that congenital limb deficiencies account for a larger percentage of children with limb loss than do acquired amputations. As mentioned earlier, for a number of years the relative frequency in new patients seen in a nationwide network of cooperative child amputee clinics has been reported as approximately 60 per cent congenital and 40 per cent acquired.

In contrast to acquired childhood amputations, congenital limb deficiencies occur with almost equal frequency in males and females, and the upper limb is involved twice as often as the lower limb.[1, 79] Multiple limb involvement occurs in approximately 30 per cent of children with congenital limb deficiency, compared to 10 per cent of children with acquired amputations: bimembral involvement in 15 per cent, trimembral in 5 per cent, and quadrimembral in 10 per cent.

prostheses for a year or longer if prompt early fitting is employed.[5, 102, 161] Early results of new chemotherapeutic programs for malignant bone tumors indicate a marked improvement in survival rates for these lesions.[116, 135, 166] The widespread use of immediate postsurgical prosthetic fitting coupled with early definitive prosthetic fitting in children is of proven psychological and functional benefit. Many physicians and lay administrators have heeded these newer

ETIOLOGY

In order to comprehend the various theories concerning the production of skeletal limb deficiencies it is necessary to have an understanding of the normal embryologic development of the human limb.[16, 62, 123, 131, 143] At 4 postovulatory weeks the origins of the upper and lower limbs can be detected on the lateral body wall of the growing embryo as small buds of mesenchymal tissue. During the next 3 weeks these limb buds grow larger and differentiate into the distinctly identifiable limb segments of arm, forearm, and hand in the upper limb buds, and thigh, leg, and foot in the lower limb buds. The development of the various limb segments is in a proximodistal sequence, so that the arm and thigh appear before the forearm and leg, which in turn appear before the hand and foot. The mesenchymal tissue within the limb buds condenses into detectable skeletal elements which then chondrify and become cartilaginous models of individual bones. Ossification of these cartilaginous models rapidly follows in a regular sequence. Clefts occur in the cartilaginous skeleton and, with further cavitation, differentiate into articulations or joints. By 7 postovulatory weeks the embryonic skeleton is well formed and is a readily recognizable replica of the postnatal skeleton. From the foregoing it is apparent that, regardless of the nature of the factors responsible for congenital limb deficiencies, they must act upon the differentiating embryo some time between the third and the seventh postovulatory week.

Numerous theories concerning the mechanism of production of congenital defects have been proposed and a veritable host of environmental factors capable of producing such defects has been identified, both experimentally and clinically.[33, 43, 44] To review such material is beyond the scope of this discussion. Suffice it to say that most theories indicate either a mechanism responsible for an arrest in the development of the embryonic limb or some form of destructive process of structures already formed. Such mechanisms or processes must act upon the embryo during narrowly defined time limits, as noted above.

CLASSIFICATION

Beginning as early as 1837 Saint-Hilaire devised a classification of skeletal limb deficiencies and in the subsequent literature on embryology many others have been recorded. The terms used in these classifications were cumbersome and unwieldly and lent themselves very poorly to clinical application in orthopaedic surgery. It was not until 1951 when O'Rahilly[129] identified a consistent morphologic pattern in skeletal limb deficiencies that a clinically functional classification of these defects was devised. This classification was further expanded in the classic publication by Frantz and O'Rahilly in 1961[54] and has remained the most widely used classification in the United States for skeletal limb deficiencies. The Frantz and O'Rahilly classification will be used in this chapter. In this classification only *absent* skeletal parts are described. Deficiencies are divided into two major types: (1) *terminal,* where there are no unaffected parts distal to and in line with the deficient portion, and (2) *intercalary,* where the middle part of a limb component is deficient but those portions proximal and distal to it are present. Each of these main groups is in turn divided into two groups: (1) *transverse,* where the defect extends transversely across the entire width of the limb, or (2) *longitudinal* (paraxial), where only the preaxial or postaxial portion of the limb component is absent.

Terminology used to describe the various anomalies employs seven terms of Greek derivation, three based on the word *melos* (limb) combined with familiar medical prefixes: *amelia* refers to complete absence of a limb, *hemimelia* (literally "half a limb") refers to absence of the major portion of a limb, and *phocomelia* (seal-limb) exists when the terminal portion of a limb (hand or foot) is attached more or less directly to the trunk in a foreshortened manner. The remaining four terms are *acheiria* (absent hand), *apodia* (absent foot), *adactylia* (absent digit), and *aphalangia* (absent phalanx).

Hemimelia is further subdivided into *complete hemimelia,* where the entire distal half of a limb is absent; *incomplete hemimelia,* where the greater portion of the distal half of a limb is absent; and *paraxial hemimelia,* where the preaxial or postaxial portion of the distal half of a limb is absent. Paraxial hemimelia may be either terminal or intercalary. (Figure 22-25 illustrates the Frantz-O'Rahilly classification of congenital limb deficiencies.)

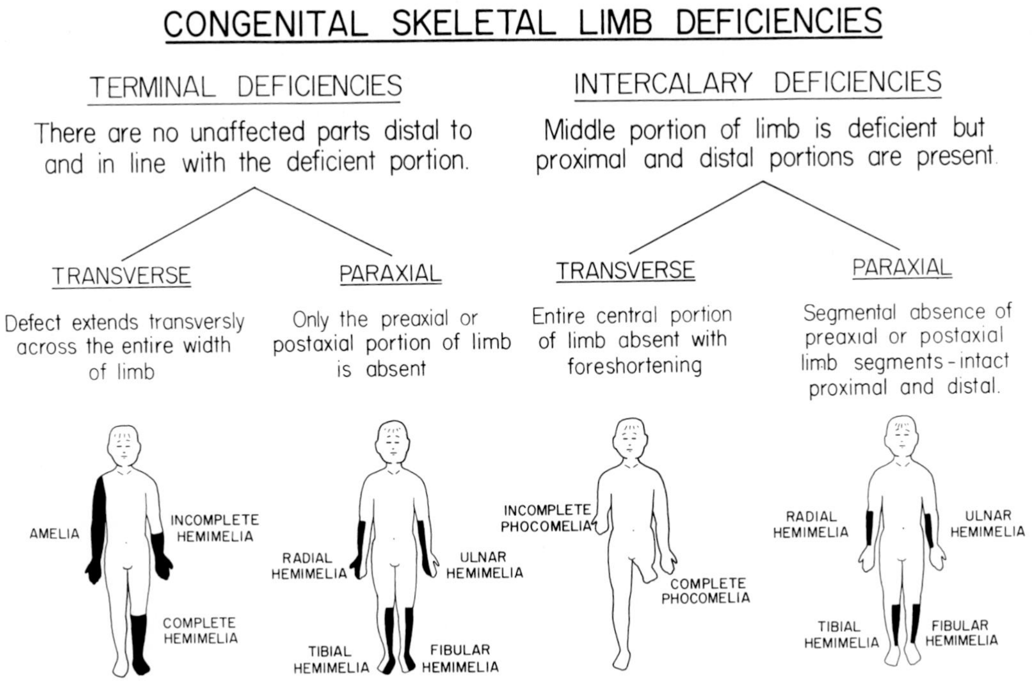

CONGENITAL SKELETAL LIMB DEFICIENCIES

TERMINAL DEFICIENCIES

There are no unaffected parts distal to and in line with the deficient portion.

TRANSVERSE

Defect extends transversly across the entire width of limb

PARAXIAL

Only the preaxial or postaxial portion of limb is absent

INTERCALARY DEFICIENCIES

Middle portion of limb is deficient but proximal and distal portions are present.

TRANSVERSE

Entire central portion of limb absent with foreshortening

PARAXIAL

Segmental absence of preaxial or postaxial limb segments - intact proximal and distal.

AMELIA

INCOMPLETE HEMIMELIA

RADIAL HEMIMELIA

ULNAR HEMIMELIA

COMPLETE HEMIMELIA

TIBIAL HEMIMELIA

FIBULAR HEMIMELIA

INCOMPLETE PHOCOMELIA

COMPLETE PHOCOMELIA

RADIAL HEMIMELIA

ULNAR HEMIMELIA

TIBIAL HEMIMELIA

FIBULAR HEMIMELIA

FIG. 22-25. The Frantz-O'Rahilly classification of congenital limb deficiencies. (Redrawn from Hall, C. B., Brooks, M. B., and Dennis, J. F.: Congenital skeletal deficiencies of the extremities. Classification and fundamentals of treatment. JAMA, *181*:590–599, 1962.)

Approximately 85 per cent of congenital limb deficiencies can be easily and accurately classified by the Frantz and O'Rahilly method.[130] However, the European orthopaedic community has evolved yet another classification,[74] and there have been several modifications of the Frantz and O'Rahilly classification in the United States.[21, 29, 63] Most recently, the International Society of Prosthetics and Orthotics sponsored a new classification based on the Frantz and O'Rahilly system which will hopefully be acceptable to both United States and European clinicians.[79, 80]

MEDICAL MANAGEMENT

In addition to the high incidence of multimembral involvement, children with congenital limb deficiencies also have a high incidence of associated congenital defects of other organ systems, such as genitourinary anomalies, cardiac defects, and cleft palate. All these children should have a complete medical evaluation to detect and treat such lesions. Musculoskeletal problems other than skeletal limb deficiencies may occur, which can alter medical and prosthetic management. One such problem is radial head dislocation, which is seen in a high percentage of children with transverse partial hemimelia of the upper limb.[94, 160] Another is idiopathic scoliosis, which has been reported in as many as 48 per cent of children with upper limb deficiencies and which is apparently unrelated to either prosthetic use or nonuse.[45, 68, 104, 115] The presence or potential development of such associated medical problems mandates clinicians to possess the knowledge that such associated conditions may occur and to maintain a continuing high index of suspicion to detect them.

Since terminal transverse deficiencies are really homologues of acquired amputations[2] and are generally treated as such,[92, 159] the medical and prosthetic management of these deficiencies will not be discussed, except for bilateral amelia. This section will deal primarily with terminal paraxial hemimelia, intercalary paraxial hemimelia, and phocomelia.

Aitken[10] has enumerated the biomechanical losses occurring in intercalary and terminal paraxial lower limb deficiencies as: (1) limb length inequality, (2) malrotation, (3) inadequate proximal musculature, and (4) unstable proximal joints. In upper limb deficiencies the same biomechanical losses are present, plus varying degrees of loss of prehension. An analysis of such deformities reveals that each deformity can be envisioned as a homologue of an acquired amputation. By determining the most distal stable joint beyond which there is adequate tissue to function as an amputation stump one may then determine the proper prosthetic fitting level (i.e., below-knee, above-knee, below-elbow, etc.). At this point a decision must be made to either proceed with prosthetic fitting, as determined above, or to perform a surgical conversion to provide a better stump and enhance prosthetic fitting. Prostheses used for anomalous limbs must often be quite atypical and frequently present problems in fabrication and in function.

SURGICAL MANAGEMENT

Surgical conversions of anomalous limbs are performed as either primary or secondary procedures.[10] Primary conversions are done in limb deficiencies whose life history is so well known that one can predict that a conversion will eventually become necessary. Secondary conversions are those performed after a period of prosthetic fitting around the deformity has proved that a conversion will undoubtedly provide better prosthetic use and overall function. Aitken feels that there are no indications for primary conversion in upper limb deficiencies, and has found that only 8 to 10 per cent of these cases need secondary conversion. However, in lower limb deficiencies there are definite indications for primary conversion, and slightly over half of these cases require either primary or secondary conversion. A clear understanding of this treatment philosophy will eliminate many frustrating uncertainties when the clinician is confronted with formulating a treatment program for the unusual and ofttimes bizarre congenital skeletal limb deficiencies.

UPPER LIMB DEFICIENCIES

Paraxial Radial Hemimelia

Radial hemimelia is second only to fibular hemimelia in frequency of occurence among congenital deficiencies of the long bones.[129] However, the condition is not often seen as a primary or solitary presenting problem in child amputee clinics because this skeletal limb deficiency is basically treated as a surgical problem rather than as a condition requiring prosthetic restoration. Furthermore, even untreated cases can develop a high degree of independent function. Nonetheless, the nature of the problem and its relative frequency appear to justify its inclusion in this section.

Radial hemimelia (often referred to as radial club hand) is characterized by radial deviation of the hand, marked shortening of the forearm, and a generalized underdevelopment of the limb.[136] The ulna is usually bowed with the concave side toward the radial side of the forearm (Fig. 22-26). Absence or abnormality of muscles, tendons, nerves, and blood vessels of the forearm are common.[152] There is often atrophy or absence of shoulder girdle muscles and the scapula and clavicle may be hypoplastic. The humerus is often short and either end may be deformed. The hand almost always exhibits absence of the thumb and first metacarpal, and the radial portion of the carpus is usually absent. The radius is completely absent in over 50 per cent of cases, but the proximal portion (and occasionally the distal portion) may be present. Over half the cases are bilateral.

Suggested treatment has varied from no treatment at all or simple casting to correct the hand deformity, to very aggressive surgical programs.[40, 52, 59, 78, 132, 136, 137] The most widely accepted treatment program at present consists of casting very early in infancy to stretch the soft tissues on the ulnar side of the wrist, followed by soft-tissue surgical releases on both the radial and ulnar sides of the wrist. A second surgical procedure is then done to centralize the carpus

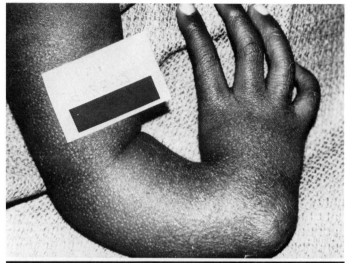

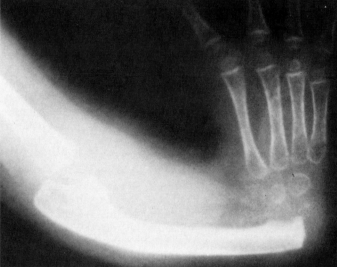

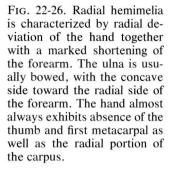

Fɪɢ. 22-26. Radial hemimelia is characterized by radial deviation of the hand together with a marked shortening of the forearm. The ulna is usually bowed, with the concave side toward the radial side of the forearm. The hand almost always exhibits absence of the thumb and first metacarpal as well as the radial portion of the carpus.

over the distal end of the radius, utilizing temporary internal fixation with Kirschner wires, followed by casting or bracing until skeletal growth is complete. Most authors also advocate tendon transfers at the wrist to provide dynamic stabilization of the hand, and osteotomy of the ulna, if indicated.[19, 22, 154] All authors emphasize that good elbow motion and satisfactory hand function are prerequisites for surgery. In bilateral cases, the ability of the child to get his hand to his mouth following surgery is of prime importance. If this cannot be accomplished, then surgery should not be done.

Paraxial Ulnar Hemimelia

Ulnar hemimelia is the second rarest type of congenital deficiency of a long bone, the rarest type being an isolated complete deficiency of the humerus (proximal phocomelia).[105, 129] The majority of cases is unilateral, and males are involved twice as often as females. Because this deficiency presents as either a terminal or an intercalary deficiency and may be partial or complete, the clinical appearance of the limb is markedly variable.[55] The hand may have five digits, but most commonly the two ulnar rays are absent. A monodigital hand is the

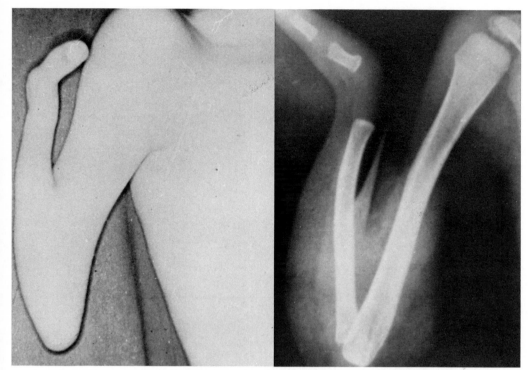

Fig. 22-27. In ulnar hemimelia the hand is frequently monodigital and, in this instance, there is a severe flexion contracture of the elbow with marked soft-tissue webbing in the antecubital area.

second most common hand deformity (Fig. 22-27). Partial deficiency of the ulna is more common than complete absence, and when incomplete the proximal remnant is usually late in ossifying. In such cases, early roentgenograms may give rise to a false diagnosis of a complete deficiency.[105] At the elbow, the proximal radius may articulate with the capitellum in a normal manner, the radiohumeral joint may be fused, or the radial head may be completely dislocated. The position of the elbow varies from fusion in full extension to a severe flexion contracture, accompanied by marked soft-tissue webbing in the antecubital area. Weakness and atrophy of the proximal arm and shoulder girdle musculature is common.

Treatment for ulnar hemimelia will obviously vary with the clinical picture presented.[55, 154] Most patients can be managed without surgery and some without any form of prosthetic fitting. Prime considerations in designing a treatment program for children with this condition are the presence of bilat-

eral involvement, the range of elbow motion, the number of digits present, and their prehensile capacity. If elbow motion of at least 90° of extension is present, fitting with a standard below-elbow prosthesis will provide prehension and equalize limb lengths. In the presence of severe antecubital soft-tissue webbing, experience has shown that surgical release of the soft tissues is ineffective in achieving functional elbow extension.[10] In such cases, where the elbow is severely flexed, the limb may be fitted prosthetically as an elbow disarticulation with the flexed forearm segment and the humerus encased within the socket and the digit or digits present used to control the elbow lock. If there is insufficient force or excursion in the digit to control the elbow lock, surgical conversion to an elbow disarticulation followed by appropriate prosthetic fitting may provide better function and cosmesis than any atypical prosthetic fitting (Fig. 22-28). In cases where the elbow is fused in extension, there are reports of per-

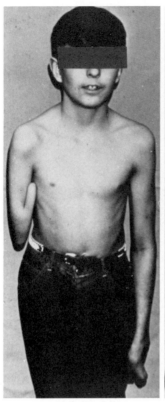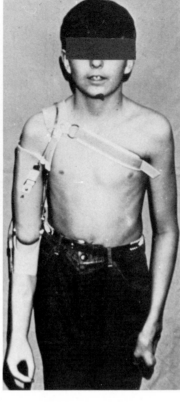

FIG. 22-28. In those instances of ulnar hemimelia with a nonfunctional monodigital hand and severe flexion contracture at the elbow, surgical conversion to an elbow disarticulation followed by appropriate prosthetic fitting may be appropriate.

forming either a resection arthroplasty of the elbow or an angulation osteotomy of the humerus to improve elbow position.[129, 154] There is no good follow-up data on the few such cases reported in the literature.

Phocomelia

Prior to the thalidomide tragedy which occurred in Europe in the latter part of the 1950s phocomelia was an uncommon congenital limb deficiency. In Schleswig-Holstein only three phocomelias occurred in 266,599 live births between 1949 and 1956. In September, 1961, at the height of occurrence of thalidomide-induced limb deformities, the rate had risen to five phocomelias per *1000* births. Upper limb phocomelia is bilateral in over 50 per cent of cases, and in cases due to thalidomide is almost always bilateral.[125] Complete phocomelia occurs more commonly than either the proximal or distal forms.

The typical clinical picture of complete upper limb phocomelia is the child with a hand attached directly to the trunk at the level of the shoulder, more often bilaterally.[10, 54, 63, 98] The hand may consist of five digits, but more frequently has less, with the thumb being the digit most often absent (Fig. 22-29). Strength and function in these hands are rarely normal, but they tend to improve with growth of the child. However, prehension is usually possible to a greater or lesser degree except, of course, in monodigital hands. The chief biomechanical deficiency in such cases is loss of limb length. In bilateral cases, the affected children commonly develop independence in feeding and in writing, but are unable to perform activities such as dressing and toileting because of the severe limb shortening. Children with proximal or distal forms of the defect obviously have less limb shortening and correspondingly less difficulty with dressing and toileting. Other skeletal limb deficiencies are frequently seen in association with phocomelia, especially amelia involving the contralateral limb.

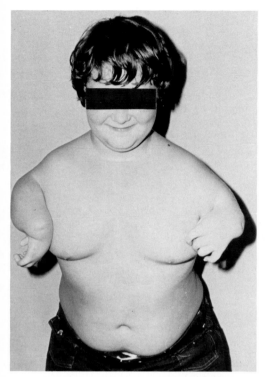

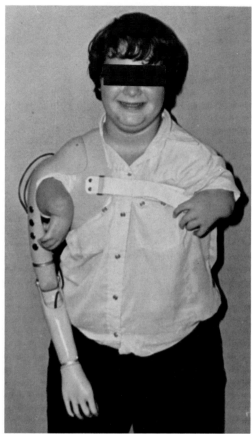

FIG. 22-29. In bilateral complete upper limb phocomelia the hands are attached directly to the trunk at the level of the shoulder. While prehension is possible, hand strength and function are rarely normal. Severe foreshortening of the limbs prevents independence in dressing and toileting.

FIG. 22-30. This child with bilateral complete upper limb phocomelia has been fitted with an electrically powered prosthesis. The phocomelic hand is used to manipulate a series of switches in the arm segment to control various prosthetic functions.

Children with unilateral phocomelia of the proximal or distal variety and a sound opposite upper limb rarely utilize prostheses.[10] Their sound upper limb is utilized for most functional activities. The comparatively long phocomelic limb is more assistive than a prosthesis and, in addition, possesses normal sensation. Unilateral prosthetic fitting of the least functional limb in bilateral cases enhances dressing and toileting and may be desirable, although most such children prefer to use assistive devices rather than a prosthesis for these activities.

Children with unilateral complete upper limb phocomelia and a sound opposite upper limb may likewise reject conventional prosthetic fitting, but often find an externally powered prosthesis of benefit. Bilateral cases require prostheses in order to achieve maximal function, although some older children prefer assistive devices rather than their prostheses. Prostheses should be fenestrated to allow maximal unrestricted use of the phocomelic hand. If conventional body-powered prostheses are used, fitting should be unilateral and the phocomelic hand utilized for elbow-lock operation, if possible.[10, 111] A few highly skillful children may successfully utilize bilateral prostheses of this type. Externally powered prostheses are highly desirable for these children. With such devices the phocomelic hand can usually manipulate several switches and thereby can control a variety of prosthetic functions (Fig. 22-30).

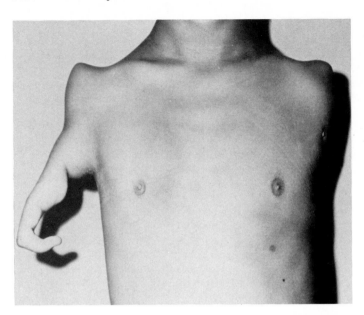

FIG. 22-31. In instances of unilateral upper limb amelia, the opposite upper limb often presents a monodigital type of phocomelia.

Amelia

Amelia is the absence of all skeletal elements of the entire limb. The shoulder girdle (both scapula and clavicle) is present and is usually normal, although often hypermobile. Excessive fat is sometimes present about the shoulder, either in the form of fat pads or as a diffuse subcutaneous collection. In other instances, there is a paucity of subcutaneous fat and the acromioclavicular joint is quite prominent. Amelia occurs somewhat more often in males, and the condition is bilateral in approximately half the cases. A phocomelia, often of the monodigital type, may involve the opposite upper limb in unilateral amelia[54] (Fig. 22-31).

Being a terminal transverse deficiency, upper limb amelia is the congenital homologue of an acquired shoulder disarticulation. Unilateral cases may be fit prosthetically as described in the section dealing with acquired amputations, bearing in mind that conventional body-powered prostheses are less efficient in the high level upper limb amputee, and that externally powered prostheses are preferable, if available.

Bilateral amelia presents the most severe functional loss of all upper limb skeletal deficiencies.[10, 98] The intelligent, highly motivated, and well-trained child with this defect can achieve near-normal levels of independence with a combination of good prosthetic management, excellent prehensile use of the feet, and certain adaptive devices such as modified clothing and dressing hooks.[4] The degree of prehensile foot capability that these children can attain is remarkable, and early and continuous use of the feet for assistance in self-care activities in the home should be encouraged.

Prosthetic fitting of the bilateral upper limb amelic is initiated by applying bilateral shoulder caps at approximately 6 months of age, or whenever sitting balance is attained.[4, 10] A passive articulated prosthesis can be applied on one side after the child becomes accustomed to the shoulder caps, and activation of the terminal device can be accomplished when the child evinces interest in attempting to insert objects into the hook—usually at 1 year of age or slightly older (Fig. 22-32). Voluntary control of the prosthetic elbow can rarely be accomplished before the age of 2 or even older. Unilateral prosthetic fitting of these children should be continued until their intellectual capacity and coordination matures enough for them to comprehend the complexity of bilateral control systems. This rarely occurs before age 6 and may never be practical with body powered prostheses.

When external power is used, bilateral

FIG. 22-32. *(A)* Bilateral upper limb amelia presents the most severe functional loss of all upper limb skeletal deficiencies. *(B)* Early prosthetic fitting is by means of shoulder caps. *(C)* Subsequent unilateral fitting with an articulated prosthesis. (Photographs courtesy of Dr. G. T. Aitken, Area Child Amputee Center, Grand Rapids, Michigan.)

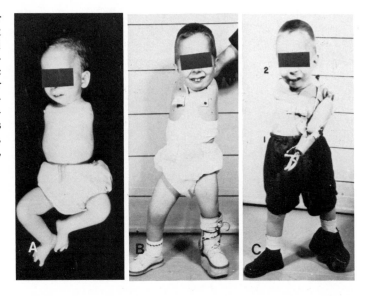

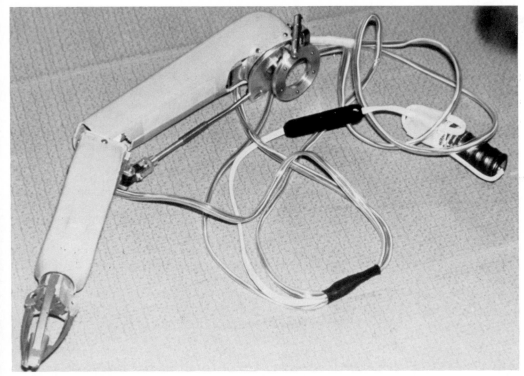

FIG. 22-33. The Ontario Crippled Children's Center coordinated electric arm is an externally powered prosthesis designed to provide coordinated feeding motions of the shoulder, elbow, forearm and terminal device.

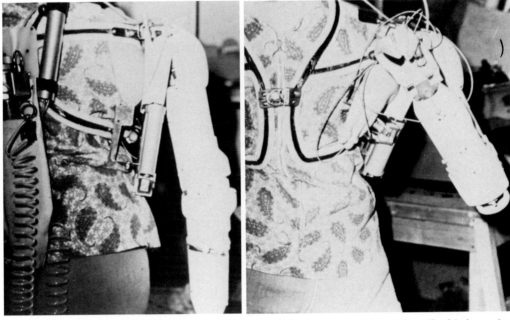

FIG. 22-34. A complex system of tubing, cylinders and pistons powered by carbon dioxide is used to provide function for this child with complete upper limb phocomelia.

fitting of extremely simple devices designed to provide two-handed clasping activity by means of powered humeral rotation has been successfully accomplished by children of 2 years of age and even younger.[117] More sophisticated powered prostheses providing elbow motion, forearm rotation, and prehension should be fitted unilaterally when the child is sufficiently mature to operate them effectively.[112, 118, 144, 151] Young children can very successfully learn to feed themselves with powered prostheses designed to provide coordinated "feeding motions" of the shoulder, elbow, forearm, and terminal device.[114] (Fig. 22-33). Selective, rather than synchronized, motions are desirable for dressing and toileting activities in the older child who has developed sufficient coordination to control such powered prostheses.

Externally Powered Upper Limb Prostheses

During the late 1950s the extensive use of thalidomide, a tranquilizing agent, by women in the early weeks of their pregnancy resulted in the birth of large numbers of infants with severe skeletal limb deficiencies, especially bilateral phocomelia. This tragic event was directly responsible for the rapid development of externally powered upper limb prostheses for children. Body powered prostheses for high level upper limb loss are functionally ineffective, especially in bilateral limb involvement. This functional ineffectiveness is most apparent in children, where both amplitude of power and cable excursion are limited.

Thalidomide was not marketed in the United States, but was widely prescribed in Europe. During the height of the thalidomide tragedy European prosthetic centers were literally inundated with children with severe upper limb skeletal deficiencies. Recognizing the limitation of body powered prostheses in providing function for the high level, bilateral upper limb amputee, many of these centers began to experiment with pneumatic prostheses. Pressurized carbon dioxide was selected as the power source, being nonflammable, inexpensive, easily stored under pressure, and reasonably available. Prosthetic systems and components were developed, control techniques designed, and training programs devised to incorporate pneumatic-powered prostheses into the management program of these children. By 1962 Marquardt reported fitting children in the second year of life with a CO_2 powered prosthetic system which provided basic two-handed clasping function—the now famous "patty-cake" prosthesis.[118] More sophisticated systems providing elbow motion, wrist rotation, and terminal device operation were developed for older children[118] (Fig. 22-34). Other centers in continental Europe, in Great Britain, and in Canada rapidly adopted the Heidleberg system, developed modifications, or designed entirely new systems for their own patients.[34, 60, 73, 96, 109, 125, 150, 151] Electricity was selected as a power source by some centers, and prostheses were designed which utilized electronic components powered by nickle-cadmium batteries (Fig. 22-35). Control of these sophisticated and sometimes complex externally powered prostheses proved to be a major problem for some of the severely limb-deficient children, and a number of investigators began using amplified electrical signals generated by muscle contraction to activate powered components—a technique termed *myoelectric control*.[30, 88, 146]

During the ensuing years each form of external power has had its proponents, and both pneumatic and electric components and control systems have been refined. Each of these systems has been at least partially effective, but all continue to exhibit shortcomings. The high cost of these devices and the relatively small market for them has hampered their widespread availability. Furthermore, these sophisticated systems are less durable than conventional prostheses and when mechanical failure occurs, very few prosthetic facilities are able to repair them. This leads to a prolonged "downtime" when the child is unable to use the prosthesis, which, in turn, produces discouragement in the child, parent, and clinic staff. These difficulties clearly illustrate the need for a network of specialized fitting centers in this country and for governmental fiscal support for treating the severely involved limb-deficient child.

A detailed discussion of externally powered prostheses is obviously beyond the scope of this chapter, but it is appropriate to briefly review the more commonly used pneumatic and electric power systems.[35, 106, 112, 113, 126, 127] Almost all pneumatic sys-

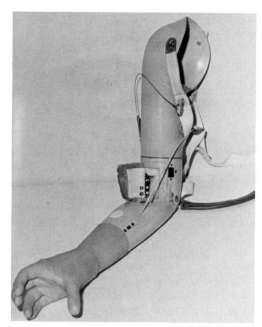

FIG. 22-35. Rechargeable nickle-cadmium batteries are the power source for both the elbow and the terminal device in this above-elbow prosthesis.

tems utilize carbon dioxide as a power source. This gas is stored in a liquid state in a small high pressure metal cylinder suspended from the prosthesis. Such small cylinders generally contain sufficient gas for a full day of prosthetic operation and are refilled from large tanks kept in the home or at treatment centers. Any of a variety of body motions of small amplitude and excursion (scapular motion, phocomelic digits, etc.) can be utilized to apply pressure or tension on valves which release CO_2 from the tank into the system. The CO_2 flows from the tank through flexible plastic tubing to the actuator, which is either a type of bellows or a piston. The pressurized gas causes the piston to move, and this motion is transmitted to the appropriate prosthetic component and results in elbow flexion, terminal device operation, or another appropriate response. Pressure or tension on other valves (or variations of pressure on the initial valve) by body motion releases gas from the system and reverses the achieved prosthetic motion (i.e., elbow extension). Pneumatic systems are attractive because of their simplicity of action, smoothness of operation, rapid response, and the relatively high horsepower they develop. On the debit side, these systems are quite bulky and the gas cylinders are heavy. Although the pistons operate very quietly, the valves produce a noisy hissing sound, which is objectionable. The inconvenience of refilling the gas cylinders each night is also a detraction.

Electrically powered prosthetic systems utilize highly efficient nickle-cadmium batteries as an energy source. These small batteries can be connected in series to provide a large amount of electrical energy in a small sized, light-weight pack which can be suspended from the prosthesis or incorporated into the prosthesis in a variety of ways. Such battery packs generally are capable of providing sufficient energy for a full day of prosthetic operation. They are easily recharged overnight by a simple recharger, which is plugged into an ordinary 110-volt household electric outlet. Either switches controlled by body motion or myoelectric control systems may be used to release energy from the battery to the prosthetic components. As with the pneumatic valves, any of a variety of body motions of small amplitude and excursion can be utilized to operate the biomechanically controlled switches. Appropriate pressure on the switch allows electrical energy to flow from the battery through wires to the actuator, which is most commonly a small 12-volt electric motor of the permanent magnet, direct current type. These motors produce the desired motion of prosthetic components through a variety of gear or screw mechanisms. When pressure is released from the switch, prosthetic motion ceases. Pressure on other switches (or variations in pressure on the initial switch) produces reverse motion of the prosthetic component. Various braking and cut-off mechanisms are incorporated into the design of these electrical components to prevent motors from burning out when switches are held down after the prosthetic component has achieved maximum excursion. Electric motors tend to be somewhat heavier, slower, and less powerful than pneumatic pistons of comparable size and they are certainly more complex. However, the great potential of electronic systems, the small and highly efficient batteries, and the ease of recharging this power source has made electrically powered prosthetic systems more popular than pneumatic systems in North America.

Control of electrically powered prostheses by means of myoelectric signals is a highly attractive option, and in certain centers in North America, Great Britain, and continental Europe it has proved to be quite effective. Most commonly, myoelectric control systems utilize surface electrodes located over muscle remnants in the amputation stumps to pick up electric signals generated when these muscle fibers are contracted at the patient's volition (Fig. 22-36). These minute electrical signals are then amplified electronically to a level that is sufficiently high to control a switch which releases a flow of current from a battery pack to an electric motor, thereby activating a prosthetic component. Usually, two separate muscles are used to produce the signals that control opposing functions of a prosthetic component (e.g., opening and closing of a prosthetic hand). However, it is possible to utilize multiple signals from the same muscle for this purpose, or even to use weak and strong signals from one muscle to control opposing functions. Furthermore, proportional control of a prosthetic component has been accomplished by using progressively more intense signals to produce more rapid motion or more powerful function. Unfortunately, the most successful applications of myoelectric control have been in that group of patients who need it least—the below-elbow amputees, with the "Russian hand" being a prime example.[108, 110, 134] High level upper limb amputees have successfully utilized such systems, but mostly in applied research settings.[37, 41, 144, 145, 153]

When external power is used in prosthetics, the need for sensory feedback becomes even more apparent than when conventional body powered systems are used. Biomechanical control of externally powered prostheses results in at least some pressure on sensitive body areas and this produces a certain amount of feedback. Visual and even auditory feedback from the noise of prosthetic operation are important cues, especially in myoelectrically controlled systems. Sophisticated research to enhance sensory feedback in prosthetic use is in progress in several centers on this continent, among them the University of New

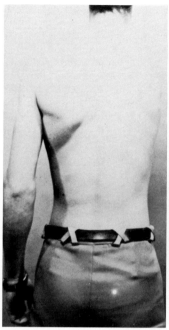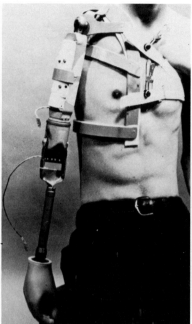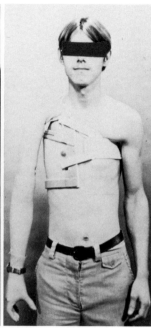

Fig. 22-36. Electromyelographic signals generated from muscle remnants are used to control the motions of the electrically powered forequarter prosthesis in this young man with an acquired forequarter amputation. The soft polyurethane foam covering of the endoskeletal system provides excellent cosmesis for the finished prosthesis.

Brunswick, Duke University, and the Massachusetts Institute of Technology.[138]

The need for and potential use of external power in children's prostheses is obviously great. Regretfully, there is a paucity of commercially available powered components in this country. Some pneumatic systems are available from Germany through a U.S. distributor. An electric elbow for children and a small sized child's electric hand are available in Canada. The newly developed electric Michigan hook is also available in a 10X size in the U.S.[50] Such excellent devices as the Michigan feeding arm, the Ontario Crippled Children's Center coordinated electric arm, and several electric elbows in children's sizes have been manufactured on a limited basis for field testing, but are not available commercially in the U.S. at this time.[67, 114, 164]

LOWER LIMB DEFICIENCIES

Paraxial Fibular Hemimelia

Fibular hemimelia is the most frequently occurring congenital deficiency of the long bones.[129, 171] The deficiency may be of either the terminal or the intercalary type, and may be either partial or complete. It is most commonly seen as a complete terminal deficiency and is more often unilateral, although a significant percentage of cases is bilateral. Males are affected almost twice as often as females in most reported series.

Although fibular hemimelia is often referred to as a congenital absence of the fibula, the condition is actually a total limb involvement rather than a simple absence of one bone.[49] While the foot may be normal in the intercalary type, the typical patient exhibits a foot in which one or more of the lateral rays are absent and the lateral tarsal bones are absent or fused. The distal tibial epiphysis is abnormal, the tibia is markedly shortened, and there is a characteristic anteromedial tibial bowing. In over half the cases there is some degree of femoral shortening, varying from minor shortening to severe proximal femoral focal deficiency (Fig. 22-37). This combination of skeletal defects results in a limb with a very characteristic clinical appearance—the leg segment is

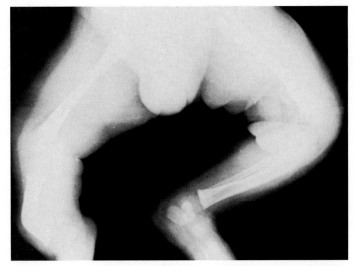

FIG. 22-37. In this roentgenogram of an infant with fibular hemimelia, not only is there an obvious complete absence of the fibula but also the marked shortening of the tibia and the characteristic anteromedial tibial bowing are clearly seen.

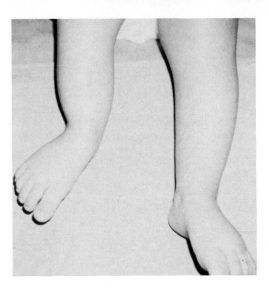

FIG. 22-38. The typical clinical appearance of fibular hemimelia is a limb in which the leg segment is quite short and bowed anteriorly and the foot is held in an equinovalgus position. The skin dimple overlying the apex of the tibial bow can be discerned in this photograph. In this instance of intercalary deficiency, all of the rays of the foot are present.

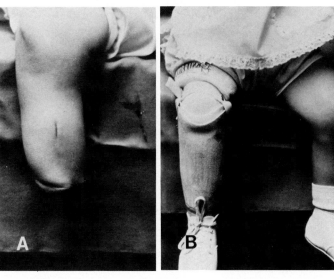

FIG. 22-39. (A) This child with fibular hemimelia has been treated by ankle disarticulation with Syme's-type closure. (B) Subsequent prosthetic fitting is with a patellar tendon-bearing prosthesis.

short and bowed and there is a skin dimple overlying the apex of the bow, the foot is fixed in a pronounced equinovalgus position, and one or two lateral rays are commonly absent in the foot (Fig. 22-38).

The major clinical problems in unilateral fibular hemimelia are: (1) the severe leg length discrepancy, and (2) the foot deformity.[49] Analyses of several large series have shown that leg length discrepancy is present in all cases and that it is progressive, the average discrepancy at skeletal maturity being approximately 5 inches.[14, 49, 93, 171] Unfortunately, those children with intercalary deficiencies who present a normal foot tend to have greater leg length inequality than children with terminal deficiencies, who, of course, have more severe foot deformities.[95] Bilateral cases present the problem of foot deformities plus disproportionate dwarfism. Most authors now agree that the tibial bowing rarely requires active treatment by osteotomy, and they find that the bowing decreases with age and is not a significant clinical problem.[14, 49] Where fibular hemimelia is associated with proximal femoral focal deficiency, the treatment should focus on the femoral deficiency rather than on the fibular hemimelia.[95]

In the past, the foot deformities seen in fibular hemimelia have been treated with various soft-tissue releases designed to place the foot beneath the tibia in a normal weightbearing position, sometimes followed by tarsal arthrodesis. The leg length inequality has been treated by leg lengthening procedures, epiphysiodesis of the sound limb, or a combination of such procedures.[17, 36, 147, 162] The end result of these multiple operations has been unsatisfactory in essentially all large review series. The leg length inequality was not adequately corrected and the foot was not often satisfactory for weightbearing. High shoe lifts, with or without braces, have been used to correct the leg length inequality. These devices are not only ungainly, but are most unsightly. In view of the present knowledge of the life history of this deficiency, the presently preferred method of treatment is early ablation of the foot by an ankle disarticulation with a Syme's-type closure.[1, 14, 49, 93, 94, 171] This produces a sturdy end-bearing stump at the below-knee level that can be nicely fit with an end-bearing below-knee prosthesis which increases function and is cosmetically pleasing (Fig. 22-39). These children can ambulate without their prostheses when necessary in the home or in an emergency situation, and their function remains excellent in adulthood. Even in the bilateral case foot ablation and prosthetic fitting is preferable to the rather severe disproportionate dwarfism that such children exhibit at skeletal maturity.

Paraxial Tibial Hemimelia

Tibial hemimelia is unique among the congenital limb deficiencies in that it is the only such skeletal deficiency with a documented familiar occurence.[142] Furthermore, approximately three-fourths of all cases have accompanying skeletal anomalies, especially central aphalangia (lobster-claw hand) and reduplication of toes.[9] As many as 20 per cent of these children have congenital hip dislocations.[10]

Exclusive of the terminal transverse deficiencies, tibial hemimelia is one of the more frequently occurring skeletal deficiencies in the lower limb. Its incidence has been estimated at one case per million persons in the United States.[25]

Tibial hemimelia may occur as either a terminal or an intercalary deficiency, and may be either complete or incomplete. Approximately 30 per cent of cases have bilateral involvement.[25] The clinical picture varies with the exact type of deficiency. In all cases, however, the leg segment is markedly shortened and the foot is fixed in a severe varus position, with the sole of the foot facing the perineum (Fig. 22-40). The knee joint is unstable, with the degree of instability related to the presence or absence of a proximal tibial remnant (incomplete or complete deficiency). In some instances there is a severe flexion contracture of the knee associated with a popliteal web. In terminal deficiencies, there is absence of one or more of the medial rays of the foot. In intercalary deficiencies, the foot may be normal or there may be reduplication with more than five rays present.

The major clinical problems in tibial hemimelia are the severe shortening of the leg segment, the malrotation of the foot, and

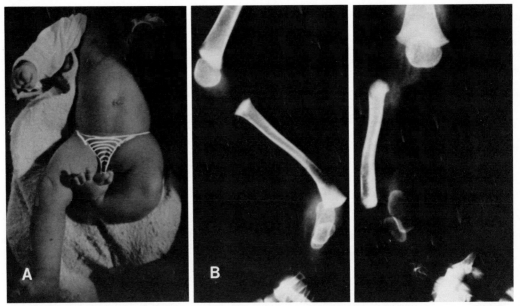

FIG. 22-40. *(A)* In tibial hemimelia, there is not only marked shortening of the leg segment, but also the foot is fixed in such a severe varus position that the sole of the foot is actually facing the perineum. Reduplication of toes is present in this particular infant. *(B)* Roentgenographically, the tibia is entirely absent, with lateral displacement of the fibula and marked varus positioning of the foot.

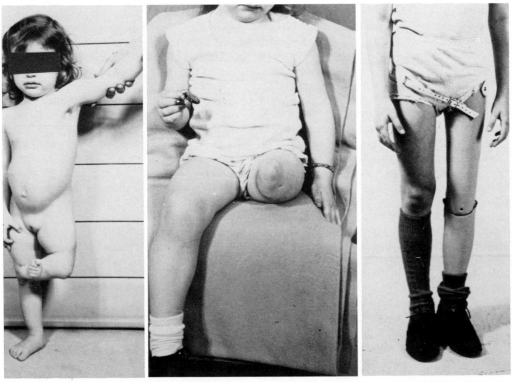

FIG. 22-41. In instances of tibial hemimelia with severe flexion contracture and webbing at the knee, knee disarticulation and fitting with a knee disarticulation prosthesis is the procedure of choice. (Photographs courtesy of Dr. G. T. Aitken, Area Child Amputee Center, Grand Rapids, Michigan.)

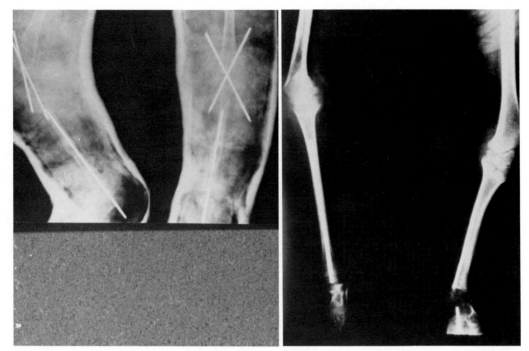

FIG. 22-42. In those instances of tibial hemimelia where the knee is not severely contracted, the upper end of the fibula may be centralized beneath the femur—the Fredrick Brown procedure. In this instance the foot was centralized beneath the fibula, but in most instances ablation of the foot is preferable because of the severe limb shortening present in this skeletal limb deficiency.

the instability and contracture of the knee. Traditional reconstructive surgical procedures are inadequate to satisfactorily correct these problems, and there is general agreement that this condition is best managed by primary surgical conversion of the defects into an acceptable amputation stump followed by appropriate prosthetic fitting. The type of surgical conversion performed is determined by the exact nature of the deformity. If there is a severe flexion contracture of the knee with popliteal webbing, knee disarticulation is the procedure of choice.[9] This is followed by prosthetic fitting with a knee-disarticulation prosthesis (Fig. 22-41).

In complete deficiencies of either the terminal or intercalary type where the knee is not severely contracted, the upper end of the fibula may be centralized beneath the femur and the foot ablated—the Fredrick Brown procedure[24] (Fig. 22-42). This is followed by fitting with a below-knee prosthesis with side joints and a thigh corset to help stabilize the knee. There is remarkable hypertrophy

of the fibula following transposition into a weightbearing position, and excellent results have been achieved with this operation in properly selected cases.[9, 158] Brown has emphasized that this surgery should be done during the first year of life and has pointed out the residual mediolateral knee instability and the tendency for recurrent knee flexion contracture that occurs following surgery.[25, 26]

In incomplete deficiencies where the proximal tibial remnant articulates with the femur, a synostosis may be performed between the distal end of the tibial remnant and the fibula, followed by ablation of the foot and fitting with a below-knee prosthesis[9, 69] (Fig. 22-43). Side joints and a thigh corset are also needed in these cases because of mediolateral knee instability.

Proximal Femoral Focal Deficiency

If terminal transverse skeletal limb deficiencies are excluded, the three most commonly encountered lower limb deficien-

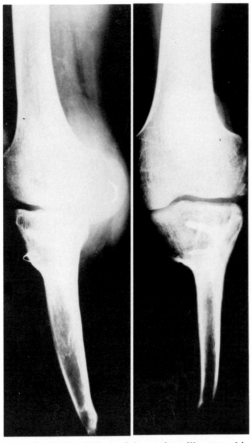

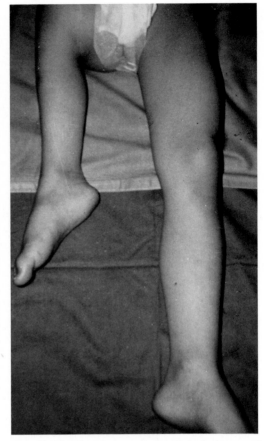

FIG. 22-43. The father of the patient illustrated in Fig. 22-42 exhibited an incomplete tibial hemimelia with preservation of the proximal end of the tibia. His limb deficiency had been treated years earlier by a synostosing operation between the fibula and the upper end of the tibia with subsequent ablation of the foot and an excellent long-term surgical result.

FIG. 22-44. The characteristic clinical picture of a child with proximal femoral focal deficiency. The thigh segment of the involved limb is quite short and is held in a flexed, abducted and externally rotated position at the hip. The bulky soft tissues of the upper thigh taper sharply toward the knee, giving rise to the so-called ship's funnel appearance. The ankle joint of the involved limb often lies at approximately the level of the knee joint of the sound side.

cies are fibular hemimelia, tibial hemimelia, and that group of deficiencies wherein there is a sharply localized absence of the proximal end of the femur involving the iliofemoral joint.[10] This latter group has been extensively analyzed by Aitken[7, 8] and others,[15, 18, 46, 86, 128] and is known as *proximal femoral focal deficiency* (PFFD). In the past, this form of skeletal deficiency was frequently confused with other types of femoral dysgenesis, such as congenital coxa vara, congenital bowing of the femur, congenital shortening of the femur, and even phocomelia. However, PFFD is now recognized as a uniquely separate and distinct type of skeletal limb deficiency.

Children with this entity present a rather characteristic clinical picture[7, 10] (Fig. 22-44). The thigh segment of the involved limb is quite short and is held in a flexed, abducted and externally rotated position at the hip. The bulky soft tissues of the upper thigh taper sharply toward the knee, giving the thigh segment a "ship's funnel" appearance. The knee is carried in flexion, but can usually be extended. Almost two-thirds of

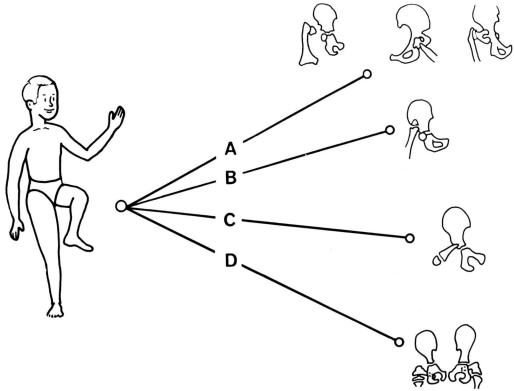

FIG. 22-45. Aitken classification of proximal femoral focal deficiency. (From Aitken, G. T.: Proximal femoral focal deficiency. Definition, classification and management. *In* A Symposium on Proximal Femoral Focal Deficiency—A Congenital Anomaly. National Academy of Sciences, Washington, D. C., 1969.)

these cases have an ipsilateral fibular hemimelia with the accompanying shortening of the leg segment and foot deformity anticipated in this condition. The foot on the affected limb usually lies at or near the level of the knee of the sound limb. Roughly 15 per cent of cases have bilateral involvement and present as instances of profound asymmetrical dwarfism, with each lower limb exhibiting the above-described appearance.

Aitken[7] has classified proximal femoral focal deficiency into four subclasses, based on the roentgenographic appearance of the lesion (Fig. 22-45). In Class A a head of the femur is present, together with an adequate acetabulum and a very short femoral segment. Initially, there is no bony connection between the shaft segment and the head of the femur. At skeletal maturity, a bony connection is present between the shaft of the femur and the head, neck, and trochanteric component. In most instances a pseudarthrosis is evident at their point of connection, and this defect does not usually heal (Fig. 22-46A). In Class B a head of the femur is present and there is an adequate acetabulum. There is a short femur, usually with a small bony tuft on its proximal end. At skeletal maturity there is no osseous connection between the femoral head and shaft (Fig. 22-46B). In Class C there is no femoral head and the acetabulum is severely dysplastic. The shaft of the femur is short with an ossified tuft at its proximal end (Fig. 22-46C). In Class D the femoral head and the acetabulum are completely absent. The femoral shaft is deformed and very short and there is no tuft of bone at its proximal end (Fig. 22-46D).

As with most skeletal limb deficiencies,

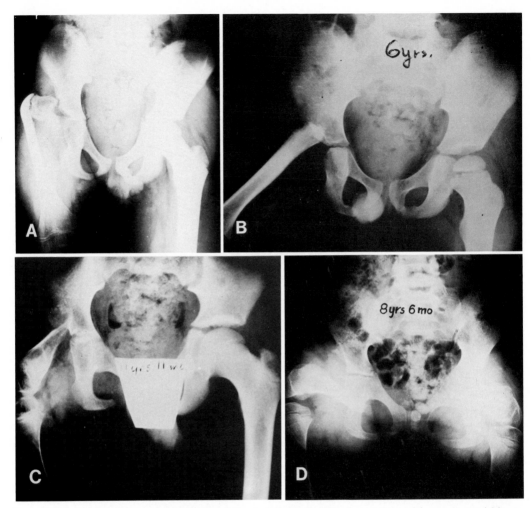

FIG. 22-46. *(A)* Type A proximal femoral focal deficiency. The femoral head is present within an adequate acetabulum and, although the femur is quite short, there is an obvious connection between the shaft segment and the head and neck of the femur. A pseudoarthrosis is evident at the point of connection. *(B)* Type B proximal femoral focal deficiency. A femoral head is present as well as an adequate acetabulum. The femur is quite short and there is a small bony tuft at the proximal end. *(C)* Type C proximal femoral focal deficiency. The femoral head is absent and the acetabulum is severely dysplastic. The shaft of the femur is quite short and there is an ossified tuft at its proximal end. *(D)* Type D proximal femoral focal deficiency. The femoral head and the acetabulum are completely absent, the femoral shaft is markedly shortened and no tuft of bone is noted at the proximal end. The majority of cases falling in the Type D category are bilateral. (Roentgenograms courtesy of Dr. G. T. Aitken, Area Child Amputee Center, Grand Rapids, Michigan.)

treatment of proximal femoral focal deficiency is determined by the specific problems presented by each individual case. However, some general rules can be given for treating each specific subtype of the deficiency. All cases of unilateral PFFD exhibit the biomechanical losses of limb length inequality, malrotation, instability of proximal joints, and inadequacy of proximal musculature.[7] Bilateral cases do not present significant limb length inequality, but manifest the other biomechanical deficiencies

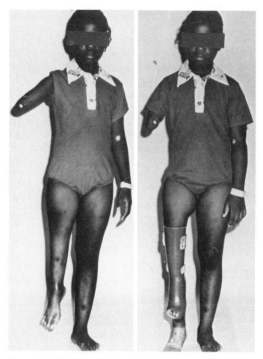

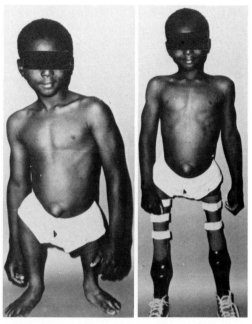

FIG. 22-47. This child with a unilateral proximal femoral focal deficiency also has a transverse terminal hemimelia of the ipsilateral upper limb. She has been fitted with a nonstandard prosthesis in order to equalize her limb lengths.

FIG. 22-48. Children with bilateral proximal femoral focal deficiency should not be treated surgically unless they have such severe foot deformities that they cannot ambulate without prostheses. Nonstandard prostheses are used outside of the home to correct the disproportionate dwarfism of these children and to raise them to peer height.

plus disproportionate dwarfism. It is of interest that almost all reported bilateral cases of PFFD are of the Class D subtype.[7]

Unilateral PFFD may be treated nonsurgically by a nonstandard prosthesis, which is fitted around the child's plantarflexed foot and which incorporates a prosthetic knee joint just beneath the anatomical foot (Fig. 22-47). Such prosthetic fitting will immediately equalize leg lengths and by appropriate fabrication and alignment can minimize limb malrotation and instability of the hip and knee. A prosthesis will obviously have no effect on the inadequate proximal musculature. Ambulation in such prostheses is reasonably good, but the cosmetic effect leaves much to be desired.

Children with bilateral PFFD generally walk quite well without any form of prosthetic restoration, and surgical procedures almost always detract from their ambulatory

independence rather than benefit them.[76] It is widely accepted that children with bilateral PFFD should not be treated surgically unless they have such severe foot deformities that they cannot ambulate without prostheses.[7, 66, 91] Nonstandard prostheses, as described above, are used outside of the home to correct the disproportionate dwarfism of these children and raise them to peer height (Fig. 22-48).

When properly selected surgical procedures are carried out in the child with unilateral PFFD, subsequent prosthetic fit and function can be significantly improved. Standard orthopaedic reconstructive procedures have proved totally ineffective in correcting the leg length inequality seen in unilateral PFFD, especially where there is an accompanying ipsilateral fibular hemimelia.[7, 121, 170] The preferred treatment is surgical conversion to the homologue of either

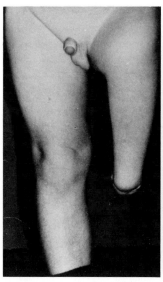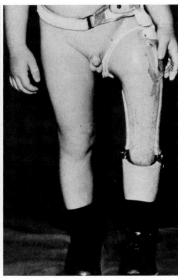

FIG. 22-49. In those children with unilateral proximal femoral focal deficiency where the ankle joint of the involved limb lies approximately at the level of the knee joint of the sound limb, surgical conversion by means of an ankle disarticulation and Syme's-type closure with subsequent prosthetic fitting with a nonstandard above-knee prosthesis is appropriate.

an acquired below-knee or an above-knee amputation with appropriate prosthetic fitting. Whether to attempt conversion and prosthetic fitting as a below-knee amputee or to convert and fit as an above-knee amputee is a decision which is best made on the basis of the anticipated leg length discrepancy at skeletal maturity. Amstutz[13] has demonstrated that there is a constant percentage of growth retardation of the involved limb. By obtaining serial leg length roentgenograms and performing the appropriate calculations, a reasonably accurate prediction of limb length discrepancy at skeletal maturity can be made in a young child. If it is anticipated that the foot of the affected limb will lie proximal to or at the level of the knee of the sound limb, then ablation of the foot by ankle disarticulation with Syme's closure and prosthetic fitting as an above-knee amputee is indicated[7, 121, 170] (Fig. 22-49). If calculations indicate that the foot of the affected limb will be significantly distal to the level of the knee of the sound limb, then consideration should be given to performing a Van Nes rotational osteotomy[167] through the leg, removing enough bone to allow a full 180° rotation of the foot without creating tension on the neurovascular structures of the leg. The ankle joint of the rotated limb should then lie at the level of the knee on the sound limb and

will function as a knee joint, while the foot will function as a below-knee amputation stump.[7, 65, 66, 89, 89a., 90] Following surgery these children are prosthetically fit as below-knee amputees, with the prosthesis having side joints and a thigh shell to encase and stabilize the true anatomic knee (Fig. 22-50). When the Van Nes procedure is performed in very young children the twisted leg muscles tend to derotate the limb and additional surgery is often necessary to restore proper rotation. For this reason Hall[89] has suggested that the Van Nes procedure not be done on children under 12 years of age.

Following either ankle disarticulation and above-knee prosthetic fitting or rotationplasty and below-knee prosthetic fitting, consideration should be given to arthrodesis of the knee in order to provide a more stable stump and enhance prosthetic fitting.[7, 13, 20, 121, 170] Proper timing and technique of knee arthrodesis is essential to ensure that the growth potential of the distal femoral and proximal tibial epiphyses is not prematurely destroyed and desirable stump length lost. Knee arthrodesis can help to overcome the flexion-abduction-external rotation deformity at the hip and, when necessary, can affect rotational loss following a Van Ness procedure in the younger child (Fig. 22-51).

FIG. 22-50. In unilateral instances of proximal femoral focal deficiency where the foot of the affected limb lies significantly distal to the level of the knee of the sound limb, a Van Nes rotational osteotomy through the leg may be performed. The foot is rotated 180° and the leg segment shortened so that the ankle joint of the involved limb lies at approximately the level of the knee joint of the sound limb. Prosthetic fitting as a below-knee amputation can then be satisfactorily accomplished. (Photographs courtesy of Dr. Al Kritter, Waukesha, Wisconsin.)

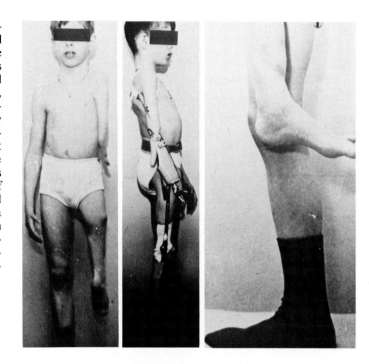

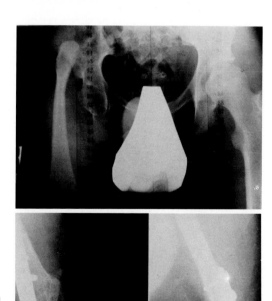

FIG. 22-51. This child with unilateral proximal femoral focal deficiency was treated by ankle disarticulation with Syme's closure and subsequent prosthetic fitting as an above-knee amputee. Subsequent arthrodesis of the knee joint of the involved limb with appropriate bone resection allowed equalization of knee centers and enhanced prosthetic fitting.

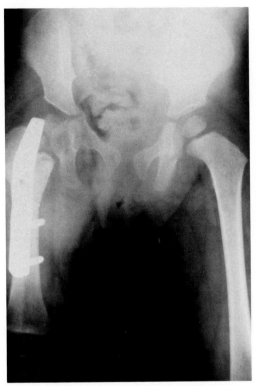

FIG. 22-52. In Type A or B proximal femoral focal deficiency, subtrochanteric osteotomy to achieve continuity between the femoral head-neck segment and the shaft segment may be beneficial.

Reconstructive surgery about the hip can improve hip stability and can enhance the function of the hip musculature. However, hip surgery should only be undertaken in those subtypes where a femoral head is present and the acetabulum is adequate—Classes A and B.[7, 13, 27, 107] Reconstructive procedures of various type in Classes C and D have rarely been successful and usually have resulted in functional loss.[20, 121, 169, 170] Subtrochanteric osteotomy of Class A and B hips has been beneficial when bony continuity between the femoral head-neck segment and the shaft segments can be obtained. (Fig. 22-52).

King[82, 83, 84, 85, 87] has achieved a significant degree of success in attaining hip stability and a single skeletal lever for prosthetic use by performing a two-stage surgical procedure in selected cases of unilateral PFFD. In Class B cases he advises performing a concomitant knee arthrodesis and subtrochanteric osteotomy by using a single intramedullary nail for internal fixation at both the knee and the hip. At a second stage the nail is removed and the foot ablated by ankle disarticulation. These children are then prosthetically fit as above-knee amputees. Surgery can be done at an early age since the knee epiphyses are not disturbed by the intramedullary nail.

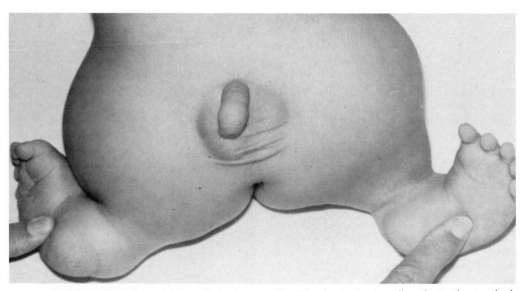

FIG. 22-53. Complete bilateral lower limb phocomelia. The foot attaches directly to the trunk, is usually deformed, and has very limited muscle function.

Fig. 22-54. In complete lower limb phocomelia, surgical removal of the foot is contraindicated, since the foot enhances socket suspension and provides sensory feedback concerning the position of the prosthesis. The socket portion of the prosthesis must be modified to accommodate for these phocomelic feet.

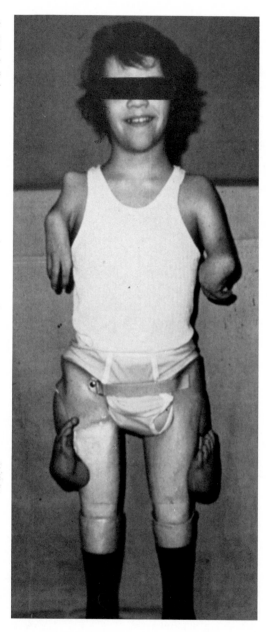

Phocomelia

In complete lower limb phocomelia all proximal portions of the limb are absent and the foot attaches directly to the trunk (Fig. 22-53). Tarsal elements may be absent or present in varying degrees in the foot, and the toes are variable in number. There is usually some degree of toe flexion present. The condition is seen more often in males and is bilateral in 20 per cent to 30 per cent of cases.[54]

Functionally, complete lower limb phocomelia may be considered the homologue of an acquired hip disarticulation and prosthetically treated with a hip disarticulation prosthesis, as discussed in the section on acquired lower limb amputation. The socket portion of the prosthesis must be appropriately modified to accomodate the phocomelic foot (Fig. 22-54). In spite of the bizarre appearance of a foot attached directly to the trunk, surgical removal of the foot is contraindicated since it affords an excellent weightbearing surface, enhances socket suspension, and provides sensory feedback concerning the position of the prosthesis.[2]

In bilateral cases, treatment measures are initiated during infancy to develop head and trunk control. At approximately age 6 months the child is placed in the upright position in a plastic laminate bucket mounted on a stable base to facilitate sitting balance. After 3 or 4 months the child has usually achieved sufficient balance to graduate to an OCCC swivel walker.[10, 67, 97, 119, 144] This device was designed at the Ontario Crippled Children's Center to provide a limited degree of ambulation by converting lateral sway motion of the child's trunk to forward progression of the swivel walker (Fig. 22-55). Initially, the pylons of the swivel walker are quite short in order to maintain the child's center of gravity close to the floor and to enhance standing stability. As the child's balance and agility increase, the pylons may be progressively lengthened to bring the child up to peer height. The child with normal upper limbs who can use crutches may be fit with standard bilateral hip disarticulation prostheses at approxi-

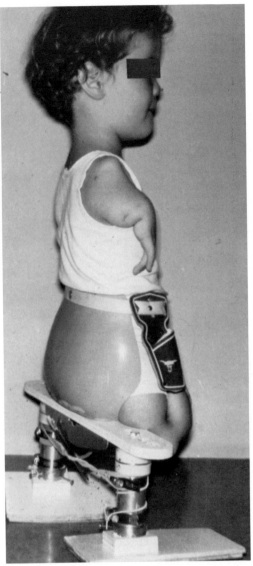

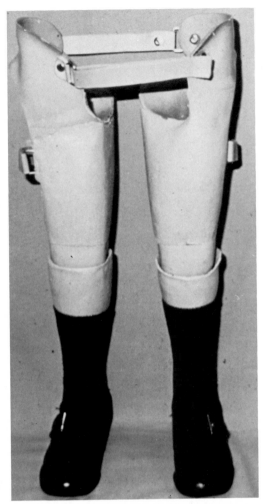

FIG. 22-56. Cosmetic articulated prostheses that incorporate swivel walker ankle joints can be fabricated for the older child with bilateral lower limb phocomelia to allow short-distance ambulation over level surfaces.

FIG. 22-55. The Ontario Crippled Children's Center swivel walker provides the bilateral lower limb phocomelic child with a limited degree of ambulation by converting lateral sway motion of the trunk to forward progression of the swivel walker.

mately 2 years of age and may be trained to walk with a swing-to or swing-through crutch gait. The child whose upper limbs will not accommodate crutches can be fit with more cosmetic articulated prostheses, incorporating swivel-walker ankle joints for short distance ambulation over level surfaces (Fig. 22-56). Such children will require some form of electrically powered cart or wheelchair for independent mobility over longer distances or over uneven surfaces.

Amelia

Lower limb amelia is the complete absence of all bony elements of the lower limb. There may be a lobule of fat or a deep dimple present on the pelvis at the normal site of

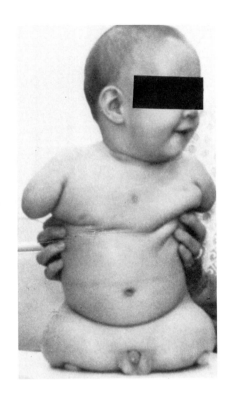

Fig. 22-57. In lower limb amelia, there is complete absence of all bony elements of the lower limb. A lobule of fat is present at the normal site of lower limb attachment and the pelvis is characteristically widened due to a local accumulation of subcutaneous fat. This child not only has bilateral lower limb amelia but also has bilateral transverse terminal hemimelia of his upper limbs.

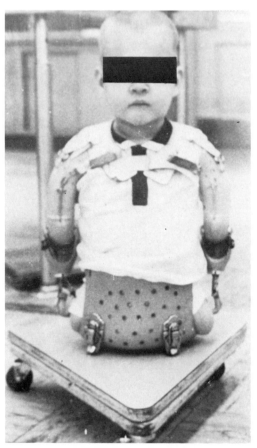

Fig. 22-58. Children with bilateral lower limb amelia are fitted with a plastic laminate "bucket" in infancy to allow them to achieve good sitting balance.

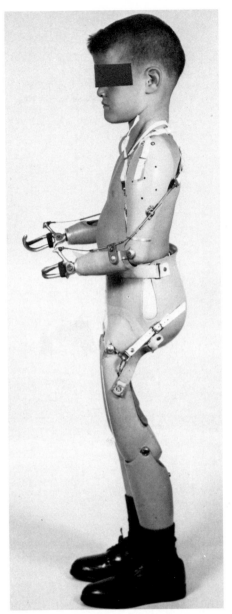

FIG. 22-59. Final prosthetic fitting of the bilateral lower limb amelic child is by means of articulated hip disarticulation prostheses.

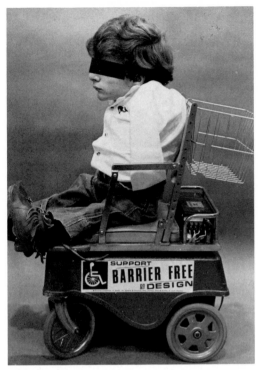

FIG. 22-60. The Child Amputee Prosthetic Project electrically powered cart provides the severely involved lower limb or multimembral amputee with independent mobility over long distances.

lower limb attachment. The pelvis is characteristically widened due to a local accumulation of subcutaneous fat (Fig. 22-57). The condition occurs more often in males and is bilateral in 50 per cent of cases.[54]

Amelia is a terminal transverse deficiency and in the lower limb is the congenital homologue of an acquired hip disarticulation. Unilateral cases are fit with a standard hip disarticulation prosthesis. As with the bilateral phocomelic, bilateral cases require the use of a stable plastic laminate bucket to achieve good sitting balance in infancy (Fig. 22-58). These children are then graduated to a swivel walker and subsequently to articulated hip disarticulation prostheses (Fig. 22-59). Those with good upper limb function will achieve a satisfactory swing-to or swing-through crutch gait, but those with upper limb deficiencies of such severity to preclude the use of crutches will require swivel walker ankle joints in their prostheses for limited walking on level surfaces and a powered cart (Fig. 22-60) or wheelchair for independent mobility over longer distances or over uneven surfaces.[10, 42, 72, 165]

REFERENCES

1. Aitken, G. T.: Amputation as a treatment for certain lower-extremity congenital abnormalities. J. Bone Joint Surg.,*41A:*1267–1285, 1959.
2. ———: Overgrowth of the amputation stump. ICIB,*1*(11):1–8, 1962.
3. ———: Surgical amputation in children. J. Bone Joint Surg.,*45A:*1735–1741, 1963.
4. ———: Management of severe bilateral upper limb deficiencies. Clin. Orthop.,*37:*53–60, 1964.
5. ———: Prosthetic fitting following amputation for bone tumors. ICIB,*3*(5):1–2, 1964.
6. ———: The child with an acquired amputation. ICIB,*7*(8):1–15, 1968.
7. ———: Proximal femoral focal deficiency—definition, classification, and management. *In* A Symposium on Proximal Femoral Focal Deficiency—A Congenital Anomaly. Washington, D.C., National Academy of Sciences, 1969.
8. ———: Proximal femoral focal deficiency. *In* Limb Development and Deformity; Problems of Evaluation and Rehabilitation. Springfield, Charles C Thomas, 1969.
9. ———: Tibial hemimelia. *In* A Symposium on Selected Lower Limb Anomalies, Surgical and Prosthetic Management. Washington, D.C., National Academy of Sciences, 1971.
10. ———: The child amputee—An overview. Orthop. Clin. North Am.,*3*(2):447–472, 1972.
11. Aitken, G. T., and Frantz, C. H.: The juvenile amputee. J. Bone Joint Surg.,*35A:*659–664, 1953.
12. ———: Management of the child amputee. AAOS Instruc. Course Lect.,*17:*246–298, 1960.
13. Amstutz, H. C.: The morphology, natural history, and treatment of proximal femoral focal deficiency. *In* A Symposium on Proximal Femoral Focal Deficiency—A Congenital Anomaly. Washington, D.C., National Academy of Sciences, 1969.
14. ———: Natural history and treatment of congenital absence of the fibula. J. Bone Joint Surg., *54A:*1349, 1972.
15. Amstutz, H. C., and Wilson, P. D., Jr.: Dysgenesis of the proximal femur (coxa vara) and its surgical management. J. Bone Joint Surg., *44A:*1–24, 1962.
16. Arey, L. B.: Developmental Anatomy. Philadelphia, W. B. Saunders, 1965.
17. Arnold, W. D.: Congenital absence of the fibula. Clin. Orthop.,*17:*20–29, 1959.
18. Badger, V. M., and Lambert, C. N.: Differential diagnosis of an apparent proximal femoral focal deficiency. ICIB,*5*(1):3–9, 1965.
19. Bayne, L. G., Lovell, W. W., and Marks, T. W.: The radial club hand. J. Bone Joint Surg., *52A:*1065, 1970.
20. Bevan-Thomas, W. H., and Millar, E. A.: A review of proximal focal femoral deficiencies. J. Bone Joint Surg.,*49A:*1378–1388, 1967.
21. Blakeslee, B.: The limb-deficient child. Berkeley, Univ. of Calif. Press, 1963.
22. Bora, F. W., Nicholson, J. T., and Cheema, H. M.: Radial meromelia: The deformity and its treatment. J. Bone Joint Surg., *52A:*966–979, 1970.

23. Brooks, M. B., and Mazet, R.: Prosthetics in child amputees. Clin. Orthop.,*9:*190–204, 1957.
24. Brown, F. W.: Construction of a knee joint in congenital total absence of the tibia (paraxial hemimelia tibia). A preliminary report. J. Bone Joint Surg.,*47A:*695–704, 1965.
25. ———: The Brown operation for total hemimelia tibia. *In* A Symposium on Selected Lower Limb Anomalies, Surgical and Prosthetics Management. Washington, D.C., National Academy of Sciences, 1971.
26. Brown, F. W., and Pohnert, W. H.: Construction of a knee joint in meromelia tibia (congenital absence of the tibia). A fifteen year follow-up study. J. Bone Joint Surg.,*54A:*1333, 1972.
27. Burgess, E.: The surgical means of obtaining hip stability with motion in congenital proximal femoral focal deficiency. ICIB,*1*(3):1–4, 1961.
28. Burgess, E. M., and Romano, R. L.: Immediate postsurgical prosthetic fitting of children and adolescents following lower-extremity amputations. ICIB,*7*(3):1–10, 1967.
29. Burtch, R. L., Fishman, S., and Kay, H. W.: Nomenclature for congenital skeletal limb deficiencies, a revision of the Frantz and O'Rahilly classification. Artif. Limbs, *10:*24–35, 1966.
30. Buttomley, A. H.: Myo-electric control of powered prostheses. J. Bone Joint Surg., *47B:*411–415, 1965.
31. Cary, J. M.: Traumatic amputation in childhood—Primary management. ICIB, *14*(6):1–10, 1975.
32. Clippinger, F. W., Jr., and Titus, B. R.: Prosthetic principles—lower limb. *In* The Child With An Acquired Amputation. Washington, D.C., National Academy of Sciences, 1972.
33. Cohlan, S. O.: Environmental factors in human teratology. *In* Normal and Abnormal Embryological Development. Washington, D.C., National Research Council, 1967.
34. Corrivean, C.: Prostheses powered by carbon-dioxide. ICIB,*7*(5):13–16, 1968.
35. ———: Prosthetic principles in upper-limb externally powered prostheses. *In* The Child With An Acquired Amputation. Washington, D.C., National Academy of Sciences, 1972.
36. Coventry, M. B., and Johnson, E. W.: Congenital absence of the fibula. J. Bone Joint Surg., *34A:*941–955, 1952.
37. Dankmeyer, C. H., Sr., Dankmeyer, C. H., Jr., and Massey, M. D.: An externally powered modular system for upper-limb prostheses. Orthot. Prosthet.,*26:*36–40, 1972.
38. Davidson, W. H., and Bohne, W. H. O.: The Syme amputation in children. J. Bone Joint Surg., *57A:*905–908, 1975.
39. Davies, E. J., Friz, B. R., and Clippinger, F. W., Jr.: Children with amputations. ICIB,*9*(3):6–19, 1969.
40. Delorme, T. D.: Treatment of congenital absence of the radius by transepiphyseal fixation. J. Bone Joint Surg.,*51A:*117–129, 1969.
41. Dorcas, D. S., Dunfield, V. A., and O'Shea, B. J.: A myoelectric prosthesis for a forequarter amputation. ICIB,*7*(11):15–20, 1968.

42. Dresher, C. S., and Macdonell, J. A.: Total amelia. J. Bone Joint Surg.,*47A:*511–516, 1965.

43. Duraiswami, P. K.: Experimental causation of congenital skeletal defects and its significance in orthopedic surgery. J. Bone Joint Surg., *34B:*646–698, 1952.

44. ———: Comparison of congenital defects induced in developing chickens by certain teratogenic agents with those caused by insulin. J. Bone Joint Surg.,*27A:*277–294, 1955.

45. Epps, C. H.: Upper-extremity limb deficiency with concomitant infantile structural scoliosis. ICIB,*5*(2):1–9, 1965.

46. ———: Proximal femoral focal deficiency: A case report of a necropsy. ICIB,*6*(5):1–6, 1967.

47. Epps, C. H., and Haile, J. H.: Experience with the Munester-type below-elbow prosthesis. ICIB, *7*(10):1–6, 1968.

48. Epps, C. H., and Vaughn, H. H.: Training the child with a lower-limb amputation. *In* The Child With An Acquired Amputation. Washington, D. C., National Academy of Sciences, 1972.

49. Farmer, A. W., and Laurin, C. A.: Congenital absence of the fibula. J. Bone Joint Surg.,*42A:*1–12, 1960.

50. Fisher, A. G., and Childress, D. S.: The Michigan electric hook: A preliminary report on a new electrically powered hook for children. ICIB, *12*(9):1–10, 1973.

51. Fishman, S., and Kay, H. W.: The Muenster-type below-elbow socket, an evaluation. Artif. Limbs, *8:*4–14, 1964.

52. Frankel, M. E., Goldner, J. L., and Stelling, F. H.: Radial club hand: Is centralization necessary: A rational surgical approach. J. Bone Joint Surg., *53A:*1026, 1971.

53. Frantz, C. H., and Aitken, G. T.: Management of the juvenile amputee. Clin. Orthop. *9:*30–47, 1959.

54. Frantz, C. H., and O'Rahilly, R.: Congenital skeletal limb deficiencies. J. Bone Joint Surg., *43A:*1202–1224, 1961.

55. ———: Ulnar hemimelia. Artif. Limbs,*15:*25–35, 1971.

56. Friedman, L.: Should the Munester below-elbow prosthesis be prescribed for children? ICIB, *11*(7):7–15, 1972.

57. Gazeley, W. E., Ey, M. D., and Sampson, W.: Follow-up experiences with Muenster prostheses. ICIB,*7*(10):7–11, 1968.

58. Glassner, J. R.: Spontaneous intra-uterine amputation. J. Bone Joint Surg.,*45A:*351–355, 1963.

59. Goldner, J. L.: Congenital absence of the radius and digital deformities: "club hand" (paraxial hemimelia radialis). ICIB,*4*(9):1–6, 1965.

60. Goldner, J. L., and Titus, B. R.: An experience with externally powered prostheses for children. ICIB,*7*(2):1–8, 1967.

61. Gorton, A.: Field study of the Muenster-type below-elbow prosthesis. ICIB,*6*(8):8–9, 1967.

62. Hall, C. B.: Recent concepts in the treatment of the limb-deficient child. Artif. Limbs, *10:*36–51, 1966.

63. Hall, C. B., Brooks, M. B., and Dennis, J. F.: Congenital skeletal deficiencies of the Extremities. Classification and fundamentals of treatment. JAMA,*181:*590–599, 1962.

64. Hall, C. B., Rosenfelder, R., and Tabloda, C.: The juvenile amputee with a scarred stump. *In* The Child With An Acquired Amputation. Washington, D.C., National Academy of Sciences, 1972.

65. Hall, J. E.: Rotation of congenitally hypoplastic lower limbs to use the ankle joint as a knee. ICIB, *6*(2):3–9, 1966.

66. Hall, J. E., and Bochmann, D.: The surgical and prosthetic management of proximal femoral focal deficiency. *In* A Symposium: Proximal Femoral Focal Deficiency—A Congenital Anomaly. Washington, D.C., National Academy of Sciences, 1969.

67. Hall, J. E., and Sauter, W. F.: Surgical and prosthetic management of three congenital child amputees. ICIB,*7*(2):9–18, 1967.

68. Hammond, N. L., III, Levitt, R. L., and Hunter, J. M.: Scoliosis combined with congenital deficiencies of the upper limb: The effect of prosthesis wearing. ICIB,*12*(3):30–32, 1972.

69. Hancock, C. I., and King, R. E.: The one-bone leg. ICIB,*7*(3):11–17, 1967.

70. Harris, R. I.: Syme's amputation. The technical details essential for success. J. Bone Joint Surg., *38B:*614–632, 1956.

71. Haslam, E. T.: Intra-uterine gangrene of the forefoot. ICIB,*3*(5):3–9, 1964.

72. Haslam, E. T., Hayden, J., and Dutro, J.: The habilitation of a congenital quadruple amputee. ICIB,*6*(9):1–11, 1967.

73. Hauberg, G., and John, H.: Treatment at Abteilung 10—Dysmelien. ICIB,*5*(6):4–10, 1966.

74. Henkel, L., and Wilbert, H. G.: Dysmelia. J. Bone Joint Surg.,*51B:*399–414, 1969.

75. Herndon, J. H., and LaNone, A. M.: Salvage of a short below-elbow amputation with pedicle flap coverage. ICIB,*12*(7):5–9, 1973.

76. Hussain, T., and Emmerson, A.: Conservative management of bilateral proximal femoral focal deficiency. ICIB,*13*(9):9–12, 1974.

77. Hutchison, J.: The training of upper-limb amputees with conventional and externally powered prostheses. *In* The Child With An Acquired Amputation. Washington, D.C., National Academy of Sciences, 1972.

78. Kato, K.: Congenital absence of the radius. J. Bone Joint Surg.,*6:*589–626, 1924.

79. Kay, H. W.: A proposed international terminology for the classification of congenital limb deficiencies. ICIB,*13*(7):1–16, 1974.

80. ———: Clinical applications of the new international terminology for the classification of congenital limb deficiencies. ICIB,*14*(3):1–24, 1975.

81. Kay, H. W., and Fishman, S.: 1018 Children With Skeletal Limb Deficiencies. New York Univ. Post-Graduate Medical School, Prosthetics and Orthotics, 1967.

82. King, R. E.: Concepts of proximal femoral focal deficiencies. ICIB,*1*(2):1–7, 1961.

83. ———: Surgical correction of proximal femoral focal deficiency, ICIB,*4*(11):1–10, 1965.

84. ———: Providing a single skeletal lever in proximal femoral focal deficiency. ICIB, *6*(2):23–28, 1966.

85. ———: Some concepts of proximal femoral focal deficiency. *In* A Symposium:. Proximal Femoral

Focal Deficiency—A Congenital Anomaly. Washington, D.C., National Academy of Sciences, 1969.

86. King, R. E., and McCraney, T.: Proximal femoral focal deficiency—Quo vadis? ICIB, *12*(8):1–8, 1973.

87. King, R. E., and Marks, T. W.: Follow-up findings on the skeletal lever in the surgical management of proximal femoral focal deficiency. ICIB, *11*(3):1–4, 1971.

88. Knowles, J. B., Stevens, B. L., and Howe, L.: Myoelectric control of a hand prosthesis. J. Bone Joint Surg., *47B:*416–420, 1965.

89. Kostuik, J. P., Gillespie, R., Hall, J. E., and Hubbard, S.: Van Nes rotational osteotomy for treatment of proximal femoral focal deficiency and congenital short femur. J. Bone Joint Surg., *57A:*1039–1046, 1975.

89a. Kritter, A. E.: Tibial rotation-plasty for proximal femoral focal deficiency. J. Bone Joint Surg., *59A:* 927–934, 1977.

90. Kritter, A., and Becker, D.: Proximal femoral focal deficiency and amelia: A case report. ICIB, *14*(4):1–6, 1975.

91. Kritter, A. E., and Gillespie, T.: Bilateral proximal femoral focal deficiency and bilateral paraxial fibular hemimelia. ICIB, *11*(12):1–8, 1972.

92. Kruger, L. M.: Classification and prosthetic management of limb-deficient children. ICIB, *7*(12):1–25, 1968.

93. ———: Fibular hemimelia. *In* A Symposium on Lower Limb Anomalies, Surgical and Prosthetic Management. Washington, D.C., National Academy of Sciences, 1971.

94. Kruger, L. M., and Bregan, N. R.: A study of radial head dislocation in children with transverse partial hemimelia of the upper limb. ICIB, *10*(1):1–4, 1970.

95. Kruger, L. M., and Talbott, R. D.: Amputation and prosthesis as definitive treatment in congenital absence of the fibula. J. Bone Joint Surg., *43A:*625–642, 1961.

96. Kuhn, G. C.: Treatment of the child with severe limb deficiencies. ICIB, *10*(3):1–26, 1970.

97. Lamb, D. W., Simpson, D. C., and Pirie, R. B.: The management of lower limb phocomelia. J. Bone Joint Surg., *52B:*688–691, 1970.

98. Lamb, D. W., Simpson, D. C., Schutt, W. H., Spiers, N. I., and Baker, G.: The management of upper limb deficiencies in the thalidomide type syndrome. J. R. Coll. Surg. Edinb., *10*(2):102, 1965.

99. Lambert, C. N.: An unusual case. ICIB, *6*(7):20, 1967.

100. ———: Amputation surgery in the child. Surg. Clin. North Am., *3*(2):473–482, 1972.

101. ———: Etiology. *In* The Child With An Acquired Amputation. Washington, D.C., National Academy of Sciences, 1972.

102. ———: Limb loss through malignancy. *In* The Child With An Acquired Amputation. Washington, D.C., National Academy of Sciences, 1972.

103. Lambert, C. N., Hamilton, R. C., and Pellicore, R. H.: The juvenile amputee program: Its social and economic value. J. Bone Joint Surg., *51A:*1135–1138, 1969.

104. Lambert, C. N., and Sciora, J.: The incidence of scoliosis in the juvenile amputee population. ICIB, *11*(2):1–6, 1971.

105. Laurin, C. A., and Farmer, A. W.: Congenital absence of ulna. Canad. J. Surg., *2:*204–207, 1959.

106. Lippay, A. L.: External power and the amputee: An engineer's view. ICIB, *7*(5):7–12, 1968.

107. Lloyd-Roberts, G. C., and Stone, K. H.: Congenital hypoplasia of the upper femur. J. Bone Joint Surg., *45B:*557–560, 1963.

108. Lozac'h, Y.: An improved and more versatile myoelectric control. ICIB, *11*(8):13–15, 1972.

109. Lundberg, C., Paul, S. W., Van Derwerker, E. E., and Allen, J. C.: Experience with carbon-dioxide-power-assisted prostheses. ICIB, *12*(1):1–6, 1972.

110. Lyttle, D., Sweitzer, R., Steinke, T, Treffler, E., and Hobson, D.: Experiences with myoelectric below-elbow fittings in teenagers. ICIB, *13*(6):11–20, 1974.

111. McKenzie, D. S.: The prosthetic management of congenital deformities of the extremities. J. Bone Joint Surg., *39B:*233–247, 1957.

112. ———: The clinical application of externally powered artificial arms. J. Bone Joint Surg., *47B:*399–410, 1965.

113. McLaurin, C. A.: External power in upper-extremity prosthetics and orthotics. ICIB, *6*(1):19–26, 1966.

114. ———: On the use of electricity in upper extremity prostheses. J. Bone Joint Surg., *47B:*448–452, 1965.

115. Makley, J. T., and Heiple, K. G.: Scoliosis associated with congenital deficiencies of the upper extremity. J. Bone Joint Surg., *52A:*279–287, 1970.

116. Malpas, J. S.: Advancements in the treatment of osteogenic sarcoma. J. Bone Joint Surg., *57B:*267, 1975.

117. Marquardt, E.: Aktive Prosthesenversorgung eines Armlosen Kleinkindes im 2. Lebensjahr. Jahrbuch dur Fursorge fur Korperbehinderte, 1962. (Reprinted in ICIB, *3*(4):1964.)

118. ———: The Heideleberg pneumatic arm prosthesis. J. Bone Joint Surg., *47B:*425–434, 1965.

119. Matlock, W. M., and Elliott, J.: Fitting and training children with swivel walker. Artif. Limbs, *10:*27–38, 1966.

120. Mazet, R., Jr.: Syme's amputation. A follow-up study of fifty-one adults and thirty-two children. J. Bone Joint Surg., *50A:*1549–1563, 1968.

121. Meyer, L. C., Friddle, D., and Pratt, R. W.: Problems of treating and fitting the patient with proximal femoral focal deficiency. ICIB, *10*(12):1–4, 1971.

122. Meyer, L. C., and Sauer, B. W.: The use of porous high-density polyethelene caps in the prevention of appositional bone growth in the juvenile amputee: A preliminary report. ICIB, *14*(9,10):1–4, 1975.

123. Milaire, J.: The contribution of histochemistry to our understanding of limb morphogenesis and some of its congenital deviations. *In* Normal and Abnormal Embryological Development. Washington, D.C., National Research Council, 1967.

124. Mongeau, M.: An approach to the rehabilitation of the child amputee. ICIB, *6*(4):1–2, 1967.

125. ———: Our experience with the thalidomide children. An interim report. ICIB, 6(4):3–7, 1967.

126. ———: New hope for the patient with several upper-extremity deficiencies: externally powered prostheses. ICIB, 7(5):1–6, 1968.

127. ———: General principles in the rehabilitation of upper-limb amputees with conventional or externally powered prostheses. *In* The Child With an Acquired Amputation. Washington, D.C., National Academy of Sciences, 1972.

128. Morgan, J. D., and Somerville, E. W.: Normal and abnormal growth at the upper end of the femur. J. Bone Joint Surg., 42B:264–272, 1960.

129. O'Rahilly, R.: Morphological patterns in limb deficiencies and duplications. Am. J. Anat. 89:135–193, 1951.

130. ———: The Nomenclature and Classification of Limb Anomalies. *In* Bergsma, D. (ed.): Limb Malformations. New York, Birth Defects Original Article Series, The National Foundation, 1969.

131. ———: Normal development of the human embryo. *In* Normal and Abnormal Embryological Development. Washington, D.C., National Research Council, 1967.

132. Pardini, A. G., Jr.: Radial dysplasia. Clin. Orthop., 57:152–177, 1968.

133. Pellicore, R. J., Mier, S., Hamilton, R. C., and Lambert, C. N.: Experiences with the Hepp-Kuhn below-elbow prosthesis. ICIB, 8(6):9–14, 1969.

134. Popov, B.: The bio-electrically controlled prosthesis. J. Bone Joint Surg., 47B:421–424, 1965.

135. Price, C. H. G. *et al:* Osteosarcoma in children. J. Bone Joint Surg., 57B:341, 1975.

136. Riordan, D. C.: Congenital absence of the radius. J. Bone Joint Surg., 37A:1129–1140, 1955.

137. ———: Congenital absence of the radius: A fifteen year follow-up. J. Bone Joint Surg., 45A, 1783, 1963.

138. Rohland, T. A.: Sensory feedback in upper-limb prosthetic systems, ICIB, 13(9):1–8, 1974.

139. Romano, R. L.: Immediate Postsurgical Prosthetic Fitting of the Child With an Acquired Amputation. Washington, D.C., National Academy of Sciences, 1972.

140. Romano, R. L., and Burgess, E. M.: Extremity growth and overgrowth following amputation in children. ICIB, 5(4):11–12, 1966.

141. ———: The immediate postsurgical prosthetic fitting technique applied to child amputees. ICIB, 9(9):1–10, 1970.

142. Russell, J. E.: Tibial hemimelia: limb deficiency in siblings. ICIB, 14(7, 8):15–23, 1975.

143. Saunders, J. W.: Control of growth patterns in limb development. *In* Normal and Abnormal Embryological Development. Washington, D.C., National Research Council, 1967.

144. Sauter, W. F.: Prostheses for the Child Amputee. Surg. Clin. North Am., 3(2):483–494, 1972.

145. Schmeisser, G., Seamone, W., and Hoshall, C. H.: Early clinical experience with the Johns Hopkins externally powered modular system for upper-limb prostheses. Orthot. Prosthet., 26:41–52, 1972.

146. Scott, R. N.: Surgical implications of myoelectric control. Clin. Orthop., 61:248–260, 1968.

147. Serafin, J.: A new operation for congenital absence of the fibula. J. Bone Joint Surg., 49B:59–65, 1967.

148. Setoguchi, Y.: School and the child amputee. *In* The Child With An Acquired Amputation. Washington, D.C., National Academy of Sciences, 1972.

149. Setoguchi, Y., Shaperman, J., and Talbert, D.: Vocational considerations. *In* The Child With An Acquired Amputation. Washington, D.C., National Academy of Sciences, 1972.

150. Simpson, D. C.: Gripping surfaces for artificial hands. ICIB, 12(6):1–4, 1973.

151. Simpson, D. C., and Lamb, D. W.: A system of powered prostheses for severe bilateral upper limb deficiency. J. Bone Joint Surg., 47B:442–447, 1965.

152. Skerik, S. K., and Flatt, A. E.: The anatomy of congenital radial dysplasia. Clin. Orthop. 66:124–143, 1969.

153. Stern, P. H., and Lanko, T.: A myoelectrically controlled prosthesis using remote muscle sites. ICIB, 12(7):1–3, 1973.

154. Straub, L. R.: Congenital absence of the radius and of the ulna. J. Bone Joint Surg., 54A:907, 1972.

155. Swanson, A. B.: The Krukenberg procedure in the juvenile amputee. J. Bone Joint Surg., 46A:1540–1548, 1964.

156. ———: Bone overgrowth in the juvenile amputee and its control by the use of silicone rubber implants. ICIB, 8(5):9–16, 1969.

157. ———: Silicone-rubber implants to control the overgrowth phenomenon in the juvenile amputee. ICIB, 11(9):5–8, 1972.

158. Swanson, A. B., Polglase, V. N., and Applegate, W.: The Brown procedure in congenital absence of the tibia: A report of two cases. ICIB, 10(11):1–12, 1971.

159. Sypniewski, B. L.: The child with terminal transverse partial hemimelia: A review of the literature on prosthetic management. Artif. Limbs, 16:20–50, 1972.

160. Tablada, C., and Clarke, S.: A fitting for the unilateral below-elbow amputee with a dislocated radial head. ICIB, 13(8):1–6, 1974.

161. Taft, C. B., and Fishman, S.: Survival and prosthetic fitting of children amputated for malignancy. ICIB, 5(5):9–28, 1966.

162. Thompson, T. C., Straub, L. R., and Arnold, W. D.: Congenital absence of the fibula. J. Bone Joint Surg., 39A:1229–1237, 1957.

163. Tooms, R. E., and Snell, R. R.: Prosthetic principles—Conventional upper-limb prostheses. *In* The Child With An Acquired Amputation. Washington, D.C., National Academy of Sciences, 1972.

164. Tooms, R. E., Snell, R., and Speltz, E.: An electrically powered elbow unit. ICIB, 6(10):1–4, 1967.

165. ———: Treating the quadrimembral amputee. ICIB, 8(2):1–5, 1968.

166. Trifard, A., and Neary, R.: Prognostic et traitement des sarcomes osteogenigues. J. Chir. 104:185–193, 1972.

167. Van Nes, C. P.: Rotation-plasty for congenital de-

fects of the femur. Making use of the ankle of the shortened limb to control the knee joint of a prosthesis. J. Bone Joint Surg., *32B:*12–16, 1950.

168. Von Soal, G.: Epiphysiodesis combined with amputation. J. Bone Joint Surg., *21:*442–443, 1939.

169. Wenzlaff, E. F.: Surgical ablation of the remaining femoral segment in proximal femoral focal deficiency. ICIB, *9*(1):1–5, 1969.

170. Westin, G. W., and Gunderson, G. O.: Proximal femoral focal deficiency—A review of treatment experiences. *In* A Symposium on Proximal Femoral Focal Deficiency—A Congenital Anomaly. National Academy of Sciences, Washington, D.C., 1969.

171. Wood, W. L., Zlotsky, N., and Westin, G. W.: Congenital absence of the fibula. Treatment by Syme amputation—indications and technique. J. Bone Joint Surg., *47A:*1159–1169, 1965.

23 *Orthotic Management*

Newton C. McCollough III, M.D.

INTRODUCTION

The term "orthosis" refers to an external orthopaedic appliance which is used to control the motion of body segments. The motion controlled may be in the sagittal, coronal, or transverse planes. The types of motion controlled are rotary, as in most joint motion, or translatory, as in vertical displacement of a fractured long bone. Motion control may be of several different types. An orthosis may eliminate motion entirely in a joint by locking it in place, or it may impose varying degrees of assistance or resistance to joint motion. Another type of motion control is axial unloading which is representative of translatory motion control, and it is frequently employed in the lower limb.

Orthoses in children, as in adults, are prescribed to accomplish one or more specific functions. They may be used to prevent deformity, correct deformity, protect a joint or segment, or to improve function. It is important to identify the purpose or purposes of orthotic control at the time of prescription.

ORTHOTIC TERMINOLOGY

Until relatively recently, orthotic terminology has been in complete disarray. Harris has stated that it has in fact resembled "a mausoleum in which to record and honor the names of the departed."* A task force of the Committee on Prosthetic and Orthotic Education of the National Academy of Sci-

---
*Harris, E.E.: Personal communication, 1973.

ences has developed a simplified and internationally accepted terminology for describing classes of orthotic devices.[19] This terminology forms the basis for the Atlas of Orthotics recently published by the Committee on Prosthetics and Orthotics of the American Academy of Orthopaedic Surgeons.[1] The type or class of orthosis is now designated by the joints or segments of the body which it encompasses. Acronyms are used to abbreviate the designation for prescription writing. Thus, the device formerly known as a short-leg brace is now called an ankle-foot orthosis (AFO). A long-leg brace is described as a knee-ankle-foot orthosis (KAFO). A lumbosacral spine orthosis is designated as an LSO. The Milwaukee brace would be classified as a CTLSO. There are obviously many variations within each class or category of devices, and specific characteristics of each must be further described in the prescription. The new terminology, however, does introduce an orderly approach to identification of devices and to orthotic prescription.

RATIONALE FOR ORTHOTIC PRESCRIPTION

Much progress can be made in understanding the principles of orthotic prescription if it is possible to ignore many of our old concepts of "bracing." To "brace" confers the intention of shoring up or supporting by static means, while the term "orthotics" is used to include static as well as dynamic control of the limb. One of the erroneous concepts of "bracing" in the past has been the tendency to lock the extremity into a rigid static device for control of a particular undesirable motion, while at the same time inhibiting some of the remaining normal functions of the limb. For example, a KAFO to control genu valgum also may eliminate knee flexion and extension and limit eversion and inversion at the subtalar joint. The ideal orthosis would control *only* the genu valgum, while permitting normal biomechanical functions to continue unimpeded in the same limb.

One of the first major departures from conventional orthotic design was the functional long-leg brace developed at the University of California at Los Angeles.[4] This device with its quadrilateral socket, offset knee joints, and hydraulic resistance to plantar flexion provided knee stability during stance phase and free knee flexion during swing phase, thereby enabling the polio patient with a flail knee and ankle to walk with a more natural and less energy-consuming gait. This orthosis was designed on sound biomechanical principles to control a specific offending motion, i.e., uncontrolled knee flexion during stance phase, but it permitted the normal and desirable function of knee motion during swing phase. Other investigational orthoses have been similarly designed to permit normal function, such as the dual axis ankle-foot orthosis developed at the University of California at Berkeley, which controls drop foot but permits subtalar motion.[22] A rational approach to orthotic prescription therefore involves approaching the problem on a biomechanical basis without preconceived ideas of conventional orthotic devices. This approach also tends to negate the concept of "disease bracing" or the automatic prescription of certain appliances identified with specific disease entities. Rather, one should approach each patient, regardless of the underlying disease, by analysis of the specific biomechanical deficits present, followed by translation of this information into the appropriate mechanical substitute.

Special forms have been developed and described elsewhere for diagramatically illustrating the biomechanical deficits of the patient's limbs or spine.[1, 29, 36] While these forms are helpful educational tools, they may be cumbersome to use for the average practitioner. However, the principle involved is an important one and serves as the basis for modern orthotic prescription. The approach to orthotic prescription should always follow a logical sequence: (1) a biomechanical analysis of the patient's deficits should be made; (2) the functional disability and the treatment objectives should be identified; (3) the desired orthotic control should be specified at each level; (4) the appropriate orthotic components should be selected to provide the desired control; and (5) the components should be combined in the prescription into an appropriate orthotic device.

ADVANCES IN ORTHOTICS

There have been many advances in orthotics over the past 10 years. Chief among them has been the increasing sophistication of the orthotic practitioner or certified orthotist, the advent of new materials for use in fabrication of orthotic devices, and the trend toward providing improved cosmesis and comfort in these devices.

New materials which have been introduced into the field of orthotics in the past 10 years are primarily plastics, including the thermosetting plastics and various thermoplastics. These plastic materials may be used alone or in combination with metal to produce lighter weight, more cosmetic, and in many instances more functional devices than we have had available in the past. Thermosetting plastics are those that require application of heat to cure or harden, but that will not soften upon further heating. An example is the familiar plastic laminate used in prosthetic sockets. This type of material is useful in orthotics for quadrilateral brims of knee-ankle-foot orthoses, patellar tendon-bearing brims of ankle-foot orthoses, and for foot orthoses or shoe-insert designs. Thermoplastic materials are those that soften each time the temperature is raised to a critical level and harden upon lowering of the temperature. The most commonly used thermoplastics in orthotics are polypropylene, polyethylene, and polycarbonate. Of these, polypropylene finds the widest application due to its unusual feature of extreme resistance to fatigue upon repeated bending. Thermoplastics are usually hand molded or vacuum molded over positive models of the limbs or trunk, giving a precise and intimate fit.

There has been an increasing trend toward providing better cosmesis and comfort in both limb and spinal orthotic devices. The more common use of plastics has had an enormous influence upon both of these factors. While the objectives of cosmesis and comfort are probably secondary to providing adequate function or efficiency of the appliance, they are nevertheless important, and no less important in the child than in the adult. We have all known patients who will even sacrifice better function for comfort or cosmesis by refusing to wear a standard metal orthosis. The seemingly minor inconvenience of not being able to change shoes when an orthotic device is used is of major concern to many children. The advent of thermoplastic materials for use in orthoses to control inadequate dorsiflexion has obviated this problem by virtue of a shoe-insert design, while at the same time it has solved the problem of cosmesis. The physician should not neglect the importance of cosmesis and comfort when prescribing an orthosis for a child, since a much higher degree of acceptance may be obtained with less psychological trauma by appropriate utilization of newer materials in the design and fabrication of the device.

PHILOSOPHY OF ORTHOTIC PRESCRIPTION

Prescription of an orthosis for a child requires careful consideration of the purposes to be achieved, the biomechanical design, the length of time required for wear, the frequency of growth adjustments or frequency of replacement of the entire orthosis due to growth, and the impact of the device upon the child and his parents. The long-term effects of wearing an unsightly appliance may be much more devastating than the trauma of corrective or reconstructive surgery, if there is a choice betwen the two methods of treatment. The prescription of an appliance just to reassure the parents that something is being done for a mild or self-correcting deformity when the efficacy of the device is questionable is not fair to the child or to the parents.

The orthotic device prescribed should be the minimum amount of hardware required to accomplish the desired objective. Frequently, surgical correction of deformity may reduce or eliminate the need for orthotic prescription. A combination of surgical and orthotic management combined with a physical therapy program is frequently the best approach to a clinical problem, particularly in neuromuscular disorders.

In all cases the feelings and emotional make-up of the child should be taken into consideration when prescribing a device. The physician should appreciate the impact on the child of having to wear an appliance for a long period of time during the formative years. Considerations as to alternative methods of treatment should be given, and if orthotic management is the treatment of choice, the device prescribed should be as unencumbering as possible, controlling insofar as is possible only the particular problem in question. Consideration should also be given in the design of the device to provide optimum cosmesis and comfort insofar as is technically feasible.

LOWER LIMB ORTHOTICS

The most common site of application of orthotic devices in children is the lower limb. The purposes of orthotic management varies widely and includes prevention of deformity, correction of deformity, protection of a joint or limb segment, and improvement in junction. Frequently, two or more of these purposes may be achieved by the same device, such as improvement in gait and prevention of ankle contracture by the use of an AFO with a 90° plantar flexion stop.

The Foot and Ankle

Orthotic control of problems about the foot and ankle is accomplished by the use of proper shoes, foot orthoses (FO) or ankle-foot orthoses (AFO). Shoes are classified as orthotic devices when they are prescribed to perform specific orthotic functions. As the foundation for many lower limb orthoses, they also may be thought of as integral parts of the orthotic system.

Metatarus Adductus. The reverse-last or

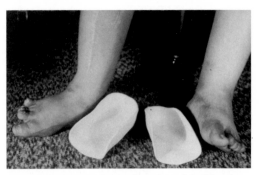

FIG. 23-1. The UCB (University of California at Berkeley) shoe insert for moderate to severe planovalgus. (Courtesy Robert O. Nitschke, Rochester, New York)

outflare shoe is indicated either as prewalker or closed-toe shoe. Shoes alone will not correct rigid deformities, but they are useful to maintain correction for a period of time following casting. Flexible deformities may be corrected over a period of several months with the use of this type of shoe worn 24 hours a day.

Pes Planovalgus. Mild degrees of flattening of the longitudinal arch do not need treatment. Children usually do not develop a longitudinal arch until they are 5 to 6 years of age, so moderate flattening of the arch early in childhood is the rule rather than the exception. Children who have flattening of the arch associated with heel valgus may be treated with an inverted or supinated last shoe to adduct the forefoot, using Thomas heels with a $^1/_8$- or $^3/_{16}$-inch medial heel wedge and a medial arch support. Such children with hypermobile flat feet will always have the tendency to planovalgus deformity no matter how long the shoes are worn, but it may be possible to reduce the ultimate degree of deformity by prolonged corrective shoe wear.

Children who have more severe degrees of pes planovalgus and who are symtomatic may be treated with special foot orthoses. Today the most commonly used devices are the molded leather shoe insert and the molded plastic shoe insert (UCB insert) developed at the University of California at Berkeley.[22] The molded leather insert is a custom-made, firm, longitudinal arch support fabricated from a cast of the foot. It provides good support for the longitudinal arch, but does not control heel valgus. The molded plastic shoe insert provides not only an arch support, but also grasps the heel of the foot to prevent heel valgus (Fig. 23-1). This device is fabricated over a positive plaster mold of the foot in the corrected position. While the molded plastic insert foot orthosis is an effective positioning device for the foot, it is not known whether or not any permanent correction can be achieved.

Pes Calcaneovalgus. This common positional foot deformity in the newborn usually requires no specific treatment other than passive exercise by the mother. If severe, the Denis Browne bar foot orthosis may be used, angled with the apex cephalad and the feet in neutral rotation to accentuate inversion of the feet at the subtalar joint. The length of the bar in this instance should not exceed the width of the pelvis. Correction is usually observed within 2 months of night wear.

Talipes Equinovarus. Orthotic management of this condition is an adjunct to other non surgical and surgical methods of treatment and is used solely to maintain the correction achieved by these other methods. There is no corrective orthotic device for this deformity. Following correction in the infant, outflare or reverse-last prewalker shoes may be attached to a Denis Browne bar which is angled with the apex caudad, the affected foot or feet being externally rotated on the bar to 70° to 80°. This arrangement produces a dorsiflexion-eversion force when the infant kicks and tends to prevent recurrent deformity. Another type of orthosis which may be used to maintain the foot in the corrected position is a single medial upright AFO with a 90° plantar flexion stop and a lateral T strap attached to a reverse-last prewalker shoe. For the ambulatory child, a reverse-last shoe with a $^1/_4$-inch lateral heel and sole wedge and a reverse Thomas heel should be used with or without the single-medial upright AFO, depending upon the degree of concern regarding recurrence.

Dorsiflexion Insufficiency. Lack of adequate dorsiflexion of the foot results in a "drop foot" with inadequate clearance of the toes during the swing phase of gait. Secondary effects on gait occur from compensatory efforts to clear the foot, and include excessive hip and knee flexion (steppage gait), vaulting on the sound side, and circumduction of the affected limb. If inadequate dorsiflexion is combined with contracture of the heel cord, a toe-heel gait during stance phase results, imparting an extension movement to the knee resulting in genu recurvatum. If a varus component is present with inadequate dorsiflexion, foot contact occurs initially on the lateral border of the feet, perhaps producing initial stance phase instability. The orthotic approach to each of these three situations differs slightly.

Isolated Dorsiflexion Insufficiency. Pure loss of dorsiflexion power requires a dorsiflexion-assist AFO. The orthoses of choice are either the double-upright spring dorsiflexion-assist orthosis,[1] or the molded plastic-AFO-insert orthosis (Fig. 23-2).[36] Either of these devices will provide dorsiflexion assistance while permitting the normal function of plantar flexion at heel strike, thus providing the most optimal gait. If one were to use an AFO with a 90° plantar flexion stop, plantar flexion at heel strike would be restricted and an undesirable flexion movement imparted to the knee by the posterior calf band.

The molded plastic-insert AFO has the advantage of being lightweight and cosmetic. However, there is no adjustability for growth, so that the maximum period of use is about 2 years. If this device is selected, the trim lines at the ankle should be sufficiently posterior to allow flexible plantar flexion at heel strike.

Dorsiflexion Insufficiency With Dynamic Equinus. If inadequate dorsiflexion of the foot is associated with mild dynamic or spastic equinus, the orthoses described above may be used. If the spasticity is moderate to severe, the orthoses of choice are either the double-upright AFO with 90° plantar flexion stop, or the molded plastic-insert AFO fabricated with the ankle trim lines sufficiently anterior to provide stiff resistance to plantar flexion (Fig. 23-3). In cases which demonstrate significant hyperextension of the knee associated with the spastic equinus, modifying the plantar flexion stop to slightly above 90° or fabricating the plastic AFO in slight dorsiflexion is indicated. This modification will provide an increased flexion

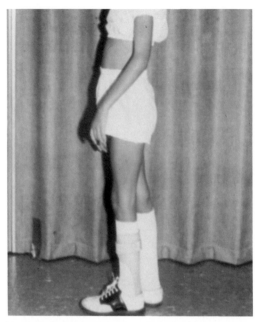

FIG. 23-2. Molded polypropylene AFO for foot and ankle control in a child with spastic left hemiparesis.

movement at the knee transmitted through the posterior calf band.

Dorsiflexion insufficiency combined with structural equinus requires surgical or serial-cast correction of the equinus deformity prior to bracing.

Dorsiflexion Insufficiency With Varus. Mild degrees of varus deformity during swing phase need no special consideration, and any orthoses used for isolated dorsiflexion insufficiency will be adequate. Moderate dynamic varus during swing phase may be controlled by the addition of a lateral T strap to the double-upright AFO. Severe varus deformity in swing phase cannot be controlled by orthotic means, and it requires surgical correction.

Dynamic Varus Deformity During Stance Phase. Orthotic management of dynamic varus deformity during stance phase of gait is difficult at best, and frequently it requires surgical correction as the preferred management. If the varus is mild during foot contact, a lateral T strap added to either a single-medial-upright or a double-upright AFO may be sufficient to provide stability in

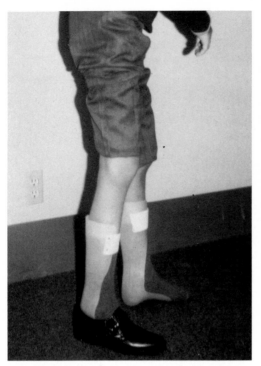

FIG. 23-3. Molded polypropylene AFO with ankle rigidity provided by extending the trim lines anterior to the malleoli.

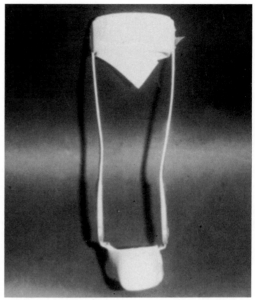

FIG. 23-4. N.Y.U. (New York University) AFO for foot and ankle control, viewed from the posterior.

conjunction with a high-top shoe. Moderate degrees of dynamic varus deformity may be controlled by either the molded insert, double-upright AFO[9] (Fig. 23-4) or the molded plastic-insert AFO with the ankle trim lines anterior to the malleoli so as to provide mediolateral stability (Fig. 23-3). Severe degrees of dynamic varus deformity or structural varus deformity are not amenable to orthotic control and surgical correction is indicated.

Plantar Flexion Insufficiency. Inadequacy of ankle plantar flexion is usually caused by paralysis of the triceps surae. The effects on gait are excessive ankle dorsiflexion during stance phase, which may be exaggerated in the presence of a weak quadriceps, and inadequate push-off. The former is subject to orthotic control, the latter is not. It is important to control excessive ankle dorsiflexion during stance phase in the growing child in order to minimize the development of the calcaneus deformity which invariably occurs.

The standard orthotic control for plantar flexion insufficiency is the double-upright AFO with 90° dorsiflexion (anterior) stops. There are two important considerations in the fabrication and application of this device. The calf band must be as high as possible to gain optimal mechanical advantage in preventing forward rotation of the tibia over the ankle. A more positive control may be gained by reversing the calf band to provide firm pressure over the proximal tibia. Secondly, in order to minimize motion between the orthosis and the shoe, an extended stirrup should be used, attached to a steel shank running the length of the shoe.

A molded plastic-insert AFO with a pretibial shell may also be used to provide control of excessive ankle dorsiflexion[17] (Fig. 23-5). The plastic material used must be of sufficient thickness to provide a rigid ankle and foot plate. This device, when properly constructed, gives excellent control of the foot and ankle and prevents excessive ankle dorsiflexion. The disadvantage of this

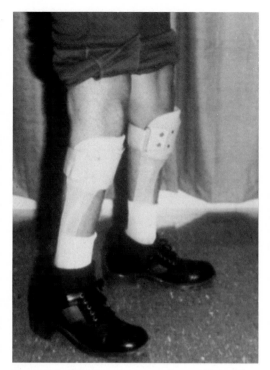

FIG. 23-5. Molded polypropylene AFO with a pretibial shell for control of excessive ankle dorsiflexion.

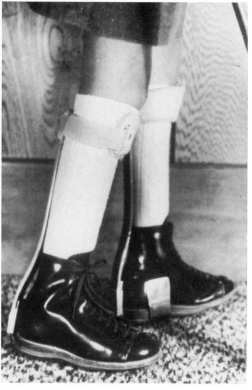

FIG. 23-6. Posterior-bar AFO for control of excessive ankle dorsiflexion. (Courtesy Robert O. Nitschke, Rochester, New York)

orthosis in the growing child is the lack of adjustability, and since the effectiveness of control depends to a considerable degree upon the height of the pretibial shell, a new orthosis may be required on a yearly basis.

The posterior-bar AFO is a relatively new device used to substitute for the plantar flexors of the ankle in preventing excessive ankle dorsiflexion (Fig. 23-6). The posterior bar may be made of spring steel or fiberglass material and must be attached securely to an extension of a steel shank in the sole of the shoe at the heel. The orthosis essentially provides a dynamic force to prevent forward rotation of the tibia over the ankle during stance phase of gait.

The Flail Foot and Ankle. Total paralysis about the foot and ankle is best managed by an orthosis which provides some resistance to both plantar flexion and dorsiflexion, while providing adequate mediolateral stability for the subtalar joint. This may be ac-

complished by the use of a double-upright AFO with anterior and posterior spring-loaded resistance (Fig. 23-7), or by the molded plastic-insert AFO utilizing sufficiently thick material to provide the desired resistance.

The molded spiral AFO[25] (Fig. 23-8) also provides resistance to plantar flexion and dorsiflexion, but experience with this device in children has been limited.

The Painful Ankle. Hemophilia, rheumatoid arthritis, osteochondritis dissecans, and other abnormalities of the ankle joint may produce symptoms or potential conditions for which orthotic protection is indicated. In such situations it may be desirable to eliminate all motion in the ankle joint, or at least reduce motion to a minimum. The molded plastic-insert AFO with trim lines which extend anterior to the malleoli (Fig.

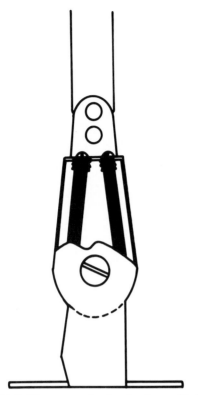

FIG. 23-7. Diagrammatic sketch of an ankle joint with anterior and posterior channels that may be used with stops or spring loaded.

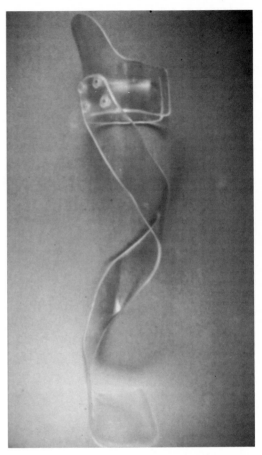

FIG. 23-8. Molded spiral AFO for resistance to both plantar flexion and dorsiflexion of the ankle.

23-3) provides relatively rigid immobilization of the ankle joint. It should be used with special shoe modifications, consisting of a soft rubber heel (SACH heel) and a rocker bar on the sole. This permits simulated ankle motion by compression of the heel at heel strike followed by rolling over the rocker bar to achieve toe-off. As an alternative to the molded plastic AFO design, one may use a double-upright, rigid-ankle AFO attached to a shoe with a steel shank and similar shoe modifications.

Axial unloading of the ankle joint, while highly desirable in many instances to relieve symptoms or to prevent joint compression, cannot be achieved effectively by orthotic means. The patellar tendon-bearing AFO[36] in theory reduces upright bearing forces on the ankle joint, but in practice it simply has not worked in the author's experience. Significant unloading of the ankle joint requires weightbearing forces about the proximal tibia and patellar tendon, which are more than the patient can tolerate.

The Leg

Tibial Torsion. Internal or external tibial torsion may occur as a developmental abnormality, but internal torsion of the tibia is by far the most common of the two. The decision to treat internal tibial torsion during infancy is highly individualized, and among orthopaedic surgeons a range of opinion can be found, from "treat none" to "treat all." Clinical experience tells us that many, but not all, of these deformities spontaneously regress by the time the child begins to walk. If the deformity appears to be significant by

FIG. 23-9. This posterior-bar KAFO with a rotational adjustment at the foot is used as a night splint for internal tibial torsion.

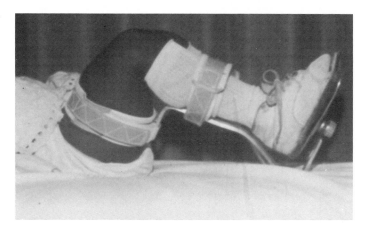

the age of 4 to 6 months, treatment with the Denis Browne bar may be undertaken, and correction is usually apparent within 3 to 6 months. Prewalker shoes (reverse-last shoes if metatarsus adductus is also present) are attached to the bar and externally rotated from 45° to 60° or to the position at which slight resistance is felt to external rotation of the leg. The length of the bar should not exceed the width of the anterior-superior spines of the ileum by more than an inch or two, or the feet will be forced into pronation and a secondary deformity will be produced. This device may be used for treatment of internal tibial torsion during the first year and one half of life. In the author's experience, it is poorly tolerated if instituted beyond that time, due to the fact that independent movement of the legs is prevented.

In the older child, a device has been developed which permits independent leg movement for the treatment of torsional deformities of the leg (Fig. 23-9). It consists of a posterior aluminum bar KAFO with a 90° bend at the knee and at the ankle. The shoe plate has a rotational adjustment permitting graduated external rotation. Placing the knee in flexion confines the rotational force to the leg segment, avoiding the dissipation of the force upward to the hip, which occurs with the Denis Browne bar. The orthosis should be adjusted in the child, externally rotating the foot until resistance is encountered, then the foot plate should be locked in position. Further adjustments into external rotation then are made monthly.

The HKAFO twister orthosis may also be used for the treatment of tibial torsion in the older child (Fig. 23-10). Since the torque force is not confined to the lower leg segment, but is dissipated upwards to the hip, it is not felt to be as effective as the orthosis just described. It consists of flexible hydraulic tubing or spring cables attached to a pelvic band and to the shoes with an adjustment to rotate the shoes outward or inward at the ankle. It produces essentially no restriction of motion of the limb other than the desired rotational control. It may be used either as a nighttime device or it may be worn during the waking hours as well. The device is well tolerated by children as a night splint, and successful results have been obtained up to 8 years of age with usage from 4 to 6 months.

Protection of the Leg. Protective orthoses for the leg segment may be indicated in the child with osteogenesis imperfecta, congenital pseudarthrosis of the tibia, or other pathologic states that compromise the integrity of bone structure. A lightweight protective device made of polypropylene and lined with polyethylene foam can be fabricated from a positive model of the leg (Fig. 23-11). It may be formed either as a leg cylinder or as an AFO, and it is of a ''clamshell'' design with anterior and posterior halves which are secured together with Velcro straps. Extension of the anterior, medial, and lateral portions to the supracondylar area of the femur will add rotational control and will still permit full flexion and extension of the knee.

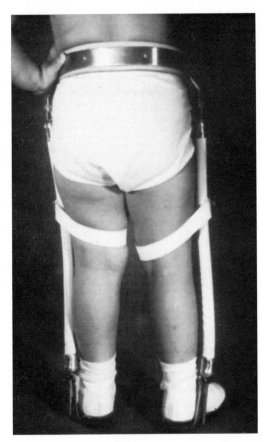

FIG. 23-10. HKAFO twister orthosis for dynamic control of limb rotation or tibial torsion. (From Staros, A., and LeBlanc, M.: Orthotic components and system. *In* American Academy of Orthopaedic Surgeons: Atlas of Orthotics. St. Louis, C. V. Mosby, 1975.)

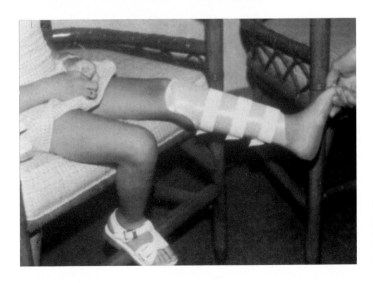

FIG. 23-11. Molded polypropylene AFO of a bivalve design with a shoe insert for protection of the tibia in a child with osteogenesis imperfecta.

In the older child, protection of the leg segment may be achieved by the use of the tibial-fracture orthosis made from Orthoplast* with a polypropylene ankle joint previously described by Sarmiento.[39] The orthosis may be split vertically to allow removal and reapplication, using Velcro straps for closure.

Fractures of the Tibia and Fibula. Although the treatment of fractures is beyond the scope of this text, it should be pointed out that fractures of the tibia and fibula in the older child and adolescent may be successfully managed by the use of fracture bracing (Fig. 23-12). The orthosis is applied after 2 weeks of immobilization in a long-leg cast, and full weightbearing is permitted, as tolerated. Angular deformities must be corrected prior to application of the orthosis.

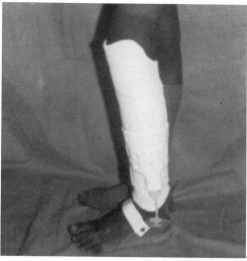

FIG. 23-12. Tibial fracture brace on a child 10 years of age.

The Knee

Genu Varum. Bowing of the legs is a normal physiological event in children up to 2 years of age and needs no treatment in this age group. Persistant genu varum which is not decreasing is pathologic in children over the age of 3, and it may be due to failure of spontaneous correction of developmental genu varum, tibia vara (Blount's disease), rickets, or other metabolic bone disease. Regardless of the cause, orthotic management is indicated in children over the age of 3 with varus deformities of the knee in excess of 15°, as measured by a standing roentgenogram. In the older child or adolescent, orthotic management is not likely to be effective and surgical correction is generally preferred.

The degree to which orthotic management is effective in the management of pathologic genu varum is open to question. In principle, one hopes to influence epiphyseal growth at the distal femoral and proximal tibial growth plates by producing tension forces on the medial side of the knee joint and compressive forces on the lateral side. The extent to which this is possible is not known, nor is it known whether actual correction or simple arrest of progression of deformity can be achieved by orthotic means. In children who are braced for genu varum, it is important to

*Johnson and Johnson, New Brunswick, New Jersey.

obtain periodic standing roentgenograms out of the brace to measure the knee angle and assess the effect of orthosis wear. It has been the author's impression that gradual correction of genu varum deformity can occur with prolonged orthotic usage, although it is impossible to rule out spontaneous correction with growth or with vitamin D therapy in the case of rickets.

It is impossible to apply a corrective force at the knee and at the same time permit free knee motion. Therefore, orthoses employed in the correction of genu varum must have locked knee joints or no knee joints at all. Therefore, it is usually desirable to permit a few hours of freedom from the orthosis every day, utilizing the device at night and about half of the waking hours.

Two orthotic designs for use in genu varum have been employed. The more conventional system is an HKAFO with free ankle joints, a single-medial lower upright connected to a single-lateral upper upright by a posterior thigh band. The two lateral uprights are joined by a pelvic band with free hip joints (Fig. 23-13). The corrective pullover pads are placed over the lateral aspect of the proximal tibiae and knee joints and anchored to the medial uprights. The second design consists of a double-lateral-upright

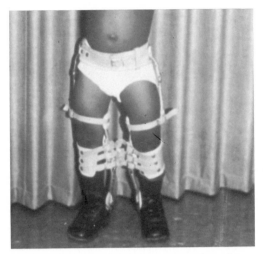

Fig. 23-13. A HKAFO for the correction of genu varum, with a pullover pad to a medial upright.

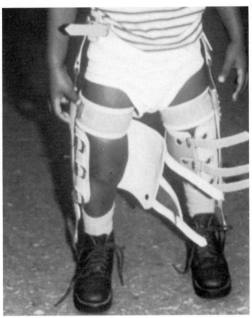

Fig. 23-14. A HKAFO for correction of genu varum, with lateral uprights and adjustable pads to provide a medially directed corrective force.

HKAFO with free ankle joints and hip joints and an adjustable pushover pad centered at the level of the knee joint (Fig. 23-14). Relief must be provided over the area of the peroneal nerve.

Salter has described a night splint for genu varum in children over the age of 2 years, consisting of a Denis Browne bar to anchor the feet and an encircling leather or fabric gauntlet about the knees to produce the corrective force.[37] In the author's personal experience, this device is too confining to be tolerated well by the child.

Genu Valgum. Physiologic genu valgum occurs in many children between the ages of 2 and 8 years. Unfortunately, there is no available statistical information regarding the natural progression and resolution of this deformity. It has been the author's policy to consider genu valgum pathologic in this age group when it exceeds 15°, as measured by a standing roentgenogram. In children over the age of 8 years, genu valgum in excess of 10° is considered abnormal. Orthotic treatment is instituted in these two categories of patients and continued until correction is achieved or until the decision is made to treat surgically.

As in the case of genu varum, no available data exists as to the efficacy of orthotic treatment in this condition. The rational for altering the deformity by orthotic means rests on the theory that it is possible to create tension forces on the lateral side of the knee joint and compressive forces on the medial side of the joint, thereby influencing epiphyseal growth. It cannot be stated with certainty that the correction observed with the use of orthoses is due entirely to the effect of the appliance, or whether some degree of natural correction with growth might be a factor. Significant correction of deformity by orthotic means in children over the age of 10 years is doubtful.

The recommended orthosis for genu valgum deformity is a single-lateral-upright KAFO with thigh and calf bands, a medial pullover pad anchored to the lateral upright, and a free ankle joint (Fig. 23-15). In order for the appliance to be effective, the knee must be maintained in full extension, so the device is fabricated either without a knee joint or with dropping knee locks. The orthoses should be worn as night splints and for one-half of the waking hours, allowing some freedom of activity for the child during the daytime.

Genu valgum also may occur in conjunction with paralytic states in which muscles about the hip and knee are inadequate, and it is frequently seen in poliomyelitis. The management of this type deformity will be discussed under "Quadriceps Insufficiency," below.

Genu Recurvatum. In children, hyperextension of the knee during the stance phase of gait is most frequently observed in association with either spastic or flaccid paralysis. In the spastic state, the cause is usually related to overactivity of the triceps surae, producing a tethering effect upon normal forward rotation of the tibia over the ankle from foot flat to midstance. The use of either a rigid molded plastic-insert AFO fabricated in 10° of dorsiflexion, or a double-upright AFO with the planter stop set at 10° above neutral frequently controls this gait defect, assuming that the quadriceps is of normal strength. If the deformity persists to a significant degree with the use of an AFO, a double-upright aluminum KAFO with free ankle and extension stops at the knees is indicated. If the quadriceps is also weak, drop-ring knee locks should be added to the orthosis to maintain knee stability.

In the case of genu recurvatum due to flaccid paralysis, the cause is usually quadriceps insufficiency, and the knee is consciously placed in the hyperextended position to achieve knee stability. After a period of time, the recurvatum increases as a result of ligamentous stretching. The increasing pressures upon the anterior portions of the epiphyseal plates at the knee may cause accentuation of the deformity with growth. In this case, treatment with the appropriate KAFO for quadriceps insufficiency permits the knee to maintain a minimally extended or slightly flexed position during stance phase.

Quadriceps Insufficiency. Inadequacy of knee extension power as an isolated defect is rare, and paralysis of the quadriceps is usually associated with weakness in other portions of the limb. However, stabilization of the knee segment is the key to ambulation in extensive lower limb paralysis. While it is possible for the child with a paralyzed quadriceps to walk without an orthosis if the hip extensors are adequate, he must maintain the knee in a hyperextended and locked po-

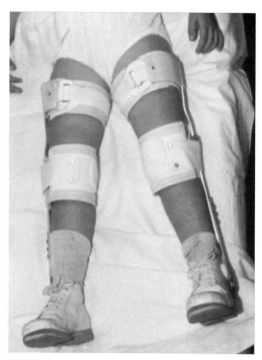

FIG. 23-15. Lateral-upright KAFO's with medial pullover pads for correction of genu valgum.

sition. Abnormal pressures are created on the epiphyseal plates at the knee which can lead to progressive deformity. Therefore, it is important to provide knee stability in these children unless the natural course of their disease renders them nonambulatory in childhood.

The conventional orthosis used for quadriceps insufficiency is a double-upright aluminum KAFO with thigh and calf bands, drop-ring knee locks, an anterior knee pad, and an ankle joint which is appropriate to the biomechanical situation at the ankle. This device provides excellent knee stability and prevents hyperextension of the knee. In the case of bilateral involvement, the use of plunger knee locks may be preferred, so that manual operation of the knee locks can be performed at the hip level. If genu valgum is associated with quadriceps insufficiency, the anterior knee pad may be modified to pull the knee toward the lateral upright, or a pressure pad centered over the medial femoral condyle may be used.

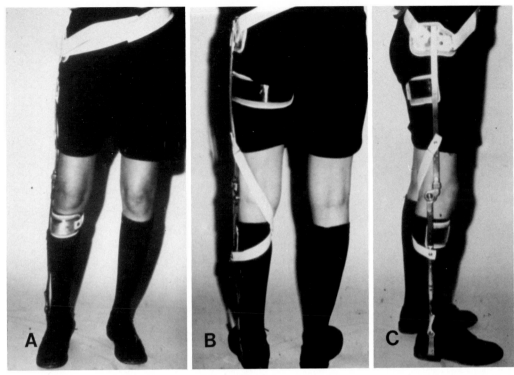

FIG. 23-16. *(A, B, and C)* Single-lateral-upright KAFO with a pretibial shell and a silesian bandage for control of knee instability and flaccid paralysis.

Excellent knee stability may also be achieved in flaccid paralysis by the use of the single-lateral-upright KAFO with a pretibial shell and a posterior popliteal strap (Fig. 23-16).[33] This device is easier to don, lighter in weight, and more cosmetic than the double-upright KAFO. It incorporates a drop-ring knee lock and an ankle joint of choice which may be attached to a shoe insert. The posterior cross strap effectively holds the knee forward into the pretibial shell, allowing the patient to kneel into the orthosis for stability. An accessory silesian belt can be added for rotational stability, if necessary. The device may be used in the case of bilateral quadriceps insufficiency as well.

A third alternative for providing knee stability in the child is the molded plastic KAFO with drop-ring knee locks, which is fabricated from a positive model of the lower limb (Fig. 23-17).[28] This device also provides excellent knee stability with the advantage of minimal weight, and it is particularly useful in situations of extreme general weakness where weight is an important consideration, such as in the muscular dystrophy patient. The disadvantage of this orthosis is the relative lack of adjustability in the growing child. The maximum period of time before a completely new orthosis is needed is 2 years. The orthosis may be used without the drop-ring knee locks for control of genu recurvatum in the presence of an adequate quadriceps.

In spastic paralysis, weakness of knee extension is frequently associated with hamstring tightness or overactivity. The double-upright KAFO is usually indicated in this situation, as the single-lateral-upright and molded plastic designs do not provide sufficient control of dynamic knee flexion. In many cases, it is preferable to improve quadricep function and knee extension by

FIG. 23-17. *(A and B)* Molded polypropylene KAFO for control of knee instability utilized in a child with muscular dystrophy.

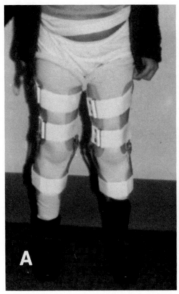
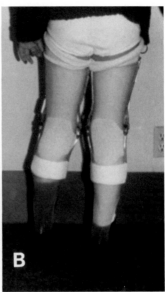

hamstring lengthening or transfer, thus reducing the orthotic requirements to that of an AFO.

Orthotic considerations with regard to hip control associated with quadricep insufficiency in cases with paralysis about the hip will be considered under "The Hip," page 1070.

Knee-flexion Contracture. The occurrence of knee-flexion contracture is common in flaccid paralysis, spastic paralysis, hemophiliac arthropathy, and rheumatoid arthritis. When a tendency to develop knee-flexion contracture is noted, the use of a night splint to control the deformity is indicated. The preferred splint is the three-point-extension knee orthosis (KO) which consists of double aluminum uprights attached to pivotal calf and thigh bands and an anterior knee pad. This device may also be used to correct mild knee-flexion deformities by gradually tightening the anterior knee pad as extension occurs.

In more severe knee-flexion deformities, attempting orthotic or plaster correction may result in posterior subluxation of the tibia on the femur. The dial-lock knee mechanism may be used on a double-upright KAFO with shallow calf band placed under the proximal tibia to resist posterior displacement of the tibia. Graduated knee extension may then be achieved by progressive adjustment of the dial lock over a period of several weeks.

A more effective method of correcting knee-flexion contractures is the use of the extension-desubluxation hinge developed at Orthopaedic Hospital in Los Angeles for use in hemophiliac arthropathy.[27, 41] This device is incorporated into a short-leg cast and a thigh cylinder, and it has adjustments to obtain knee extensionas well as to obtain desubluxation of the tibia, or to prevent subluxation of the tibia during correction of the flexion deformity (Fig. 23-18).

Protection of the Knee Joint. There are instances in which one wishes to protect the knee joint from stress by the use of an orthotic device. Examples are hemophiliac arthropathy and posttraumatic situations.

The hinged knee cage may be used to provide minimal protection against flexion and extension as well as medial and lateral stresses. The most effective knee cage is custom-made from a positive model of the leg and is comprised of polypropylene thigh and calf cuffs connected by drop-ring knee locks.[12]

The Lennox Hill knee orthosis is a special knee cage designed to prevent rotary stress

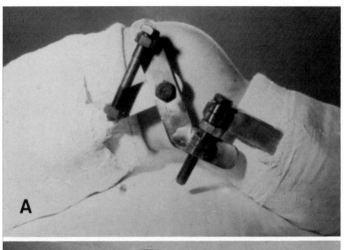

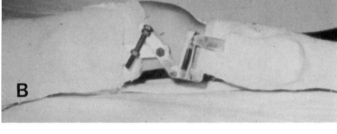

Fig. 23-18. *(A and B)* Extension-desubluxation hinge for correction of knee-flexion contracture associated with posterior subluxation of the tibia in hemophilia.

as well as valgus stress following football injuries, and it may be useful in the older child and adolescent to prevent abduction, external rotation injuries of the knee joint.[1]

Maximal protection may be afforded the knee joint by the use of a full-length KAFO of either the single- or double-upright type with a drop-ring knee lock and a free ankle. As an alternative device for complete immobilization of the knee joint, a polypropylene knee cylinder may be used. Whenever the knee joint must be protected by an orthosis for a prolonged period of time, it is essential that the knee be mobilized at least a few hours each day, and that a physical therapy program for quadriceps strengthening be instituted on a daily basis to prevent stiffness and atrophy.

The Hip

Orthotic control of hip motion in the swing phase of gait is reasonably effective, but the control of hip motion during stance phase to provide stability of the trunk on the femoral head is relatively ineffective. Stabilization of the trunk on the femur in both the anterioposterior and mediolateral directions can only be achieved by joining a lower limb orthosis to a spinal orthosis with an adequate hip lock. This situation renders the child so completely immobile as to defeat the purpose of orthotic use, which is to provide an ambulatory capacity. Children with extensive lower limb paralysis involving the hip who maintain a free range of hip motion can usually stabilize their hip joints by hyperextension, if knee stability is provided by the appropriate KAFO. Orthotic stabilization of the knees allows the child to shift his center of gravity posteriorly so that the floor reaction line is posterior to the hip joint, permitting stabilization of the hip by tension on the anterior capsule.

Adduction-Abduction Control. In flaccid paralytic states involving the musculature about the hip, a common gait defect is flailing of the lower limbs during swing phase dur to inadequate control by the hip abductors and adductors to maintain the limb in the line of progression. An HKAFO consisting of a pelvic band with free hip points in the sagittal plane attached to either a double- or single-upright KAFO controls unwanted adduction-abduction during the swing phase of gait. Hip rotation during swing phase is also prevented by this device. If some degree of flexion-extension control is also desirable, a hip lock may be used.

In the case of spastic paralysis, excessive adduction or "scissoring" is frequently present during swing phase, which may seriously interfere with the child's ability to walk. If knee instability is also present, the use of a similar HKAFO is indicated for control of excessive hip adduction. If knee stability is adequate, adduction control may be achieved by the use of the Rancho Los Amigos hip-control orthosis (Fig. 23-19).[1] This orthosis is designed to allow free hip flexion, extension and abduction, but it provides an adjustable stop against adduction. The advantage of using this device, even if AFO's are required, is that knee motion is preserved and a more natural gait can be achieved.

Stabilization of the pelvis on the femur during stance phase to prevent downward tilt of the pelvis is very difficult to achieve by orthotic means. Partial control may be obtained with a polypropylene girdle attached to a polypropylene thigh cylinder by a heavy-duty hip joint.

Rotational Control. Control of unwanted rotation of the limbs during swing phase may be accomplished by use of the HKAFO with a pelvic band. If adequate knee stability is present and hip abduction-adduction control is adequate, a twister-cable orthosis from a pelvic band may be attached directly to the shoes or to the lateral uprights of the AFO's. This system selectively controls hip rotation while allowing all other hip motion and knee motion to remain free.

Flexion-Extension Control. Orthotic control of hip flexion and extension is frequently desirable in severe paralysis of the lower limbs, such as that which occurs in poliomyelitis and myelomeningocele, when the patient is unable to lock his hips by hyperextension. As has been noted previously, optimal control of undesired flexion of the hips due to extensor insufficiency during stance phase is difficult to achieve with-

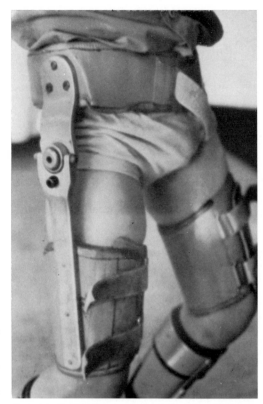

FIG. 23-19. HO for control of hip adduction in cerebral palsy. (From Staros, A., and LeBlanc, M.: Orthotic components and system. *In* American Academy of Orthopaedic Surgeons: Atlas of Orthotics. St. Louis, C. V. Mosby, 1975.)

out rendering the patient completely immobile. Some degree of free hip flexion must be available to the child if he is to be able to advance the limbs in an alternating gait. This gait pattern can be achieved if the child has some strength in his hip flexors. Therefore, hip locks, when used to control flexion of the hips, should be modified to allow 10° to 15° of flexion-extension movement in children with available hip-flexion power to permit an alternating gait pattern.

In patients who exhibit excessive forward rotation of the pelvis and increased lumbar lordosis (commonly seen in myelomeningocele), the addition of a buttock sling to a modified pelvic band helps to reduce the tendency to hip flexion and improves the standing position (Fig. 23-20).

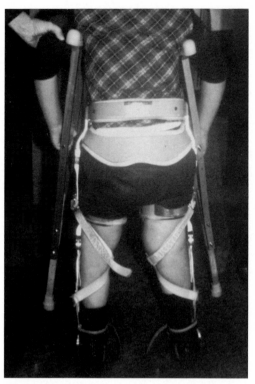

FIG. 23-20. HKAFO of single-lateral-upright design utilized in a child with myelomeningocele and absent hip extensors.

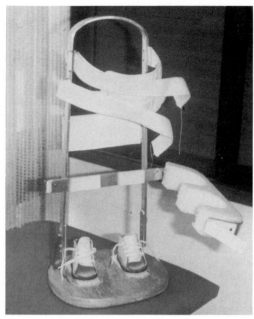

FIG. 23-21. Simple standing frame utilized for children ages 1 to 3 with extensive lower extremity paralysis.

For children who have no motor power about the hips and who are unable to stabilize their hips by hyperextension to permit ambulation with KAFO's, complete immobilization of the hips for stability is indicated. This requires bracing of the trunk as well and limits ambulation to a swing-to type of gait. Children generally do not develop sufficient balance and coordination to perform this type of gait until they are 4 to 5 years of age. From the age of 1 to 5, an orthosis is used principally for standing rather than walking. The orthosis of choice is a standing frame of some type which may be fitted between 1 and 2 years of age (Fig. 23-21). As the child approaches 4 to 5 years of age, the parapodium may be used for standing as well as for developing a swing-to gait. (Fig. 23-22) The child learns this gait pattern on the parallel bars and then on crutches, and must be taught how to fall and protect himself with his sound upper limbs so that he loses the fear of falling. When the swing-to gait has been mastered in the parapodium, an HKAFO can be prescribed with rigid hip locks and a spinal extension. Although the child may continue to ambulate with the parapodium, this device has the disadvantage of having to be worn over the clothing, which usually becomes objectionable by the age of 7 or 8 years. It should be emphasized that children who have such a severe level of paralysis are primarily wheelchair patients, and ambulation, such as it is, is purely for physiologic and psychologic reasons. Nearly all children will discard their orthoses in favor of the wheelchair by the time of early adolescence.

Femoral Anteversion. The entity of increased femoral anteversion, or excessive internal femoral torsion, is of clinical significance because it produces an intoeing gait. The long-terms effects upon the hip and knee joint are not known. Popular methods of treatment for this condition include various shoe modifications in an attempt to produce an outtoeing gait, and orthotic devices for the purpose of producing external rotation of the limb such as the Denis Browne bar and the "twister" torsion orthosis. Although such devices may produce a change in the habit pattern of walking, there is no evidence that they have any effect upon the reduction of femoral torsion. Iabry and his associates have shown that little spontaneous reduction of increased femoral anteversion can be expected in children with a toe-in gait, and in fact shoes, bars, and twisters have had no measurable effect upon femoral torsion after 5$\frac{1}{2}$ years.[15]

In the case of the twister orthosis and the Denis Browne bar, the external rotation force applied to the foot is dissipated through the subtalar, ankle, and knee joints and there is probably very little in the way of torque produced upon the femur. Therefore, until recently, it has been our policy either to not treat femoral anteversion by orthotic devices and allow compensatory mechanisms to develop which eventually reduce intoeing, or, in the severe cases, to perform derotational femoral osteotomy.

A device developed at the University of Miami for use as a nighttime orthosis for femoral anteversion has been in use for the past 3 years. The "twister" principle is used, but the torsion force is confined to the femur by design of the orthosis. It consists of a pelvic band and twister cables attached to knee cages of thermoplastic design, which maintain the knees in the position of 20° to 30° of flexion (Fig. 23-23). In order to properly adjust this HKO on initial application, the femora are manually externally rotated until resistance is met, and the twister cables are locked in that position on the knee cages, thus preventing any further internal rotation. The orthosis is readjusted into further external rotation on a monthly basis, always locking the orthosis when resistance is met. Thus, a small amount of external torsional force is applied to the femur and across the femoral epiphyseal plates. After 6 to 12 months of night wear, a measurable increase in external rotation of the hips and a corresponding decrease in internal rotation will be noted, coinciding with reduction of the intoeing gait. This orthosis has been used in children up to 8 years of age with satisfactory results.

Legg-Calvé-Perthes Disease. There is now nearly universal agreement that a basic prin-

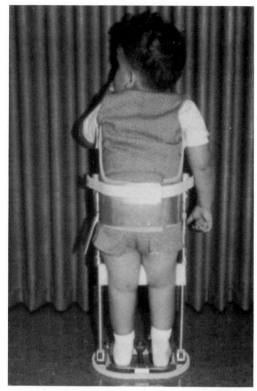

Fig. 23-22. Parapodium utilized for standing, as well as for a swing-to type of ambulation, in older children with extensive lower limb paralysis.

ciple in the orthotic management of Legg-Calvé-Perthes disease is concentric containment of the femoral head within the acetabulum.[7, 11, 20, 23, 34, 38, 43] There is less agreement upon whether or not femoral head containment with weightbearing or without weightbearing is preferred. In order to produce adequate containment of the femoral head within the acetabulum, so as to achieve equal distribution of pressures upon the head, the orthotic device used must position the hip in abduction and some degree of internal rotation. The old ischial weightbearing ring caliper with patten shoe has been condemned as not only being ineffective, but also it is probably injurious to the femoral head due to its failure to position the hip in abduction and internal rotation.[10]

The earliest abduction ambulatory device used for treatment of Legg-Calvé-Perthes

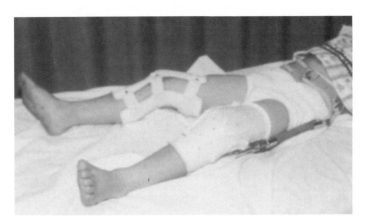

FIG. 23-23. HKO twister orthosis utilized as a night splint for control of internal femoral torsion.

disease was the "broomstick plaster" described by Petrie.[34] Bilateral long-leg walking casts were connected by two broomsticks to fix the hips in 45° of abduction and 5° to 10° of internal rotation. The child ambulated with the use of crutches, and new plasters were applied every 3 to 4 months. The "Toronto orthosis" described by Bobechko and his associates[7] obviates the need for casts and cast changes; it positions the hips in a similar degree of abduction and internal rotation (Fig. 23-24). Since the knees are permitted to flex in this device, the effects of prolonged joint immobility are eliminated, and it is possible to sit comfortably. A similar bilateral hip-abduction orthosis developed by Curtis and his associates at Newington Children's Hospital has recently been reported as giving 68 per cent of patients with Perthes disease good results, with an average of 20 months' usage.[11] It should be emphasized that all of the devices mentioned above provide excellent positioning of the hips in abduction and internal rotation with full weightbearing permitted. The disadvantages of this method of treatment are that both lower extremities must be braced and crutches must be used to assist ambulation, which is awkward at best. In addition, unless adequate medial support is provided at the knees, genu valgum can be a complication due to forces upon the epiphyseal plates of the distal femur and proximal tibia.

Non-weightbearing hip-abduction, internal rotation orthoses have been described by Harrison and Sanders and their associates.[20] Both of these devices position the femoral head within the acetabulum and maintain the knee on the affected side in about 90° of flexion. The opposite limb remains free, and a three-point gait is utilized with crutches. Due to the fact that the affected hip is positioned by fixing the relationship between the femur and the trunk, the hip is effectively immobilized. Although the forces of weightbearing are eliminated upon the hip, the loss of hip motion is not conducive to the physiologic requirements of the joint, and this may be a theoretical disadvantage to this type of orthosis.

The trilateral-socket hip-abduction orthosis described by Tachdjian and Jouett is an attempt to combine a reduction in weightbearing upon the femoral head with adequate positioning of the head for acetabular containment.[43] This is achieved in unilateral cases with a unilateral KAFO consisting of a trilateral socket of plastic laminate and a medial upright extending to a foot plate which suspends the limb from contact with the floor (Fig. 23-25). An elevated shoe is used on the sound side. Abduction is maintained by the shape of the socket and the ischial shelf, which is formed so as to be horizontal with the floor when the limb is in 30° of abduction. The advantages of this orthosis are that weightbearing upon the femoral head is reduced while it is maintained in a position of containment, the

FIG. 23-24. Toronto-design KAFO for use in providing hip abduction and internal rotation in Legg-Calvé-Perthes disease. (From Staros, A., and LeBlanc, M.: Orthotic components and systems. *In* American Academy of Orthopaedic Surgeons: Atlas of Orthotics. St. Louis, C. V. Mosby, 1975.)

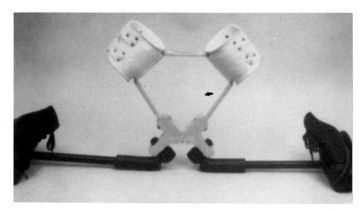

sound leg is not confined by the orthosis, and crutches are not required, allowing freedom of upper limb activity. The disadvantage of the device is that it does not provide as much abduction as the other devices mentioned, and unless carefully constructed and maintained, it may not provide consistent femoral head containment.

Recently, the Scottish Rite Hospital orthosis for Legg-Calvé-Perthes disease has been introduced by Lovell, Hopper, and Purvis. This device, while maintaining sufficient abduction for femoral head containment, does not provide internal rotation of the hip (Fig. 23-26). Preliminary results, however, are encouraging.

In selecting the proper orthosis for the treatment of Legg-Calvé-Perthes disease, the physician must consider the relative importance of the amount of weightbearing upon the femoral head, the degree of motion permitted at the hip, the degree of femoral head containment, the degree of freedom of activity permitted, and the psychologic impact of the device upon the child. It is the orthopaedic surgeon's assessment of the relative importance of these parameters, combined with his assessment of the individual patient, that dictates the orthotic prescription. Whatever device is selected, adequate containment of the femoral head within the acetabulum is an essential prerequisite to optimal treatment. Periodic roentgenograms of the hip with the child standing in his orthosis should be obtained

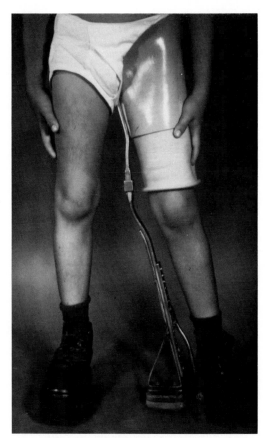

FIG. 23-25. Trilateral-socket hip-abduction orthosis for use in Legg-Calvé-Perthes disease. (From Staros, A., and LeBlanc, M.: Orthotic components and systems. *In* American Academy of Orthopaedic Surgeons: Atlas of Orthotics. St. Louis, C. V. Mosby, 1975.)

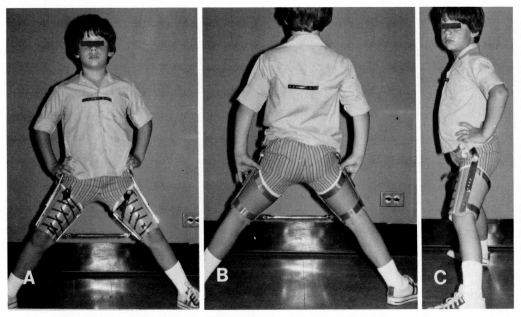

FIG. 23-26. The Scottish Rite Hospital orthosis for Legg-Calvé-Perthes disease.

to assess the femoral head coverage.

Congenital Dislocation of the Hip. Orthotic devices have a prominent place in the early treatment of congenital dislocations of the hip. Many types of devices have been described, but all are designed to position the hip in flexion, abduction, and external rotation. Varying degrees of freedom of motion of the hip are permitted, for even the static-type splints provide only relative immobilization of the hip joint.

There are two primary indications for the use of the hip orthosis in the management of congenital dislocation of the hip. The first and most common indication is for the treatment of hip dysplasia in the newborn period. Prompt recognition of the disorder, followed by adequate positioning of the affected hip or hips by a splint of suitable design, usually results in a normal hip by 8 to 12 weeks of age.[6, 44] The second indication for use of an orthotic device in children with congenital dislocation of the hip is to reduce the period of cast immobilization following closed reduction of the dislocation in the older infant or child. Since the period of plaster immobilization may be 6 to 8 months in the child whose dislocation was recog-

nized and treated at 6 months of age, the use of a suitable orthosis, in lieu of plaster, after the first 2 or 3 months of immobilization is felt to be highly desirable.[21]

The simplest splint for management of congenital dysplasia of the hip in the newborn is the pillow splint originally described by Frejka.[16] Commercially available, it is a waterproof pillow designed to be secured between the legs over the diapers so as to prevent adduction, extension, and internal rotation of the hips. Since it must be removed at each diaper change, it is recommended only for dysplastic and for subluxed hips, not for the treatment of truly dislocated hips in the newborn. A more modern version of the Frejka pillow is the Craig abduction splint which is made of padded semirigid plastic, also worn over the diapers, necessitating removal with diaper change.[8]

A second class of orthotic devices developed for management of congenital dislocation of the hip in the infant is represented by the splints described by Von Rosen[44] and by Barlow.[5] Both of these devices are made of thin, malleable aluminum strips which are covered by rubber or leather. They are designed so that the bulk of the splint cradles the child's back, and the terminal portions of the aluminum splints contour about the infant's thighs and shoulders, holding the hips in 90° of flexion, abduction, and external rotation. The degree of abduction as well as flexion can be adjusted by manual bending of the aluminum strips. Both of these splints, by their design, permit some motion of the hip joints, but prevent an undesirable degree of extension, adduction, and internal rotation. Also, they have the advantage that the splint need not be removed when the diapers are changed; bathing the infant is even possible while the device is in place. Thus, they may be used effectively for dislocated hips, which when placed in the position of flexion, abduction and external rotation are stable.

A third class of devices permits more active motion of the hips, but confines the hip motion to a range which will not permit subluxation or dislocation of the hips. The device described by Ilfeld consists of two metallic thigh cuffs with washable covers attached to an adjustable bar by universal joints.[21] The design permits change of diapers without device removal, sitting, standing and walking with adequate positional control of the hips. It has been used in children from 1½ to 30 months of age, and for dislocation as well as for dysplasia. Ilfeld also reports good results with use after casting for 6 to 8 weeks following reduction of dislocations in the older infant, thus markedly reducing the time of plaster immobilization. Another dynamic type of splint which restricts, but does not severely inhibit, motion of the hips while retaining adequate position is the Pavlik harness.[14] This device consists of a system of adjustable straps secured to the trunk and attached to padded stirrups for the feet which limit hip extension, adduction, and internal rotation. Diapers and clothing may be changed without having to remove the harness (Fig. 23-27).

The use of abduction bars between the feet is not recommended for treatment of congenital dislocation of the hip, since unless the degree of abduction is extremely wide, as described by Ponseti,[35] the child will be able to flex and adduct the hips to an undesirable degree. Such devices also tend to keep the hips in extension most of the time, which is not the optimal position for

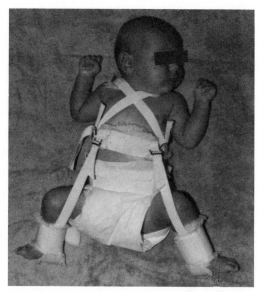

FIG. 23-27. Pavlik harness for control of hip extension and adduction in congenital dislocation of the hip.

centralization of the femoral head within the acetabulum in infants.

Perhaps with the exception of the Ilfeld splint, orthotic treatment of congenital dysplasia or dislocation of the hip is not sufficiently effective beyond the age of 18 months to merit use. Surgical approaches to centralization of the hip beyond this age are generally recommended.

UPPER LIMB ORTHOTICS

As in the lower limb, the application of orthotic devices in the upper limb may be used to prevent deformity, correct deformity, or improve function.

Prevention of deformity or protection of joint segments is usually accomplished by the use of static splinting devices designed of metal or thermoplastic material. Joint positioning prevents contracture, and in some instances it may, in and of itself, improve function to a degree, such as positioning of the thumb in opposition. Static splints find their greatest use in the prevention of deformities following peripheral nerve injury and in temporary spastic states, as well as in

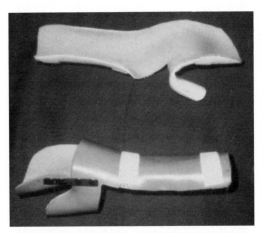

FIG. 23-28. Dorsal and volar WHO's for splinting of the wrist and hand.

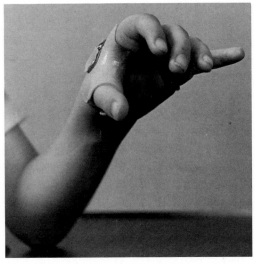

FIG. 23-29. Short opponens orthosis used for positioning the thumb in the functional position of opposition for grasp. (Courtesy Thorkild Engen, C. O., Houston, Texas)

prevention of deformity due to juvenile rheumatoid arthritis.

Correction of deformity may be accomplished by adjustable static splints or by dynamic devices employing elastic or spring force of mild but constant degree. Recent joint contractures associated with paralysis, arthritis, or hemarthrosis may be effectively corrected by such measures, but old or well-established contractures generally require surgical correction.

The task of restoring function by orthotic means to the defective upper limb has historically been fraught with difficulty. The problem of reduplicating mechanically the highly refined system of joints, levers, and motors present in the normal upper limb is enormous when compared to the lower limb. Added to this dilemma is the seemingly impossible task of providing an adequate sensory feedback system to allow coordination of motor skills to a degree necessary to restore upper limb function. Augmentation or restoration of motor power in the upper limb by orthotic means is gross at best, and when combined with a severe sensory deficit it may be of little practical use to the patient. Substitution of motor activity may be accomplished by mechanical, electrical, or pneumatic devices subject to these limiting factors.

A major consideration in the use of upper limb orthoses in children is the degree of pa-

tient acceptance or tolerance of the device. If the orthosis is to be successful, it must be worn. Any orthosis which significantly impairs function rather than assisting it, or any orthosis that gets in the way when performing certain activities will be doomed to failure. Children have very little "gadget tolerance" and reject a device if it is too encumbering or restrictive. Therefore, every effort should be made to keep the orthotic design simple, lightweight, and of a design which interferes as little as possible with remaining normal motor and sensory functions.

Upper limb orthoses are also designated by the joint levels which they encompass, ie., hand orthosis (HO), wrist-hand orthosis (WHO), and elbow orthosis (EO).

The Hand and Wrist

Prevention of Deformity. Orthoses designed to prevent deformity are most commonly utilized about the hand and wrist following musculoskeletal trauma, peripheral nerve injury, burns, and in rheumatoid arthritis. Usually they may be removed for several hours a day to permit therapy, bathing, and some freedom of activity. They

FIG. 23-30. Long opponens orthosis (WHO) for wrist stabilization as well as thumb opposition. (Courtesy Thorkild Engen, C. O., Houston, Texas)

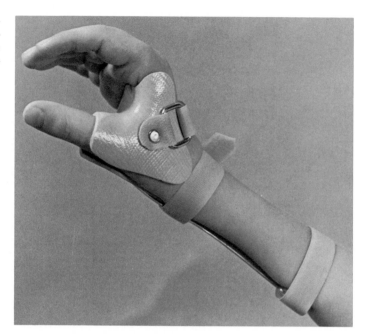

are also considered relatively temporary devices, seldom having to be worn for more than a few months.

Basic positioning splints for the hand and wrist to maintain a functional position may be made of thermoplastic material, using either a dorsal or volar forearm section (Fig. 23-28). These splints are intended primarily for night use and limited daytime use, since they are relatively encumbering. They are commonly indicated in juvenile rheumatoid arthritis.

Loss of thumb opposition and abduction requires the use of a short opponens splint which maintains the thumb in a position of opposition and prevents contracture of the web space (Fig. 23-29). This splint also enhances function in cases of thenar paralysis, since it provides positioning for pinch activities. If wrist stabilization is also required, the long opponens splint may be used, which also provides splinting and immobilization of the wrist (Fig. 23-30). In combined median and ulnar nerve loss with total loss of the intrinsic musculature, a dorsal bar over the proximal phalanges may be attached to maintain flexion of the metacarpophalangeal joints and prevent an intrinsic minus contracture (extension contracture of the metacarpophalangeal joints). Associated flexion contractures of the interphalangeal joints may be prevented by the addition of an outrigger to this system to support rubberband slings for finger extension.

Loss of extensor power secondary to radial nerve palsy may be managed by use of the long opponens splint with a dorsal outrigger to provide rubberband, sling extension assist to the metacarpophalangeal joints. The addition of a thumb-extension assist to the opposition post maintains the thumb in adequate position for a pinch type of grasp.

Detailed descriptions of these devices may be found in the recent Atlas of Orthotics published by the American Academy of Orthopaedic Surgeons.[1]

Correction of Deformity. Correction of mild deformities of the hand and wrist is possible by the use of orthotic devices, provided that the contractures are of relatively recent origin. A family of dynamic splints designed by the late Sterling Bunnel are available commercially as off-the-shelf items.* Included are extension and flexion assists for the in-

---

*H. Weniger, Inc., 70 12th Street, San Francisco, California.

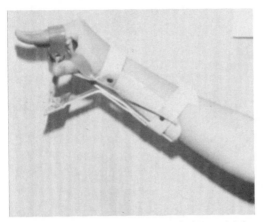

FIG. 23-31. Dynamic metacarpophalangeal joint flexion assist.

terphalangeal joints and for the metacarpophalangeal joints. Dynamic extension assists for the metacarpophalangeal joints may also be provided by the use of rubberband slings for the fingers from an outrigger, which is based upon a dorsal or long opponens wrist splint. Dynamic flexion assists for the metacarpophalangeal joints may be provided in a similar manner from an outrigger attachment based upon a volar wrist splint. (Fig. 23-31). In the case of extension contractures of the metacarpophalangeal joints

and flexion contractures of the interphalangeal joints associated with burns of the hand, this system may be modified by attaching the rubberbands to small metallic hooks which are glued to the fingernails. In this manner, direct contact of the slings with the burned fingers is avoided.

Flexion deformities of the wrist may best be corrected by serial casting into extension, or by the use of a remoldable thermoplastic volar splint, which is periodically removed and heated, gradually bringing the wrist up into further extension.

Restoration of Function. Restoration of function about the hand and wrist may be accomplished by the use of simple positioning orthoses, by mechanical harnessing of wrist extensor power to provide two-digit flexion to a fixed thumb, or by the use of external power to drive a prehension-type orthosis. Regardless of the method used, the function provided by such devices is that of relatively gross prehension and release. There is no orthotic device at present which can provide the function of manipulation within the grasp.

Loss of wrist stability due to lack of extensor power or due to intrinsic joint disease will result in a weak and inefficient grasp. Wrist stabilization orthoses are indicated in this situation, and they considerably improve the strength of grip. The orthosis

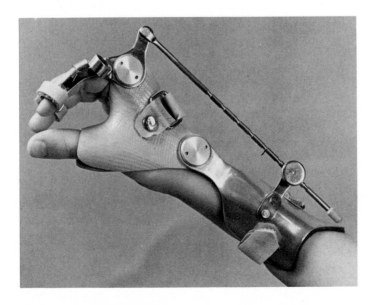

FIG. 23-32. The wrist-driven flexor-hinge orthosis converts the excursion of active wrist extension to finger flexion against the fixed thumb in opposition. The primary indication for this orthosis is in a child with a C6 quadriplegia. (Courtesy Thorkild Engen, C. O., Houston, Texas)

FIG. 23-33. Wrist-driven flexor-hinge orthosis utilizing external power by means of a carbon dioxide artificial muscle. This device is indicated in quadriplegia when active wrist extension is absent but sufficient proximal arm control is present, as in the C5 quadriplegic. (Courtesy Thorkild Engen, C. O., Houston, Texas)

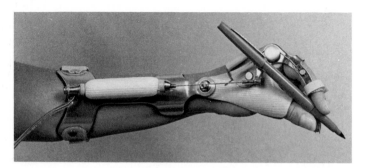

should be based dorsally on the wrist and forearm, and the palmar support section should be narrow so as to interfere minimally with the closing capacity of the hand and palmar sensation. The most effective wrist position for maximum strength of grasp is 35° of dorsiflexion. However, most day-to-day activities involving prehension are performed with the wrist in the neutral position.[24] Therefore, for optimal functional restoration, the wrist-hand orthosis should stabilize the wrist in the neutral or slightly dorsiflexed position.

Loss of thumb opposition, such as that seen in median nerve injuries and polio, is a severe functional handicap. Positioning of the thumb in opposition by means of an appropriate orthosis can restore fine prehension to a degree by allowing the mobile index and long fingers to approximate the fixed thumb. If wrist stability and extensor power are present, a short opponens splint is indicated (Fig. 23-29). If the wrist is unstable, or if wrist extensor power is inadequate, a long opponens splint should be used (Fig. 23-30). Opponens splints may be made of aluminum,[3] plaster laminate,[13] or thermoplastic material. In the case of the younger child, custom-fabricated splints of thermoplastic material are generally required.

Loss of function of the thumb and the fingers, typified by the quadriplegia patient, is an even more severe disability, since grasp of any type is lacking. In those patients who retain wrist extension (for example, the C6 quadriplegic) gradual contracture of the finger flexors may provide return of gross grasp by a tenodesis effect. Finer prehension of a pinch type may be achieved by the use of the wrist-driven flexor-hinge orthosis,

or the "tenodesis splint."[3, 13] This device utilizes a mechanical linkage to convert the excursion of wrist extension to flexion of the index and long fingers against the thumb, which is fixed in the position of opposition (Fig. 23-32). Thus a "three-jawed chuck" type of prehension is produced by extension of the wrist, and release is accomplished by passive wrist flexion. It should be emphasized that while this type of prehension is useful for some activities, it is not useful for all, and the gross, natural tenodesis type of grasp is preferred much of the time. Wearing the orthosis also inhibits such activities as dressing and wheeling a wheelchair. Younger children tend to reject this orthosis due to these factors, while older children use it for selected activities requiring a pinch type of prehension.

Combined loss of function of the thumb, fingers, and wrist, as exemplified by the C5 quadriplegic, requires the use of external power to restore the ability to grasp. In this situation, the basic wrist-driven flexor-hinge orthosis is used, but an external power source is used to activate the wrist extension mechanism of the orthosis (Fig. 23-33). The power source may be either electrical or pneumatic. In the case of electronically driven orthoses, a worm-gear mechanism is used, and in the case of the pneumatically driven orthosis, the carbon dioxide artificial muscle is used.[3, 13] Effective use of prehension-type orthoses requires sufficient proximal control of the limb segments to permit positioning of the hand in space, so that high-level quadriplegics who are devoid of shoulder and elbow movement are unable to benefit from this type of device. This device has application primarily in the older

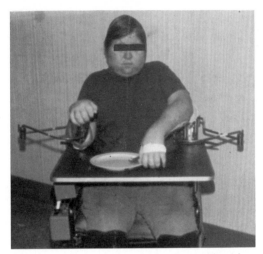

FIG. 23-34. Mobile arm supports as utilized in a child with severe Guillain-Barré syndrome.

child who has sufficient coordination and skill developed in the proximal musculature and sufficient concentration and learning ability to be able to utilize the orthosis.

The Elbow and Shoulder

Prevention of Deformity. The majority of day-to-day activities are performed with the elbow flexed by 10° to 20° on either side of the 90° position. Therefore, splinting of the elbow is usually done with the elbow flexed at 90°. Various types of thermoplastic materials may be used to fabricate temporary elbow splints. A posterior splint is generally used, but anterior splints are useful in preventing flexion contracture in the burned child. Following injury of any type, the elbow joint tends to become stiff rapidly, so that whenever splinting of the elbow is utilized for immobilization alone it is of the utmost importance that it be removed periodically for therapy and range-of-motion exercises.

Static splinting of the shoulder in abduction and external rotation may be accomplished by the "airplane splint." Such a position is commonly desirable in the management of children with burns involving the axilla to prevent the development of adduction and internal rotation contracture.

The orthosis may be fabricated of aluminum covered by leather or it may be made of thermoplastic material. In either case, the orthosis must derive its support from the iliac crest on the same side. Failure to base the device on the iliac crest results in instability and discomfort.

Correction of Deformity. Regaining lost elbow motion as a result of contracture is difficult and requires a combination of physical therapy and orthotic management. In contractures of long standing, surgical release of the contracture is usually indicated.

The simplest type of orthotic device employed is the thermoplastic splint, which may be reheated and reformed to maintain the maximum correction that is obtained by physical therapy. The three-point extension orthosis may be used to gradually stretch the elbow into extension by progressive tightening of the elbow pad. The pivoted arm and forearm cuffs rotate to accommodate to the changing elbow position.

Hinged elbow orthoses may also be used in effecting reduction of either flexion or extension contractures. A turnbuckle may provide the corrective force, or dial-lock joints may be preferred. Dynamic hinged elbow orthoses have also been used to achieve elbow flexion, with rubber tubing or elastic straps providing the dynamic force.

Whenever an elbow orthosis is used for the purpose of correcting deformity, the correction should occur gradually over a long period of time, so that only minimal force is employed and there is no discomfort produced by wearing the orthosis. A physical therapy program consisting of gentle passive and active assisted range of motion should be used concurrently.

Restoration of Function. Paralysis of elbow flexion may be substituted for by a dynamic elbow-flexion assist orthosis with arm and forearm cuffs connected by a single axis joint and elastic straps positioned anterior to the axis of the elbow joint.[26] The triceps is used to provide elbow extension against the dynamic flexion force.

When there is severe weakness of musculature about the shoulders and elbows, but some residual strength remains in the poor-muscle-grade range, the mobile arm support is a most useful device.[2, 26] This or-

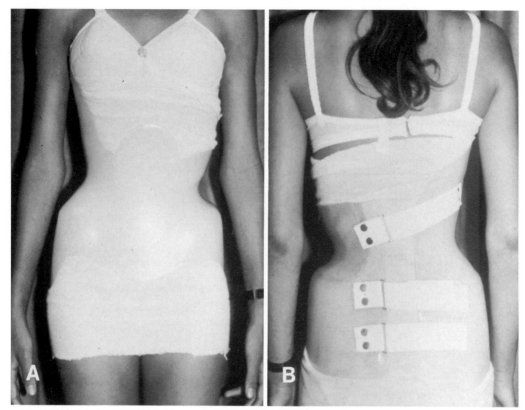

FIG. 23-35. *(A)* Anterior view of a molded polypropylene TLSO for control of idiopathic lumbar scoliosis. *(B)* Posterior view of a polypropelene TLSO with a built-in corrective lumbar pad.

thotic device is used primarily for wheelchair-confined patients with proximal upper limb weakness, as is seen frequently in polio, muscular dystrophy and related disorders. It provides a support system for the upper limb, which counteracts and balances the forces of gravity, allowing the weakened muscles to function more efficiently by gravity assistance. The system is attached to the child's wheelchair, and it consists of a forearm trough which is balanced at an appropriate pivotal joint on freely movable linkage rods. The pivotal joint of attachment on the forearm trough is crucial to optimal function. With the system ideally balanced, weak external rotators and adductors of the shoulder produce elbow flexion and some supination, and weak internal rotators of the shoulder are capable of providing elbow extension, pronation,

and a downward type of reach (Fig. 23-34).

For the severely paralyzed shoulder and elbow, such as is seen in brachial plexus palsy or in poliomyelitis, restoration of function by orthotic means is essentially impossible. Elaborate orthotic devices have been described such as the ratchet-type functional-arm orthosis[3] and the electric arm orthosis,[32] but the amount of gadgetry required to accomplish relatively simple motion control is immense. Such orthoses are not well tolerated by children, and are seldom tolerated even by adults, since the functional gains are minimal in comparison to the inconvenience of wearing the device.

THE SPINE

As in the extremities, orthoses for the spine are used to prevent and correct defor-

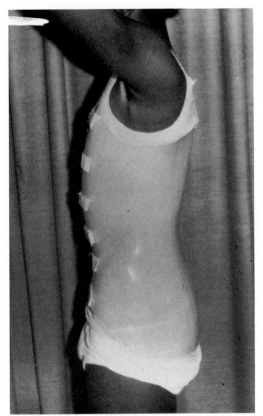

FIG. 23-36. Postoperative scoliosis jacket of polypropylene made from a positive plaster model.

mity. They may also be used to improve or restore function by stabilizing a collapsing paralytic spine, which in turn aids sitting balance and frees the arms from having to support the trunk.

Spinal orthoses in use for children today are vastly improved over those used 10 years ago, due to the emergence of new materials and technology. Thermoplastics such as polypropylene, polyethylene, vitrathene and Orthoplast are being used in the fabrication of the Milwaukee brace, LSO flexion jackets and TLSO scoliosis jackets (Fig. 23-35). Postoperative scoliosis jackets made of thermoplastic material reduce the length of time in body casts, and due to the intimate and total contact type of fit achieved, they provide excellent immobilization (Fig. 23-36).

In this text, the details of spinal orthotics in children may be found in Chapter 16.

REFERENCES

1. American Academy of Orthopaedic Surgeons. Atlas of Orthotics: Biomechanical principle and application. St. Louis, C. V. Mosby, 1975.
2. Anderson, M. H.: Functional Bracing of the Upper Extremities. Springfield, Charles C Thomas, 1958.
3. _____: Upper Extremity Orthotics. Springfield, Charles C Thomas, 1965.
4. Anderson, M. H., and Bray, J. J.: Biomechanical considerations in the design of a functional long leg brace. Biomed. Sci. Instrum., *1:*385, 1963. (Reprinted Orthot. Prosthet. Appl. J., *18:*273, 1964.)
5. Barlow, T. G.: Early diagnosis and treatment of congenital dislocation of the hip. J. Bone Joint Surg., *44B:*292-301, 1962.
6. _____: Congenital dislocation of the hip: early diagnosis and treatment. Lond. Clin. Med. J., *5:*47-58, 1964.
7. Bobechko, W. P., McLaurin, C. A., and Motlock, W. M.: Toronto orthosis for Legg-Perthes disease. Artif. Limbs, *12:*36-41, 1968.
8. Coleman, S. S.: Treatment of congenital dislocation of the hip in the infant. J. Bone Joint Surg., *47A:* 590-601, 1965.
9. Committee on Prosthetics Research and Development, National Academy of Sciences: A clinical evaluation of four lower limb orthoses. (Report E-5), Washington D.C., 1972.
10. Committee on Prosthetics Research and Development, National Academy of Sciences: Report of a workshop on the child with an orthopaedic disability: his orthotic needs, and how to meet them. Washington, D.C., 1973.
11. Curtis, B. H., Gunther, S. T., Gossling, H. R., and Paul, S. W.: Treatment for Legg-Perthes disease with the Newington ambulation-abduction brace. J. Bone Joint Surg., *56A:*1135-1146, 1974.
12. Dixon, M. A., and Palumbo, R. L.: Polypropelene knee orthosis with latex suprapatellar strap suspension. Orthot. Prosthet., *29:*29-31, 1975.
13. Engen, T. J.: Development of upper extremity orthotics, I, and II. Orthot. Prosthet., [March and June] 1970.
14. Erlacher, P. J., Early treatment of dysplasia of the hip. J. Internat. Col. Surgeons, *38:*348-353, 1962.
15. Fabry, G., MacEwen, D., and Shands, A. R., Jr.: Torsion of the femur. J. Bone Joint Surg., *55A:*1726-1737, 1973.
16. Frejka, M. B.: Treatment of congenital dislocation of the hip. Unpublished paper presented at the Annual Meeting of the American Academy of Orthopaedic Surgeons, Chicago, 1947.
17. Glancy, J., and Lindseth, R. E.: The polypropelene solid ankle orthosis. Orthot. Prosthet. *26:*14, 1972.
18. Hall, J. E., Miller, W. E., Schumann, W., and Stanish, W.: A refined concept in the orthotic management of scoliosis: a preliminary report. Orthot. Prosthet., *29(4):*7-13, 1975.
19. Harris, E. E.: A new orthotic terminology. Orthot. Prosthet. *27:*6, 1973.

20. Harrison, M. H. M., Turner, M. H., and Nicholson, T. J.: Coxa plana—results of a new form of splinting. J. Bone Joint Surg., *51A*:1057-1069, 1969.

21. Ilfeld, F. W.: The management of congenital dislocation and dysplasia of the hip by means of the special splint. J. Bone Joint Surg., *39A*:99-109, 1957.

22. Inman, V. T.: UC-BL dual axis control system and UC-BL shoe insert. Bull. Prosthet. Res., *10:*11, 1969.

23. Karadinas, John E.: Conservative treatment of coxa plana: a comparison of the early results of different methods. J. Bone Joint Surg., *53A:*315-325, 1971.

24. Klopsteg, P. E., and Wilson, P. D.: Human limbs and their substitutes. New York, Hafner, 1968.

25. Lehneis, H. R.: New developments in lower limb orthotics through bioengineering. Arch. Phys. Med. Rehab., *53(7):*303-310, 1972.

26. Long, C.: Upper Limb Bracing in Orthotics Etcetera. Baltimore, Waverly Press, 1966.

26a. Lovell, W. W.: Personal communication, 1978.

27. McCollough, N. C. III: Comprehensive management of musculoskeletal disorders in hemophilia. Committee on Prosthetics Research and Development, National Academy of Sciences, Washington, D.C., 1973.

28. _____: Current status of lower limb orthotics. Orthop. Digest, *3:*17-29, 1975.

29. _____: Rationale for orthotic prescription in the lower extremity. Clin. Orthop., *102:*32-45, 1974.

30. McCollough, N. C. III, Fryer, C. M., and Glancy, J.: A new approach to patient analysis for orthotic prescription. Arti. Limbs, *14:*68, 1970.

31. McIlmurray, W. J., and Greenbaum, W.: A below knee weight bearing brace. Orthop. Prosthet. Appl. J., *12(2):*81-82, 1958.

32. Nickel, V. L., Allen, J. R., and Karchak, A., Jr.: Control systems for externally powered orthotic devices, final project report. Rancho Los Amigos Hospital, Downey, California, May 1, 1960 to July 31, 1970, Professional Staff Association.

33. Nitschke, R. O.: A single bar above knee orthosis. Orthot. Prosthet., *25:*4-25, 1971.

34. Petrie, J. G., and Bitenc, I.: The abduction weight-bearing treatment in Legg Perthes disease. J. Bone Joint Surg., *53B:*54-62, 1971.

35. Ponseti, I.: Causes of failure in the treatment of congenital dislocation of the hip. J. Bone Joint Surg., *26:*775-792, 1944.

36. Rubin, G., and Dixon, M.: The modern ankle foot orthoses (AFO's). Bull. Prosthet. Res., *10-19:*20-41, 1973.

37. Salter, R. B.: Textbook of Disorders and Injuries of the Musculo-skeletal System. Baltimore, Williams & Wilkens, 1970.

38. Sanders, J. A.: A long term follow up on coxa plana at the Alfred I. Dupont Institute. South. Med. J., *62:*1042-47, 1969.

39. Sarmiento, A.: A functional below the knee brace for tibial fractures. J. Bone Joint Surg., *52A:*295, 1970.

40. Schultz, M., and McCollough, N. C., III: Polypropylene in spinal orthotics. Orthot. Prosthet., *28(3):*43-48, 1974.

41. Smith, C. F.: Long term management and rehabilitation in hemophilia. Project Report. Orthopaedic Hospital, Los Angeles, 1969.

42. Smith, E. M., and Juvinall, R. C.: Theory of feeder mechanics. Am. J. Phys. Med., *42:*3, 1963.

43. Tachdjian, M. O., and Jouett, L. O.: Trilateral socket hip abduction orthosis for the treatment of Legg-Perthes disease. Orthot. Prosthet., *22(2):*49-62, 1968.

44. VonRosen, S.: Diagnosis and treatment of congenital dislocation of the hip joint in the new born. J. Bone Joint Surg., *44B:*284-291, 1962.

Index

Vol. 1: pp. 1-532; Vol. 2: pp. 533-1086